THE COMPLETE FOOD COUNTER

With more than 4 million copies of their bestselling *Counter* books in print, Annette B. Natow and Jo-Ann Heslin tell readers everything they want to know about making the best food choices when snacking, shopping, cooking, and eating out.

The nutrition experts have completely updated, revised, and expanded this one-volume, easy-to-use, and easy-to-carry reference that has every nutrition count you'll ever need:

- Calories
- Fat
- Cholesterol
- Protein
- Carbohydrate
- Fiber
- Sodium

Books by Annette B. Natow and Jo-Ann Heslin

The Calorie Counter (Third Edition)

The Cholesterol Counter (Sixth Edition)

The Complete Food Counter (Second Edition)

The Diabetes Carbohydrate and Calorie Counter
(Second Edition)

Eating Out Food Counter

The Fat Counter (Sixth Edition)

The Food Shopping Counter (Second Edition)

The Healthy Heart Food Counter

The Most Complete Food Counter

The Pocket Fat Counter (Second Edition)

The Pocket Protein Counter

The Protein Counter (Second Edition)

The Ultimate Carbohydrate Counter

The Vitamin and Mineral Food Counter

Published by POCKET BOOKS

THE
COMPLETE
FOOD COUNTER

Second Edition

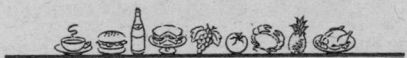

**Annette B. Natow, Ph.D.
and Jo-Ann Heslin, M.A., R.D.**

with the assistance of Karen J. Nolan, Ph.D.

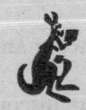

POCKET BOOKS
New York   London   Toronto   Sydney

POCKET BOOKS, a division of Simon & Schuster, Inc.
1230 Avenue of the Americas, New York, NY 10020

Copyright © 1999, 2003, 2006 by Annette B. Natow and Jo-Ann Heslin

Originally published as a trade paperback in 1999 by Pocket Books. The 1999 edition of this work was titled *The Most Complete Food Counter.*

All rights reserved, including the right to reproduce this book or portions thereof in any form whatsoever. For information address Pocket Books, 1230 Avenue of the Americas, New York, NY 10020

ISBN-13: 978-1-4165-0981-3
ISBN-10:   1-4165-0981-X

First Pocket Books paperback printing of this revised edition January 2006

10   9   8   7   6

POCKET and colophon are registered trademarks of Simon & Schuster, Inc.

Cover design by Anna Dorfman

Manufactured in the United States of America

For information regarding special discounts for bulk purchases, please contact Simon & Schuster Special Sales at 1-800-456-6798 or business@simonandschuster.com

ACKNOWLEDGMENTS

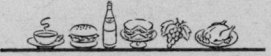

For graciously sharing her knowledge: Karen J. Nolan, Ph.D.

For all her continuous support and help, our agent, Nancy Trichter.

For her suggestions and editing skills, Sara Clemence.

For his creative computer programming and technical support, Brian Robinson.

Without the tireless cooperation of Stephen Llano and the production department at Pocket Books, *The Complete Food Counter, Second Edition,* would never have been completed.

A special thank you to our editor, Micki Nuding.

". . . foods, though so numerous and so varied in form, can be reduced to rather simple terms."

Mary Swartz Rose, Ph.D.
Feeding the Family
The Macmillan Company, 1919

CONTENTS

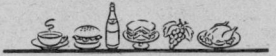

PART ONE

Brand Name, Nonbranded (Generic), and Take-Out Foods

PART TWO

Restaurant Chains

INTRODUCTION

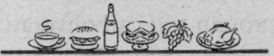

Calories, fat, cholesterol, protein, carbohydrate, fiber, sodium—the list is long. Because your body is working all the time (even when you're sleeping), you need a source of calories and other nutrients to keep you going. Different foods have different assortments of nutrients. Some foods, like meat and cheese, are high in protein; fruits are high in carbohydrates; and whole wheat bread has lots of fiber. When you eat a variety of foods, it balances out so that you get all the nutrients you need. *The Complete Food Counter, Second Edition,* is the most comprehensive source to make sure you get everything you need, listing nutrition values for over 17,000 foods.

Calories (CALS)

Calories are calories, whether they come from apples or chocolate fudge. All foods, except water, have some. Every time you eat, you take in calories. Your body is a machine that uses food calories as fuel. When the amount of fuel you take in equals the amount of fuel you need for your body to run, your weight remains constant. Eat too many calories, and your body uses what it needs and stores the remainder for future use. You see the storage on your thighs, hips, and waist. Eat too few calories, and your body draws on its fuel reserves.

Your thighs, hips, and waist get slimmer as the surplus is depleted.

Calories come from the fat, protein, and carbohydrate in foods. Fat has the most calories of the three—more than twice as many as protein and carbohydrate. One teaspoon of fat has 40 calories, while a teaspoon of either carbohydrate or protein has only 16 calories.

Over and over, studies have shown that if you cut calories, you lose weight. If you eat too many calories—even from healthy foods—you gain weight. It doesn't matter if those calories come from bread, meat, or salad dressing. The key to long-term weight control is to burn as many calories as you eat.

Smart Stuff

According to a recent government survey, the average woman eats 1,850 calories a day; the average man eats 2,550.

Fat

Fat has a bad reputation that is undeserved. It's important for providing energy, supplying essential fatty acids that the body cannot make, insulating the body and protecting vital organs, carrying fat-soluble vitamins, and becoming part of cell membranes. And, just as important, fat makes food taste good.

Fats (or *lipids,* as scientists refer to them) is actually an umbrella term for several similar substances. You get fats from the foods you eat, and your body can also make some fats. Food fats are made up of strands of *fatty acids.* You can think of these fatty acids as strands of beads that vary in combination and number of beads depending on their chemical composition.

There are 3 main types of fatty acids—saturated, monounsaturated, and polyunsaturated. Foods contain combinations of all three, but we label foods as sources of saturated (butter), monounsaturated (olive oil), or polyunsaturated (corn oil) based on the predominant fat in the food. Recent research suggests that the *type* of fat you eat may be more important than the *amount* of fat you eat.

Experts recommend that your daily fat intake make up 20% to 35% of your total calories. This means that if you regularly eat 1,800 calories a day, somewhere between 360 (20%) and 630 (35%) calories should come from fat. To convert fat calories into grams of fat, all you need to know is that 1 gram of fat = 9 calories. Using the example of 1,800 calories, the grams of fat each day would range from 40 to 70.

$$360 \text{ fat calories } (20\%) \div 9 = 40 \text{ grams of fat}$$
$$630 \text{ fat calories } (35\%) \div 9 = 70 \text{ grams of fat}$$

But we need to set the record straight. Even though current research suggests that a moderate fat intake may be healthy, no one is suggesting a *high* fat intake is good for you.

Smart Stuff

A recent study found that dieters who were given 35% of their daily calories as fat found it easier to stick with their weight-loss plan and kept their weight off longer.

Cholesterol (CHOL)

Cholesterol is a white, waxy, fatlike substance found in every cell in your body. It insulates nerve cells and helps skin cells retain moisture. Cholesterol makes up a major part of your brain. It's the main building block from which vitamin D and essential hormones such as cortisone, estrogen, and testosterone are made. But having too much cholesterol in your blood is unhealthy. The excess can be deposited onto your artery walls, narrowing them and interfering with normal blood flow.

You get cholesterol every time you eat animal foods—meat, poultry, fish, eggs, milk, yogurt, cheese, or butter. There is no cholesterol in foods that grow in the ground. Vegetables, fruits, nuts, seeds, cereals, and grains have none. Cholesterol can also be made in the body. In fact, most people make three times more cholesterol than they eat in their food.

Smart Stuff

It's simple. If a food grows in the ground, it has no cholesterol. If a food has a face, it has cholesterol.

On average, American men eat about 330 milligrams of cholesterol a day; women eat about 240 milligrams. The federal government's National Cholesterol Education Program recommends no more than 200 milligrams of cholesterol a day. The American Heart Association (AHA) recommends that you limit cholesterol to less than 300 milligrams a day; 200 milligrams if you already have heart disease.

Your daily cholesterol intake should be based on the results of your latest blood test. If your total cholesterol and LDL (low density lipoproteins) levels are within the desirable range, limit your cholesterol to less than 300 milligrams a day. If your numbers are up, reduce your daily intake to 200 milligrams a day.

Protein (PROT)

Your body loses millions of cells each day. They are used up, worn out, rubbed off, and even cut off (such as your beard or fingernails). You need a source of protein to replace these lost cells.

Protein is found in every cell, tissue, and substance in your body, except for urine and bile. Bones, teeth, muscles, enzymes, skin, and blood all contain protein. Active tissues, such as muscles and glands, are high in protein, while less active tissues, such as fat, have less.

Protein is made up of small building blocks called *amino acids*. There are 20 amino acids that the body uses to build different proteins, just like the letters in the alphabet are used to make different words. Of the 20 different amino acids found in food, 9 are known as *essential. These 9 must be obtained directly from the food you eat.* The remaining 11 can be made in the body. When you eat many different foods, you get varying amounts of protein and varying amounts of the different amino acids. That is one of the reasons it's important to eat a variety of foods. Almost all foods you eat contain protein—some more, some less. Fruits have very little protein compared to meat, milk, cheese, beans, grains, and vegetables, all of which have more.

When your body is stressed in any way, physically or mentally, protein is lost. When it's too hot or too cold, you need extra protein. More protein is needed to replace nitrogen lost during heavy sweating. Exercise, fever, surgery, injury, infection, and broken bones all increase your need for protein. Even emotional stress, such as losing your job or taking an exam, causes protein loss.

A quick way to estimate your daily protein need is to divide your weight by 2.2. For example, if you weigh 150 pounds, you should be eating 68 grams of protein a day (150 ÷ 2.2 = 68). Most people eat more than their recommended level of protein daily.

Smart Stuff

The top 10 sources of protein eaten in the U.S. are: beef, poultry, milk, yeast bread, cheese, fish, eggs, fresh pork, ham, and pasta.

Carbohydrate (CARB)

Carbohydrates include sugars, starches, and fibers found in foods. All plant foods—fruits, vegetables, beans, and grains—are rich in carbohydrates. Fruits have more sugar. Vegetables, beans, and grains have more starch. Both have some fiber.

Sugars and starches are your body's main source of energy, or calories. When the food you eat is digested, sugar molecules move easily into the blood stream and travel to cells. There they are burned for needed energy to keep your body working. Starch molecules are more complex. They are made up of many sugar molecules bound together. During digestion, these larger starch molecules are slowly broken apart to yield smaller sugar fragments, which are sent to the cells to be converted into energy. If you eat more carbohydrate calories than your body needs for energy, the leftover is stored as fat.

Smart Stuff

Simple carbohydrates *are foods that contain a lot of sugar—syrups, jelly, honey, soda, and molasses.*
Complex carbohydrates *are foods that contain a lot of starch—whole grains, cereals, beans, and vegetables. These foods are also rich in vitamins, minerals, and fiber.*

Years ago, you were told to eat all the carbohydrates you wanted. In fact, most Americans get 50% or more of their daily calories as carb. Today, however, carbs are being blamed for many of our health concerns, especially obesity. So, how much carb should you be eating?

The National Academy of Sciences' Recommended Dietary Allowance (RDA) for carbohydrate is 130 grams a day. This recommendation ensures that your body has the minimum amount of carbohydrate needed to function properly. Most of us eat far more. The Food and Drug Administration (FDA) has set 300 grams of carb as the Daily Value (DV)—the amount needed by the "typical" American consumer. This recommendation comes closer to the usual daily carbohydrate intake of most adults.

You can estimate what your individual carb intake should be by first deciding what amount of carb you want to eat each day. Most food professionals consider a diet with 40% or less of your daily calories coming from carbohydrates to be a low-carb diet.

Let's use 40% carbohydrate as an example. If you eat 1,800 calories a day:

40% of 1,800 calories = 720 carb calories per day

To figure out how many grams of carbs to eat each day, you need to know that 1 gram of carb = 4 calories. Continuing to use the example above:

720 carb calories per day ÷ 4 = 180 grams of carb per day

These values more than meet the RDA recommendation of at least 130 grams of carbohydrate a day. To make good carb choices, choose more foods that are higher in starch and fiber, and fewer foods that are higher in sugar.

Fiber

Fiber is a type of carbohydrate that your body doesn't digest and that provides no calories. But it is important. Fiber aids in losing weight, helps to manage diabetes, relieves constipation, and protects against colon cancer. It may even lower your risk for heart disease.

Yet most of us eat too little of it. We average about 15 grams of fiber a day, far less than we should be eating.

Smart Stuff

Experts recommend the following amounts of fiber daily:

Men

19–50 years old	38 grams of fiber
50 and older	30 grams of fiber

Women

19–50 years old	25 grams of fiber
50 and older	21 grams of fiber
Pregnant	28 grams of fiber

Add foods rich in fiber to your diet slowly—beans, berries, bran, fruits, oatmeal, vegetables, and whole grains. Don't go overboard, because it takes your body a little time to adjust to the extra bulk passing through your digestive tract. And drink plenty of fluids. Fiber soaks up fluids like a sponge. This not only helps you feel fuller longer but helps form soft, easily passed stools.

Sodium (SOD)

Most of us eat 2,300 to 4,700 milligrams of sodium a day. Experts recommend 1,500 milligrams for adults, less for older adults. In fact, many experts believe that healthy adults could do nicely on as little as 500 milligrams of sodium a day.

Smart Stuff

What the experts are saying:

Americans eat too much salt.
Adults aged 19–50 should get no more than
1,500 milligrams of sodium a day; those between
50 and 70 should get 1,300 milligrams; and people
over 70 should get 1,200 milligrams.
The upper limit of intake for all adults
should not exceed 2,300 milligrams.

Sodium regulates your body's fluid level, both outside and inside cells. This monitors your blood volume, blood pressure, and the acidity of your body. The movement of sodium into and out of cells allows other important substances to make this journey, too, helping to transmit the nerve impulses and electrical messages vital to your body's minute-by-minute functioning.

Most people associate too much sodium with high blood pressure. This assumption has been proven by studies done throughout the world. In places where little salt is used, blood pressure does not go up with age as it does in the U.S. Reducing sodium can lower high blood pressure in people who have it, and even, to a lesser extent, in people who have normal blood pressure. About 10% to 15% of all people with high blood pressure are very sensitive to salt. If they reduce the amount of salt they eat, their blood pressure goes down. People who are not salt-sensitive will not see as dramatic results, but their blood pressure does go down. It's wise to eat less salt because keeping your blood pressure values within normal range reduces your risk for heart attacks, strokes, and kidney disease.

When people are told to eat less sodium, most stop salting their food. That's actually not the best approach, because your total daily sodium intake comes from:

Salt-added and **sodium**-containing additives used in food processing	77%
Sodium found naturally occurring in food	12%
Salt added in cooking or at the table	11%

USING YOUR COMPLETE FOOD COUNTER

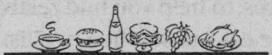

The Complete Food Counter, Second Edition, lists the portion size, calories, fat, cholesterol, protein, carbohydrate, fiber, and sodium values for more than 17,000 foods. These are key nutrients for you to consider when choosing foods. Fat, cholesterol, and sodium are nutrients you may want to limit. You can be more liberal with the others, aiming for moderate amounts of calories, protein, and carbohydrate, and higher amounts of fiber. Recommended intakes for all nutrients provided are given in the introduction. There are still other nutrients needed for good health, but when you eat a variety of foods containing the nutrients listed in this counter, you will automatically get the others.

Now you can compare the values in your favorite foods and, when necessary, choose substitutes before you go out to shop or eat. This will save you time and help you decide what to buy.

The counter section of the book is divided into two parts: Part One: Brand Name, Nonbranded (Generic), and Take-Out Foods; and Part Two: Restaurant Chains. Each part lists foods or restaurant chains alphabetically.

In Part One, for each category, you will find nonbranded (generic) foods listed first, in alphabetical order, followed by an alphabetical listing of brand name foods. The nonbranded listings will help you estimate calorie values when you don't see your favorite. They can also help you to evaluate store brands. Large categories are divided into subcategories, such as canned, fresh, frozen, and ready-to-eat, to make it easier to find what you're looking for. Some categories have "see" and "see also" references, to help you find related items.

Because people eat out so often, we listed more than 500 take-out foods in Part One. These are found in the take-out subcategory in many categories throughout this section. Look there for foods you take out or order in, because these foods are not nutrition labeled.

Most foods are listed alphabetically. But in some cases, foods are grouped by category. For example, a tuna sandwich is found in the SANDWICH category. Other group categories include:

ASIAN FOOD   **Page 24**
    includes all types of Asian foods
    except egg rolls and sushi, which are
    found in separate categories

DELI MEATS/COLD CUTS   **Page 230**
    includes all sandwich meats except
    chicken, ham, and turkey, which are
    found in separate categories

DINNER   **Page 233**
    includes all by brand name, except
    pasta dinners, which are found in
    a separate category

LIQUOR/LIQUEUR   **Page 354**
    includes all alcoholic beverages
    and mixed drinks except beer,

champagne, and wine, which
are found in separate categories

In Part Two, Restaurant Chains, 91 national and regional restaurants are listed, including candy, coffee, doughnut, ice cream, pizza, burger, seafood, sandwich, and ethnic food chains. Brand name foods are required by federal law to have nutrition information on labels. Restaurants, however, provide this information voluntarily.

With *The Complete Food Counter, Second Edition,* as your guide, you have at your fingertips the most thorough guide to the calories and important nutrients in the foods you eat.

DEFINITIONS

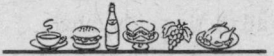

as prep (as prepared): refers to food that has been prepared according to package directions

lean and fat: describes meat with some fat on its edges that is not cut away before cooking, or poultry prepared with skin and fat as purchased

lean only: refers to lean meat that is trimmed of all visible fat, or poultry without skin

shelf stable: refers to prepared products found on the supermarket shelf that are ready-to-eat or are ready to be heated and do not require refrigeration

take-out: describes prepared dishes that you purchase ready-to-eat; those included serve as a guide to the calories, fat, cholesterol, protein, carbohydrate, fiber, and sodium values of similar products you may purchase.

ABBREVIATIONS

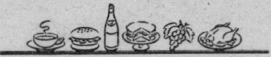

avg	=	average
diam	=	diameter
fl	=	fluid
frzn	=	frozen
g	=	gram
in	=	inch
lb	=	pound
lg	=	large
med	=	medium
mg	=	milligram
oz	=	ounce
pkg	=	package
pt	=	pint
prep	=	prepared
qt	=	quart
reg	=	regular
sec	=	second
serv	=	serving
sm	=	small
sq	=	square
tbsp	=	tablespoon
tr	=	trace
tsp	=	teaspoon
w/	=	with
w/o	=	without
<	=	less than

NOTES

Cals = Calories

Prot = Protein
  All protein values are given in grams (g).

Fat = Fat
  All fat values of foods are given in grams (g).

Carb = Carbohydrate
  All carbohydrate values are given in grams (g).

Chol = Cholesterol
  All cholesterol values are given in milligrams (mg).

Sod = Sodium
  All sodium values are given in milligrams (mg).

Fiber = Fiber
  All fiber values are given in grams (g).

tr (trace) = less than 1 gram of protein, fat, carbohydrate, or fiber, and less than 1 milligram of cholesterol or sodium.

— (dash) indicates data was not available.

0 (zero) indicates that there is none of the nutrient in that food.

Discrepancies in figures are due to rounding, product reformulation, and reevaluation. Labeling law allows rounding of values. Because much of the data is analysis data, obtained directly from manufacturers, not from labels, in some cases our values may not be exactly the same as label information because our values have not been rounded.

PART ONE

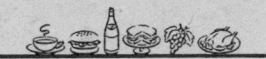

Brand Name, Nonbranded (Generic), and Take-Out Foods

FOOD	PORTION	CALS	PROT	FAT	CHOL	CARB	FIBER	SOD
ABALONE								
fresh fried	3 oz	161	17	6	80	9	–	502
raw	3 oz	89	15	1	72	5	–	255
ACEROLA								
fresh	1	2	tr	tr	0	tr	–	0
ACEROLA JUICE								
juice	1 cup	51	1	1	0	12	1	7
ADZUKI BEANS								
canned sweetened	1 cup	702	11	tr	0	163	–	645
dried cooked	1 cup	294	17	tr	0	57	17	18
AKEE								
fresh	3.5 oz	223	5	20	0	5	–	–
ALCOHOL (see BEER AND ALE, CHAMPAGNE, LIQUOR/LIQUEUR, MALT, WINE)								
ALE (see BEER AND ALE)								
ALFALFA								
sprouts	1 cup	40	1	tr	0	1	1	2
sprouts	1 tbsp	1	tr	tr	0	tr	tr	0
ALLIGATOR								
cooked	3 oz	126	28	2	57	0	0	66
ALLSPICE								
ground	1 tsp	5	tr	tr	0	1	–	1
ALMONDS								
almond butter honey & cinnamon	1 tbsp	96	3	8	0	4	–	2
almond butter w/ salt	1 tbsp	101	2	9	0	3	–	75
almond butter w/o salt	1 tbsp	101	2	10	0	3	–	2
almond meal	1 oz	116	11	5	0	8	–	2
almond paste	1 oz	127	3	8	0	12	–	3
dried unblanched	1 oz	167	6	15	0	6	–	3
dry roasted unblanched	1 oz	167	5	15	0	7	–	3

FOOD	PORTION	CALS	PROT	FAT	CHOL	CARB	FIBER	SOD
dry roasted unblanched salted	1 oz	167	5	15	0	7	—	260
dry roasted w/ salt	24 nuts (1 oz)	170	6	15	0	6	3	100
jordan almonds	10 (1.4 oz)	190	4	7	0	28	1	0
oil roasted blanched	1 oz	174	16	16	0	5	3	3
oil roasted blanched salted	1 oz	174	5	16	0	5	—	3
oil roasted unblanched	1 oz	176	6	16	0	5	—	3
praline	17 pieces (1.4 oz)	210	5	12	0	21	3	45
toasted unblanched	1 oz	167	6	14	0	7	3	3
American Almond								
Almond Paste	2 tbsp	140	4	9	0	13	2	0
Marzipan	2 tbsp	130	2	5	0	19	1	0
Roasted Butter	2 tbsp	180	6	16	0	6	3	55
Judy's								
Sugar Free Coconut Almond Brittle	¼ piece (1 oz)	90	1	5	0	2	1	0
Keto								
Chocolatey Covered	1 oz	169	6	13	—	7	5	—
Low Carb Creations								
Soft Almond Brittle	2 pieces (1 oz)	170	6	12	0	17	2	170
Mama Mellace's								
Butter Rum	1 oz	150	4	10	0	13	2	0
Cinnamon Roasted	1 oz	140	4	9	0	14	2	0
Maranatha								
Almond Butter	2 tbsp	220	8	18	0	6	3	0
Raw Almond Butter	2 tbsp	190	7	17	0	7	4	0
Tamari Almonds	¼ cup	160	6	14	0	6	3	140
Sweet Delights								
Almond Roasters	⅓ pkg (1 oz)	190	6	14	0	6	3	200
AMARANTH								
leaves cooked	1 cup	28	3	tr	0	5	—	28
uncooked	1 cup (6.8 oz)	729	28	13	0	129	30	41

FOOD	PORTION	CALS	PROT	FAT	CHOL	CARB	FIBER	SOD
ANCHOVY								
canned in oil	1 can (1.6 oz)	95	13	4	–	0	–	1651
canned in oil	5	42	6	2	–	0	–	734
fresh fillets	3 (0.4 oz)	21	2	1	–	tr	–	–
fresh raw	3 oz	62	17	4	–	0	–	88
ANGLERFISH								
raw	3.5 oz	72	15	1	–	0	–	109
ANISE								
seed	1 tsp	7	tr	tr	0	1	–	tr
ANTELOPE								
roasted	3 oz	127	25	2	107	0	–	46
APPLE								
CANNED								
sliced sweetened	1 cup	137	tr	1	0	34	4	7
Del Monte								
Fruit Pleasures Pie Spiced Apples	½ cup (4.1 oz)	70	0	0	0	18	1	10
Luck's								
Fried Apples	½ cup (4.7 oz)	130	0	0	0	33	2	0
DRIED								
cooked w/ sugar	1 cup	232	1	tr	0	58	5	53
cooked w/o sugar	1 cup	145	1	tr	0	39	5	51
rings	10	155	1	tr	0	42	6	56
Del Monte								
Dried Apples	¼ cup	110	1	0	0	26	3	250
FRESH								
apple	1 sm	63	tr	tr	0	16	3	0
apple	1 lg	125	tr	1	0	32	6	0
apple	1 med	81	tr	tr	0	21	4	1
w/o skin sliced	1 cup	63	tr	tr	0	16	2	0
w/o skin sliced & cooked	1 cup	91	tr	tr	0	23	4	1
w/o skin sliced & microwaved	1 cup	95	tr	tr	0	25	5	1
Chiquita								
Apple	1 med (5.4 oz)	80	0	0	0	22	5	0

FOOD	PORTION	CALS	PROT	FAT	CHOL	CARB	FIBER	SOD
Cool Cut								
Apples & Caramel Dip	1 pkg (4.25 oz)	180	1	5	5	32	3	80
FROZEN								
sliced w/o sugar	1 cup	83	tr	1	0	21	3	5
TAKE-OUT								
baked	1 (5.3 oz)	126	tr	tr	0	33	3	1
baked no sugar	1 (5.9 oz)	82	tr	1	0	21	3	6
APPLE JUICE								
frzn as prep	1 cup	111	tr	tr	0	28	–	17
frzn not prep	1 can (6 oz)	350	1	1	0	87	–	54
juice + vitamin C	1 cup	117	tr	tr	0	29	tr	7
mulled cider	1 serv	265	1	1	0	42	6	12
Apple & Eve								
100% Juice	8 fl oz	110	1	0	0	26	–	5
Cider	8 fl oz	110	1	0	0	27	–	10
Eden								
Organic Juice	8 oz	80	0	0	0	23	0	0
Hansen's								
Junior Juice 100%	1 box (4.23 oz)	60	0	0	0	15	1	0
Langers								
100% Cider	8 oz	120	0	0	0	28	–	0
100% Juice	8 oz	120	0	0	0	28	–	0
Diet Cocktail	8 oz	60	0	0	0	14	–	10
Low Carb Creations								
Apple Cider as prep	1 serv	10	0	0	0	2	0	5
Mott's								
100% Juice	1 box (8 oz)	120	0	0	0	29	–	15
100% Juice	8 fl oz	120	0	0	0	29	0	20
100% Natural	8 fl oz	120	0	0	0	29	0	20
Naked Juice								
Just Apple	8 oz	120	0	0	0	29	0	5
Ocean Spray								
100% Juice	8 oz	110	0	0	0	28	0	35
Odwalla								
Spiced Harvest Cider	8 fl oz	130	0	0	0	30	0	20
Robert & James								
100% Juice	8 oz	110	0	0	0	28	–	35

FOOD	PORTION	CALS	PROT	FAT	CHOL	CARB	FIBER	SOD
Snapple								
Diet	8 oz	15	0	0	0	4	–	10
Snapple Apple	8 fl oz	120	0	0	0	30	–	10
Swiss Miss								
Hot Apple Cider Mix	1 serv	84	tr	tr	0	20	1	58
Hot Apple Cider Mix Low Calorie	1 serv	14	0	0	0	3	0	78
Turkey Hill								
Herbal Cider w/ Chamomile & Lemongrass	1 cup	100	–	0	0	24	–	–
Zeigler's								
Old Fashioned Cider	8 oz	120	0	0	0	30	0	25
APPLESAUCE								
sweetened	½ cup	97	tr	tr	0	25	2	4
unsweetened	½ cup	52	tr	tr	0	14	2	2
Eden								
Organic	½ cup	50	0	0	0	15	2	15
Organic Sweet Cinnamon	½ cup	50	0	0	0	19	4	0
Jok'n'Al								
Low Carb	1 tbsp	10	0	0	0	2	–	0
Mott's								
Single-Serve Cinnamon	1 pkg (4 oz)	100	0	0	0	26	–	0
Single-Serve Natural	1 pkg (4 oz)	50	0	0	0	12	–	0
Single-Serve Original	1 pkg (4 oz)	100	0	0	0	24	–	0
Musselman's								
Apple Sauce	1 pkg (4 oz)	80	0	0	0	20	2	10
Vermont Village								
Organic Unsweetened	½ cup	80	tr	0	0	19	2	1
APRICOT JUICE								
nectar	1 cup	141	1	tr	0	36	2	9
Ceres								
Apricot	8 oz	120	0	0	0	30	0	10

FOOD	PORTION	CALS	PROT	FAT	CHOL	CARB	FIBER	SOD
APRICOTS								
CANNED								
halves heavy syrup pack w/ skin	1 cup (9.1 oz)	214	1	tr	0	55	–	10
halves water pack w/ skin	1 cup (8.5 oz)	65	2	tr	0	16	–	7
halves water pack w/o skin	1 cup (8 oz)	51	2	tr	0	12	–	25
heavy syrup	3 halves	99	1	tr	0	26	2	6
juice pack	3 halves	51	1	tr	0	13	2	3
puree from heavy syrup pack w/ skin	¾ cup (9.1 oz)	214	1	tr	0	55	–	10
puree from light pack w/ skin	¾ cup (8.9 oz)	160	1	tr	0	42	–	10
puree from water pack w/ skin	¾ cup (8.5 oz)	65	2	tr	0	16	–	7
puree juice pack w/ skin	1 cup (8.7 oz)	119	2	tr	0	31	–	9
water pack	3 halves	30	1	tr	0	7	2	3
Del Monte								
Halves Unpeeled Lite	½ cup (4.3 oz)	60	0	0	0	16	1	10
Orchard Select Halves Unpeeled	½ cup (4.4 oz)	80	0	0	0	21	1	10
DRIED								
halves	4	32	tr	tr	0	9	1	0
halves cooked w/o sugar	½ cup	153	2	tr	0	40	6	4
FRESH								
apricots	1	17	tr	tr	0	4	1	0
Chiquita								
Apricots	3 med (4 oz)	60	0	1	0	11	1	0
FROZEN								
sweetened	½ cup	119	1	tr	0	30	3	5
ARROWHEAD								
corm boiled	1 med	9	1	tr	0	2	–	2
flour	1 cup	457	tr	tr	0	113	4	3

FOOD	PORTION	CALS	PROT	FAT	CHOL	CARB	FIBER	SOD
ARTICHOKE								
CANNED								
Progresso								
Hearts	2 pieces (2.9 oz)	30	2	0	0	6	1	240
Hearts Marinated	2 pieces (1.1 oz)	170	0	5	0	2	0	110
S&W								
Marinated Hearts	2 pieces (1 oz)	20	0	2	0	2	1	80
FRESH								
cooked	1 med	60	4	tr	0	13	7	114
hearts cooked	½ cup	42	3	tr	0	9	5	80
FROZEN								
cooked	1 pkg (9 oz)	108	7	1	0	22	11	127
Birds Eye								
Hearts	½ cup	40	–	0	0	–	6	45
ARUGULA								
fresh	½ cup	3	tr	tr	0	tr	tr	3
ASIAN FOOD *(see also* DINNER, EGG ROLLS, SUSHI*)*								
CANNED								
chow mein chicken	1 cup	95	7	tr	8	18	–	725
Chun King								
Beef Pepper Oriental BiPack	1 cup (8.8 oz)	98	10	2	14	13	3	865
Chow Mein Beef BiPack	1 cup (8.6 oz)	78	8	1	6	11	3	718
Chow Mein BiPack Chicken	1 cup (8.8 oz)	98	8	3	6	11	3	1123
Chow Mein Pork BiPack	1 cup (8.6 oz)	78	7	2	10	9	2	1183
Hot & Spicy Chicken BiPack	1 cup (8.6 oz)	98	8	3	19	11	1	857
Sweet & Sour Chicken BiPack	1 cup (8.9 oz)	161	7	2	25	29	3	687
La Choy								
Beef Pepper Oriental BiPack	1 cup (8.8 oz)	98	10	2	14	13	3	865

FOOD	PORTION	CALS	PROT	FAT	CHOL	CARB	FIBER	SOD
Chow Mein Beef BiPack	1 cup (8.6 oz)	78	8	1	6	11	3	718
Chow Mein Chicken PiBack	1 cup (8.9 oz)	98	8	3	6	11	3	1123
Chow Mein Shrimp BiPack	1 cup (8.6 oz)	52	4	1	4	9	3	965
Main Entree Chow Mein Chicken	1 cup (9.3 oz)	80	8	4	9	6	3	1325
Oriental Beef w/ Noodles BiPack	1 cup (8.8 oz)	156	18	3	17	18	4	896
Oriental Chicken w/ Noodles BiPack	1 cup (8.7 oz)	154	14	4	23	18	2	1100
Sweet & Sour Chicken BiPack	1 cup (8.9 oz)	161	7	2	25	29	3	687
Teriyaki Chicken BiPack	1 cup (8.6 oz)	109	8	3	20	15	3	1230
FRESH								
wonton wrappers	1	23	1	tr	1	5	–	46
Azumaya								
Round Wraps	10	160	6	1	10	31	1	370
Square Wraps	6	160	6	1	10	31	1	370
Wrappers Large Square	3	170	7	1	10	35	1	410
Nasoya								
Egg Roll Wrapper	3	170	7	1	10	35	1	410
Won Ton Wrappers	8	160	6	1	10	31	1	370
FROZEN								
Amy's								
Bowls Teriyaki	1 pkg (10 oz)	300	10	2	0	59	3	780
Skillet Meals Teriyaki Stir Fry	1 cup	320	9	3	0	64	4	590
Stir Fry Asian Noodle	1 pkg (10 oz)	240	12	5	0	41	6	680
Stir Fry Thai	1 pkg (9.5 oz)	270	7	11	0	36	2	420
Banquet								
Fried Rice w/ Chicken & Egg Rolls	1 meal (8.5 oz)	330	12	9	60	51	5	1270

FOOD	PORTION	CALS	PROT	FAT	CHOL	CARB	FIBER	SOD
Birds Eye								
Easy Recipe Creations Oriental Lo Mein	2¼ cups	230	8	4	5	40	2	1200
Easy Recipe Creations Sesame Ginger Teriyaki	2¼ cups	140	6	2	0	24	4	1230
Easy Recipe Creations Spicy Szechuan Cashews	2¼ cups	180	6	5	0	29	4	1410
La Choy								
Beef Pepper Oriental	1 cup (7.1 oz)	151	8	1	10	30	2	714
Chow Mein Vegetable	1 cup (8.9 oz)	108	2	2	0	20	5	1135
Lean Cuisine								
Everyday Favorites Oriental Style Dumplings	1 pkg (9 oz)	300	10	6	20	51	2	520
Everyday Favorites Teriyaki Stir Fry	1 pkg (10 oz)	290	18	4	20	45	4	590
MIX								
Annie Chun's								
Meal Kit Black Bean	1 serv	230	8	3	0	42	2	670
Meal Kit Garlic Scallion	1 serv	230	7	5	0	39	2	780
Meal Kit Soy Ginger	1 serv	220	8	2	0	42	3	850
TAKE-OUT								
buddha's delight w/ cellophane noodles fat choi jai	1 serv (7.6 oz)	211	7	4	tr	44	2	772
cashew chicken	1 serv	406	–	29	61	–	–	988
cha siu bao steamed buns w/ chicken filling	1 (2.3 oz)	160	5	3	15	26	tr	300

FOOD	PORTION	CALS	PROT	FAT	CHOL	CARB	FIBER	SOD
chop suey cantonese chicken	1 serv	570	–	17	70	–	–	1070
chop suey w/ beef & pork	1 cup	300	26	17	68	13	–	1053
chop suey w/ pork	1 cup	375	19	29	62	29	2	1378
chow mein chicken	1 cup	255	31	10	75	10	–	718
chow mein pork	1 cup	425	32	24	89	21	3	1673
chow mein shrimp	1 cup	221	13	10	55	21	3	1658
chow mein vegetable	1 serv (8 oz)	90	3	3	0	15	4	1010
filipino chicken adobo	1 serv (15 oz)	555	33	26	116	45	1	468
fried rice chicken	1 serv	314	–	89	5	–	–	972
fried rice vegetable	1 cup	210	3	9	0	30	1	520
fried rice w/ egg	6.7 oz	395	8	20	–	49	2	–
general tsao's chicken	1 serv	723	–	35	143	–	–	1775
kung pao chicken	1 cup	409	–	29	60	–	–	988
kung pao chicken w/ rice	1 serv (1.75 cups)	240	12	3	25	42	4	800
lo mein pork	1 serv	323	–	40	7	–	–	1337
moo goo gai pan chicken	1 cup	272	–	35	31	–	–	305
phad thai	1 serv (9.2 oz)	232	11	9	0	30	1	426
sesame seed paste bun	1 (2.5 oz)	220	5	6	0	39	2	53
shrimp & snow peas	1 cup	220	–	148	12	–	–	1067
shrimp chips	1¼ cups (1 oz)	140	2	6	0	19	0	240
shu mai chicken & vegetable dumplings	6 (3.6 oz)	160	10	5	35	18	1	910
soba noodles w/ vegetables	1 serv	276	–	39	8	–	–	1092
spring roll	1 (3.5 oz)	112	12	2	–	37	5	670
stir fry beef & broccoli	2 cup	512	–	202	39	–	–	1473

FOOD	PORTION	CALS	PROT	FAT	CHOL	CARB	FIBER	SOD
stir fry garlic green beans	1 serv	68	–	0	1	–	–	357
stir fry vegetable	1 serv	235	–	70	11	–	–	1900
sweet & sour chicken w/o rice	1 serv	416	–	95	6	–	–	442
sweet & sour pork	1 serv (8 oz)	250	6	8	30	37	2	1500
sweet red bean bun	1 (2.5 oz)	130	4	1	0	38	2	95
szechuan chicken w/ lo mein	1 cup (5.3 oz)	190	10	1	5	35	0	560
szechuan cold noodles	1 serv	334	–	0	7	–	–	1531
tempura seafood & vegetable	1 serv	590	–	185	32	–	–	1660
tempura vegetables	5 pieces (4 oz)	270	2	15	0	31	2	210
teriyaki beef w/ sticky rice	1 serv	664	–	105	14	–	–	898
teriyaki chicken plain	¾ cup	399	30	27	92	7	–	2190
teriyaki chicken w/ rice	1 serv (11 oz)	430	19	6	25	77	1	1210
wonton fried	½ cup (1 oz)	111	2	8	31	8	1	147

ASPARAGUS
CANNED

FOOD	PORTION	CALS	PROT	FAT	CHOL	CARB	FIBER	SOD
spears	½ cup	23	3	1	0	3	2	347
Del Monte								
Cuts & Tips	½ cup (4.4 oz)	20	2	0	0	3	1	420
Spears Extra Long	½ cup (4.4 oz)	20	2	0	0	3	1	420
Spears Tender Young	½ cup (4.4 oz)	20	2	0	0	3	1	420
Tips Hand Selected	½ cup (4.4 oz)	20	2	0	0	3	1	420
S&W								
Green	6 pieces (4.5 oz)	15	2	0	0	4	1	260

FOOD	PORTION	CALS	PROT	FAT	CHOL	CARB	FIBER	SOD
FRESH								
cooked	½ cup	22	2	tr	0	4	1	10
cooked	4 spears	14	2	tr	0	3	1	7
raw	4 spears	15	tr	tr	0	1	tr	0
raw	½ cup	16	2	tr	0	3	1	2
FROZEN								
cooked	1 pkg (10 oz)	82	9	1	0	14	5	12
cooked	4 spears	17	2	tr	0	3	1	2
Birds Eye								
Cuts	½ cup	25	–	0	0	–	2	5
Jumbo Spears	3 oz	20	–	0	0	–	1	5
ATEMOYA								
fresh	½ cup	94	1	1	–	24	–	2
AVOCADO								
fresh mashed	1 cup	407	5	40	0	16	11	28
fresh peeled california	1	306	4	30	0	12	9	21
fresh peeled florida	1	340	5	27	0	27	16	15
Brooks Tropical								
Lite SlimCado	1 tbsp	35	0	3	0	3	tr	–
Chiquita								
Fresh	⅓ med (1 oz)	55	1	5	0	3	3	0
TAKE-OUT								
guacamole	1 serv (2.2 oz)	105	1	10	0	5	2	187
BACON								
breakfast strips cooked	3 strips	156	10	12	36	tr	0	714
gammon lean & fat grilled	4.2 oz	274	35	15	–	0	0	–
pan fried	3 strips	109	6	9	16	tr	0	303
Armour								
Star cooked	1 strip	38	–	3	6	–	–	185
Health Is Wealth								
Uncured Sliced	2 slices (0.5 oz)	70	3	7	10	0	–	380

FOOD	PORTION	CALS	PROT	FAT	CHOL	CARB	FIBER	SOD
Ready Crisp								
Fully Cooked	3 slices (0.5 oz)	70	4	6	15	0	—	270
BACON SUBSTITUTES								
meatless	1 strip	16	1	1	0	tr	tr	73
Bac-Os								
Chips or Bits	1½ tbsp (7 g)	30	3	2	0	2	0	120
Lightlife								
Fakin' Bacon Bits	1 tsp	45	1	1	0	1	0	25
Smart Bacon	2 strips (0.8 oz)	45	6	2	0	2	0	360
Morningstar Farms								
Breakfast Strips	2 (0.5 oz)	60	2	5	0	2	tr	220
BAGEL								
cinnamon raisin	1 lg	359	13	2	0	72	3	422
cinnamon raisin toasted	1 lg	363	13	2	0	73	3	426
egg	1 lg	364	14	3	31	69	3	662
egg	1 mini	72	3	1	6	14	1	131
mini onion	1 (1.4 oz)	100	4	0	0	20	1	90
oat bran	1 lg	334	14	2	0	70	5	664
onion	1 lg	363	13	2	0	71	3	706
plain	1 mini	72	3	tr	0	14	1	139
plain	1 lg	360	13	2	0	70	3	700
poppy seed	1 lg	360	14	2	0	70	3	700
Atkins								
Cinnamon Raisin	1	200	20	4	0	20	11	290
Onion	1	190	19	5	0	19	11	290
Plain	1	190	20	5	0	18	11	310
Natural Ovens								
Blueberry	1 (3 oz)	190	9	2	0	40	4	220
Cinnamon Raisin	1 (3 oz)	180	9	1	0	40	5	240
Golden Crunch	1 (3 oz)	190	15	11	0	15	8	200
Hearty Grains & Onion	1 (3 oz)	190	10	4	0	37	7	250
Raspberry	1 (3 oz)	180	7	2	0	38	5	110
Whole Grain	1 (3 oz)	170	9	3	0	35	6	200

FOOD	PORTION	CALS	PROT	FAT	CHOL	CARB	FIBER	SOD
Pepperidge Farm								
Mini	1 (1.4 oz)	110	4	1	0	22	1	200
Plain	1 (3.5 oz)	290	11	1	0	60	2	480
Sara Lee								
Blueberry	1 (2.8 oz)	210	8	1	0	41	2	570
Cinnamon Raisin	1 (2.8 oz)	220	8	1	0	45	3	320
Egg	1 (2.8 oz)	210	7	1	0	44	2	460
Oat Bran	1 (2.8 oz)	210	8	1	0	42	3	570
Onion	1 (2.8 oz)	210	7	0	0	44	2	540
Plain	1 (2.8 oz)	210	8	1	0	43	2	500
Poppy Seed	1 (2.8 oz)	210	8	1	0	41	2	570
Sesame Seed	1 (2.8 oz)	210	8	2	0	42	2	530
Thomas'								
Carb Counting Whole Wheat	1 (2.2 oz)	140	11	2	0	22	6	330
Everything	1 (3.6 oz)	300	10	4	0	56	3	510
Multi-Grain	1 (3.6 oz)	280	11	2	0	55	4	460
Plain	1 (3.6 oz)	280	10	2	0	56	2	530
Uncle B's								
Plain	1 (2.8 oz)	210	8	1	0	41	2	310
Weight Watchers								
Original	1 (2.8 oz)	190	10	2	0	44	10	520
BAKING POWDER								
baking powder	1 tsp	2	0	0	0	1	–	488
low sodium	1 tsp	5	0	0	0	2	–	4
Clabber Girl								
Baking Powder	1 tsp	0	tr	0	0	1	–	435
Davis								
Baking Powder	1 tsp	0	0	0	0	0	–	380
Rumford								
Aluminum Free	⅛ tsp	0	0	0	0	tr	–	110
BAKING SODA								
baking soda	1 tsp	0	0	0	0	0	–	1259
BALSAM PEAR (BITTER GOURD)								
leafy tips cooked	½ cup	10	1	tr	0	2	1	4
leafy tips raw	½ cup	7	1	tr	0	1	–	3
pods cooked	½ cup	12	1	tr	0	3	1	4

FOOD	PORTION	CALS	PROT	FAT	CHOL	CARB	FIBER	SOD

BAMBOO SHOOTS
canned sliced	1 cup	25	2	1	0	4	2	9
fresh	½ cup	21	2	tr	0	1	2	3
fresh cooked	½ cup	12	1	tr	0	2	—	5
Chun King								
Bamboo Shoots	2 tbsp (0.8 oz)	3	tr	tr	0	1	tr	0
La Choy								
Bamboo Shoots	2 tbsp (0.8 oz)	3	tr	tr	0	1	tr	0

BANANA
banana chips	1 oz	147	1	10	0	17	2	2
fresh	1 med	109	1	tr	0	28	3	1
fresh mashed	1 cup	207	2	1	0	53	5	2
fresh sliced	1 cup	138	2	1	0	35	4	2
powder	1 tbsp	21	tr	tr	0	5	1	0
whole dried	1 piece (1.2 oz)	130	1	1	0	33	2	0
Chiquita								
Fresh	1 med (4.4 oz)	110	1	0	0	29	4	0

BARBECUE SAUCE
barbecue	1 cup	188	5	5	0	32	—	2038
Atkins								
Barbecue Sauce	1 tbsp	15	0	1	0	tr	0	180
Bull's Eye								
Original	2 tbsp	50	—	0	0	—	—	—
Carb Options								
Original	2 tbsp	10	0	0	0	3	0	340
Hunt's								
Hickory	2 tbsp	45	0	0	0	11	tr	290
Hickory & Brown Sugar	2 tbsp	70	0	0	0	16	1	360
Honey Hickory	2 tbsp (1.2 oz)	50	0	0	0	12	tr	380
Honey Mustard	2 tbsp	50	0	0	0	12	1	310
Hot & Spicy	2 tbsp	45	0	0	0	11	tr	440
Mesquite	2 tbsp	40	0	0	0	9	tr	360
Original	2 tbsp	45	1	0	0	11	tr	290

FOOD	PORTION	CALS	PROT	FAT	CHOL	CARB	FIBER	SOD
Muir Glen								
Garlic Mesquite	2 tbsp (1.3 oz)	40	0	0	0	6	tr	265
Hot & Smoky	2 tbsp (1.2 oz)	40	0	0	0	6	tr	265
Original	2 tbsp (1.2 oz)	40	0	0	0	6	tr	265
Steel's								
Sugar Free	2 tbsp	15	0	0	0	2	0	200
BARLEY								
flour	1 cup	511	15	2	0	110	15	6
malt flour	1 cup	585	17	3	0	127	12	18
pearled cooked	1 cup (5.5 oz)	193	4	1	0	44	6	5
pearled uncooked	1 cup	704	20	2	0	155	31	18
Mother's								
Quick Cooking	⅓ cup	170	5	1	0	37	5	0
BARRACUDA								
fresh	3 oz	122	14	8	66	0	0	57
BASIL								
fresh chopped	2 tbsp	1	tr	tr	0	tr	tr	0
ground	1 tsp	4	tr	tr	0	1	–	tr
leaves fresh	5	1	tr	tr	0	tr	tr	0
BASS								
freshwater raw	3 oz	97	16	3	58	0	–	59
sea cooked	3 oz	105	20	2	45	0	–	74
sea raw	3 oz	82	16	2	35	0	–	58
striped baked	3 oz	105	19	3	87	0	–	75
striped bass farm raised	4 oz	110	20	3	90	0	0	80
BAY LEAF								
crumbled	1 tsp	2	tr	tr	0	tr	–	tr
BEANS (see also individual names)								
CANNED								
baked beans plain	½ cup	118	6	1	0	26	6	504
baked beans vegetarian	½ cup	118	6	1	0	26	6	504
baked beans w/ beef	½ cup	161	8	5	29	22	–	632

FOOD	PORTION	CALS	PROT	FAT	CHOL	CARB	FIBER	SOD
baked beans w/ franks	½ cup	184	9	9	8	20	9	551
baked beans w/ pork	½ cup	134	7	2	9	25	7	522
baked beans w/ pork & sweet sauce	½ cup	140	7	2	9	26	7	423
baked beans w/ pork & tomato sauce	½ cup	124	7	1	9	24	7	554
refried beans	½ cup	134	8	1	—	23	—	534
Amy's								
Vegetarian Baked	½ cup	120	5	5	0	24	6	480
B&M								
Barbeque Baked	½ cup (4.6 oz)	210	8	1	0	42	9	570
Maple Baked	½ cup	150	6	1	0	28	6	340
Vegetarian 99% Fat Free	½ cup	150	6	1	0	28	6	340
Bush's								
Barbecue	½ cup (4.6 oz)	160	6	1	0	32	6	510
Country Style	½ cup	170	7	1	0	33	7	680
Homestyle	½ cup	150	6	2	5	28	8	480
Maple Cured Bacon	½ cup	150	7	1	0	28	7	620
Original	½ cup	150	7	1	0	29	7	550
Vegetarian	½ cup (4.6 oz)	130	6	0	0	24	6	550
Campbell's								
Pork & Beans	½ cup	140	6	1	<5	27	7	460
Eden								
Organic Baked w/ Sorghum & Mustard	½ cup (4.6 oz)	150	8	0	0	27	7	130
Gebhardt								
Chili	½ cup (4.6 oz)	134	7	1	0	31	7	630
Refried Jalapeno	½ cup (4.5 oz)	105	7	3	1	19	6	380

FOOD	PORTION	CALS	PROT	FAT	CHOL	CARB	FIBER	SOD
Refried No Fat	½ cup (4.5 oz)	92	7	tr	0	20	6	480
Refried Traditional	½ cup (4.5 oz)	109	6	3	1	20	6	497
Refried Vegetarian	½ cup (4.5 oz)	118	8	2	tr	21	7	550
Heinz								
Vegetarian	1 cup	250	11	1	0	48	9	840
Hunt's								
Big John's Beans & Fixin's	½ cup (4.7 oz)	127	7	4	3	23	6	590
Homestyle Country Kettle	½ cup (4.6 oz)	152	7	2	1	31	7	425
Homestyle Special Recipe	½ cup (4.7 oz)	185	7	3	1	36	8	687
Mix & Serve	½ cup (4.7 oz)	125	2	3	1	30	8	575
Pork & Beans	½ cup (4.5 oz)	130	6	1	tr	28	4	516
Old El Paso								
Refried Fat Free	½ cup	100	6	0	0	18	6	580
Open Range								
Ranch	½ cup (4.4 oz)	124	6	3	1	23	8	628
Pringles								
Vegetarian	1 cup (7.9 oz)	250	11	1	0	48	9	840
Rosarita								
3 Bean Recipe Bacon & Jalapeno	½ cup (4.6 oz)	117	8	2	1	22	5	543
3 Bean Recipe Chilies & Chicken	½ cup (4.6 oz)	115	7	1	1	22	4	517
3 Bean Recipe Chilies & Chorizo	½ cup (4.6 oz)	111	8	2	1	19	4	591
3 Bean Recipe Onions & Peppers	½ cup (4.6 oz)	104	7	1	1	20	5	539
Fiesta Beans Bacon & Jalapenos	½ cup (4.6 oz)	117	8	2	1	22	5	543

FOOD	PORTION	CALS	PROT	FAT	CHOL	CARB	FIBER	SOD
Fiesta Beans Chicken & Chilies	½ cup (4.6 oz)	115	7	1	1	22	4	517
Fiesta Beans Chilies & Chorizo	½ cup (4.6 oz)	110	8	2	1	19	4	591
Fiesta Beans Onions & Peppers	½ cup (4.6 oz)	104	8	1	1	20	5	539
Refried Bacon	½ cup (4.5 oz)	116	6	3	1	19	8	489
Refried Green Chile	½ cup (4.5 oz)	110	6	3	1	20	7	495
Refried Low Fat Black	½ cup (4.5 oz)	107	8	1	0	23	7	569
Refried Nacho Cheese	½ cup (4.5 oz)	108	8	2	2	19	6	574
Refried No Fat	½ cup	90	7	0	0	17	5	590
Refried No Fat Green Chiles & Lime	½ cup (4.5 oz)	101	8	tr	0	22	8	565
Refried No Fat w/ Zesty Salsa	½ cup (4.5 oz)	105	6	tr	0	24	6	599
Refried Onion	½ cup (4.5 oz)	114	6	3	1	21	6	508
Refried Spicy	½ cup (4.5 oz)	118	7	3	0	22	6	574
Refried Traditional	½ cup (4.5 oz)	108	5	1	0	19	5	510
Refried Vegetarian	½ cup (4.5 oz)	237	15	5	tr	42	13	1101
S&W								
Barbecue Beans Ranch Recipe	½ cup (4.5 oz)	100	6	2	0	25	8	640
Van Camp								
Baked Fat Free	½ cup (4.6 oz)	132	6	tr	0	29	5	505
Baked Original	½ cup	140	7	1	0	30	6	540
Baked Southern Style Sauteed Onion	½ cup (4.8 oz)	145	6	1	1	35	8	555
Baked Sweet Hickory & Bacon	1 can (4.8 oz)	143	6	1	tr	32	6	471

FOOD	PORTION	CALS	PROT	FAT	CHOL	CARB	FIBER	SOD
Beanee Weenee Baked	1 cup (9.1 oz)	410	18	14	40	58	10	1210
Beanee Weenee BBQ	1 cup (7.7 oz)	290	14	12	35	36	7	970
Beanee Weenee Microwave	1 cup (7.5 oz)	260	14	11	35	29	6	1020
Beanee Weenee Original	1 cup (9.1 oz)	320	16	14	40	35	8	1240
Beanee Weenee Zestful	1 cup (7.7 oz)	300	14	12	35	40	7	1030
Brown Sugar	½ cup (4.6 oz)	170	7	3	5	31	6	410
Pork And Beans	½ cup (4.6 oz)	110	6	2	0	23	6	490
Vegetarian	½ cup (4.6 oz)	110	6	1	0	23	5	400

FROZEN
Natural Touch

FOOD	PORTION	CALS	PROT	FAT	CHOL	CARB	FIBER	SOD
Nine Bean Loaf	1 in slice (3 oz)	160	8	8	<5	13	5	350

TAKE-OUT

FOOD	PORTION	CALS	PROT	FAT	CHOL	CARB	FIBER	SOD
baked beans	½ cup	161	8	5	29	22	—	632
barbecue beans	3.5 oz	120	4	tr	0	26	—	460
four bean salad	3.5 oz	100	4	tr	0	20	—	280
frijoles w/ cheese	1 cup	225	—	8	37	—	—	882
refried beans	½ cup	43	2	2	2	5	—	104
three bean salad	¾ cup	230	5	11	0	31	1	500

BEAN SPROUTS (see ALFALFA, SPROUTS)

BEAR

FOOD	PORTION	CALS	PROT	FAT	CHOL	CARB	FIBER	SOD
simmered	3 oz	220	28	11	—	0	—	—

BEAVER

FOOD	PORTION	CALS	PROT	FAT	CHOL	CARB	FIBER	SOD
roasted	3 oz	140	30	6	—	0	—	50
simmered	3 oz	141	23	5	—	0	—	39

BEECHNUTS

FOOD	PORTION	CALS	PROT	FAT	CHOL	CARB	FIBER	SOD
dried	1 oz	164	2	14	0	10	—	—

FOOD	PORTION	CALS	PROT	FAT	CHOL	CARB	FIBER	SOD
BEEF *(see also* BEEF DISHES, VEAL*)*								
CANNED								
corned beef	3 oz	85	10	5	–	0	–	–
Treet								
Luncheon Loaf	2 oz	130	6	11	50	3	0	740
Luncheon Loaf 50% Less Fat	2 oz	110	6	8	45	4	0	750
FRESH								
bottom round lean & fat trim 0 in braised	3 oz	193	26	26	82	0	–	43
bottom round lean & fat trim 0 in Choice roasted	3 oz	172	24	8	66	0	–	56
bottom round lean & fat trim 0 in Select braised	3 oz	171	27	6	82	0	–	43
bottom round lean & fat trim 0 in Select roasted	3 oz	150	24	24	66	0	–	56
bottom round lean & fat trim ¼ in Choice braised	3 oz	241	24	15	81	0	–	42
bottom round lean & fat trim ¼ in Choice roasted	3 oz	221	22	14	68	0	–	53
bottom round lean & fat trim ¼ in Select braised	3 oz	220	25	13	81	0	–	42
bottom round lean & fat trim ¼ in Select roasted	3 oz	199	23	11	68	0	–	54

FOOD	PORTION	CALS	PROT	FAT	CHOL	CARB	FIBER	SOD
brisket flat half lean & fat trim 0 in braised	3 oz	183	26	8	81	0	–	53
brisket flat half lean & fat trim ¼ in braised	3 oz	309	21	24	81	0	–	48
brisket point half lean & fat trim 0 in braised	3 oz	304	20	24	78	0	–	57
brisket point half lean & fat trim ¼ in braised	3 oz	343	19	29	79	0	–	55
brisket whole lean & fat trim 0 in braised	3 oz	247	23	17	79	0	–	55
brisket whole lean & fat trim ¼ in braised	3 oz	327	27	27	80	0	–	52
chuck arm pot roast lean & fat trim 0 in braised	3 oz	238	25	14	85	0	–	53
chuck arm pot roast lean & fat trim ¼ in braised	3 oz	282	23	20	85	0	–	51
chuck blade roast lean & fat trim 0 in braised	3 oz	284	23	21	88	0	–	56
chuck blade roast lean & fat trim ¼ in braised	3 oz	293	23	22	88	0	–	55
corned beef brisket cooked	3 oz	213	15	16	83	tr	–	964
eye of round lean & fat trim 0 in Choice roasted	3 oz	153	24	5	59	0	–	53
eye of round lean & fat trim 0 in Select roasted	3 oz	137	24	4	59	0	–	53

FOOD	PORTION	CALS	PROT	FAT	CHOL	CARB	FIBER	SOD
eye of round lean & fat trim ¼ in Choice roasted	3 oz	205	23	12	62	0	—	50
eye of round lean & fat trim ¼ in Select roasted	3 oz	184	23	10	61	0	—	51
flank lean & fat trim 0 in braised	3 oz	224	23	14	62	0	—	60
flank lean & fat trim 0 in broiled	3 oz	192	22	11	58	0	—	69
ground extra lean broiled medium	3 oz	217	22	14	71	0	—	59
ground extra lean broiled well done	3 oz	225	24	14	84	0	—	70
ground extra lean fried medium	3 oz	216	21	14	69	0	—	59
ground extra lean fried well done	3 oz	224	24	14	79	0	—	69
ground extra lean raw	4 oz	265	21	19	78	0	—	75
ground lean broiled medium	3 oz	231	21	16	74	0	—	65
ground lean broiled well done	3 oz	238	24	15	86	0	—	76
ground regular broiled medium	3 oz	246	20	18	76	0	—	70
ground regular broiled well done	3 oz	248	23	17	86	0	—	79
ground 97% fat free irradiated	4 oz	160	22	8	70	0	0	85
ground low-fat w/ carrageenan raw	4 oz	160	20	7	53	tr	—	70
porterhouse steak lean & fat trim ¼ in Choice broiled	3 oz	260	21	19	70	0	—	52
porterhouse steak lean only trim ¼ in Prime broiled	3 oz	185	24	9	68	0	—	56

FOOD	PORTION	CALS	PROT	FAT	CHOL	CARB	FIBER	SOD
rib eye small end lean & fat trim 0 in Choice broiled	3 oz	261	21	19	70	0	—	54
rib large end lean & fat trim 0 in roasted	3 oz	300	20	24	72	0	—	55
rib large end lean & fat trim ¼ in broiled	3 oz	295	18	24	69	0	—	54
rib large end lean & fat trim ¼ in roasted	3 oz	310	19	25	72	0	—	54
rib small end lean & fat trim 0 in broiled	3 oz	252	21	18	70	0	—	54
rib small end lean & fat trim ¼ in broiled	3 oz	285	20	22	71	0	—	53
rib small end lean & fat trim ¼ in roasted	3 oz	295	19	24	71	0	—	53
rib whole lean & fat trim ¼ in Choice broiled	3 oz	306	19	25	70	0	—	53
rib whole lean & fat trim ¼ in Choice roasted	3 oz	320	19	27	72	0	—	53
rib whole lean & fat trim ¼ in Prime roasted	3 oz	348	19	30	72	0	—	54
rib whole lean & fat trim ¼ in Select broiled	3 oz	274	19	21	69	0	—	54
rib whole lean & fat trim ¼ in Select roasted	3 oz	286	19	23	71	0	—	54
shank crosscut lean & fat trim ¼ in Choice simmered	3 oz	224	26	12	68	0	—	52

FOOD	PORTION	CALS	PROT	FAT	CHOL	CARB	FIBER	SOD
short loin top loin lean & fat trim 0 in Choice broiled	1 steak (5.4 oz)	353	43	19	119	0	—	104
short loin top loin lean & fat trim 0 in Choice broiled	3 oz	193	23	10	65	0	—	57
short loin top loin lean & fat trim 0 in Select broiled	1 steak (5.4 oz)	309	44	14	119	0	—	104
short loin top loin lean & fat trim ¼ in Choice braised	3 oz	253	22	18	68	0	—	54
short loin top loin lean & fat trim ¼ in Choice broiled	1 steak (6.3 oz)	536	46	38	143	0	—	114
short loin top loin lean & fat trim ¼ in Prime broiled	1 steak (6.3 oz)	582	46	43	143	0	—	114
short loin top loin lean & fat trim ¼ in Select broiled	1 steak (6.3 oz)	473	46	31	140	0	—	114
short loin top loin lean only trim 0 in Choice broiled	1 steak (5.2 oz)	311	43	14	113	0	—	101
short loin top loin lean only trim ¼ in Choice broiled	1 steak (5.2 oz)	314	42	15	112	0	—	100
shortribs lean & fat Choice braised	3 oz	400	18	36	80	0	—	43
t-bone steak lean & fat trim ¼ in Choice broiled	3 oz	253	21	18	70	0	—	52
t-bone steak lean only trim ¼ in Choice broiled	3 oz	182	24	9	68	0	—	56
tenderloin lean & fat trim 0 in Select broiled	3 oz	194	23	11	72	0	—	52

FOOD	PORTION	CALS	PROT	FAT	CHOL	CARB	FIBER	SOD
tenderloin lean & fat trim ¼ in Choice broiled	3 oz	259	21	19	73	0	—	50
tenderloin lean & fat trim ¼ in Choice roasted	3 oz	288	20	22	73	0	—	55
tenderloin lean & fat trim ¼ in Choice broiled	3 oz	208	23	12	72	0	—	52
tenderloin lean & fat trim ¼ in Prime broiled	3 oz	270	21	20	73	0	—	50
tenderloin lean & fat trim ¼ in Select roasted	3 oz	275	21	21	73	0	—	48
tenderloin lean only trim 0 in Select broiled	3 oz	170	24	7	71	0	—	54
tenderloin lean only trim ¼ in Choice broiled	3 oz	188	24	10	71	0	—	54
tenderloin lean only trim ¼ in Select broiled	3 oz	169	24	7	71	0	—	54
tip round lean & fat trim 0 in Choice roasted	3 oz	170	24	8	69	0	—	54
tip round lean & fat trim 0 in Select roasted	3 oz	158	24	6	69	0	—	55
tip round lean & fat trim ¼ in Choice roasted	3 oz	210	23	13	70	0	—	53
tip round lean & fat trim ¼ in Prime roasted	3 oz	233	22	15	70	0	—	53
tip round lean & fat trim ¼ in Select roasted	3 oz	191	23	10	70	0	—	53

FOOD	PORTION	CALS	PROT	FAT	CHOL	CARB	FIBER	SOD
top round lean & fat trim 0 in Choice braised	3 oz	184	30	6	77	0	—	38
top round lean & fat trim 0 in Select braised	3 oz	170	30	5	77	0	—	38
top round lean & fat trim ¼ in Choice braised	3 oz	221	29	11	77	0	—	38
top round lean & fat trim ¼ in Choice broiled	3 oz	190	26	9	72	0	—	51
top round lean & fat trim ¼ in Choice fried	3 oz	235	28	13	82	0	—	58
top round lean & fat trim ¼ in Prime broiled	3 oz	195	26	9	72	0	—	51
top round lean & fat trim ¼ in Select braised	3 oz	199	29	8	77	0	—	38
top round lean & fat trim ¼ in Choice braised	3 oz	175	26	7	72	0	—	51
top sirloin lean & fat trim 0 in Choice broiled	3 oz	194	25	10	76	0	—	55
top sirloin lean & fat trim 0 in Select broiled	3 oz	166	25	6	76	0	—	55
top sirloin lean & fat trim ¼ in Choice broiled	3 oz	228	23	14	76	0	—	53
top sirloin lean & fat trim ¼ in Choice fried	3 oz	277	24	19	83	0	—	59
top sirloin lean & fat trim ¼ in Select broiled	3 oz	208	24	12	76	0	—	54
tripe raw	4 oz	111	16	4	107	0	—	52

FOOD	PORTION	CALS	PROT	FAT	CHOL	CARB	FIBER	SOD
Laura's Lean								
Eye Of Round Steak Or Roast	4 oz	140	–	4	50	–	–	55
Flank Steak	4 oz	140	–	5	50	–	–	55
Ground 92% Lean	4 oz	160	–	9	60	–	–	70
Ground Round 96% Lean	4 oz	140	–	5	60	–	–	50
Ribeye Steak	4 oz	145	–	5	55	–	–	50
Sirloin Steak	4 oz	140	–	5	60	–	–	55
Sirloin Tip Steak Or Roast	4 oz	120	–	3	60	–	–	55
Strip Steak	4 oz	140	–	4	55	–	–	60
Tenderloin Filet	4 oz	140	–	5	55	–	–	55
Top Round Steak Or Roast	4 oz	130	–	3	55	–	–	55
Maverick Ranch								
Filet Mignon	4 oz	120	22	4	60	0	0	55
Ground	4 oz	130	22	5	60	0	0	65
Ground Round	4 oz	130	24	4	60	0	0	65
Ground Sirloin & Chuck	4 oz	130	22	5	60	0	0	65
NY Strip Steak	4 oz	150	22	7	55	0	0	55
Rib Eye Steak	4 oz	170	20	10	50	0	0	55
Top Round Steak & Roast	4 oz	110	24	4	50	0	0	55
Top Sirloin	4 oz	160	20	8	55	0	0	60
FROZEN								
patties broiled medium	3 oz	240	21	17	80	0	–	66
READY-TO-EAT								
dried beef	5 slices (21 g)	35	–	tr	–	tr	–	–
smoked beef cooked	1 sausage (1.4 oz)	134	–	12	29	–	–	–
Alpine Lace								
Roast Beef 97% Fat Free	2 oz	70	13	2	40	1	0	200
Boar's Head								
Corned Beef Brisket	2 oz	80	12	4	40	0	0	460

FOOD	PORTION	CALS	PROT	FAT	CHOL	CARB	FIBER	SOD
Eye Round Pepper Seasoned	2 oz	90	14	3	40	0	0	130
Italian Style Oven Roasted Top Round	2 oz	80	12	2	40	2	0	350
Roast Beef Cajun	2 oz	80	14	3	35	0	0	200
Top Round Deluxe	2 oz	90	14	3	30	0	0	80
Top Round Oven Roasted No Salt Added	2 oz	90	14	3	30	0	0	40
TAKE-OUT								
roast beef medium	2 oz	70	12	2	30	0	—	210
roast beef rare	2 oz	70	12	2	30	0	—	210
BEEF DISHES								
CANNED								
corned beef hash	3 oz	155	10	10	—	9	—	—
Mary Kitchen								
Corned Beef Hash 50% Reduced Fat	1 cup	280	19	12	65	25	3	1070
FROZEN								
Banquet								
Sandwich Toppers Creamed Chipped Beef	1 pkg (4 oz)	120	7	6	25	8	0	700
Sandwich Toppers Gravy & Salisbury Steak	1 pkg (5 oz)	210	9	16	25	8	2	790
Sandwich Toppers Gravy & Sliced Beef	1 pkg (4 oz)	70	8	2	25	5	0	440
Boston Market								
Meatloaf w/ Mashed Potatoes & Gravy	1 pkg (16 oz)	880	23	55	100	55	3	2720
REFRIGERATED								
Hormel								
Beef Roast Au Jus	1 serv (5 oz)	200	28	9	75	3	—	450
Beef Tips w/ Gravy	½ cup	160	20	7	55	5	1	760

FOOD	PORTION	CALS	PROT	FAT	CHOL	CARB	FIBER	SOD
Morton's Of Omaha								
Beef Pot Roast w/ Gravy	1 serv (3 oz)	160	27	5	55	2	0	310
Smithfield								
Beef Tips w/ Gravy	½ cup	170	23	5	50	6	tr	390
Tyson								
Roast Beef In Brown Gravy	1 serv + gravy (3.5 oz)	160	22	6	55	3	0	1210
SHELF-STABLE								
TastyBite								
Beef Roganjosh	1 pkg (9.5 oz)	270	18	15	25	19	3	1000
Meatballs Vindaloo	1 pkg (9.5 oz)	270	12	18	25	17	4	900
TAKE-OUT								
beef bourguignon	1 serv (7 oz)	254	23	16	128	3	1	212
bubble & squeak	5 oz	186	2	13	–	16	3	–
bulgoghi korean grilled beef	1 serv (5.2 oz)	256	23	15	67	5	tr	834
cornish pasty	1 (8 oz)	847	20	52	–	79	3	–
greek moussaka	1 serv (8.5 oz)	450	24	33	179	12	1	763
irish stew	1 cup (7 oz)	280	23	16	–	10	–	–
kebab indian	1 (5.4 oz)	553	47	40	–	2	–	–
kheena	6.7 oz	781	34	71	–	1	tr	–
koftas	5	280	18	22	–	3	tr	–
peppered steak	1 cup	331	–	73	21	–	–	650
pot roast w/ gravy	1 serv (6 oz)	320	54	10	110	4	0	620
samosa	2 (4 oz)	652	6	62	–	20	2	–
shepherds pie	1 serv (7 oz)	282	16	16	70	20	2	840
steak & kidney pie w/ top crust	1 slice (5 oz)	400	21	26	–	23	1	–
stew	6 oz	208	17	13	–	6	1	–
stew w/ vegetables	1 cup	220	16	11	71	15	–	292
stroganoff	¾ cup	260	14	19	69	43	–	503
swiss steak	4.6 oz	214	23	9	61	10	2	139
toad in the hole	1 (4.7 oz)	383	10	29	–	23	1	–

FOOD	PORTION	CALS	PROT	FAT	CHOL	CARB	FIBER	SOD
BEEFALO								
roasted	3 oz	160	26	5	49	0	–	70
BEER AND ALE								
alcohol free beer	7 fl oz	50	1	tr	–	11	–	3
ale brown	10 oz	77	1	0	0	8	0	–
ale pale	10 oz	88	1	0	0	12	0	–
beer light	12 oz can	100	tr	0	0	5	0	10
beer regular	12 oz can	146	1	0	0	13	tr	19
black & tan	1 serv (12 oz)	146	1	0	0	13	1	18
boilermaker	1 serv	216	1	0	0	13	1	18
lager	10 oz	80	1	0	0	4	0	–
mead	1 serv	250	1	0	0	13	1	18
pilsener lager beer	7 fl oz	85	1	tr	–	13	–	4
shandy	1 serv	125	1	0	0	12	1	16
stout	10 oz	102	1	0	0	6	0	–
Amstel								
Light	1 bottle (12 oz)	95	0	0	0	5	–	–
Anchor								
Liberty Ale	1 bottle (12 oz)	188	–	0	0	–	–	–
Porter	1 bottle (12 oz)	205	–	0	0	–	–	–
Steam	12 oz	152	–	0	0	–	–	–
Beamish								
Stout	12 oz	131	–	–	–	–	–	–
Beck's								
Béer	1 bottle (12 oz)	143	–	0	0	–	–	–
Blue Moon								
White	1 bottle (12 oz)	171	–	0	0	13	–	–
Bud								
Ice Light	1 bottle (12 oz)	110	–	0	0	7	–	–
Budweiser								
Beer	1 bottle (12 oz)	143	–	0	0	11	–	–

FOOD	PORTION	CALS	PROT	FAT	CHOL	CARB	FIBER	SOD
Ice	1 bottle (12 oz)	148	–	0	0	9	–	–
Light	1 bottle (12 oz)	110	–	0	0	7	–	–
Busch								
Beer	1 bottle (12 oz)	133	–	0	0	10	–	–
Ice	1 bottle (12 oz)	173	–	0	0	13	–	–
Light	1 bottle (12 oz)	110	–	0	0	7	–	–
Clausthaler								
Beer	1 bottle (12 oz)	96	–	0	0	6	–	–
Colt 45								
Malt Liquor	1 bottle (12 oz)	172	–	0	0	–	–	–
Coors								
Extra Gold	1 bottle (12 oz)	147	–	0	0	11	–	–
Light	1 bottle (12 oz)	102	–	0	0	5	–	–
Nonalcoholic	1 bottle (12 oz)	73	–	0	0	14	–	–
Original	1 bottle (12 oz)	148	–	0	0	11	–	–
Corona								
Extra	1 bottle (12 oz)	148	–	0	0	–	–	–
Light	1 bottle (12 oz)	109	–	0	0	7	–	–
Deschutes								
Bachelor ESB	1 bottle (12 oz)	180	–	0	0	–	–	–
Black Butt Porter	1 bottle (12 oz)	185	–	0	0	–	–	–
Cascade Ale	1 bottle (12 oz)	140	–	0	0	–	–	–

FOOD	PORTION	CALS	PROT	FAT	CHOL	CARB	FIBER	SOD
Mirror Pond Pale	1 bottle (12 oz)	175	–	0	0	–	–	–
Edison								
Light	1 bottle	109	–	0	0	7	–	–
Genesee								
12 Horse	1 bottle (12 oz)	152	–	0	0	14	–	–
Genny Light	1 bottle (12 oz)	96	–	0	0	6	–	–
Guinness								
Draught	1 bottle (12 oz)	125	–	0	0	10	–	–
Foreign Extra Stout	1 bottle (12 oz)	176	–	0	0	14		
Hamm's								
Beer	1 bottle (12 oz)	144	–	0	0	12	–	–
Light	1 bottle (12 oz)	110	–	0	0	7	–	–
Heineken								
Beer	1 bottle (12 oz)	166	–	0	0	10	–	–
I.C.								
Light	1 bottle (12 oz)	96	–	0	0	3	–	–
Icehouse								
5.0	1 bottle (12 oz)	132	–	0	0	9	–	–
5.5	1 bottle (12 oz)	149	–	0	0	10	–	–
J.W. Dundee								
Honey Brown	1 bottle (12 oz)	150	–	0	0	14	–	–
Keystone								
Light	1 bottle (12 oz)	100	–	0	0	5	–	–

FOOD	PORTION	CALS	PROT	FAT	CHOL	CARB	FIBER	SOD
Kilarney's								
Red Lager	1 bottle (12 oz)	197	–	0	0	23	–	–
Killian's								
Beer	1 bottle (12 oz)	163	–	0	0	14	–	–
Lowenbrau								
Beer	1 bottle (12 oz)	160	–	0	0	–	–	–
Michelob								
Ultra Low Carbohydrate	1 bottle (12 oz)	95	1	0	0	3	–	–
Weinhard's								
Ale	1 bottle (12 oz)	147	–	0	0	13	–	–
Amber Ale	1 bottle (12 oz)	169	–	0	0	14	–	–
Dark	1 bottle (12 oz)	150	–	0	0	13	–	–
Hefeweizen	1 bottle (12 oz)	128	–	0	0	9	–	–
BEET JUICE								
juice	7 oz	72	2	0	0	16	–	400
BEETS								
CANNED								
harvard	½ cup	89	1	tr	0	22	–	199
pickled	½ cup	75	1	tr	0	19	–	301
sliced	½ cup	27	1	tr	0	6	–	–
Del Monte								
Pickled Crinkle Style Sliced	½ cup (4.5 oz)	80	1	0	0	19	2	380
Sliced	½ cup (4.3 oz)	35	1	0	0	8	2	290
Whole	½ cup (4.3 oz)	35	1	0	0	8	2	290
Greenwood								
Harvard	1 serv (4.4 oz)	100	1	0	0	27	1	370
Pickled	1 oz	25	0	0	0	6	0	100

FOOD	PORTION	CALS	PROT	FAT	CHOL	CARB	FIBER	SOD
S&W								
Julienne	½ cup (4.3 oz)	30	1	0	0	7	1	230
Pickled Sliced	1 oz	15	0	0	0	4	1	50
Pickled Whole	1 oz	15	0	0	0	4	1	50
Sliced	½ cup (4.3 oz)	30	1	0	0	7	1	230
Whole Small	½ cup (4.3 oz)	30	1	0	0	7	1	230
Veg-All								
Small Sliced	½ cup	40	tr	0	0	8	1	300
FRESH								
greens cooked	½ cup	20	2	tr	0	4	—	173
greens raw	½ cup	4	tr	tr	0	1	—	38
greens raw chopped	½ cup	4	tr	tr	0	1	—	38
raw sliced	½ cup (2.4 oz)	29	1	tr	0	7	—	53
sliced cooked	½ cup (3 oz)	38	1	tr	0	9	—	65
whole cooked	2 (3.5 oz)	44	2	tr	0	10	—	77
whole raw	2 (5.7 oz)	70	3	tr	0	16	—	126

BEVERAGES (see BEER AND ALE, CHAMPAGNE, COFFEE, DRINK MIXERS, ENERGY DRINKS, FRUIT DRINKS, ICED TEA, LIQUOR/LIQUEUR, MALT, MILKSHAKE, SODA, TEA/HERBAL TEA, WATER, WINE)

BISCUIT

FOOD	PORTION	CALS	PROT	FAT	CHOL	CARB	FIBER	SOD
MIX								
buttermilk	1 (2 oz)	191	4	7	—	28	1	544
plain	1 (2 oz)	191	4	7	—	28	1	544
Bisquick								
Buttermilk	½ cup	150	2	6	0	21	—	320
Cheese Garlic	½ cup	160	2	7	0	22	—	360
Cinnamon Swirl	½ cup	150	2	4	0	30	—	330
Mix	⅓ cup (1.4 oz)	160	3	6	0	25	—	400
Reduced Fat	⅓ cup	140	3	3	0	27	tr	500
Kentucky Kernel								
Biscuit	¼ cup (1 oz)	171	3	5	0	28	1	659
MiniCarb								
Buttery as prep	1	255	10	21	145	3	2	290

FOOD	PORTION	CALS	PROT	FAT	CHOL	CARB	FIBER	SOD
REFRIGERATED								
buttermilk	1 (1 oz)	98	2	4	0	14	–	341
plain	1 (1 oz)	98	2	4	–	14	tr	341
Hungry Jack								
Butter Tastin' Flaky	1 (1.2 oz)	100	2	5	0	14	0	350
Cinnamon & Sugar	1 (1.2 oz)	110	2	4	0	17	tr	280
Flaky	1 (1.2 oz)	100	2	5	0	14	0	360
Flaky Buttermilk	1 (1.2 oz)	100	2	5	0	14	0	360
TAKE-OUT								
buttermilk	1 (2 oz)	212	4	10	2	27	–	348
oatcakes	2 (4 oz)	115	3	5	–	16	1	–
plain	1 (35 g)	276	4	34	5	13	–	584
tea biscuit	1 (3 oz)	210	5	3	0	30	1	370
w/ egg	1 (4.8 oz)	316	11	20	233	24	–	654
w/ egg & bacon	1 (5.2 oz)	458	17	31	353	29	1	999
w/ egg & ham	1 (6.7 oz)	442	20	27	300	30	4	1382
w/ egg & sausage	1 (6.3 oz)	581	19	39	302	41	1	1141
w/ egg & steak	1 (5.2 oz)	410	18	28	272	21	–	888
w/ egg cheese & bacon	1 (5.1 oz)	477	16	31	261	33	–	1260
w/ ham	1 (4 oz)	386	13	18	25	44	1	1433
w/ sausage	1 (4.4 oz)	485	12	32	35	40	1	1071
w/ steak	1 (4.9 oz)	455	13	26	25	44	–	795
BISON								
roasted	3 oz	122	24	2	70	0	–	48
BLACK BEANS								
dried cooked	1 cup	227	15	1	0	41	15	1
Bean Cuisine								
Pasta & Beans Mediterranean Black Beans & Fusilli	1 serv	210	7	1	0	30	4	10
Eden								
Organic	½ cup (4.6 oz)	100	7	0	0	18	6	15
Progresso								
Black Beans	½ cup (4.6 oz)	110	7	1	0	17	7	400

FOOD	PORTION	CALS	PROT	FAT	CHOL	CARB	FIBER	SOD
BLACKBERRIES								
canned in heavy syrup	½ cup	118	2	tr	0	30	–	3
fresh	½ cup	37	1	tr	0	9	3	0
unsweetened frzn	1 cup	97	2	1	0	24	–	2
BLACKBERRY JUICE								
Clear Fruit								
Blackberry Rush	8 oz	90	0	0	0	23	–	0
Everfresh								
Clear Fruit Blackberry Rush	8 oz	90	0	0	0	23	–	0
BLACKEYE PEAS								
CANNED								
w/pork	½ cup	199	7	4	17	40	–	840
Eden								
Organic	½ cup (4.6 oz)	90	6	1	0	16	4	25
DRIED								
cooked	1 cup	198	13	1	0	36	16	6
FROZEN								
Birds Eye								
Blackeye Peas	½ cup	110	7	1	0	21	4	10
BLINTZE								
Cohen's & Wilton								
Cheese	1	80	5	3	13	10	0	140
Golden								
Cheese	1 (2.1 oz)	80	6	2	15	13	2	135
Potato	1	90	3	4	5	15	2	170
Vegetable	1	110	2	5	5	15	0	230
Ratner's								
Cheese	1 (2.2 oz)	90	5	2	30	14	tr	160
TAKE-OUT								
cheese	1 (2.7 oz)	160	5	9	65	15	tr	240
BLUEBERRIES								
canned in heavy syrup	1 cup	225	2	1	0	56	–	9
fresh	1 cup	82	1	1	0	20	–	9
unsweetened frzn	1 cup	78	1	1	0	19	–	1

FOOD	PORTION	CALS	PROT	FAT	CHOL	CARB	FIBER	SOD
A&L Farms								
Bleuets Fresh	1 pt	80	1	0	0	19	5	0
Tree Of Life								
Organic	1 cup (5 oz)	80	1	0	0	20	2	0
BLUEFIN								
fillet baked	4.1 oz	186	30	6	88	0	–	90
BLUEFISH								
fresh baked	3 oz	135	22	5	64	0	–	65
BOAR								
wild roasted	3 oz	136	24	4	–	0	–	–
BOK CHOY (see CABBAGE)								
BONITO								
fresh	3 oz	117	20	4	–	0	0	–
BORAGE								
fresh chopped	½ cup	9	1	tr	0	1	–	35
fresh chopped cooked	3½ oz	25	2	1	0	4	–	88
BOTTLED WATER (see WATER)								
BOYSENBERRIES								
in heavy syrup	1 cup	226	3	tr	0	57	–	9
unsweetened frzn	1 cup	66	1	tr	0	16	–	2
BRAINS								
beef pan-fried	3 oz	167	11	13	1696	0	–	134
beef simmered	3 oz	136	9	11	1746	0	–	102
lamb braised	3 oz	124	11	9	1737	0	–	114
lamb fried	3 oz	232	14	19	2128	0	–	133
pork braised	3 oz	117	10	8	2169	0	0	77
veal braised	3 oz	115	10	8	2635	0	–	133
veal fried	3 oz	181	12	14	1802	0	–	150
BRAN								
corn	1 cup (2.7 oz)	170	6	1	0	65	65	5
oat	½ cup (1.6 oz)	116	8	3	0	31	7	2
oat cooked	½ cup (3.8 oz)	44	4	1	0	13	3	1
rice	½ cup (2.1 oz)	187	8	12	0	29	12	3
wheat	½ cup (2 oz)	63	5	1	0	19	12	1

FOOD	PORTION	CALS	PROT	FAT	CHOL	CARB	FIBER	SOD
Hodgson Mill								
Oat	¼ cup	120	6	3	0	23	6	3
Wheat Unprocessed	¼ cup	30	2	0	0	10	7	0
BRAZIL NUTS								
dried unblanched	1 oz	186	4	19	0	4	—	0
BREAD								
CANNED								
boston brown	1 slice (1.6 oz)	88	2	1	—	20	2	284
FROZEN								
Marie Callender's								
Cornbread & Honey Butter	1 piece + butter	210	2	11	15	28	1	370
Original Garlic	1 piece	190	4	8	<5	23	2	330
Parmesan & Romano Garlic	1 piece	200	5	10	5	23	2	430
MIX								
cornbread	1 piece (2 oz)	189	4	6	37	29	1	467
Atkins								
Caraway Rye as prep	1 slice	150	12	0	0	8	5	150
Country White as prep	1 slice	70	12	0	0	8	5	135
Sourdough as prep	1 slice	70	12	0	0	8	5	170
Buitoni								
Focaccia Rosemary & Garlic	1 piece (1 oz)	110	4	1	0	22	1	250
Foccacia Italian Herb & Cheese	1 slice	110	3	2	0	21	0	390
Carbolite								
Bread Mix as prep	1 slice	45	6	5	0	4	—	130
Hodgson Mill								
European Cheese & Herb	¼ cup (1.2 oz)	130	5	1	0	21	tr	250
Honey Whole Wheat	¼ cup (1.2 oz)	120	5	1	0	22	2	160

FOOD	PORTION	CALS	PROT	FAT	CHOL	CARB	FIBER	SOD
Keto								
Quick Bread All Flavors as prep	1 slice	55	5	0	0	3	–	95
MiniCarb								
Country White as prep	1 slice	80	9	3	0	7	4	115
Sassafras								
12 Grain & Sunflower	1 slice (1.4 oz)	150	5	2	0	28	1	160
READY-TO-EAT								
baguette parisian	2 oz	120	5	0	0	26	tr	270
baguette whole wheat	2 oz	140	6	0	0	29	1	360
challah	1 slice (2 oz)	160	3	3	0	29	1	250
cracked wheat	1 slice	65	2	1	–	12	1	135
egg	1 slice (1.4 oz)	115	4	2	20	19	–	197
french	1 slice (1 oz)	78	3	1	0	15	1	172
french	1 loaf (1 lb)	1270	43	18	0	230	–	2633
gluten	1 slice	47	2	tr	0	8	–	104
italian	1 slice (1 oz)	81	3	1	0	15	1	175
italian	1 loaf (1 lb)	1255	41	4	0	256	–	2656
navajo fry	1 (10.5 in diam)	527	11	15	0	85	–	1112
navajo fry	1 (5 in diam)	296	6	9	0	48	–	625
oat bran	1 slice	71	3	1	0	12	1	122
oat bran reduced calorie	1 slice	46	2	1	0	10	–	81
oatmeal	1 slice	73	2	1	–	13	1	162
oatmeal reduced calorie	1 slice	48	2	1	0	10	–	89
pita	1 sm (1 oz)	78	3	tr	0	16	1	152
pita	1 reg (2 oz)	165	5	1	0	33	1	322
pita whole wheat	1 reg (2 oz)	170	6	2	0	35	5	340
pita whole wheat	1 sm (1 oz)	76	3	1	0	16	2	151
potato scallion	1 slice (2 oz)	120	4	1	0	24	0	340
protein	1 slice	47	2	tr	0	8	–	104

FOOD	PORTION	CALS	PROT	FAT	CHOL	CARB	FIBER	SOD
pumpernickel	1 slice	80	3	1	0	15	2	215
raisin	1 slice	71	2	1	0	14	–	101
rice bran	1 slice	66	1	1	0	12	–	119
rye	1 slice	83	3	1	0	16	2	211
rye reduced calorie	1 slice	47	2	1	0	9	–	93
seven grain	1 slice	65	3	1	0	12	2	127
sourdough	1 slice (1 oz)	78	3	1	0	15	1	172
vienna	1 slice (1 oz)	78	3	1	0	15	1	172
wheat reduced calorie	1 slice	46	2	1	–	10	3	117
wheat berry	1 slice	65	2	1	0	12	1	132
wheat bran	1 slice	89	3	1	0	17	3	175
wheat germ	1 slice	74	3	1	–	14	–	157
white	1 slice	67	2	1	0	12	1	135
white reduced calorie	1 slice	48	2	1	0	10	2	104
white toasted	1 slice	67	2	1	0	13	–	136
white cubed	1 cup	80	2	1	0	15	–	154
whole wheat	1 slice	70	3	1	–	13	2	149
Arnold								
Bran'nola Country Oat	1 slice (1.3 oz)	110	4	2	0	20	3	160
Carb Counting Multigrain	1 slice	60	5	–	–	9	3	–
Country White	1 slice (1.3 oz)	110	3	2	0	21	tr	250
Country Classics Buttermilk	1 slice	110	4	2	0	19	tr	180
Country Classics Wheat	1 slice (1.3 oz)	110	4	2	0	19	2	190
Natural 100% Whole Wheat	1 slice (1.3 oz)	90	4	1	0	16	3	170
Raisin Cinnamon	1 slice (1 oz)	80	2	2	0	15	1	95
Atkins								
Rye	1 slice	60	7	1	5	8	5	110
White	1 slice	60	7	1	5	8	5	115
Beefsteak								
Rye Soft	1 slice	70	2	1	0	14	0	200

FOOD	PORTION	CALS	PROT	FAT	CHOL	CARB	FIBER	SOD
Bread Du Jour								
French	3 in slice (2 oz)	140	5	1	0	26	1	310
Damascus								
Pita	1 (2 oz)	130	6	0	0	29	2	150
Pita Whole Wheat	1 (2 oz)	160	6	0	0	32	3	230
Wraps Honey Wheat	½ wrap (2 oz)	130	5	0	0	28	1	150
Wraps Plain	½ wrap (2 oz)	130	5	0	0	29	1	150
Wraps Spinach	1 (4 oz)	280	10	0	0	52	2	460
Wraps Tomato	1 12-inch (4 oz)	240	10	0	0	58	2	440
Ecce Panis								
Country Wheat	1 slice (2 oz)	150	4	0	0	32	2	320
European Baguette	2 oz	150	5	0	0	34	1	370
Freihofer's								
100% Whole Wheat	1 slice	90	45	2	0	17	3	160
Whole Wheat Light	2 slices	80	5	1	0	19	5	160
Gold Medal								
100% Whole Wheat	1 slice	70	2	2	0	13	2	180
Home Pride								
Carb Action Multigrain	1 slice	60	6	–	–	8	1	–
Carb Action White Fiber	1 slice	60	4	–	–	10	4	–
Wheat	1 slice (1 oz)	80	2	1	0	14	1	190
La Mexicana								
Wraps Chocolate	1 (1.3 oz)	120	4	3	0	18	1	360
Wraps Southwestern Mild Chili	1 (1.3 oz)	120	4	4	0	18	1	360
Wraps Spinach	1 (1.3 oz)	120	4	4	0	18	1	360
Wraps Tomato Basil	1 (1.3 oz)	120	4	4	0	18	1	360
Milton's								
Healthy Multi-Grain	1 slice (1.4 oz)	110	3	1	0	24	3	150

FOOD	PORTION	CALS	PROT	FAT	CHOL	CARB	FIBER	SOD
Natural Ovens								
100% Whole Grain	1 slice	60	4	1	0	14	5	80
7 Grain Herb	1 slice	70	4	1	0	16	4	70
Better White	1 slice	80	4	1	0	19	2	75
Cracked Wheat	1 slice	80	4	1	0	16	3	70
English Muffin Bread	1 slice	80	4	1	0	16	2	70
Glorious Cinnamon Raisin	1 slice	70	3	1	0	15	2	70
Happiness Raisin Pecan	1 slice	70	3	1	0	15	3	70
Health Max	1 slice	80	3	1	0	16	3	80
Hunger Filler	1 slice	60	4	1	0	13	4	90
Lo Carb Golden Crunch	1 slice	70	8	4	0	7	4	80
Lo Carb Original	1 slice	60	7	2	0	8	5	70
Mild Rye	1 slice	70	3	1	0	13	4	70
Multi-Grain Stay Slim	1 slice	60	3	1	0	14	5	90
Nutty Natural	1 slice	70	3	1	0	16	5	70
Right Wheat	1 slice	60	2	1	0	13	5	90
Soft Wheat	1 slice	70	3	1	0	15	3	70
Sunny Millet	1 slice	60	3	1	0	14	4	80
Pepperidge Farm								
Apple Cinnamon	1 slice (1 oz)	80	4	2	0	15	1	120
Deli Rye Seedless	1 slice	80	3	1	0	15	1	210
Deli Swirl Rye & Pump	1 slice	80	3	1	0	15	1	220
Farmhouse Butter Topped Wheat	1 slice	110	4	2	0	21	2	210
Farmhouse Country Wheat	1 slice	110	4	2	0	21	2	190
Farmhouse Hearty White	1 slice (1.5 oz)	110	5	2	<5	20	tr	260
Farmhouse Sesame Wheat	1 slice	110	4	2	0	19	2	190
Farmhouse Soft Oatmeal	1 slice	110	4	1	0	21	1	200
Farmhouse Sourdough	1 slice (1.5 oz)	110	4	2	0	20	1	220

FOOD	PORTION	CALS	PROT	FAT	CHOL	CARB	FIBER	SOD
Jewish Rye	1 slice	80	3	1	0	15	2	210
Natural Whole Grain Whole Wheat	1 slice (1.2 oz)	90	4	1	0	16	2	135
Natural Whole Grain Honey Oat	1 slice (1.2 oz)	90	4	2	0	15	2	135
Swirl Cinnamon	1 slice (1 oz)	90	2	3	0	15	1	110
Swirl French Vanilla	1 slice	140	4	4	0	23	tr	190
Swirl Raisin Cinnamon	1 slice (1 oz)	80	3	2	0	14	1	105
Stroehmann								
Honey Cracked Wheat	1 slice	90	3	1	0	16	1	140
New York Rye	1 slice (1 oz)	80	3	1	0	15	1	150
TastyBite								
Nan Kontos Massala	½ loaf (1.4 oz)	120	7	3	0	15	1	160
Nan Kontos Onion	½ loaf (1.4 oz)	120	7	4	0	15	1	160
Nan Kontos Roghani	½ loaf (1.4 oz)	125	4	3	0	19	1	240
Nan Kontos Tandoori	½ loaf (1.4 oz)	120	4	3	0	19	1	240
Roti Kontos Missy	½ loaf (1.4 oz)	125	5	4	0	18	2	185
Thomas'								
Toasting Cinnamon Raisin	1 slice	120	3	3	0	22	1	170
Toasting Bread Cinnamon	1 slice	130	3	5	0	20	1	170
Toufayan								
Wraps Sundried Tomato Basil	1 (2 oz)	183	6	5	0	30	2	537
Wraps Wheat	1 (2 oz)	183	6	5	0	29	3	354
TAKE-OUT								
chapatis as prep w/ fat	1 bread (1.6 oz)	95	3	2	3	18	3	180
chapatis as prep w/o fat	1 (2½ oz)	141	5	1	—	31	5	—

FOOD	PORTION	CALS	PROT	FAT	CHOL	CARB	FIBER	SOD
cornbread	2 in x 2 in (1.4 oz)	107	4	2	28	18	–	276
cornstick	1 (1.3 oz)	101	2	4	30	13	tr	195
focaccia	1 piece (2 oz)	130	4	3	0	23	1	310
focaccia onion	1 piece (4.6 oz)	282	6	10	0	43	2	536
focaccia rosemary	1 piece (3.5 oz)	251	6	7	0	40	2	535
focaccia tomato olive	1 piece (4.7 oz)	270	6	8	0	42	2	683
garlic bread	2 slices (2 oz)	190	3	8	0	27	1	290
irish soda bread	1 slice (2 oz)	174	4	3	11	34	–	239
naan	1 bread (3.5 oz)	286	7	9	46	43	2	546
papadums fried	2 (1.5 oz)	81	4	4	–	9	2	–
paratha	1 bread (2.1 oz)	201	4	10	27	23	2	268

BREAD COATING
Don's Chuck Wagon

FOOD	PORTION	CALS	PROT	FAT	CHOL	CARB	FIBER	SOD
Chicken Baking Mix	¼ cup (1 oz)	95	3	0	0	21	1	850
Fish & Chips Mix	¼ cup (1 oz)	100	3	0	0	21	1	740
Fish Mix	¼ cup (1 oz)	95	4	0	0	21	1	940
Mushroom Batter Mix	¼ cup (1 oz)	95	3	0	0	21	1	990
Onion Ring Mix	¼ cup (1 oz)	100	3	0	0	21	1	690
Seafood Bake & Fry Mix	¼ cup (1 oz)	95	2	0	0	21	1	990

Luzianne

FOOD	PORTION	CALS	PROT	FAT	CHOL	CARB	FIBER	SOD
Cajun Chicken Coating Mix	2 tbsp (1 oz)	100	3	1	0	20	1	1260

BREAD MACHINE MIX
Betty Crocker

FOOD	PORTION	CALS	PROT	FAT	CHOL	CARB	FIBER	SOD
Harvest Wheat	⅟₁₁ loaf	140	4	3	0	25	2	220
Home-Style White	⅟₁₁ loaf	130	4	2	0	25	0	220

Carbsense

FOOD	PORTION	CALS	PROT	FAT	CHOL	CARB	FIBER	SOD
Harvest Wheat as prep	1 slice	60	11	0	0	4	1	120

FOOD	PORTION	CALS	PROT	FAT	CHOL	CARB	FIBER	SOD
Keto								
Cinnamon Raisin as prep	1 slice	79	13	0	0	6	3	95
French Loaf as prep	1 slice	79	13	0	0	5	3	95
Sourdough Rye as prep	1 slice	79	13	1	–	5	3	95
Ketogenics								
Low Carb Honey Wheat as prep	1 slice	80	0	1	0	7	5	60
Low Carb Original White as prep	1 slice	62	13	0	0	2	–	277
Low Carb Pumpernickel Rye as prep	1 slice	80	11	2	0	7	5	–
BREADCRUMBS								
dry	1 cup	426	14	6	–	78	5	930
dry seasoned	1 cup (4 oz)	441	17	3	–	85	5	3180
fresh	⅔ cup	76	4	1	0	14	1	153
Arnold								
Italian	¼ cup	110	4	2	0	19	1	560
Keto								
Low Carb Cajun	½ cup	185	13	1	–	13	9	595
Low Carb Italian	½ cup	185	13	1	–	13	9	480
Low Carb Original	½ cup	185	13	1	–	13	9	480
Progresso								
Garlic & Herb	¼ cup (1 oz)	100	4	2	0	18	1	530
Italian Style	¼ cup (1 oz)	110	4	2	0	20	1	430
Parmesan	¼ cup (1 oz)	100	4	2	0	17	1	870
Plain	¼ cup (1 oz)	110	4	2	0	19	1	210
Ronzoni								
Italian Flavored	¼ cup	120	4	2	0	21	2	330
BREADFRUIT								
fresh	¼ small	99	1	tr	0	26	–	2
seeds cooked	1 oz	48	2	1	0	9	–	–
seeds raw	1 oz	54	2	2	0	8	–	–
seeds roasted	1 oz	59	2	tr	0	11	–	–

FOOD	PORTION	CALS	PROT	FAT	CHOL	CARB	FIBER	SOD
BREADNUT TREE SEEDS								
dried	1 oz	104	2	tr	0	23	–	–
BREADSTICKS								
onion poppyseed	1	64	2	1	10	11	–	69
plain	1 sm	25	1	1	0	4	–	66
plain	1	41	1	1	0	7	–	66
Angonoa								
Deli Style Sesame	3 (0.5 oz)	730	2	3	0	10	tr	110
Bread Du Jour								
Original	1 (1.9 oz)	130	5	1	0	25	1	290
Sourdough	1 (1.9 oz)	130	5	1	0	25	1	280
John Wm Macy's								
CheeseSticks Original Cheddar	3 (1 oz)	130	6	6	11	14	1	190
Pepperidge Farm								
Snack Sticks Wheat	9 (1 oz)	130	3	4	0	22	1	370
Stella D'Oro								
Original	1 (0.4 oz)	45	1	1	0	7	0	40
Roasted Garlic	1	45	1	1	0	8	0	230
Snack Stix Cracked Pepper	4 (0.5 oz)	70	2	2	0	11	0	290
BREAKFAST BARS (see CEREAL BARS, ENERGY BARS)								
BREAKFAST DRINKS								
orange drink powder	3 rounded tsp	93	0	0	0	24	–	4
orange drink powder as prep w/water	6 oz	86	0	0	0	22	–	9
Carnation								
Instant Breakfast French Vanilla as prep w/ 2% milk	1 serv	250	13	5	–	40	–	220
Instant Breakfast French Vanilla as prep w/ fat free milk	1 serv	220	13	1	–	40	–	230

FOOD	PORTION	CALS	PROT	FAT	CHOL	CARB	FIBER	SOD
Instant Breakfast French Vanilla as prep w/ whole milk	1 serv	280	13	8	–	39	–	220

BROAD BEANS
canned	1 cup	183	14	1	0	32	–	1161
dried cooked	1 cup	186	13	1	0	33	–	8
fresh cooked	3½ oz	56	5	tr	0	10	–	41

BROCCOFLOWER
fresh raw	½ cup (1.8 oz)	16	1	tr	0	3	–	12

BROCCOLI
FRESH
chinese broccoli (gai lan) cooked	1 cup (3.1 oz)	19	1	1	0	3	2	6
chopped cooked	½ cup	22	2	tr	0	4	2	20
raw chopped	½ cup	12	1	tr	0	2	1	12

FROZEN
chopped cooked	½ cup	25	3	tr	0	5	–	22
spears cooked	½ cup	25	3	tr	0	5	3	22
spears cooked	10 oz pkg	69	8	tr	0	13	4	60

Birds Eye
Chopped	⅓ cup	25	–	0	0	–	2	15
Cuts	½ cup	25	–	0	0	–	3	30
Florets	1 cup	25	2	0	0	4	2	35
In Cheese Sauce	½ cup	70	3	4	5	7	2	500

Fresh Like
Spear	3.5 oz	26	3	tr	–	5	1	32

Health Is Wealth
Broccoli Munchees	2 (1 oz)	60	2	2	0	10	1	170

Tree Of Life
Cuts	1 cup (3.1 oz)	25	2	0	0	4	2	20

BROWNIE
FROZEN
Greenfield
Fat Free Homestyle	1 (1.3 oz)	110	2	0	0	27	0	60

FOOD	PORTION	CALS	PROT	FAT	CHOL	CARB	FIBER	SOD
MIX								
plain	1 (1.2 oz)	139	1	7	9	20	1	83
plain low calorie	1 (0.8 oz)	84	1	2	0	16	1	21
Atkins								
Kitchen Fudge as prep	1 (2 inch)	60	3	0	0	17	4	80
Aunt Paula's								
Low Carb Chef Fudge Brownie as prep	1 (2.5 inch)	89	7	5	3	9	2	–
Betty Crocker								
Chocolate Chunk as prep	1	180	1	9	21	25	–	90
Dark Chocolate Fudge as prep	1	170	1	7	21	24	–	120
Dark Chocolate w/ Syrup as prep	1	170	2	7	21	25	–	105
Fudge as prep	1	170	1	7	21	23	–	100
German Chocolate Coconut Pecan Filling as prep	1	200	1	8	21	29	1	115
Hot Fudge as prep	1	170	2	8	21	23	–	105
Original as prep	1	180	1	6	21	27	–	135
Peanut Butter as prep	1	180	3	8	21	23	–	105
Stir'n Bake w/ Mini Kisses as prep	1 serv	220	2	7	0	38	1	160
Turtle w/ Caramel & Pecans as prep	1	170	1	8	21	25	–	95
Walnut as prep	1	180	2	9	21	23	–	90
Big Train								
Low Carb Chocolate Chip as prep	1 (2 inch)	140	2	9	42	15	4	45
Keto								
Chocolate Fudge as prep	1	59	6	3	–	2	1	50

FOOD	PORTION	CALS	PROT	FAT	CHOL	CARB	FIBER	SOD
MiniCarb								
Chocolate Brownie as prep	1	220	5	17	50	10	8	75
No Pudge!								
All Flavors	1	100	2	0	0	21	tr	90
Sweet Rewards								
Low Fat Fudge as prep	1	130	2	3	0	27	1	115
Reduced Fat Supreme as prep	1	140	2	3	21	27	—	110
READY-TO-EAT								
plain	1 sm (1 oz)	115	1	5	5	18	1	88
plain	1 lg (2 oz)	227	3	9	10	36	1	175
w/ nuts	1 (1 oz)	100	1	4	14	16	—	59
Greenfield								
Blondie Fat Free Apple Spice	1 (1.3 oz)	110	2	0	0	26	0	60
REFRIGERATED								
Toll House								
Brownie Dough	½ pkg (1.5 oz)	180	2	7	15	26	2	160
TAKE-OUT								
plain	one 2-in sq (2.1 oz)	243	3	10	10	39	—	153
BRUSSELS SPROUTS								
FRESH								
cooked	1 sprout	8	1	tr	0	2	—	4
cooked	½ cup	30	2	tr	0	7	3	17
raw	1 sprout	8	1	tr	0	2	1	5
raw	½ cup	19	1	tr	0	4	—	11
FROZEN								
cooked	½ cup	33	3	tr	0	6	—	18
Birds Eye								
Brussels Sprouts	11 sprouts	35	3	0	0	7	3	15
BUCKWHEAT								
groats roasted cooked	1 cup (5.9 oz)	647	6	1	0	34	5	7
groats roasted uncooked	1 cup (5.7 oz)	567	19	4	0	123	17	18

FOOD	PORTION	CALS	PROT	FAT	CHOL	CARB	FIBER	SOD
BUFFALO								
burger	4 oz	150	24	5	50	1	0	80
water buffalo roasted	3 oz	111	23	2	52	0	–	48
BULGUR								
cooked	1 cup (6.3 oz)	151	7	tr	0	34	8	9
uncooked	1 cup (4.9 oz)	479	17	2	0	106	26	24
TAKE-OUT								
tabbouleh	½ cup	120	–	4	0	–	–	252
BURBOT (FISH)								
fresh baked	3 oz	98	65	1	65	0	–	106
BURDOCK ROOT								
cooked	1 cup	110	3	tr	0	26	–	5
fresh	1 cup	85	2	tr	0	20	–	6
BUTTER								
clarified butter	3½ oz	876	tr	99	256	0	–	–
ghee cow's milk	1 tbsp	126	–	14	39	–	0	0
ghee vegetable oil	1 tbsp	126	–	14	0	–	0	0
stick	1 pat (5 g)	36	tr	4	11	tr	–	41
stick	1 stick (4 oz)	813	1	92	248	tr	–	937
whipped	1 tbsp	70	0	7	20	0	0	0
whipped	1 pat (4 g)	27	tr	3	8	tr	–	31
whipped	4 oz	542	1	61	165	tr	–	625
Breakstone's								
Salted	1 tbsp (0.5 oz)	100	0	11	30	0	–	85
Cabot								
Butter	1 tbsp	100	0	11	30	0	0	90
Unsalted	1 tbsp	100	0	11	30	0	0	0
Corman								
Light	1 tbsp	55	tr	6	5	0	0	60
Hotel Bar								
Stick	1 tbsp (0.5 oz)	100	0	11	30	0	–	90

FOOD	PORTION	CALS	PROT	FAT	CHOL	CARB	FIBER	SOD
Keller's								
European	1 tbsp (0.5 oz)	100	0	11	30	0	0	0
Land O Lakes								
Salted	1 tbsp (0.5 oz)	100	0	11	30	0	–	85
Ultra Creamy Salted	1 tbsp (0.5 oz)	110	0	12	30	0	–	85
BUTTER BEANS								
CANNED								
Van Camp								
Butter Beans	½ cup (4.6 oz)	110	8	1	0	22	7	430
FROZEN								
Birds Eye								
Speckled	½ cup	100	6	0	0	20	4	130
BUTTER SUBSTITUTES								
stick	1 stick	811	1	91	99	1	–	1013
Keto								
Butta	1 tsp	43	0	5	0	0	0	0
Molly McButter								
Natural Butter	1 tsp	5	0	0	0	1	–	180
Natural Cheese	1 tsp	5	0	0	0	1	–	125
Roasted Garlic	1 tsp	5	0	0	0	1	–	125
Olivio								
Spread	1 tbsp	80	0	8	0	0	0	95
BUTTERBUR								
canned fuki chopped	1 cup	3	tr	tr	0	tr	–	5
fresh fuki	1 cup	13	tr	tr	0	3	–	7
BUTTERFISH								
baked	3 oz	159	19	9	71	0	–	97
fillet baked	1 oz	47	6	3	21	0	–	29
BUTTERNUTS								
dried	1 oz	174	7	16	0	3	–	0

FOOD	PORTION	CALS	PROT	FAT	CHOL	CARB	FIBER	SOD
BUTTERSCOTCH (see also CANDY)								
Hershey's								
Chips	1 tbsp	80	tr	4	0	10	–	10
Nestle								
Morsels	1 tbsp	80	0	4	0	9	0	15
CABBAGE (see also COLESLAW)								
chinese bok choy shredded cooked	½ cup	10	1	tr	0	2	–	29
chinese pak-choi raw shredded	½ cup	5	1	tr	0	1	–	23
chinese pe-tsai raw shredded	1 cup	12	1	tr	0	2	–	7
chinese pe-tsai shredded cooked	1 cup	16	2	tr	0	3	–	11
danish raw	1 head (2 lbs)	228	13	2	0	49	18	164
danish raw shredded	½ cup (1.2 oz)	9	1	tr	0	2	tr	6
danish shredded cooked	½ cup (2.6 oz)	17	1	tr	0	3	1	6
green raw	1 head (2 lbs)	228	12	2	0	49	18	164
green raw shredded	½ cup (1.2 oz)	9	1	tr	0	2	tr	6
green shredded cooked	½ cup (2.6 oz)	17	1	tr	0	3	1	6
napa cooked	1 cup (3.8 oz)	13	1	tr	0	2	0	12
red raw shredded	½ cup	10	tr	tr	0	2	1	4
red shredded cooked	½ cup	16	1	tr	0	3	–	6
savoy raw shredded	½ cup	10	1	tr	0	2	–	10
savoy shredded cooked	½ cup	18	1	tr	0	4	–	17
Greenwood								
Sweet & Sour Red	½ cup	100	1	0	0	24	0	380
Lohmann								
Red Cabbage Sweet & Sour	¼ cup	40	0	0	0	10	0	110

FOOD	PORTION	CALS	PROT	FAT	CHOL	CARB	FIBER	SOD
TAKE-OUT								
korean kimchee	½ cup	22	2	tr	0	4	4	–
northern white kimchi	½ cup	79	3	1	0	18	7	–
stuffed cabbage	1 (6 oz)	373	25	22	95	18	–	1007
sweet & sour red cabbage	4 oz	61	1	3	–	8	3	–
CACTUS								
napoles fresh sliced	½ cup (1.5 oz)	7	1	tr	0	1	–	9
pricklypear fresh	1 cup (5.3 oz)	56	2	1	0	13	4	–
CAKE (see also CAKE MIX)								
angelfood	1 cake (11.9 oz)	876	20	3	0	197	5	2548
battenburg cake	1 slice (2 oz)	204	3	10	–	28	1	–
boston cream pie frzn	⅙ cake (3.2 oz)	232	2	8	34	40	1	132
carrot w/ cream cheese icing home recipe	1 cake 10 in diam	6175	63	328	1183	775	–	4470
cheesecake 9 in diam	1 cake	3350	60	213	2053	317	–	2464
cheesecake	⅙ cake (2.8 oz)	256	4	18	44	20	2	165
cherry fudge w/ chocolate frosting	⅛ cake (2.5 oz)	187	2	9	–	27	–	160
coffeecake fruit	⅛ cake (1.8 oz)	156	3	5	–	26	–	192
cream puff shell	1 (2.3 oz)	239	6	17	129	15	–	368
crumpet	1 (2.3 oz)	131	4	1	0	31	2	535
devil's food cupcake w/ chocolate frosting	1	120	2	4	19	20	–	92
devil's food w/ creme filling	1 (1 oz)	105	1	4	15	17	–	105
eccles cake	1 slice (2 oz)	285	2	16	–	36	1	–
eclair	1 (1.4 oz)	149	2	10	–	15	tr	–

FOOD	PORTION	CALS	PROT	FAT	CHOL	CARB	FIBER	SOD
fruitcake	1 piece (1.5 oz)	139	1	4	2	27	–	116
fruitcake dark home recipe	1 cake 7½ in x 2¼ in	5185	74	228	640	738	–	2123
jelly roll lemon filled	1 slice (3 oz)	210	3	2	35	48	tr	300
madeira cake	1 slice (1 oz)	98	1	4	–	15	1	–
pound	¹⁄₁₀ cake (1 oz)	117	2	6	66	15	–	119
pound	1 cake (8½ x 3½ x 3 in	1935	26	94	1100	257	–	1857
pound fat free	1 cake (12 oz)	961	18	4	0	208	–	1158
pound cake home recipe	1 loaf 8½ in x 3½ in	1935	33	94	1100	265	–	1645
sheet cake w/ white frosting home recipe	1 cake 9 in sq	4020	37	129	636	694	–	2488
sheet cake w/o frosting home recipe	⅑ cake	315	4	12	61	48	–	258
sheet cake w/o frosting home recipe	1 cake 9 in sq	2830	35	108	552	434	–	2331
sour cream pound	¹⁄₁₀ cake (1 oz)	117	1	5	17	16	tr	120
sponge	¹⁄₁₂ cake (1.3 oz)	110	2	1	39	23	–	93
sponge cake dessert shell	1 (0.8 oz)	70	1	2	20	12	0	150
sponge w/ creme filling	1 (1.5 oz)	155	1	5	7	27	–	155
tiramisu	1 cake (4.4 lbs)	5732	101	421	2395	439	3	1107
toaster pastry apple	1 (1¾ oz)	204	2	5	–	37	–	218
toaster pastry blueberry	1 (1¾ oz)	204	2	5	–	37	–	218

FOOD	PORTION	CALS	PROT	FAT	CHOL	CARB	FIBER	SOD
toaster pastry brown sugar cinnamon	1 (1¾ oz)	206	3	7	–	34	–	212
toaster pastry cherry	1 (1¾ oz)	204	2	5	–	37	–	218
toaster pastry strawberry	1 (1¾ oz)	204	2	5	–	37	–	218
treacle tart	1 slice (2.5 oz)	258	3	10	–	42	1	–
vanilla slice	1 slice (2½ oz)	248	3	13	–	30	1	–
white w/ white frosting	1 cake 9 in diam	4170	43	148	46	670	–	2827
white w/ white frosting	⅟₁₆ cake	260	3	9	3	42	–	176
yellow w/ chocolate frosting	1 cake 9-in diam	3895	40	175	609	620	–	3080
yellow w/ chocolate frosting	⅛ cake (2.2 oz)	242	2	11	35	36	1	216
Amy's								
Toaster Pops Apple	1	140	5	3	0	26	tr	130
Toaster Pops Strawberry	1	140	5	3	0	26	tr	130
Baby Watson								
Cheesecake	1 slice (3 oz)	260	4	18	65	19	tr	150
Drake's								
Coffee Cake Low Fat	1 (1.1 oz)	110	1	2	10	21	0	110
Coffee Cakes	1 (1.2 oz)	140	1	6	5	20	0	100
Yodel's	1 (1 oz)	150	2	9	5	16	–	65
Entenmann's								
Apple Puffs	1 (3 oz)	270	2	13	0	37	1	230
Coffee Cake Cheese Filled Crumb	1 serv (1.9 oz)	200	4	10	35	25	tr	190
Coffee Cake Crumb	1 serv (2 oz)	250	3	12	10	33	1	210

FOOD	PORTION	CALS	PROT	FAT	CHOL	CARB	FIBER	SOD
Light Loaf Cake Fat Free	⅛ cake (1.7 oz)	120	2	0	0	27	0	190
Loaf All Butter	⅙ cake (2.4 oz)	220	3	9	0	31	0	290
Louisiana Crunch	⅛ cake (2.9 oz)	330	3	14	45	49	tr	35
Ultimate Crumb Cake	⅒ cake	250	2	13	15	32	tr	280
Fillo Factory								
Apple Turnovers Vegan	5 (5 oz)	270	5	5	0	53	2	125
Goody Man								
Happy Birthday Cupcake Chocolate	1 (1.75 oz)	200	2	6	20	34	tr	190
Happy Birthday Cupcake White	1 (1.75 oz)	190	2	5	20	36	0	230
Greenfield								
Blondie Fat Free Chocolate Chip	1 (1.3 oz)	110	2	0	0	27	0	60
Hostess								
Crumb Cake Light	1 (1 oz)	100	1	2	0	18	0	130
Jell-O								
Dessert Delights Cheesecake	1 bar (1.4 oz)	160	2	7	5	20	tr	100
Dessert Delights Chocolate Fudge Pudding	1 bar (1.4 oz)	150	2	6	0	23	1	80
Low Carb Creations								
Cheesecake Blueberry Swirl	1 slice (3 oz)	220	5	16	95	21	0	150
Cheesecake Chocolate	1 slice (3 oz)	250	6	20	115	19	0	180
Cheesecake Key Lime	1 slice (3 oz)	250	6	20	115	19	0	180
Cheesecake New York	1 slice (3 oz)	250	6	15	85	19	0	140
Cheesecake Pumpkin Swirl	1 slice (3 oz)	220	5	16	90	22	0	140

FOOD	PORTION	CALS	PROT	FAT	CHOL	CARB	FIBER	SOD
Marie Callender's								
Cobbler Apple	1 serv (4.25 oz)	370	2	20	0	45	2	170
Cobbler Berry	1 serv (4.25 oz)	370	3	21	<5	41	1	220
Cobbler Cherry	1 serv (4.25 oz)	380	3	19	5	50	0	240
Cobbler Peach	1 serv (4.25 oz)	380	3	18	0	47	0	240
Natural Touch								
Toaster Square Blueberry	1 (2.8 oz)	180	6	2	0	33	6	65
Toaster Squares Date Walnut	1 (2.8 oz)	200	6	3	0	36	8	50
Sara Lee								
Cheesecake 25% Reduced Fat	¼ cake (4.2 oz)	310	9	13	70	40	2	310
Cheesecake Cherry Cream	¼ cake (4.7 oz)	350	6	12	35	55	2	310
Cheesecake Chocolate Chip	¼ cake (4.2 oz)	410	8	21	65	47	2	300
Cheesecake French	⅙ cake (3.9 oz)	350	5	21	20	24	1	280
Cheesecake French Strawberry	⅙ cake (4.3 oz)	320	4	14	20	43	1	230
Cheesecake Strawberry Cream	¼ cake (4.7 oz)	330	6	12	40	49	2	330
Coffee Cake Butter Streusel	⅙ cake (1.9 oz)	220	4	12	35	25	1	240
Coffee Cake Crumb	⅛ cake (2 oz)	220	3	9	15	32	1	210
Coffee Cake Pecan	⅙ cake (1.9 oz)	230	4	12	25	24	1	170
Coffee Cake Raspberry	⅙ cake (1.9 oz)	220	3	8	15	27	1	220
Coffee Cake Reduced Fat Cheese	⅙ cake (1.9 oz)	180	3	6	20	28	0	230

FOOD	PORTION	CALS	PROT	FAT	CHOL	CARB	FIBER	SOD
Layer Cake Coconut	⅛ cake (2.8 oz)	260	2	14	15	33	1	210
Layer Cake Double Chocolate	⅛ cake (2.8 oz)	260	3	13	10	33	2	230
Layer Cake Fudge Golden	⅛ cake (2.8 oz)	260	2	13	15	34	1	200
Layer Cake German Chocolate	⅛ cake (2.9 oz)	280	3	14	15	35	1	250
Layer Cake Vanilla	⅛ cake (2.8 oz)	260	2	14	15	32	0	210
Original Cheesecake	¼ cake (4.2 oz)	350	7	18	50	39	1	320
Pound Cake All Butter	¼ cake (2.7 oz)	320	4	16	85	38	1	280
Pound Cake Chocolate Swirl	¼ cake (2.9 oz)	330	5	16	75	42	tr	350
Pound Cake Family Size	⅙ cake (2.7 oz)	310	4	17	75	36	1	360
Pound Cake Reduced Fat	¼ cake (2.7 oz)	280	4	11	65	42	tr	350
Pound Cake Strawberry Swirl	¼ cake (2.9 oz)	290	4	11	60	44	tr	140
Strawberry Shortcake	⅛ cake (2.5 oz)	180	2	7	15	27	1	140
Snack & Smile								
Mini Loaf Apple Cinnamon	1 loaf (2 oz)	190	2	8	10	29	0	260
Mini Loaf Banana	1 loaf (2 oz)	200	2	8	10	30	0	260
Mini Loaf Blueberry	1 loaf (2 oz)	190	2	8	10	29	tr	260
Mini Loaf Carrot	1 loaf (2 oz)	200	2	8	10	30	0	260
Super								
Bun	1 (2.5 oz)	270	5	16	10	24	tr	230
Tastykake								
Koffee Kake Cream Filled	2 (2 oz)	240	2	10	30	35	0	130
Koffee Kakes	1 (2 oz)	210	2	7	30	34	tr	160
Krimpets Butterscotch Iced	2 (2 oz)	210	2	5	60	38	0	250

FOOD	PORTION	CALS	PROT	FAT	CHOL	CARB	FIBER	SOD
TAKE-OUT								
angelfood	1/12 cake (1 oz)	73	2	tr	0	16	1	212
apple crisp	1/2 cup (5 oz)	230	37	5	0	46	–	257
baklava	1 oz	126	2	9	23	10	1	78
basbousa namoura	1 piece (1 oz)	60	2	3	0	–	2	144
boston cream pie	1/6 cake (3.3 oz)	293	4	12	43	43	1	309
cannoli w/ cannoli cream	1	369	6	21	–	42	–	–
carrot w/ cream cheese icing	1/12 cake (3.9 oz)	484	5	29	60	52	–	273
cheesecake w/ cherry topping	1/12 cake (5 oz)	359	6	23	106	33	–	254
chocolate w/ chocolate frosting	1/8 cake (2.2 oz)	235	3	11	–	35	2	213
coffeecake cheese	1/6 cake (2.7 oz)	258	5	12	–	38	1	257
coffeecake crumb topped cheese	1/6 cake (2.7 oz)	258	5	12	–	38	1	257
coffeecake crumb topped cinnamon	1/9 cake (2.2 oz)	263	4	15	20	29	2	221
cream puff w/ custard filling	1 (4.6 oz)	336	9	20	174	30	–	444
dutch honey cake	1 slice (0.8 oz)	70	1	0	0	17	0	25
eclair w/ chocolate icing & custard filling	1	205	–	10	35	–	–	–
french apple tart	1 (3.5 oz)	302	4	15	60	37	2	326
fruitcake	1/36 cake (2.9 oz)	302	3	10	24	54	3	121
gingerbread	1/9 cake (2.6 oz)	264	3	12	24	36	2	242
panettone	1/12 cake (2.9 oz)	300	6	12	90	43	2	120
petit fours	2 (0.9 oz)	120	1	7	0	15	0	15

FOOD	PORTION	CALS	PROT	FAT	CHOL	CARB	FIBER	SOD
pineapple upside down	⅑ cake (4 oz)	367	4	14	25	58	—	367
pound fat free	1 oz	80	2	tr	0	17	—	96
pound cake	1 slice (1 oz)	120	2	5	32	15	—	96
sacher torte	1 slice (2.2 oz)	240	4	11	50	30	4	120
sheet cake w/ white frosting	⅑ cake	445	4	14	70	77	—	275
strudel apple	1 piece (2½ oz)	195	2	8	—	29	2	191
tiramisu	1 piece (5.1 oz)	409	7	30	171	31	tr	79
torte chocolate ganache	1 slice (3.5 oz)	400	7	26	90	40	6	120
trifle w/ cream	6 oz	291	4	16	—	34	1	—
yellow w/ vanilla frosting	⅛ cake (2.2 oz)	239	2	9	—	38	—	220
CAKE ICING								
chocolate ready-to-use	½₂ pkg (1.3 oz)	151	tr	7	0	24	—	70
glaze home recipe	½₂ recipe (1 oz)	97	tr	2	1	20	—	25
vanilla ready-to-use	½₂ pkg (1.3 oz)	159	tr	6	0	26	—	34
Betty Crocker								
HomeStyle Mix Coconut Pecan as prep	2 tbsp	160	tr	2	0	21	tr	5
HomeStyle Mix White Fluffy as prep	6 tbsp	100	tr	0	0	24	—	60
Party Frosting Chocolate w/ Stars	2 tbsp (1.2 oz)	140	0	5	0	22	—	90
Rich & Creamy Butter Cream	2 tbsp (1.3 oz)	140	0	5	0	23	—	75
Rich & Creamy Cherry	2 tbsp (1.2 oz)	140	0	5	0	23	—	75
Rich & Creamy Chocolate	2 tbsp (1.2 oz)	130	0	5	0	21	—	90

FOOD	PORTION	CALS	PROT	FAT	CHOL	CARB	FIBER	SOD
Rich & Creamy Cream Cheese	2 tbsp (1.2 oz)	140	0	5	0	23	–	80
Rich & Creamy Dark Chocolate	2 tbsp (1.3 oz)	130	1	6	0	23	1	90
Rich & Creamy French Vanilla	2 tbsp (1.2 oz)	140	0	5	0	23	–	70
Rich & Creamy Milk Chocolate	2 tbsp (1.3 oz)	130	0	5	0	21	–	90
Rich & Creamy Rainbow Chip	2 tbsp (1.2 oz)	140	0	5	0	23	–	65
Rich & Creamy Vanilla	2 tbsp (1.2 oz)	140	0	5	0	23	–	70
Toppers Milk Chocolate	2 tbsp (1.2 oz)	130	0	5	0	22	–	85
Toppers Vanilla	2 tbsp (1.2 oz)	140	0	5	0	24	–	70
Sweet Rewards								
Ready-To-Spread Reduced Fat Chocolate	2 tbsp (1.2 oz)	120	tr	2	0	24	–	55
Ready-To-Spread Reduced Fat Vanilla	2 tbsp (1.2 oz)	130	0	2	0	27	–	60
CAKE MIX								
angelfood	½₂ cake (1.8 oz)	129	3	tr	0	29	1	255
angelfood	10 in cake (20.9 oz)	1535	36	2	0	350	9	3036
carrot w/o frosting	½₂ cake (2.5 oz)	239	4	11	–	33	–	249
carrot w/o frosting	2 layers (29.6 oz)	2886	43	133	–	395	–	3001
chocolate pudding type w/o frosting	½₂ cake (2.7 oz)	270	4	14	–	34	–	402
chocolate pudding type w/o frosting	2 layers (32.4 oz)	3234	43	172	–	409	–	4815

FOOD	PORTION	CALS	PROT	FAT	CHOL	CARB	FIBER	SOD
chocolate w/o frosting	½ cake (2.3 oz)	198	4	8	35	32	—	370
chocolate w/o frosting	2 layers (26.8 oz)	2393	44	92	425	384	—	4464
coffeecake crumb topped cinnamon	⅛ cake (2 oz)	178	3	5	28	30	2	236
devil's food w/o frosting	½ cake (2.3 oz)	198	4	8	35	32	—	370
devil's food w/ chocolate frosting	⅟₁₆ cake	235	3	8	37	40	—	181
devil's food w/ chocolate frosting	1 cake 9-in diam	3755	49	136	598	645	—	2900
fudge w/o frosting	½ cake (2.3 oz)	198	4	8	35	32	—	370
gingerbread	⅑ cake (2.4 oz)	207	3	7	24	34	2	307
gingerbread 8 in sq	1 cake	1575	18	39	6	291	—	1733
white w/o frosting	½ cake (2.2 oz)	190	3	5	—	34	—	301
white w/o frosting	2 layer cake (26 oz)	2265	30	57	—	410	—	3593
yellow w/ chocolate frosting	⅟₁₆ cake	235	3	8	36	40	—	157
yellow w/ chocolate frosting	1 cake 9-in diam	3895	40	175	609	620	—	3080
yellow w/o frosting	½ cake (2.2 oz)	202	3	6	37	34	—	299
yellow w/o frosting	2 layers (26.5 oz)	2415	35	71	437	411	—	3580
Betty Crocker								
Angel Food Fat Free	½ cake	140	3	0	0	32	—	320
Angel Food Fat Free Confetti as prep	½ cake	150	3	0	0	34	—	320
Cheesecake Chocolate Chip as prep	⅛ cake	410	3	28	99	32	1	230

FOOD	PORTION	CALS	PROT	FAT	CHOL	CARB	FIBER	SOD
Cheesecake Original as prep	1/8 cake	400	2	27	102	30	–	240
Cheesecake Strawberry Swirl as prep	1/8 cake	380	2	25	96	32	–	220
Pineapple Upside Down as prep	1/6 cake	420	2	14	36	64	–	280
Quick Bread Banana	1/12 cake	170	2	7	36	25	–	190
Quick Bread Cinnamon Streusel as prep	1/14 cake	180	3	7	30	26	–	150
Quick Bread Cranberry Orange as prep	1/12 cake	170	2	6	36	29	–	170
Quick Bread Lemon Poppy Seed as prep	1/12 cake	170	2	7	36	25	–	150
Stir'n Bake Carrot Cake w/ Cream Cheese Frosting as prep	1/6 cake	260	2	7	–	46	–	290
Stir'n Bake Coffee Cake w/ Cinnamon Streusel as prep	1/6 cake	230	2	2	12	36	–	120
Stir'n Bake Devils Food w/ Chocolate Frosting as prep	1/6 cake	240	2	7	0	42	1	270
Stir'n Bake Yellow w/ Chocolate Frosting as prep	1/8 cake	240	2	7	9	43	1	240
SuperMoist Butter Pecan as prep	1/12 cake	240	1	10	54	35	–	260
SuperMoist Butter Yellow as prep	1/12 cake	260	2	11	75	36	–	270

FOOD	PORTION	CALS	PROT	FAT	CHOL	CARB	FIBER	SOD
SuperMoist Carrot as prep	1/10 cake	320	2	15	63	42	—	340
SuperMoist Cherry Chip	1/10 cake	300	2	13	63	41	—	330
SuperMoist Chocolate Fudge as prep	1/12 cake	270	2	12	54	35	1	320
SuperMoist Golden Vanilla as prep	1/12 cake	240	1	10	54	35	—	270
SuperMoist Lemon as prep	1/12 cake	240	1	10	54	35	—	270
SuperMoist Milk Chocolate as prep	1/12 cake	240	2	10	54	34	1	290
SuperMoist Pineapple as prep	1/12 cake	250	1	7	54	25	—	270
SuperMoist Spice as prep	1/12 cake	240	1	10	54	36	—	270
SuperMoist Strawberry as prep	1/12 cake	250	1	10	39	35	—	260
SuperMoist White as prep	1/12 cake	230	2	14	0	34	—	290
SuperMoist White Light as prep	1/10 cake	210	2	3	0	43	—	380
Bisquick								
Mix	1/3 cup (1.4 oz)	160	3	6	0	25	—	400
Reduced Fat	1/3 cup (1.4 oz)	140	3	3	0	27	tr	500
Carbolite								
Cheesecake Chocolate as prep	1/8 cake	260	6	25	280	2	—	80
Carbsense								
Zero Carb Baking Mix	1 oz	110	22	1	0	4	4	380

FOOD	PORTION	CALS	PROT	FAT	CHOL	CARB	FIBER	SOD
Hodgson Mill								
Gingerbread Whole Wheat	¼ cup (1 oz)	110	2	0	0	24	2	260
MiniCarb								
Carrot as prep	1 slice	280	16	20	45	10	6	190
Chocolate as prep	1 slice	230	8	18	60	16	12	110
Zero Carb Baking Mix not prep	½ cup	55	10	1	0	2	2	160
Sweet Rewards								
Reduced Fat White as prep	1/12 cake	180	2	3	0	36	–	300
Reduced Fat Yellow as prep	1/12 cake	200	2	5	30	37	–	280
CALABAZA								
fresh	½ cup	32	1	tr	–	8	–	3
CALZONE								
TAKE-OUT								
beef and cheese	1	330	–	35	11	–	–	1120
cheese	1 (12 oz)	1020	48	54	100	86	8	1760
pepperoni	1	450	–	19	10	–	–	930
CANADIAN BACON								
grilled	1 pkg (6 oz)	257	34	12	81	2	0	2149
Boar's Head								
Canadian Bacon	2 oz	70	12	3	30	1	0	560
Hormel								
Sandwich Style	3 slices (2 oz)	70	10	3	30	0	0	640
Jones								
Slices	3	70	11	3	30	0	0	590
Real Canadian Bacon								
Peameal	4 oz	130	16	5	40	4	–	1120
Yorkshire Farms								
Uncured	3 oz	100	17	4	44	9	–	350
CANADIAN BACON SUBSTITUTES								
Yves								
Canadian Veggie Bacon	1 serv (2 oz)	80	17	1	0	1	1	480

FOOD	PORTION	CALS	PROT	FAT	CHOL	CARB	FIBER	SOD
CANDY								
boiled sweets	¼ lb	327	0	0	–	87	0	–
butterscotch	1 piece (6 g)	24	0	tr	1	6	–	3
butterscotch	1 oz	112	0	1	3	27	–	12
candied cherries	1 (4 g)	12	0	tr	0	3	–	–
candied citron	1 oz	89	tr	tr	0	23	–	82
candied lemon peel	1 oz	90	tr	tr	0	23	–	14
candied orange peel	1 oz	90	tr	tr	0	23	–	14
candied pineapple slice	1 slice (2 oz)	179	tr	tr	0	45	–	–
candy corn	1 oz	105	tr	0	0	27	–	57
caramels	1 piece (8 g)	31	tr	1	1	6	–	20
caramels	1 pkg (2.5 oz)	271	3	6	5	55	–	174
caramels chocolate	1 bar (2.3 oz)	231	1	2	0	56	–	–
caramels chocolate	1 piece (6 g)	22	tr	tr	0	6	–	–
carob bar	1 (3.1 oz)	453	11	28	–	42	–	–
crisped rice bar almond	1 bar (1 oz)	130	2	6	0	18	1	66
crisped rice bar chocolate chip	1 bar (1 oz)	115	4	4	0	21	1	79
dark chocolate	1 oz	150	1	10	0	16	–	5
fondant	1 piece (0.6 oz)	57	0	0	0	15	–	6
fondant chocolate coated	1 lg (1.2 oz)	128	1	3	0	28	–	9
fondant chocolate coated	1 sm (0.4 oz)	40	tr	1	0	9	–	3
fondant mint	1 oz	105	tr	0	0	27	–	57
fruit pastilles	1 tube (1.4 oz)	101	2	0	–	25	–	–
fudge brown sugar w/ nuts	1 piece (0.5 oz)	56	tr	1	1	11	–	14
fudge chocolate marshmallow	1 piece (0.7 oz)	84	1	3	5	14	–	21

FOOD	PORTION	CALS	PROT	FAT	CHOL	CARB	FIBER	SOD
fudge chocolate marshmallow w/ nuts	1 piece (0.8 oz)	96	1	4	5	15	–	21
fudge chocolate w/ nuts	1 piece (0.7 oz)	81	1	3	3	14	–	11
fudge peanut butter	1 piece (0.6 oz)	59	1	1	1	13	–	12
fudge vanilla w/ nuts	1 piece (0.5 oz)	62	tr	2	2	11	–	9
gumdrops	10 sm (0.4 oz)	135	0	0	0	35	–	15
gumdrops	10 lg (3.8 oz)	420	0	0	0	108	–	48
hard candy	1 oz	106	0	0	0	28	–	11
jelly beans	10 sm (0.4 oz)	40	0	tr	0	10	–	3
jelly beans	10 lg (1 oz)	104	0	tr	0	26	–	7
lollipop	1 (6 g)	22	0	0	0	6	–	2
marzipan	1 oz	128	3	7	0	15	2	5
milk chocolate	1 bar (1.55 oz)	226	3	14	10	26	–	36
milk chocolate crisp	1 bar (1.45 oz)	203	3	11	8	28	–	59
milk chocolate w/ almonds	1 bar (1.45 oz)	215	4	14	8	22	–	30
nougat nut cream	0.5 oz	49	1	4	–	8	–	–
peanut bar	1 (1.4 oz)	209	6	14	–	19	–	91
peanut brittle	1 oz	128	2	5	4	20	–	128
peanuts chocolate covered	10 (1.4 oz)	208	5	13	4	20	–	16
peanuts chocolate covered	1 cup (5.2 oz)	773	19	50	13	74	–	61
praline	1 piece (1.4 oz)	177	1	10	0	24	–	24
pretzels chocolate covered	1 (0.4 oz)	50	1	2	–	8	–	10
pretzels chocolate covered	1 oz	130	2	5	–	20	–	–
sesame crunch	20 pieces (1.2 oz)	181	4	12	0	18	–	–

FOOD	PORTION	CALS	PROT	FAT	CHOL	CARB	FIBER	SOD
sesame crunch	1 oz	146	3	9	0	14	–	–
sweet chocolate	1 oz	143	1	10	0	17	–	5
sweet chocolate	1 bar (1.45 oz)	201	2	14	0	25	–	7
taffy	1 piece (0.5 oz)	56	0	1	1	14	–	13
toffee	1 piece (0.4 oz)	65	tr	4	13	8	–	22
truffles	4 pieces (1.1 oz)	190	2	14	0	14	1	20
truffles	1 piece (0.4 oz)	59	1	4	6	5	–	8
100 Grand								
Bar	1 bar (1.5 oz)	200	2	8	10	30	tr	75
5th Avenue								
Bar	1 (0.56 oz)	80	1	4	0	10	–	25
Almond Joy								
Bar	1 (0.68 oz)	90	1	5	0	11	–	30
Altoids								
All Flavors	3 pieces	10	0	0	0	2	–	0
At Last!								
Chocolate Almond	1 bar	120	2	10	0	13	6	20
Chocolate Crisp	1 bar	110	3	9	0	14	6	40
Chocolate Mint	1 bar	110	2	10	0	15	7	25
Chocolate Peanut Butter	1 bar	120	2	11	0	14	5	20
Atkins								
Endulge Caramel Nut Chew	1 bar (1.23 oz)	140	6	9	5	17	tr	70
Endulge Chocolate Bar	1 bar (1.1 oz)	150	1	12	5	2	3	5
Endulge Chocolate Crunch	1 bar (1 oz)	150	3	12	<5	15	3	7
Endulge Peanut Butter Cups	3 pieces	160	3	13	0	17	0	70

FOOD	PORTION	CALS	PROT	FAT	CHOL	CARB	FIBER	SOD
Baby Ruth								
Bar	1 bar (2.1 oz)	270	4	13	0	36	2	130
Fun Size	1 bar (1 oz)	130	3	6	0	17	tr	60
Bittyfinger								
Bars	2	170	2	7	0	27	tr	85
Body Smarts								
Chocolate Peanut Crunch	2 bars (1.8 oz)	210	5	6	<5	34	2	70
Butterfinger								
Bar	1 (2.1 oz)	270	3	11	0	42	1	130
BB's	1 pkg (1.7 oz)	230	2	9	0	33	1	95
Fun Size	1 bar	100	1	4	0	15	0	45
Cadbury								
Milk Chocolate Roast Almond	10 blocks (1.4 oz)	220	4	13	10	21	1	80
Cape Cod Provisions								
Cranberry Bog Frogs	3 pieces (1.9 oz)	250	3	12	7	34	tr	65
Carbolite								
Caramel	1 bar	100	1	5	5	18	0	10
CarbAway	1 bar	100	1	5	5	17	0	15
CarboSnack	1 bar	110	1	6	5	20	1	15
Chocolate Truffle	1 bar (1 oz)	122	2	8	<5	17	1	54
Chocolate Almond	1 bar (1.75 oz)	298	9	21	7	3	2	57
Chocolate Crisp	1 bar (1.75 oz)	256	7	14	14	3	1	0
Chocolate Peanut Butter	1 bar (1.75 oz)	256	–	21	7	3	0	50
Crisy Caramel	1 bar (1 oz)	130	3	9	5	17	0	50
Milk Chocolate	1 bar (1.75 oz)	263	7	18	7	1	1	6
Peanut Butter Cup	1	170	3	14	5	17	1	35
Pecan Cluster	1 bar	120	1	8	5	15	1	10
CarbSlim								
Crunch Bites Chocolate Caramel	1 pkg	122	6	14	3	21	9	78

FOOD	PORTION	CALS	PROT	FAT	CHOL	CARB	FIBER	SOD
Crunch Bites Peanut Butter	1 pkg	171	8	14	2	21	9	123
Carmello								
Snack Size	1 (0.66 oz)	90	1	4	<5	12	–	20
Cary's Of Oregon								
English Toffee Milk Chocolate Almond	1 piece (0.75 oz)	110	1	8	10	12	tr	65
Charleston Chew								
Chocolate	½ bar	120	–	3	–	–	–	–
Strawberry	½ bar	120	–	3	–	–	–	–
Vanilla	½ bar	120	–	3	–	–	–	–
Chunky								
Bar	1 (1.4 oz)	210	3	11	5	24	1	20
Classic Caramels								
Chocolate Creme Filled	3 pieces	80	tr	3	<5	13	–	30
Soft & Chewy	3 pieces	80	tr	2	<5	13	–	45
Cloud Nine								
Australian Orange Peel	½ bar (1.5 oz)	220	2	13	0	25	2	5
Butter Nut Toffee	½ bar (1.5 oz)	230	3	14	5	25	1	30
Cool Mint Crisp	½ bar (1.5 oz)	220	2	13	5	26	2	5
Espresso Bean Crunch	½ bar (1.5 oz)	220	2	14	0	23	2	5
Malted Milk Crunch	½ bar (1.5 oz)	230	3	14	5	26	1	40
Milk Chocolate	½ bar (1.5 oz)	230	3	15	5	25	1	25
Oregon Red Raspberry	½ bar (1.5 oz)	230	2	15	0	25	2	5
Peanut Butter Brittle	½ bar (1.5 oz)	230	3	15	5	24	1	40
Sundried Cherry	½ bar (1.5 oz)	230	3	13	5	26	1	25
Toasted Coconut Crisp	½ bar (1.5 oz)	230	2	14	5	25	2	45
Vanilla Dark	½ bar (1.5 oz)	230	3	15	0	25	2	10

FOOD	PORTION	CALS	PROT	FAT	CHOL	CARB	FIBER	SOD
Crunch								
Fun Size	4 bars	210	2	11	10	26	tr	60
Daboga								
Organic Milk Chocolate	1 bar (2 oz)	318	4	20	10	30	6	60
Del Monte								
Radical Raizins Cinnamon	1 pkg (0.7 oz)	70	0	0	0	18	0	0
Radical Raizins Rainbow	1 pkg (0.7 oz)	70	0	0	0	18	0	0
Doctor's CarbRite								
Sugar Free Dark Chocolate	1 oz	124	2	8	–	2	2	0
Sugar Free Dark Chocolate With Almonds	4 sq (1 oz)	132	8	10	0	16	4	20
Sugar Free Milk Chocolate	1 oz	128	0	9	–	0	0	0
Sugar Free Milk Chocolate With Peanuts	4 sq (1 oz)	132	8	10	4	12	0	20
Sugar Free Milk Chocolate With Soy Crisps	4 sq (1 oz)	120	4	8	4	12	2	40
Sugar Free Mint Chocolate	1 oz	128	0	9	–	0	0	0
Fauchon								
Chocolate Assortment	3 pieces (1.1 oz)	170	3	11	<5	19	2	15
Ferrero Rocher								
Candy	3 pieces (1.3 oz)	140	4	15	0	17	1	35
Godiva								
Chocolatier Dark Chocolate w/ Raspberry	1 bar (1.5 oz)	220	2	11	3	28	0	10
Chocolatier Milk Chocolate	1 bar (1.5 oz)	230	3	13	10	26	0	30

FOOD	PORTION	CALS	PROT	FAT	CHOL	CARB	FIBER	SOD
Chocolatier Milk Chocolate w/ Almonds	1 bar (1.5 oz)	230	5	15	5	20	0	20
Mochaccino Mousse	2 pieces (1.25 oz)	210	2	15	4	17	0	10
Truffles Assorted	2 pieces (1.5 oz)	220	2	13	10	24	0	15
Goetze's								
Cow Tales	1 pkg (1 oz)	110	1	3	tr	20	tr	40
Gol D Lite								
Milk Chocolate Crisp	1 bar	125	1	9	6	15	0	18
Seashell Truffle	1 piece	54	1	3	0	6	1	0
Goldenberg's								
Peanut Chews	3 pieces	180	4	8	0	22	1	40
Golightly								
Sugar Free Caramels	5 pieces	150	1	6	10	31	—	30
Sugar Free Doublers Chews Peach & Creme	7 pieces	150	0	7	10	31	tr	0
Sugar Free Fudgie Rolls	6 pieces	130	1	5	5	28	—	25
Sugar Free Hard Candy	4 pieces	45	0	0	0	15	—	0
Goobers								
Peanuts	1 pkg (1.38 oz)	210	4	13	5	20	1	15
Good & Plenty								
Snack Size	1 box (0.6 oz)	60	0	0	0	14	—	40
Good 'N Fruity								
Snack Size	1 box (0.6 oz)	60	0	0	0	15	—	10
Heath								
Snack Size	1 bar (0.3 oz)	50	0	3	<5	6	—	35
Hershey's								
Bites Almond Joy	8 pieces	100	tr	6	<5	10	—	5
Bites Cookies 'N' Creme	8 pieces	90	2	5	0	10	—	35

FOOD	PORTION	CALS	PROT	FAT	CHOL	CARB	FIBER	SOD
Bites Milk Chocolate w/ Almond	7 pieces	90	2	6	<5	8	–	10
Bites Reese's	7 pieces	90	2	5	0	10	–	30
Bites York	9 pieces	90	0	2	0	19	–	10
Candy Coated Milk Chocolate Eggs	4 pieces	90	1	5	<5	12	–	10
Hugs	1 piece	25	0	2	0	3	–	0
Kisses	1	25	0	2	0	3	–	0
Kisses w/ Almonds	1 piece	25	0	2	0	3	–	0
Milk Chocolate	1 bar (0.6 oz)	90	1	5	<5	10	0	15
Milk Chocolate w/ Almonds	1 bar (0.6 oz)	100	2	6	<5	9	–	10
Miniature Special Dark	1 (0.3 oz)	45	0	3	0	3	–	0
Nuggets Cookies 'N' Creme	1	50	tr	3	0	5	–	20
Nuggets Dark Chocolate w/ Almonds	4	220	3	14	<5	20	3	0
Nuggets Milk Chocolate	4	230	3	13	10	24	1	35
Nuggets Milk Chocolate w/ Almonds	1	60	tr	4	0	5	–	5
Nuggets Milk Chocolate w/ Almonds & Toffee	1	50	tr	4	<5	5	–	10
Nuggets Milk Chocolate w/ Raisins & Almonds	1	50	tr	3	0	6	–	10
Pot Of Gold	3 pieces	130	1	5	<5	21	tr	45
Sweet Escapes Caramel & Peanut Butter Crispy	1 bar	80	1	3	0	13	–	70
Sweet Escapes Crispy Caramel Fudge	1 bar	70	tr	2	0	13	–	50

FOOD	PORTION	CALS	PROT	FAT	CHOL	CARB	FIBER	SOD
Sweet Escapes Crunchy Peanut Butter	1 bar (0.7 oz)	90	2	3	0	13	–	40
Sweet Escapes Triple Chocolate Wafer	1 bar	80	tr	3	0	13	–	30
Take 5	2 pkg (1.5 oz)	220	4	11	<5	25	1	180
Tastetations Butterscotch	3 pieces	60	0	2	<5	12	–	85
Tastetations Caramel	3 pieces	60	0	2	<5	12	–	85
Tastetations Chocolate	3 pieces	60	0	21	<5	12	–	30
Hint Mint								
All Flavors	2 pieces	10	0	0	0	2	–	0
Jolly Rancher								
All Flavors	3 pieces	70	0	0	0	17	–	10
Lollipops All Flavors	1 (0.6 oz)	60	0	0	0	16	–	10
Joyva								
Halvah Chocolate Covered	1 serv (2 oz)	380	5	25	0	20	3	95
Halvah Marble	1 serv (2 oz)	390	6	25	0	18	2	120
Judy's								
Sugar Free Almond Caramel Cluster	1 piece (1.5 oz)	200	5	15	<5	10	2	0
Sugar Free Cashew Caramel Cluster	1 pieces (1.5 oz)	190	2	14	5	12	1	5
Sugar Free English Toffee	1 piece (1.5 oz)	220	4	17	5	9	3	25
Sugar Free Macadamia Caramel Cluster	1 piece (1.5 oz)	220	2	20	<5	9	2	0
Sugar Free Peanut Brittle	¾ cup	100	3	6	0	2	tr	70

FOOD	PORTION	CALS	PROT	FAT	CHOL	CARB	FIBER	SOD
Sugar Free Pecan Almond Cluster	1 piece (1.5 oz)	220	2	19	<5	9	2	0
Junior Mints								
Snack Size	1 box (0.7 oz)	75	tr	1	0	16	tr	5
Kit Kat								
Bar	1 (0.6 oz)	80	tr	4	0	10	–	10
Klein								
Sugar Free Hard Candy All Flavors	3 pieces	12	0	0	0	5	0	0
Krackel								
Bar	1 (0.6 oz)	90	tr	4	0	12	–	20
Miniature	1	45	tr	3	0	5	–	5
Lambertz								
Petits Soleils Chocolate Coated Gingerbread	1 piece (0.4 oz)	47	1	2	0	7	tr	8
Landies Candies								
Sugar Free Almond Clusters	2 pieces (1.5 oz)	240	7	17	<5	17	2	105
Sugar Free Bon Bons Peanut Butter	2 (1.5 oz)	240	7	17	<5	17	tr	150
Sugar Free Coconut Clusters	2 pieces (1.5 oz)	250	5	18	10	18	1	120
Sugar Free Cookies & Cream	2 pieces (1.5 oz)	240	4	15	5	23	tr	150
Sugar Free Dark Almond Bark	1 piece (1.5 oz)	230	3	15	<5	23	2	85
Sugar Free Dark Miniature Bars	7 pieces (1.5 oz)	230	2	14	<5	26	2	0
Sugar Free Milk Miniature Bars	7 pieces (1.5 oz)	240	6	15	5	21	tr	140
Sugar Free Mint Discs	7 pieces (1.5 oz)	240	6	15	5	21	tr	140
Sugar Free Peanut Clusters	2 (1.5 oz)	240	7	17	<5	17	2	100
Sugar Free White Almond Bark	1 piece (1.5 oz)	230	2	15	<5	21	tr	90

FOOD	PORTION	CALS	PROT	FAT	CHOL	CARB	FIBER	SOD
Sugar Free White Caps	6 pieces (1.5 oz)	230	3	15	5	24	0	85
Lean Protein Bites								
Milk Chocolate	1 pkg (1 oz)	120	14	6	3	1	0	180
Peanut Butter	1 pkg (1 oz)	120	14	5	1	1	0	200
White Chocolate	1 pkg (1 oz)	120	16	4	3	2	0	200
Lifesavers								
Gummi Shapes Barnum's Animals	1 pkg (0.8 oz)	70	1	0	0	18	–	0
Lindt								
Dark Chocolate 70% Cocoa	4 blocks (1.4 oz)	220	3	17	0	13	2	20
Lindor Truffles Dark Chocolate	3 pieces	220	2	18	5	15	0	10
Lindor Truffles Milk Chocolate	3 pieces	220	2	17	5	16	0	20
Low Carb Chef								
Gummi Bears	14 pieces	138	0	0	0	30	0	0
Jelly Beans	37 pieces	120	0	0	0	36	0	10
Sugar Free Caramel Marshmallow Treats	3 pieces	140	1	7	<5	28	0	15
Sugar Free Cherry Cordials	3 pieces	250	tr	8	<5	28	tr	10
Sugar Free Coconut Clusters	4 pieces	210	2	18	<5	19	3	15
Sugar Free Milk Chocolate Covered Vanilla Caramels	3 pieces	160	1	8	10	27	0	10
Sugar Free Peanut Butter Cups	1 piece	200	3	16	<5	19	1	5
Sugar Free Peanut Butter Truffles	2 pieces	200	3	16	<5	19	1	5
Sugar Free Peanut Clusters	4 pieces	210	5	17	<5	16	2	5
Sugar Free Pecan Turtles	1 pieces	120	1	13	5	20	1	10
Sugar Free Peppermint Patties	3 pieces	150	tr	9	10	28	3	50

FOOD	PORTION	CALS	PROT	FAT	CHOL	CARB	FIBER	SOD
M&M's								
Plain	1 pkg (1.7 oz)	240	2	10	5	34	1	30
Maple Grove Farms								
Maple Sugar Candy	5 pieces (1.3 oz)	140	0	0	0	36	—	0
Mauna Loa								
Kona Coffee Crunch Chocolate	1 bar (1.8 oz)	270	3	16	—	29	4	0
Macadamia Crisp Milk Chocolate	1 bar (1.8 oz)	270	4	17	10	29	tr	55
Macadamia Milk Chocolate	1 bar (1.8 oz)	280	4	18	10	27	1	45
Mon Cheri								
Hazelnut	4 pieces	260	4	18	5	20	1	25
Mounds								
Bar	1 (0.7 oz)	90	tr	5	0	11	—	30
Mr. Goodbar								
Bar	1 (0.6 oz)	100	2	6	0	9	—	5
Miniatures	1 (0.3 oz)	45	tr	3	0	5	—	5
Necco								
Bridge Mix	¼ cup (1.5 oz)	180	2	9	5	27	tr	35
Chocolate Covered Raisins	30 pieces (1.5 oz)	170	1	7	0	30	1	35
Malted Milk Balls	11 pieces (1.5 oz)	180	1	6	0	28	tr	35
Mint	1 piece	12	—	tr	0	—	—	—
SkyBar	1 bar (1.5 oz)	190	2	9	5	28	0	45
Nestle								
Buncha Crunch	1 pkg (1.4 oz)	90	2	10	10	26	tr	60
Crunch	1 bar (1.55 oz)	230	2	12	10	29	tr	65
Crunch Disk	1 (1.2 oz)	180	2	9	5	22	tr	50
Crunchkins	5 pieces	190	2	10	5	24	tr	45
Jingles Milk Chocolate Butterfinger	5 pieces	180	2	8	<5	26	tr	55
Jingles Milk Chocolate Crunch	7 pieces	220	2	11	10	28	tr	65

FOOD	PORTION	CALS	PROT	FAT	CHOL	CARB	FIBER	SOD
Jingles White Crunch	7 pieces	230	3	14	10	24	0	80
Milk Chocolate	1 bar (1.45 oz)	220	2	13	10	26	tr	25
Nesteggs Milk Chocolate Butterfinger	5 pieces	210	3	10	5	28	tr	55
Nesteggs Milk Chocolate Crunch	5 pieces	190	2	10	5	24	tr	45
Nesteggs White Crunch	7 pieces	230	3	14	10	24	0	75
Pearson's Egg Nog	2 pieces	60	0	2	0	11	0	40
Toll House Brownie Bar	2 pieces (2 oz)	250	2	12	5	36	1	240
Toll House Cookie Bar	1 piece (1 oz)	130	tr	6	<5	18	tr	90
Treasures Butterfinger	3 pieces	180	2	9	5	24	tr	40
Treasures Crunch	4 pieces (1.4 oz)	210	2	11	10	26	tr	60
Treasures Peanut Butter	4 pieces	250	4	17	5	23	1	90
Turtles Bite Size	4 pieces	210	2	12	5	25	tr	45
Turtles Bite Size	1 piece (0.4 oz)	50	1	2	1	6	tr	11
White Crunch	1 bar (1.4 oz)	220	3	13	10	23	0	70
Newman's Own								
Organic Peanut Butter Cups Dark Chocolate	3 pieces (1.2 oz)	180	3	12	0	18	tr	55
Organic Peanut Butter Cups Milk Chocolate	3 pieces (1.2 oz)	180	4	12	0	18	tr	70
Organic Peppermint Cups	3 pieces (1.2 oz)	180	2	12	0	20	tr	15
Nibs								
Licorice	9 pieces	35	0	0	0	9	—	60
Nips								
Butter Rum	2 pieces	60	0	2	0	11	0	40

FOOD	PORTION	CALS	PROT	FAT	CHOL	CARB	FIBER	SOD
Caramel	2 pieces	60	0	2	0	11	0	40
Chocolate	2 pieces	60	0	2	0	11	0	40
Chocolate Parfait	2 pieces	60	0	2	0	10	0	30
Coffee	2 pieces	50	0	2	0	10	0	40
Vanilla Almond Cafe	2 pieces	50	0	1	0	10	0	40
Oh Henry!								
Bar	1 (1.8 oz)	120	2	5	<5	16	0	60
Payday								
Snack Size	1 (0.7 oz)	90	2	5	0	10	—	65
Pearson's								
Irish Cream Parfait	2 pieces	60	0	2	0	10	0	30
Mint Patties	1	30	tr	1	0	6	tr	14
Perlege								
Sugar Free Belgium Chocolate All Flavors	1 bar (3.5 oz)	532	14	42	—	14	3	112
Sugar Free Cream Filled Belgian Chocolate All Flavors	1 bar (1.5 oz)	226	2	16	14	22	0	32
Pez								
Candy	1 roll (0.3 oz)	35	0	0	0	9	—	0
Candy Sugar Free	1 roll (0.3 oz)	30	0	0	0	8	—	0
Planters								
Original Peanut Bar	1 pkg (1.6 oz)	230	6	14	0	22	2	70
Pure De-Lite								
Caramel	1 bar	120	2	5	3	19	1	110
Caramel Crisp	1 bar	120	3	6	3	18	1	115
Caramel Nougat	1 bar	110	2	5	3	20	1	146
Caramel Peanut Butter	1 bar	120	2	6	2	17	1	58
Caramel Pecan	1 bar	130	2	7	3	17	1	94
Sugar Free Dark Chocolate	1 bar	173	2	14	1	1	4	37
Sugar Free Milk Choclate w/ Mint	1 bar	187	3	14	8	3	1	32

FOOD	PORTION	CALS	PROT	FAT	CHOL	CARB	FIBER	SOD
Sugar Free Milk Chocolate	1 bar	187	3	14	8	3	1	32
Sugar Free Milk Chocolate w/ Almonds	1 bar	190	3	14	8	4	2	30
Sugar Free Milk Chocolate w/ Coconut	1 bar	190	3	14	8	4	1	31
Sugar Free Milk Chocolate w/ Orange	1 bar	187	3	14	8	3	1	32
Sugar Free Milk Chocolate w/ Peanuts	1 bar	190	3	14	9	4	1	30
Sugar Free White Chocolate	1 bar	187	2	14	26	3	0	96
Truffle Bar Caramel	1 bar	140	2	8	5	16	0	25
Truffle Bar Dark Mint	1 bar	160	2	12	5	13	1	20
Truffle Bar Hazelnut	1 bar	160	2	12	10	12	1	20
Truffle Bar Peanut Butter	1 bar	160	2	11	5	13	1	20
Raisinets								
Candy	1 pkg (1.58 oz)	200	2	8	<5	31	1	15
Fun Size	3 pkg	200	2	8	5	43	2	15
Reese's								
Nutrageous	1 bar (0.6 oz)	95	2	6	0	9	1	25
Peanut Butter Cups	1 (0.28 oz)	40	tr	3	0	4	—	20
Peanut Butter Eggs	1	90	2	5	0	9	—	60
Pieces	25	90	3	5	0	11	—	40
Ritter Sport								
Dark Chocolate Whole Hazelnuts	6 pieces (1.3 oz)	210	2	15	<2	16	7	<5
Robin Eggs								
Large	2 pieces	70	0	2	0	14	—	40
Medium	4 pieces	90	0	3	0	16	—	45
Mini	10 pieces	70	0	3	0	13	—	40

FOOD	PORTION	CALS	PROT	FAT	CHOL	CARB	FIBER	SOD
Rokeach								
Cotton Candy	2 cups (1 oz)	110	0	0	0	28	0	0
Rolo								
Caramels In Milk Chocolate	3 pieces (0.64 oz)	90	tr	3	<5	12	–	35
Russell Stover								
Low Carb Pecan Delights	1 pkg (1 oz)	130	2	9	0	16	tr	25
Peanut Butter & Grape Jelly	1 piece (0.8 oz)	100	2	6	<5	10	tr	30
Peanut Butter & Red Raspberry Cups	2 (1.2 oz)	140	3	9	<5	14	tr	40
Pecan Delights	1 pkg (2 oz)	280	3	18	10	27	tr	65
Pecan Roll	1 (1.75 oz)	260	3	18	<5	23	2	80
S'mores	3 (1.4 oz)	210	2	12	<5	22	tr	80
Sugar Free Peanut Butter Cups	4 pieces (1.3 oz)	200	5	13	0	17	2	140
Sugar Free Pecans & Caramel	2 pieces (1.2 oz)	170	2	12	0	17	0	30
Sixlets								
Sixlets	3 tubes	90	0	4	0	14	–	50
Smucker's								
Fruit Fillers Strawberry	1 pkg (0.9 oz)	80	1	0	0	19	–	25
Snickers								
Almond	1 bar (1.76 oz)	240	3	11	5	32	1	80
Bar	1 (2.07 oz)	280	4	14	5	35	1	140
Cruncher	1 bar (1.56 oz)	230	4	13	5	25	1	140
Sno Caps								
Candies	1 pkg (2.3 oz)	300	2	13	0	48	3	0
Speakeasy								
Organic Mints All Flavors	4 pieces (2 g)	10	0	0	0	2	–	0
Steel's								
Salt Water Taffy Assorted	3 pieces (1 oz)	90	0	1	0	22	0	50

FOOD	PORTION	CALS	PROT	FAT	CHOL	CARB	FIBER	SOD
Sugar Babies								
Tidbits	1 pkg	180	–	2	–	–	–	–
Symphony								
Bar	1 (0.6 oz)	90	1	5	<5	10	–	15
The Chocolate Traveler								
Carb Controlled Wedges Bittersweet	4 pieces	120	1	9	0	12	0	20
Carb Controlled Wedges Dark Chocolate Coffee	4 pieces	110	1	8	0	15	2	0
Carb Controlled Wedges Dark Chocolate Mint	4 pieces	110	1	8	0	15	2	0
Carb Controlled Wedges Milk Chocolate	4 pieces	120	1	8	5	15	tr	0
Wedges Bittersweet	4 pieces	130	3	10	0	10	4	20
Wedges Dark Chocolate Coffee	4 pieces	130	1	8	0	15	2	0
Wedges Dark Chocolate Mint	4 pieces	130	1	8	0	15	2	0
Wedges Milk Chocolate	4 pieces	130	1	8	5	15	0	10
Tobler								
Orange Dark Chocolate	5 pieces (1.5 oz)	240	2	13	<5	28	3	10
Toblerone								
Bittersweet Chocolate w/ Honey & Almond Nugget	½ bar (1.2 oz)	170	1	9	<5	20	2	5
Milk Chocolate w/ Honey & Almond Nougat	½ bar (1.76 oz)	170	2	9	10	21	tr	15
Tootsie								
Pop	1	60	0	0	0	12	–	10
Torras								
Sugar Free Dark Chocolate	1 oz	136	2	10	2	15	0	0

FOOD	PORTION	CALS	PROT	FAT	CHOL	CARB	FIBER	SOD
Sugar Free Milk Chocolate	1 oz	140	2	10	8	17	0	0
Sugar Free Milk Chocolate w/ Almonds	1 oz	146	2	10	6	15	0	0
Sugar Free Milk Chocolate w/ Hazelnuts	1 oz	148	2	11	6	15	0	0
Sugar Free White Chocolate	1 oz	138	2	10	6	17	0	0
Tropical Source								
Butterscotch Dream	4 pieces (0.5 oz)	60	0	0	0	14	0	30
Chocolate Dairy Free California Raisin & Currant	½ bar (1.5 oz)	230	3	13	0	25	1	15
Chocolate Dairy Free Hazelnut Espresso Crunch	½ bar (1.5 oz)	250	3	17	0	21	1	15
Chocolate Dairy Free Maple Almond Granola	½ bar (1.5 oz)	230	3	15	0	24	1	15
Chocolate Dairy Free Mint Candy Crunch	½ bar (1.5 oz)	220	2	13	0	24	1	15
Chocolate Dairy Free Red Raspberry Crush	½ bar (1.5 oz)	230	2	15	0	22	1	15
Chocolate Dairy Free Sundried Jungle Banana	½ bar (1.5 oz)	230	2	13	0	26	2	15
Chocolate Dairy Free Toasted Almond	½ bar (1.5 oz)	250	3	17	0	21	1	15
Chocolate Dairy Free Wild Rice Crisp	½ bar (1.5 oz)	230	3	14	0	26	1	15
Cool Peppermint	4 pieces (0.5 oz)	60	0	0	0	14	0	0

FOOD	PORTION	CALS	PROT	FAT	CHOL	CARB	FIBER	SOD
Lollipops All Flavors	1	24	0	0	0	6	0	0
Mango Papaya	4 pieces (0.5 oz)	60	0	0	0	14	0	1
Twizzlers								
Cherry	1 piece	30	0	0	0	8	—	25
Chocolate	1	25	0	0	0	6	—	20
Licorice	1 piece	30	0	0	0	7	—	45
Pull'N'Peel Cherry	1 piece	100	1	0	0	25	—	85
Strawberry Snack Size	3 pkgs	130	1	1	0	30	—	100
Unique Origin								
Guaranda Dark Chocolate	1 piece (0.3 oz)	54	1	4	0	4	1	2
Werther's								
Original	3 pieces (0.5 oz)	60	0	1	<5	13	0	60
Whatchamacallit								
Bar	1 (0.57 oz)	80	1	4	0	10	—	50
Whitman's								
Sampler	3 pieces (1.4 oz)	190	2	10	5	24	tr	55
Whoppers								
Malted Milk Balls	9 pieces	90	tr	4	0	15	tr	65
Yamate Chocolatier								
No Sugar Almonds & Caramel	1 piece (0.6 oz)	70	1	6	0	9	1	0
York								
Peppermint Patty	1 (0.49 oz)	50	0	1	0	11	—	0
Zagnut								
Snack Size	1 piece	70	tr	3	0	9	—	25
Zero								
Bar	1	70	tr	3	0	12	—	35
CANTALOUPE								
dried	3.5 pieces (1.4 oz)	140	0	0	0	34	1	110
fresh cubed	1 cup	57	1	tr	0	13	1	14
fresh half	½	94	2	1	0	22	2	23

FOOD	PORTION	CALS	PROT	FAT	CHOL	CARB	FIBER	SOD
Chiquita								
Wedge	¼ med (4.7 oz)	50	0	0	0	12	1	25
CARAWAY								
seed	1 tsp	7	tr	tr	0	1	–	tr
CARDAMOM								
ground	1 tsp	6	tr	tr	0	1	–	tr
CARDOON								
fresh cooked	3½ oz	22	1	tr	0	5	–	176
fresh shredded	½ cup	36	1	tr	0	4	–	151
CARIBOU								
roasted	3 oz	142	25	4	93	0	–	51
CARISSA								
fresh	1	12	tr	tr	0	3	–	1
CAROB								
carob mix	3 tsp	45	tr	0	0	11	–	12
carob mix as prep w/ whole milk	9 oz	195	8	8	33	23	–	132
flour	1 cup	185	5	1	0	92	–	36
flour	1 tbsp	14	tr	tr	0	7	–	3
Sunspire								
Carob Chips Unsweetened	13 pieces (0.5 oz)	70	2	3	0	8	0	65
Carob Chips Vegan	13 pieces (0.5 oz)	70	0	3	0	11	0	5
CARP								
fresh	3 oz	108	15	5	56	0	–	42
fresh cooked	3 oz	138	19	6	72	0	–	54
fresh cooked	1 fillet (6 oz)	276	39	12	143	0	–	107
roe raw	1 oz	37	7	tr	103	tr	–	–
roe salted in olive oil	2 tbsp (1 oz)	40	–	–	100	6	0	1400
CARROT JUICE								
canned	6 oz	73	2	tr	0	17	–	54
Naked Juice								
Just Carrot	8 oz	80	2	0	0	13	0	90

FOOD	PORTION	CALS	PROT	FAT	CHOL	CARB	FIBER	SOD

CARROTS
CANNED

FOOD	PORTION	CALS	PROT	FAT	CHOL	CARB	FIBER	SOD
slices	½ cup	17	tr	tr	0	4	1	176
slices low sodium	½ cup	17	tr	tr	0	4	1	31
Del Monte								
Sliced	½ cup (4.3 oz)	35	0	0	0	8	3	300
S&W								
Julienne	½ cup (4.3 oz)	30	1	0	0	5	2	390
Sliced	½ cup (4.3 oz)	30	1	0	0	5	2	390
Whole Small	½ cup (4.3 oz)	30	1	0	0	5	2	390
FRESH								
baby raw	1 (½ oz)	6	tr	tr	0	1	–	5
raw	1 (2.5 oz)	31	1	tr	0	7	2	25
raw shredded	½ cup	24	1	tr	0	6	2	19
slices cooked	½ cup	35	1	tr	0	8	–	52
Bolthouse Farms								
Baby	1 pkg (2.25 oz)	25	1	0	0	7	2	33
Dole								
Shredded	1 cups (3 oz)	40	1	0	0	9	2	45
Earthbound Farms								
Organic Mini Peeled	½ cup	30	1	0	0	7	3	30
FROZEN								
slices cooked	½ cup	26	1	tr	0	6	–	43
Birds Eye								
Baby Whole	½ cup	40	–	0	0	–	2	45
Sliced	½ cup	35	–	0	0	–	3	45
Fresh Like								
Carrots Slice	3.5 oz	42	1	tr	–	10	–	42

CASABA

FOOD	PORTION	CALS	PROT	FAT	CHOL	CARB	FIBER	SOD
cubed	1 cup	45	2	tr	0	11	–	20
fresh	⅟₁₀	43	1	tr	0	10	–	20

FOOD	PORTION	CALS	PROT	FAT	CHOL	CARB	FIBER	SOD
CASHEWS								
cashew butter w/o salt	1 tbsp	94	3	8	0	4	–	2
dry roasted salted	1 oz	163	4	13	0	9	–	213
dry roasted w/ salt	18 nuts (1 oz)	160	4	13	0	9	1	180
oil roasted	1 oz	163	5	14	0	8	–	5
oil roasted salted	1 oz	163	5	14	0	8	–	209
Bowlby's								
Bits Cashew	½ cup	200	4	19	0	5	1	95
Frito Lay								
Salted	1 oz	180	5	15	0	7	1	190
Maranatha								
Cashew Butter	2 tbsp	190	5	15	0	11	2	5
Tamari Cashews	¼ cup	160	5	13	0	9	1	142
Sweet Delights								
Cashew Roasters	⅓ pkg (1 oz)	170	4	14	0	10	2	220
CASSAVA								
fresh	3½ oz	120	3	tr	0	27	–	8
CATFISH								
channel breaded & fried	3 oz	194	15	11	69	7	–	238
channel raw	3 oz	99	15	4	49	0	–	54
CAULIFLOWER								
FRESH								
cooked	½ cup (2.2 oz)	14	1	tr	0	3	1	9
flowerets cooked	3 (2 oz)	12	1	tr	0	2	1	8
flowerets raw	3 (2 oz)	14	1	tr	0	3	1	17
green cooked	1½ cup (3.2 oz)	29	3	tr	0	6	3	21
green raw	1 head 7 in diam (18 oz)	158	15	2	0	31	16	118
green raw	1 cup (2.2 oz)	20	2	tr	0	4	2	15
green raw floweret	1 (0.9 oz)	8	1	tr	0	2	1	6
raw	½ cup (1.8 oz)	13	1	tr	0	3	1	15

FOOD	PORTION	CALS	PROT	FAT	CHOL	CARB	FIBER	SOD
FROZEN								
cooked	½ cup	17	1	tr	0	3	–	16
Birds Eye								
Cauliflower	½ cup	20	–	0	0	–	2	15
Fresh Like								
Florets	3.5 oz	26	2	tr	–	5	1	48
CAVIAR								
black	1 tbsp	40	4	3	94	1	–	240
red	1 tbsp	40	4	3	94	1	–	240
CELERIAC								
fresh cooked	3½ oz	25	1	tr	0	6	–	61
raw	½ cup	31	1	tr	0	7	–	78
CELERY								
diced cooked	½ cup	13	1	tr	0	3	–	68
fresh	1 stalk (1.3 oz)	6	tr	tr	0	1	1	35
raw diced	½ cup	10	tr	tr	0	2	1	52
seed	1 tsp	8	tr	tr	0	1	–	3
Dole								
Stalks	2 med (3 oz)	15	1	0	0	3	2	100
CELTUCE								
raw	3½ oz	22	1	tr	0	4	–	11
CEREAL								
bran flakes	¾ cup (1 oz)	90	4	1	0	22	–	264
corn flakes	1¼ cup (1 oz)	110	2	tr	0	24	–	351
corn flakes low sodium	1 cup (0.9 oz)	100	2	tr	0	22	tr	3
corn grits white regular & quick as prep w/ water & salt	¾ cup (6.4 oz)	109	3	tr	0	24	tr	406
corn grits white regular or quick as prep	¾ cup (6.4 oz)	109	3	tr	0	24	tr	0

FOOD	PORTION	CALS	PROT	FAT	CHOL	CARB	FIBER	SOD
corn grits yellow regular & quick as prep w/ water & salt	¾ cup (6.4 oz)	109	3	tr	0	24	tr	406
corn grits yellow regular & quick not prep	1 cup (5.5 oz)	579	14	2	0	124	3	2
crispy rice	1 cup (1 oz)	111	2	tr	0	25	tr	206
crispy rice low sodium	1 cup (0.9 oz)	105	1	tr	0	23	tr	3
farina as prep w/ water	¾ cup (6.1 oz)	88	2	tr	0	19	2	0
farina not prep	1 tbsp (0.4 oz)	40	1	tr	0	9	tr	0
granola	½ cup (2.1 oz)	285	9	15	0	32	6	15
oatmeal instant w/ cinnamon & spice as prep w/ water	1 pkg (5.6 oz)	177	5	2	0	35	3	280
oatmeal instant w/ raisins & spice as prep w/ water	1 cup (5.5 oz)	161	4	2	0	32	2	226
oatmeal instant w/ bran & raisins as prep w/ water	1 pkg (6.8 oz)	158	5	2	0	30	6	248
oatmeal instant as prep w/ water	1 cup (8.2 oz)	138	6	2	0	24	4	377
oatmeal regular & quick as prep w/ water	¾ cup (6.1 oz)	149	5	2	0	19	3	2
oatmeal regular & quick not prep	½ cup (0.9 oz)	104	4	2	0	18	3	1
oatmeal instant cooked w/o salt	1 cup	145	6	2	0	25	—	2
oatmeal quick cooked w/o salt	1 cup	145	6	2	0	25	—	2

FOOD	PORTION	CALS	PROT	FAT	CHOL	CARB	FIBER	SOD
oatmeal regular cooked w/o salt	1 cup	145	6	2	0	25	—	2
puffed rice	1 cup (0.5 oz)	56	1	tr	0	13	tr	0
puffed wheat	1 cup (0.4 oz)	44	2	tr	0	10	1	0
shredded mini wheats	1 cup (1.1 oz)	107	3	1	0	24	3	3
shredded wheat rectangular	1 biscuit (0.8 oz)	85	3	tr	0	19	2	0
shredded wheat round	2 biscuits (1.3 oz)	136	4	1	0	31	4	1
sugar-coated corn flakes	¾ cup (1 oz)	110	1	1	0	26	—	230
whole wheat hot natural as prep w/ water	¾ cup (6.4 oz)	113	4	1	0	25	3	0
Albers								
Hominy Quick Grits uncooked	¼ cup	140	3	1	0	31	1	0
Alpen								
Corn Flakes	1 serv (1 oz)	110	2	tr	—	25	tr	2
No Salt No Sugar	1 serv (2 oz)	200	7	3	—	34	6	35
Regular	1 serv (2 oz)	200	7	3	—	37	4	100
Atkins								
Banana Nut Harvest	⅔ cup	100	12	3	0	11	6	100
Blueberry Bounty w/ Almonds	⅔ cup	100	13	2	0	10	6	105
Crunchy Almond Crisp	⅔ cup	100	15	2	0	8	5	100
Aunt Paula's								
Hot Flax Cereal	1 serv (1½ oz)	100	10	5	0	8	5	140
Back To Nature								
Hi-Protein	⅔ cup	140	12	1	0	25	3	130
Muesli	½ cup	160	3	3	0	32	4	70
Puff Wheat	½ cup	160	3	3	0	32	4	70
Ultra Flax	¾ cup	150	7	2	0	28	3	0

FOOD	PORTION	CALS	PROT	FAT	CHOL	CARB	FIBER	SOD
Barbara's Bakery								
Apple Cinnamon O's	¾ cup	110	3	1	0	24	2	90
Bite Size Shredded Oats	1¼ cups (2 oz)	220	6	3	0	46	6	260
Cinnamon Puffins	1¼ cup (2 oz)	100	2	1	0	26	6	150
Cocoa Crunch Stars	1 cup (1 oz)	110	2	1	0	26	1	140
Frosted Corn Flakes	1 cup (1 oz)	110	2	1	0	27	4	100
Fruit Juice Sweetened Breakfast O's	1 cup (1 oz)	120	5	2	0	22	3	115
Fruit Juice Sweetened Brown Rice Crisps	1 cup (1 oz)	120	2	1	0	25	1	125
Fruit Juice Sweetened Corn Flakes	1 cup (1 oz)	110	2	0	0	26	2	130
GrainShop	⅔ cup (1 oz)	90	3	1	0	24	8	110
Honey Crunch Stars	1 cup (1 oz)	110	2	0	0	26	2	50
Honey Nut Toasted O's	¾ cup	120	3	2	0	23	2	90
Organic Fruity Punch	1 cup (1 oz)	110	2	1	0	26	0	120
Organic Soy Essence	¾ cup (1 oz)	100	3	1	0	25	5	110
Puffins	¾ cup (0.9 oz)	90	2	1	0	23	5	190
Shredded Spoonfuls	¾ cup	120	4	2	0	24	4	200
Shredded Wheat	2 biscuits (1.4 oz)	140	4	1	0	31	5	0
Carbsense								
Hot Cereal Country Spice not prep	½ cup	130	14	6	0	15	12	130
Hot Cereal Roasted Hazelnut not prep	½ cup	140	25	9	0	15	12	140

FOOD	PORTION	CALS	PROT	FAT	CHOL	CARB	FIBER	SOD
Country Choice								
Instant Oatmeal Apples 'N' Cinnamon	1 pkg	140	4	2	0	27	3	85
Instant Oatmeal Maple Syrup	1 pkg	170	6	2	0	32	4	80
Instant Oatmeal Organic Plus French Vanilla	1 pkg	180	7	3	0	32	3	140
Instant Oatmeal Organic Plus Golden Brown Sugar	1 pkg	180	7	3	0	32	3	140
Instant Oatmeal Regular	1 pkg	110	4	1	0	19	3	0
Oatmeal Steel Cut not prep	½ cup	150	5	3	0	27	4	0
Oats Old Fashioned not prep	½ cup	150	5	3	0	27	4	0
Oats Quick not prep	½ cup	150	5	3	0	27	4	0
Organic Multi Grain Hot Cereal not prep	½ cup	130	6	2	0	29	5	0
Deliciously Slim								
Granola Cranberry Cashew	¾ cup	230	9	13	0	29	12	100
Granola Strawberry Almond	¾ cup	230	9	13	0	29	12	100
Erewhon								
Apple Stroodles	¾ cup	110	3	1	0	25	1	15
Aztec	1 cup	110	2	0	0	26	1	70
Banana O's	¾ cup	110	2	0	0	26	2	15
Brown Rice Cream	¼ cup	170	5	1	0	36	1	30
Corn Flakes	1¼ cups	210	5	3	0	45	3	100
Crispy Brown Rice	1 cup	110	2	0	0	25	1	180
Crispy Brown Rice No Salt Added	1 cup	110	2	0	0	25	1	10
Fruit'n Wheat	¾ cup	170	51	2	0	39	5	105
Kamut Flakes	⅔ cup	110	5	0	0	25	4	75

FOOD	PORTION	CALS	PROT	FAT	CHOL	CARB	FIBER	SOD
Raisin Bran	1 cup	170	5	1	0	40	6	100
Rice Twice	¾ cup	120	2	0	0	28	0	80
Whole Wheat Flakes	1 cup	180	6	1	0	42	6	135
Expert Foods								
Low Carb Hot Cereal Sub	½ cup	24	4	0	0	2	—	65
General Mills								
Basic 4	1 cup (1.9 oz)	200	4	2	0	42	3	320
Boo Berry	1 cup (1 oz)	120	1	1	0	27	—	210
Cheerios	1 cup (1 oz)	110	3	2	0	22	3	280
Cheerios Apple Cinnamon	¾ cup	120	2	2	0	25	1	115
Cheerios Frosted	1 cup (1 oz)	120	2	1	0	25	1	210
Cheerios Honey Nut	1 cup (1 oz)	120	3	2	0	24	2	270
Cheerios Multi Grain	1 cup (1 oz)	110	3	1	0	24	3	200
Cheerios Team	1 cup (1 oz)	120	2	1	0	25	1	210
Chex Corn	1 cup (1 oz)	110	2	0	0	26	0	280
Chex Honey Nut	¾ cup	120	1	1	0	26	—	220
Chex Morning Mix Cinnamon	1 pkg (1.1 oz)	130	2	4	0	24	1	180
Chex Morning Mix Fruit & Nut	1 pkg (1.1 oz)	180	2	4	0	24	1	190
Chex Morning Mix Honey Nut	1 pkg (1.1 oz)	130	2	4	0	24	1	190
Chex Multi-Bran	1 cup (2 oz)	200	4	2	0	49	8	380
Chex Rice	1¼ cup (1.1 oz)	120	2	0	0	27	0	290
Cinnamon Grahams	¾ cup (1 oz)	120	1	1	0	26	1	240
Cinnamon Toast Crunch	¾ cup (1 oz)	130	1	4	1	24	1	210
Cocoa Puffs	1 cup (1 oz)	120	1	1	0	26	—	170
Cookie Crisp	1 cup (1 oz)	120	1	1	0	26	0	180
Count Chocula	1 cup (1 oz)	120	1	1	0	26	0	180
Country Corn Flakes	1 cup (1 oz)	120	2	0	0	26	—	270
Fiber One	½ cup (1 oz)	60	2	1	0	24	14	130
Franken Berry	1 cup (1 oz)	120	1	1	0	27	—	210
French Toast Crunch	¾ cup (1 oz)	120	1	1	0	26	0	180

FOOD	PORTION	CALS	PROT	FAT	CHOL	CARB	FIBER	SOD
Gold Medal Raisin Bran	1⅓ cups (1.9 oz)	170	5	2	0	41	6	330
Golden Grahams	¾ cup (1 oz)	120	1	1	0	25	1	270
Harmony	1¼ cups (1.9 oz)	200	5	4	0	44	2	350
Honey Nut Clusters	1 cup (1.9 oz)	210	4	3	0	46	3	270
Kaboom	1¼ cup (1 oz)	120	2	1	0	24	1	290
Kix	1⅓ cup (1 oz)	120	2	1	0	26	1	270
Kix Berry Berry	¾ cup (1 oz)	120	1	2	0	26	0	180
Lucky Charms	1 cup (1 oz)	120	2	1	0	25	1	210
Nature Valley Low Fat Fruit Granola	⅔ cup (1.9 oz)	210	4	3	0	44	3	210
Newquick	¾ cup (1 oz)	120	1	2	0	25	–	190
Oatmeal Crisp Almond	1 cup (1.9 oz)	220	5	5	0	42	4	240
Oatmeal Crisp Apple Cinnamon	1 cup (1.9 oz)	210	5	2	0	45	4	250
Oatmeal Crisp Raisin	1 cup (1.9 oz)	210	5	2	0	44	4	220
Para Su Familia Cinnamon Stars	1 cup (1 oz)	120	1	1	0	28	–	240
Para Su Familia Fruitis	1 cup (1 oz)	120	1	1	0	25	–	210
Para Su Familia Raisin Bran	1¼ cups (2 oz)	170	5	2	0	41	6	320
Raisin Nut Bran	¾ cup (1.9 oz)	200	4	4	0	41	4	250
Reese's Puffs	¾ cup	130	2	3	0	23	0	170
Snack'N Dash Cinnamon Toast Crunch	1 pkg (1.2 oz)	140	2	4	0	27	1	230
Snack'N Dash Honey Nut Cheerios	1 pkg (1 oz)	110	3	1	0	23	2	250
Snack'N Dash Lucky Charms	1 pkg (1 oz)	110	2	1	0	24	1	100

FOOD	PORTION	CALS	PROT	FAT	CHOL	CARB	FIBER	SOD
Sunrise Organic	¾ cup (1 oz)	110	1	1	0	26	1	190
Total Brown Sugar & Oat	¾ cup (1 oz)	110	2	1	0	23	1	200
Total Protein	¾ cup	120	13	4	0	11	3	270
Total Raisin Bran	1 cup	170	4	1	0	41	5	240
Total Whole Grain	¾ cup (1 oz)	110	2	1	0	23	3	190
Trix	1 cup (1 oz)	120	1	1	0	27	1	190
Wheat Hearts	¼ cup (1.3 oz)	130	5	1	0	26	2	0
Wheaties	1 cup (1 oz)	110	3	1	0	24	3	220
Wheaties Energy Crunch	1 cup (1.9 oz)	210	6	3	0	42	4	310
Wheaties Frosted	¾ cup (1 oz)	110	1	1	0	27	–	200
Wheaties Raisin Bran	1 cup (1.9 oz)	180	4	1	0	45	5	250
Grainfield's								
Brown Rice	1 serv (1 oz)	110	3	1	–	24	tr	4
Crisp Rice	1 serv (1 oz)	112	3	tr	–	25	tr	3
Raisin Bran	1 serv (1 oz)	90	2	2	–	20	2	4
Wheat Flakes	1 serv (1 oz)	100	3	1	–	20	2	2
Gram's Gourmet								
Cream Of Flax not prep	½ cup	142	18	5	0	11	8	305
Crunch Granolas All Flavors	½ cup	349	10	30	2	10	6	40
Hansen's								
Orange & Chocolate	½ cup	230	11	14	0	35	4	200
Strawberry & Yogurt	½ cup	230	6	9	0	30	6	220
Toasted Nut Crunch	½ cup	230	6	6	0	39	7	75
Tropical Cluster	½ cup	210	5	5	0	36	6	140
Hi-Lo								
Low Carb Cereal	½ cup	90	12	2	0	11	6	150
Hodgson Mill								
Bulgur Wheat w/ Soy Grits	¼ cup	116	10	1	0	22	3	0
Cracked Wheat	¼ cup	110	4	1	0	26	8	3
Multi Grain w/ Flaxseed & Soy	⅓ cup	160	7	3	0	25	6	0

FOOD	PORTION	CALS	PROT	FAT	CHOL	CARB	FIBER	SOD
Kashi								
Breakfast Pilaf as prep	½ cup (4.9 oz)	170	6	3	0	30	6	15
Go Apple Spice	½ cup (4.9 oz)	270	7	3	0	56	6	0
Go Banana Almond	½ cup (4.9 oz)	280	7	4	0	57	6	5
Go Blueberry Bliss	½ cup (4.9 oz)	260	7	3	0	55	6	5
Go Cherry Vanilla	½ cup (4.9 oz)	260	7	3	0	54	6	15
Go Just Peachy	½ cup (4.9 oz)	260	7	3	0	54	6	0
GoLean	1 cup	140	13	1	0	30	10	85
Good Friends	1 cup	170	5	2	0	43	12	130
Heart To Heart	¾ cup	110	4	2	0	25	5	90
Honey Puffed	1 cup (1 oz)	120	3	1	0	25	2	6
Medley	½ cup (1 oz)	100	4	1	0	20	2	50
Organic Promise Cranberry Sunshine	1 cup	110	2	1	0	26	2	100
Pillows Apple	¾ cup (1.9 oz)	200	3	1	0	45	2	30
Pillows Chocolate	¾ cup (1.9 oz)	200	3	1	0	45	2	50
Pillows Strawberry Crisp	¾ cup (1.9 oz)	200	3	1	0	46	2	25
Puffed	1 cup (0.9 oz)	70	3	tr	0	13	2	0
Kellogg's								
Corn Pops K-Sentials	1 oz	100	1	0	0	25	0	110
Froot Loops K-Sentials	1 oz	100	2	1	0	24	0	130
Smart Start	1 cup	190	3	1	0	43	3	280
Keto								
Cocoa Crisp	½ cup	110	21	2	0	4	1	370
Frosted Flakes All Flavors	¾ cup	110	17	1	0	9	2	180
Hot Cereal Apple Cinnamon	2 scoops	150	17	4	0	12	9	210

FOOD	PORTION	CALS	PROT	FAT	CHOL	CARB	FIBER	SOD
Hot Cereal Strawberry & Creme	2 scoops	150	17	4	0	12	9	210
Low Carb Crispy Soy	¾ cup	110	22	2	–	2	0	370
Oatmeal Old Fashioned	2 scoops	150	17	4	0	12	9	210
Liquid Cereal								
Apple & Cinnamon	1 can (11 oz)	160	7	1	5	32	1	170
Chocolate	1 can (11 oz)	170	7	1	5	33	1	125
Fruit	1 can (11 oz)	150	7	0	5	31	tr	135
Peanut Butter	1 can (11 oz)	170	7	2	5	32	1	110
Lundberg								
Purely Organic Hot'n Creamy Rice	⅓ cup	190	4	2	0	43	3	0
McCann's								
Irish Oatmeal Instant Apples & Cinnamon	1 pkg (1 oz)	130	3	2	0	26	2	130
Irish Oatmeal Instant Maple & Brown Sugar	1 pkg (1 oz)	160	4	2	0	32	3	220
Irish Oatmeal Instant Regular	1 pkg (1 oz)	100	4	2	0	18	3	80
MiniCarb								
Milk Chocolate Hot Cereal not prep	½ cup	140	12	6	10	17	13	170
Mother's								
Cinnamon Oat Crunch	1 cup	230	6	3	0	48	5	250
Cocoa Bumpers	1 cup	120	2	1	0	29	1	170
Groovy Grahams	¾ cup	100	2	1	0	24	1	240
Honey Round-Ups	¾ cups	110	2	1	0	25	1	160
Multigrain Hot Cereal	½ cup	130	5	1	0	29	5	0
Oat Bran Hot Cereal	½ cup	150	7	3	0	25	6	0
Oatmeal Instant	½ cup	150	5	3	0	27	4	0

FOOD	PORTION	CALS	PROT	FAT	CHOL	CARB	FIBER	SOD
Peanut Butter Bumpers	1 cup	130	3	3	0	26	1	270
Rolled Oats	½ cup	150	5	3	0	27	4	0
Toasted Oat Bran	¾ cup	120	4	2	0	24	3	200
Whole Wheat Hot Cereal	½ cup	130	5	1	0	30	4	0
Natural Ovens								
Great Granola	¼ cup	110	5	4	0	18	5	10
Paul's Oatmeal not prep	⅓ cup	120	4	3	0	22	3	100
Post								
Alpha-Bits Marshmallow	1 cup (1 oz)	120	2	1	0	25	0	160
Grape-Nuts	½ cup	200	7	1	0	47	6	310
Grape-Nuts Flakes	¾ cup (1 oz)	100	3	1	0	24	3	140
Great Grains Raisins Dates Pecans	½ cup	210	4	5	0	40	4	130
Selects Blueberry Morning	¾ cup (1.3 oz)	140	2	2	0	30	2	150
Shredded Wheat Spoon Size	1 cup	170	6	1	0	40	6	0
Quaker								
Oatmeal Instant Apples & Cinnamon	1 pkg (1.2 oz)	130	3	2	0	27	3	170
Oatmeal Instant Cinnamon & Spice	1 pkg (1.6 oz)	170	4	2	0	35	3	250
Oatmeal Instant Maple & Brown Sugar	1 pkg (1.5 oz)	160	4	2	0	32	3	260
Oatmeal Instant Supreme Banana Walnut	1 pkg (1.4 oz)	150	4	3	0	28	3	280
Oatmeal Nutrition for Women Golden Brown Sugar	1 pkg (1.6 oz)	170	5	2	0	33	3	310

FOOD	PORTION	CALS	PROT	FAT	CHOL	CARB	FIBER	SOD
Old Fashion Oats not prep	½ cup	150	5	3	0	27	4	0
Ralston								
Raisin Bran	1 cup	200	6	2	0	47	8	370
Sunbelt								
Berry Basic	½ cup (1.9 oz)	220	6	6	0	40	5	200
Granola Cinnamon Raisins	½ cup (1.9 oz)	200	5	3	0	42	4	80
Muesli 5 Whole Grains	½ cup (1.9 oz)	210	4	2	0	44	3	70
Uncle Sam								
Cereal	1 cup (1.9 oz)	190	7	1	0	38	10	135
Weetabix								
Cereal	2 biscuits (1.2 oz)	100	3	1	–	21	3	106
Wheatena								
Cereal	⅓ cup (1.4 oz)	150	5	1	0	33	5	0

CEREAL BARS (see also ENERGY BARS)

FOOD	PORTION	CALS	PROT	FAT	CHOL	CARB	FIBER	SOD
granola	1 (1 oz)	134	3	7	0	18	2	83
Barbara's Bakery								
Nature's Choice Apple Cinnamon	1 bar (1.3 oz)	120	2	2	0	27	2	75
Nature's Choice Blueberry	1 bar (1.3 oz)	120	2	2	0	27	2	75
Nature's Choice Cherry	1 bar (1.3 oz)	120	2	2	0	27	2	75
Nature's Choice Granola Carob Chip	1 bar (0.7 oz)	80	2	2	0	16	2	5
Nature's Choice Granola Cinnamon & Raisin	1 bar (0.7 oz)	80	2	2	0	16	3	5
Nature's Choice Granola Oats 'N Honey	1 bar (0.7 oz)	80	2	2	0	15	2	5

FOOD	PORTION	CALS	PROT	FAT	CHOL	CARB	FIBER	SOD
Nature's Choice Granola Peanut Butter	1 bar (0.7 oz)	80	2	3	0	14	2	5
Nature's Choice Raspberry	1 bar (1.3 oz)	120	2	2	0	27	2	75
Nature's Choice Strawberry	1 bar (1.3 oz)	120	2	2	0	27	2	75
Nature's Choice Triple Berry	1 bar (1.3 oz)	120	2	2	0	27	2	75
Entenmann's								
Multi-Grain Chocolate Chip	1	140	2	3	0	28	2	100
Multi-Grain Rainbow Chip	1	180	1	8	5	26	tr	100
Multi-Grain Real Raspberry	1	140	1	3	0	26	1	110
General Mills								
Milk 'N Cereal Bars Chex	1 bar (1.6 oz)	160	6	4	0	26	—	150
Milk 'N Cereal Bars Cinnamon Toast Crunch	1 bar (1.6 oz)	180	6	4	0	30	1	160
Oatmeal Crisp Apple	1 bar (1.4 oz)	150	2	2	0	31	1	110
Oatmeal Crisp Strawberry	1 bar (1.4 oz)	140	3	2	0	30	1	115
Glenny's								
Chocolate Crunch Creamy Low Fat	1 bar (1.75 oz)	190	3	3	0	36	4	113
Chocolate Crunch Roasted Peanut	1 bar (1.75 oz)	200	4	4	0	36	6	100
Chocolate Crunch Toasted Almond	1 bar (1.75 oz)	200	4	4	0	36	6	100
Hershey's								
Crispy Rice Peanut Butter	1 bar (0.5 oz)	60	tr	2	0	9	—	55
Crispy Rice Snacks Peanut Butter	1 bar (0.5 oz)	60	1	2	0	9	tr	57
Kellogg's								
Special K Blueberry	1 bar	90	2	2	0	18	tr	95

FOOD	PORTION	CALS	PROT	FAT	CHOL	CARB	FIBER	SOD
Special K Cranberry Apple	1 bar	90	2	2	0	17	tr	90
Kudos								
Apple Nut Crunch	1	90	1	3	0	15	1	65
Chocolate Chip	1	120	1	5	0	20	1	85
Peanut Butter	1	190	2	6	0	18	1	90
Snickers	1	100	1	4	0	16	0	105
With M&M's	1	100	1	9	0	17	0	115
Nabisco								
Nutter Butter Granola Bar	1 (1 oz)	120	2	8	0	21	tr	45
Oreo Granola Bar	1 (1 oz)	120	2	4	0	21	1	65
Natural Ovens								
Great Granola Chocolate Almond	1 bar	150	4	6	0	23	3	110
Great Granola Fruit & Lemon	1 bar	130	4	3	0	24	3	140
Great Granola Mixed Fruit	1 bar	130	4	3	0	24	3	140
Nature Valley								
Chewy Trail Mix Fruit & Nut	1 bar	140	3	4	0	25	2	95
Nutri-Grain								
Fruit-full Squares Apple	1 (1.7 oz)	180	3	4	0	35	1	95
Fruit-full Squares Banana	1 (1.7 oz)	190	3	5	0	35	1	95
Fruit-full Squares Cinnamon Raisin	1 (1.7 oz)	180	3	4	0	35	1	95
Minis Strawberry	1 pkg (1.5 oz)	160	2	3	0	32	1	115
Twists Low Fat Apple Cinnamon	1 (1.3 oz)	140	1	3	0	27	1	105
Twists Low Fat Banana Strawberry	1 (1.3 oz)	140	1	3	0	26	1	100
Twists Low Fat Strawberry Blueberry	1 (1.3 oz)	140	1	3	0	27	1	110

FOOD	PORTION	CALS	PROT	FAT	CHOL	CARB	FIBER	SOD
Quaker								
Chewy Chocolate Chip	1 (1 oz)	120	2	4	0	21	1	70
Chewy Cookies 'n Cream	1 (1 oz)	110	2	3	0	22	1	80
Chewy Peanut Butter Chocolate Chunk	1 (1 oz)	120	2	3	0	20	1	105
Chewy Graham Slam Chocolate Chip	1 (1 oz)	110	2	2	0	22	1	75
Chewy Graham Slam Peanut Butter	1 (1 oz)	110	2	2	0	22	1	80
Chewy Low Fat Chocolate Chunk	1 (1 oz)	110	2	2	0	22	1	80
Chewy Low Fat Oatmeal Raisin	1 (1 oz)	110	1	2	0	22	1	70
Chewy Low Fat S'mores	1 (1 oz)	110	1	2	0	22	1	80
Fruit & Oatmeal Bites Apple Crisp	1 pkg	140	2	3	0	27	1	85
Fruit & Oatmeal Bites Strawberry	1 pkg	140	2	3	0	27	1	120
Fruit & Oatmeal Bites Very Berry	1 pkg	140	2	3	0	27	1	110
Fruit & Oatmeal Cranberry Orange Muffin	1 (1.3 oz)	130	1	3	0	27	1	95
Fruit & Oatmeal Low Fat Cherry Cobbler	1 (1.3 oz)	140	2	3	0	26	1	95
Fruit & Oatmeal Low Fat Strawberry	1 (1.3 oz)	140	2	3	0	26	1	125
Fruit & Oatmeal Low Fat Strawberry Banana	1 (1.3 oz)	130	1	3	0	26	tr	100

FOOD	PORTION	CALS	PROT	FAT	CHOL	CARB	FIBER	SOD
Fruit & Oatmeal Low Fat Strawberry Cheesecake	1 (1.3 oz)	130	2	3	0	26	tr	125
Rice Krispies								
Treats Peanut Butter Chocolate	1 (0.8 oz)	110	2	4	0	16	0	100
Treats Cocoa	1 (0.8 oz)	100	1	4	0	16	0	105
Treats Original	1 (0.8 oz)	90	1	2	0	18	0	100
Skippy								
Peanut Butter	1 bar	180	4	11	0	18	1	95
Peanut Butter & Fudge	1 bar	190	4	12	0	18	1	95
Peanut Butter & Marshmallow	1 bar	140	4	12	0	14	1	170
Peanut Butter & Strawberry	1 bar	170	4	12	0	14	1	170
Sunbelt								
Apple	1 (1.3 oz)	130	1	3	0	28	tr	75
Blueberry	1 (1.3 oz)	130	1	3	0	28	tr	75
Chewy Granola Almond	1 (1 oz)	130	2	7	0	17	1	65
Chewy Granola Apple Cinnamon	1 (1.2 oz)	140	2	3	0	28	2	105
Chewy Granola Chocolate Chip	1 (1.2 oz)	160	2	7	0	23	2	70
Chewy Granola Oatmeal Raisin	1 (1.2 oz)	130	2	3	0	27	1	100
Chewy Granola Oats & Honey	1 (1 oz)	120	2	5	0	19	1	65
CHAMPAGNE								
mimosa	1 serv	117	1	tr	0	12	tr	1
punch	1 serv	113	0	0	0	5	0	tr
sekt german champagne	3.5 fl oz	84	tr	0	0	5	–	–
Andre								
Blush	4 fl oz	88	0	0	0	4	–	4
Brut	4 fl oz	84	0	0	0	4	–	4

FOOD	PORTION	CALS	PROT	FAT	CHOL	CARB	FIBER	SOD
Cold Duck	4 fl oz	100	0	0	0	8	–	4
Extra Dry	4 fl oz	92	0	0	0	4	–	4
Ballatore								
Spumante	4 fl oz	92	0	0	0	8	–	8
Eden Roc								
Brut	4 fl oz	92	0	0	0	4	–	4
Brut Rosé	4 fl oz	99	0	0	0	8	–	4
Extra Dry	4 fl oz	84	0	0	0	4	–	4
Tott's								
Blanc de Noir	4 fl oz	88	0	0	0	8	–	4
Brut	4 fl oz	80	0	0	0	tr	–	4
Extra Dry	4 fl oz	84	0	0	0	4	–	4

CHAYOTE

FOOD	PORTION	CALS	PROT	FAT	CHOL	CARB	FIBER	SOD
fresh cooked	1 cup	38	1	1	0	8	–	1
raw	1 (7 oz)	49	2	1	0	11	–	8
raw cut up	1 cup	32	1	tr	0	7	–	198

CHEESE (see also CHEESE DISHES, CHEESE SUBSTITUTES, COTTAGE CHEESE, CREAM CHEESE, NEUFCHATEL)

FOOD	PORTION	CALS	PROT	FAT	CHOL	CARB	FIBER	SOD
american	1 oz	93	6	7	18	2	–	337
american cheese food	1 pkg (8 oz)	745	45	56	145	17	–	2700
american cheese spread	1 jar (5 oz)	412	23	30	78	12	–	1910
american cold pack	1 pkg (8 oz)	752	45	56	144	19	–	2193
american cheese spread	1 oz	82	5	6	16	2	–	381
beaufort	1 oz	115	8	9	34	tr	0	128
bel paese	1 oz	112	7	9	–	0	–	–
blue	1 oz	100	6	8	21	1	–	396
blue crumbled	1 cup (4.7 oz)	477	29	39	102	3	–	1884
brick	1 oz	105	7	8	27	1	–	159
brie	1 oz	95	8	8	28	tr	–	178
cacio di roma sheep's milk cheese	1 oz	130	8	10	30	0	–	170
caerphilly	1.4 oz	150	9	13	–	0	0	–

FOOD	PORTION	CALS	PROT	FAT	CHOL	CARB	FIBER	SOD
camembert	1 wedge (1⅓ oz)	114	8	9	27	tr	–	320
camembert	1 oz	85	6	7	20	tr	–	239
cantal	1 oz	105	7	9	26	tr	0	269
caraway	1 oz	107	7	8	–	1	–	196
chabichou	1 oz	95	6	8	23	tr	0	189
chaource	1 oz	83	5	7	20	tr	0	230
cheddar	1 oz	114	7	9	30	tr	–	176
cheddar low fat	1 oz	49	9	2	6	1	–	174
cheddar low sodium	1 oz	113	7	9	28	1	–	6
cheddar reduced fat	1.4 oz	104	13	6	–	0	0	–
cheddar shredded	1 cup	455	28	37	119	1	–	701
cheshire	1 oz	110	7	9	29	1	–	198
cheshire reduced fat	1.4 oz	108	13	6	–	tr	0	–
colby	1 oz	112	7	9	27	1	–	171
colby low fat	1 oz	49	9	2	6	1	–	174
colby low sodium	1 oz	113	7	9	28	1	–	6
comte	1 oz	114	8	9	34	tr	0	105
coulommiers	1 oz	88	6	7	23	tr	0	195
crottin	1 oz	105	6	9	23	tr	0	133
derby	1.4 oz	161	10	14	–	0	0	–
edam	1 oz	101	7	8	25	tr	–	274
edam reduced fat	1.4 oz	92	13	4	–	tr	0	–
emmentaler	1 oz	115	8	9	26	tr	–	129
feta	1 oz	75	4	6	25	1	–	316
fontina	1 oz	110	7	9	33	tr	–	–
frais	1.6 oz	51	3	3	–	3	0	–
gjetost	1 oz	132	3	8	–	12	–	170
gloucester double	1.4 oz	162	10	14	–	0	0	–
goat fresh	1 oz	23	1	2	5	tr	0	18
goat hard	1 oz	128	9	10	30	1	–	98
goat semisoft	1 oz	103	6	8	22	1	–	146
goat soft	1 oz	76	5	6	13	tr	–	104
gorgonzola	1 oz	107	5	9	–	tr	–	–
gouda	1 oz	101	7	8	32	1	–	232
gruyere	1 oz	117	8	9	31	tr	–	95
lancashire	1.4 oz	149	9	12	–	0	0	–

FOOD	PORTION	CALS	PROT	FAT	CHOL	CARB	FIBER	SOD
leicester	1.4 oz	160	10	14	—	0	0	—
limburger	1 oz	93	8	8	26	tr	—	227
lymeswold	1.4 oz	170	6	16	—	tr	0	—
maroilles	1 oz	97	6	8	26	tr	0	300
monterey jack	1 oz	106	7	9	—	tr	—	152
morbier	1 oz	99	7	8	23	tr	0	283
mozzarella	1 lb	1276	88	98	356	10	—	1692
mozzarella	1 oz	80	6	6	22	1	—	106
mozzarella fresh	1 oz	80	6	6	20	tr	0	160
mozzarella low moisture	1 oz	90	6	7	25	1	—	118
mozzarella part skim	1 oz	72	7	5	16	1	—	132
muenster	1 oz	104	7	9	27	tr	—	178
parmesan grated	1 oz	129	12	9	22	1	—	528
parmesan grated	1 tbsp (5 g)	23	2	2	4	tr	—	93
parmesan hard	1 oz	111	10	7	19	1	—	454
picodon	1 oz	99	6	8	23	tr	0	—
pimento	1 oz	106	6	9	27	tr	—	405
pont l'eveque	1 oz	86	6	7	20	tr	0	191
port du salut	1 oz	100	7	8	35	tr	—	151
provolone	1 oz	100	7	8	20	1	—	248
pyrenees	1 oz	101	6	8	26	tr	0	235
quark 20% fat	1 oz	33	4	1	5	1	—	10
quark 40% fat	1 oz	48	3	3	11	1	—	10
quark made w/ skim milk	1 oz	22	4	tr	tr	1	—	11
queso anego	1 oz	106	6	9	30	1	—	321
queso asadero	1 oz	101	6	8	30	1	—	186
queso chichuahua	1 oz	106	6	8	30	2	—	175
queso fresco	1 oz	41	4	2	—	1	0	—
queso manchego	1 oz	107	8	8	27	tr	0	341
queso panela	1 oz	74	6	5	—	1	0	—
raclette	1 oz	102	7	8	26	tr	0	217
reblochon	1 oz	88	6	7	23	tr	0	240
ricotta part skim	½ cup (4.4 oz)	171	14	10	38	6	—	155
ricotta part skim	1 cup (8.6 oz)	340	28	19	76	13	—	307

FOOD	PORTION	CALS	PROT	FAT	CHOL	CARB	FIBER	SOD
ricotta whole milk	½ cup (4.4 oz)	216	14	16	63	4	–	104
ricotta whole milk	1 cup (8.6 oz)	428	28	32	124	7	–	207
romadur 40% fat	1 oz	83	7	6	–	tr	–	–
romano	1 oz	110	9	8	29	1	–	340
roquefort	1 oz	105	6	9	26	1	–	513
rouy	1 oz	95	7	8	23	tr	0	138
saint marcellin	1 oz	94	5	8	23	tr	0	171
saint nectaire	1 oz	97	6	8	23	tr	0	169
saint paulin	1 oz	85	7	6	20	tr	0	174
sainte maure	1 oz	99	6	8	23	tr	0	411
selles sur cher	1 oz	93	5	8	20	tr	0	181
stilton blue	1.4 oz	164	9	14	–	0	0	–
stilton white	1.4 oz	145	8	13	–	0	0	–
swiss	1 oz	107	8	8	26	1	–	74
swiss cheese food	1 pkg (8 oz)	734	50	55	186	10	–	3523
swiss processed	1 oz	95	7	7	24	1	–	388
tilsit	1 oz	96	7	7	29	1	–	213
tome	1 oz	92	6	7	23	tr	0	231
triple creme	1 oz	113	3	11	34	tr	0	86
vacherin	1 oz	92	5	8	23	tr	0	129
wensleydale	1.4 oz	151	9	13	–	0	0	–
whey cheese	1 oz	126	4	8	–	9	0	146
yogurt cheese	1 oz	80	6	7	15	0	0	60
Alouette								
Garlic & Herbs	2 tbsp (0.8 oz)	70	1	7	30	1	0	135
Alpine Lace								
American Jalapeno Peppers	1 slice (1 oz)	80	6	6	20	2	0	260
American Less Fat Less Sodium White	1 slice (1 oz)	50	6	6	20	2	0	200
American Less Fat Less Sodium Yellow	1 slice (1 oz)	80	6	6	20	2	0	200
Cheddar Reduced Fat	1 slice (1 oz)	70	8	5	15	1	0	170

FOOD	PORTION	CALS	PROT	FAT	CHOL	CARB	FIBER	SOD
Colby Reduced Fat	1 slice (1 oz)	80	9	5	15	1	0	115
Fat Free Parmesan	2 tsp (5 g)	10	1	0	0	0	0	65
Feta Reduced Fat	1 oz	50	5	3	10	1	0	370
Feta Reduced Fat Sun Dried Tomato & Basil	1 oz	50	5	3	10	1	0	370
Goat Reduced Fat	1 oz	40	2	3	5	tr	0	130
Mozzarella Reduced Fat	1 oz	70	8	3	10	1	0	200
Muenster Reduced Sodium	1 slice (1 oz)	100	7	9	25	1	0	85
Provolone Smoked Reduced Fat	1 slice (1 oz)	70	9	5	15	1	0	120
Swiss Reduced Fat	1 slice (1 oz)	90	8	6	20	1	0	35
Athenos								
Feta	1 oz	80	5	6	20	tr	0	320
Boar's Head								
American	1 oz	100	6	9	25	1	0	380
Baby Swiss	1 oz	110	7	9	25	tr	0	135
Canadian Cheddar	1 oz	110	7	10	35	0	0	170
Double Glouster Yellow	1 oz	110	7	10	35	0	0	200
Feta	1 oz	60	5	4	10	1	0	370
Havarti	1 oz	110	6	10	35	0	0	210
Havarti w/ Dill	1 oz	110	6	10	35	0	0	210
Havarti w/ Jalapeno	1 oz	110	6	10	35	0	0	210
Lacey Swiss	1 oz	90	9	6	15	0	0	35
Longhorn Colby	1 oz	110	7	9	30	tr	0	170
Monterey Jack	1 oz	100	6	9	25	0	0	170
Monterey Jack w/ Jalapeno	1 oz	100	6	9	25	0	0	170
Mozzarella	1 oz	90	6	7	25	tr	0	140
Muenster	1 oz	100	6	8	25	0	0	180
Muenster Low Sodium	1 oz	100	6	8	20	0	0	75
Provolone Picante Sharp	1 oz	100	7	8	25	1	0	250

FOOD	PORTION	CALS	PROT	FAT	CHOL	CARB	FIBER	SOD
Swiss	1 oz	110	8	8	20	tr	0	65
Swiss No Salt Added	1 oz	110	8	8	25	tr	0	10
Bonbel								
Mini Babybel	1 piece (0.7 oz)	70	5	6	20	0	0	170
Borden								
Lite Line Sharp Cheddar	1 oz	50	–	2	–	–	–	–
Lite Line Swiss	1 oz	50	–	2	–	–	–	–
Boursin								
Garlic & Fine Herbs	2 tbsp	120	2	13	35	tr	–	180
Cabot								
American	1 slice (0.7 oz)	80	7	7	20	1	0	270
Cheddar	1 oz	110	7	9	30	tr	0	180
Cheddar Smoked	1 oz	110	7	9	30	tr	0	180
Cheddar Light 50% Reduced Fat	1 oz	70	8	5	15	1	0	170
Cheddar Light 50% Reduced Fat Jalapeno	1 oz	70	8	5	15	1	0	170
Cheddar Light 75% Reduced Fat	1 oz	60	9	3	10	tr	0	200
Colby Jack	1 oz	110	1	9	30	7	0	170
Fancy Blend Shredded	¼ cup	100	7	7	20	1	0	180
Monterey Jack	1 oz	110	7	9	30	tr	0	170
Mozzarella Shredded	¼ cup	80	8	6	15	1	0	170
Pepper Jack	1 oz	110	7	9	30	tr	0	170
Swiss Slices	1 slice (1 oz)	110	9	8	30	1	0	60
Cedar Grove								
Marble Colby	1 oz	110	7	9	30	0	0	185
Organic Tomato Basil Cheddar	1 oz	110	7	9	30	0	0	185
Chavrie								
Goat's Milk	2 tbsp	50	3	4	20	1	0	120
Connoisseur								
Asiago Spread	1 tbsp	90	5	7	20	2	0	240

FOOD	PORTION	CALS	PROT	FAT	CHOL	CARB	FIBER	SOD
Cracker Barrel								
Sharp Cheddar 2% Milk	1 oz	90	7	6	20	tr	0	240
Finlandia								
Muenster	1 slice (1.1 oz)	120	8	10	30	tr	0	200
Fleurs De France								
Brie	3.5 oz	311	21	25	—	tr	tr	200
Hollow Road Farms								
Sheep's Milk	1 oz	45	3	3	15	1	—	65
Land O Lakes								
American	1 slice (0.7 oz)	80	4	6	20	1	0	320
American Jalapeno	1 slice (0.6 oz)	70	3	6	15	1	0	320
American Light	1 oz	70	7	5	20	2	0	400
American Reduced Salt	1 oz	110	6	9	30	tr	0	270
American Sharp	2 slices (1 oz)	100	5	9	30	1	0	420
American & Swiss	1 slice (0.6 oz)	70	4	5	15	1	0	310
Baby Swiss	1 oz	110	6	9	25	0	0	125
Chedarella	1 oz	100	7	8	25	0	0	200
Cheddar	1 oz	100	6	9	30	tr	0	180
Cheddar Extra Sharp	1 oz	110	6	8	30	tr	0	360
Cheddar Sharp	1 oz	110	7	9	30	tr	0	180
Cheese Spread Golden Velvet	1 oz	80	5	6	20	2	0	370
Colby	1 oz	110	7	9	30	tr	0	180
Jalapeno Light	1 oz	70	7	4	15	1	0	400
Monterey Jack	1 oz	110	6	8	30	tr	0	170
Monterey Jack Hot Pepper	1 oz	110	6	8	30	tr	0	140
Mozzarella	1 oz	80	7	6	15	tr	0	190
Muenster	1 oz	100	6	8	25	0	0	220
Parmesan Grated	1 tbsp	35	3	4	10	0	0	95
Provolone	1 oz	100	7	8	20	tr	0	240

FOOD	PORTION	CALS	PROT	FAT	CHOL	CARB	FIBER	SOD
Swiss	1 oz	110	8	8	25	tr	0	75
Swiss Light	1 oz	80	9	4	15	tr	0	60
Northfield								
Naturally Slender	1 oz	90	–	7	10	–	–	–
Polly-O								
Ricotta Lite	¼ cup	70	8	3	10	3	0	80
String-Ums	1 stick (1 oz)	80	7	6	20	tr	0	220
President								
Feta	1 inch cube (1 oz)	90	5	7	15	2	0	410
Rouge Et Noir								
Breakfast	1 oz	86	5	7	–	1	–	–
Brie	1 oz	86	5	7	–	1	–	–
Camembert	1 oz	86	5	7	–	1	–	–
Schloss	1 oz	86	5	7	–	1	–	–
Sargento								
Blue Crumbled	¼ cup (1 oz)	100	6	8	20	1	0	380
Cheddar Extra Sharp	1 oz	110	7	9	30	1	0	180
Cheddar Shredded	¼ cup (1 oz)	110	6	9	30	1	0	160
Cheese For Nachos & Tacos Shredded	¼ cup (1 oz)	110	6	9	25	1	0	240
Cheese For Pizza Shredded	¼ cup (1 oz)	90	7	6	20	0	0	210
Cheese For Tacos Shredded	¼ cup (1 oz)	110	6	9	25	1	0	220
Colby	1 slice (1 oz)	110	6	9	30	0	0	190
Colby-Jack Shredded	¼ cup (1 oz)	110	6	9	25	tr	0	190
Jarlsberg	1 slice (1.2 oz)	120	9	9	20	1	0	160
Monterey Jack	1 slice (1 oz)	100	6	9	30	0	0	190
Monterey Jack Shredded	¼ cup (1 oz)	100	6	9	30	0	0	190
MooTown Snackers Cheddar	1 piece (0.8 oz)	100	5	8	25	1	0	130
MooTown Snackers Cheddar Mild Light	1 piece (0.8 oz)	60	7	4	10	tr	0	170
MooTown Snackers Cheese & Pretzels	1 pkg (0.9 oz)	90	3	3	10	12	0	320

FOOD	PORTION	CALS	PROT	FAT	CHOL	CARB	FIBER	SOD
MooTown Snackers Colby-Jack	1 piece (0.8 oz)	90	5	8	20	tr	0	160
MooTown Snackers Pizza Cheese & Sticks	1 pkg (1 oz)	100	3	4	10	13	0	260
MooTown Snackers String Light	1 piece (0.8 oz)	60	7	3	10	tr	0	200
Mozzarella	1 slice (1.5 oz)	130	11	9	25	2	0	230
Mozzarella Shredded	¼ cup (1 oz)	80	7	6	15	1	0	150
Muenster	1 slice (1 oz)	100	6	9	25	tr	0	200
Parmesan Grated	1 tbsp (5 g)	25	2	2	<5	0	0	75
Parmesan Shredded	¼ cup (1 oz)	110	9	7	25	1	0	300
Parmesan & Romano Shredded	¼ cup (1 oz)	110	9	7	25	1	0	340
Parmesan & Romano Grated	1 tbsp (5 g)	25	2	2	<5	0	0	70
Pizza Double Cheese Shredded	¼ cup (1 oz)	90	7	6	20	1	0	150
Preferred Light Cheddar Mild Shredded	¼ cup (1 oz)	70	8	5	10	tr	0	200
Preferred Light Mozzarella	1 slice (1.5 oz)	90	11	5	15	0	0	230
Preferred Light Mozzarella Shredded	¼ cup (1 oz)	70	8	3	10	tr	0	140
Preferred Light Swiss	1 slice (1 oz)	80	9	4	15	tr	0	50
Provolone	1 slice (1 oz)	100	7	8	25	0	0	190
Recipe Blend 4 Cheese Mexican Shredded	¼ cup (1 oz)	110	6	9	25	tr	0	200
Recipe Blend 6 Cheese Italian Shredded	¼ cup (1 oz)	90	7	7	20	0	0	180
Reduced Fat 4 Cheese Mexican Shredded	¼ cup (1 oz)	80	8	6	20	tr	0	200

FOOD	PORTION	CALS	PROT	FAT	CHOL	CARB	FIBER	SOD
Ricotta Light	¼ cup (2.2 oz)	60	5	3	15	3	0	55
Ricotta Old Fashioned	¼ cup (2.2 oz)	90	7	6	25	3	0	75
Ricotta Part-Skim	¼ cup (2.2 oz)	80	7	5	20	2	0	75
String	1 piece (0.8 oz)	70	6	5	15	tr	0	200
Swiss	1 slice (0.7 oz)	80	6	6	20	0	0	30
Swiss Shredded	¼ cup (1 oz)	110	8	8	30	0	0	40
Swiss Wafer Thin	2 slices (1 oz)	110	5	9	25	0	0	40
Sorrento								
Mozzarella Part Skim Jalapeno	1 oz	80	8	5	15	1	0	180
Mozzarella w/ Tomato & Basil Shredded	¼ cup	80	8	5	15	1	0	180
Pizza Cheese Shredded	¼ cup	90	7	7	20	1	0	200
Stringsters	1 stick (1 oz)	80	8	5	15	1	0	170
Suisse Delicat								
Healthy Swiss	1 oz	90	9	6	25	0	0	82
Tree Of Life								
Cheddar 33% Reduced Fat Organic Milk	1 oz	90	8	6	15	1	—	135
Colby	1 oz	110	7	9	30	1	—	170
Colby Organic Milk	1 oz	120	7	10	30	1	—	190
Farmer Part Skim Organic Milk	1 oz	90	7	6	15	1	—	110
Jalapeno Organic Milk	1 oz	110	6	9	20	1	—	190
Monterey Jack 35% Reduced Fat Organic Milk	1 oz	80	8	5	15	1	—	190
Monterey Jack Organic Milk	1 oz	100	6	8	20	1	—	185

FOOD	PORTION	CALS	PROT	FAT	CHOL	CARB	FIBER	SOD
Mozzarella Organic Milk	1 oz	80	8	5	16	1	—	170
Muenster Organic Milk	1 oz	100	6	8	25	1	—	185
Provolone	1 oz	100	7	8	20	1	—	250
Wholesome Valley								
Organic American Reduced Fat	1 slice (0.7 oz)	50	4	3	10	2	0	290

CHEESE DISHES
FROZEN
Banquet

FOOD	PORTION	CALS	PROT	FAT	CHOL	CARB	FIBER	SOD
Mozzeralla Nuggets	6	260	9	18	40	19	1	1060
Fillo Factory								
Tyropita Cheese Fillo Appetizers	5 (5 oz)	340	14	12	30	44	2	480
Health Is Wealth								
Mozzarella Stick	2 (1.3 oz)	120	5	5	15	14	0	250
TAKE-OUT								
fondue	½ cup (3.8 oz)	247	15	15	49	4	—	142
fried mozzarella sticks	9	840	—	—	—	—	—	—
souffle	1 serv (7 oz)	504	23	38	370	18	1	848
welsh rarebit	1 slice	228	8	16	—	14	1	—

CHEESE SUBSTITUTES

FOOD	PORTION	CALS	PROT	FAT	CHOL	CARB	FIBER	SOD
mozzarella	1 oz	70	3	3	0	7	—	194
Sargento								
Cheddar Shredded	¼ cup (1 oz)	90	5	7	0	2	0	420
Mozzarella Shredded	¼ cup (1 oz)	80	6	6	0	tr	0	320
Yves								
Good Slice American	1 slice (0.7 oz)	35	4	2	0	0	0	290
Good Slice Cheddar	1 slice (0.7 oz)	35	4	2	0	1	1	280
Good Slice Jalapeno Jack	1 slice (0.7 oz)	35	4	2	0	0	0	250

FOOD	PORTION	CALS	PROT	FAT	CHOL	CARB	FIBER	SOD
Good Slice Mozzarella	1 slice (0.7 oz)	30	4	2	0	0	0	270
Good Slice Swiss	1 slice (0.7 oz)	35	4	2	0	1	0	260

CHERIMOYA

FOOD	PORTION	CALS	PROT	FAT	CHOL	CARB	FIBER	SOD
fresh	1	515	7	2	0	131	—	—

CHERRIES
CANNED

FOOD	PORTION	CALS	PROT	FAT	CHOL	CARB	FIBER	SOD
sour in heavy syrup	½ cup	232	2	tr	0	60	—	18
sour in light syrup	½ cup	189	2	tr	0	49	—	18
sour water packed	1 cup	87	2	tr	0	22	—	17
sweet in heavy syrup	½ cup	107	1	tr	0	27	—	3
sweet in light syrup	½ cup	85	1	tr	0	22	—	3
sweet juice pack	½ cup	68	1	tr	0	17	—	3
sweet water pack	½ cup	57	1	tr	0	15	—	2
Del Monte								
Dark Pitted In Heavy Syrup	½ cup (4.2 oz)	100	1	0	0	24	1	10
DRIED								
bing unsulfured	¼ cup	130	0	0	0	31	2	10
montmorency tart pitted	⅓ cup	160	2	1	0	36	2	0
rainier unsulfured	⅓ cup	140	1	1	0	32	2	0
yogurt covered	¼ cup	170	1	6	0	29	5	20
FRESH								
sour	1 cup	51	1	tr	0	13	—	3
sweet	10	49	1	1	0	11	—	0
Chiquita								
Cherries	21	90	2	1	0	22	9	0
Super Cherry								
Rainier	21	90	1	0	0	19	3	0
FROZEN								
dark sweet unsweetened	1 cup	110	1	1	0	25	3	0
sour unsweetened	1 cup	72	1	1	0	17	—	1
sweet sweetened	1 cup	232	3	tr	0	58	—	3

FOOD	PORTION	CALS	PROT	FAT	CHOL	CARB	FIBER	SOD
CHERRY JUICE								
Eden								
Montmorency Juice	8 oz	140	1	1	0	33	0	30
Juicy Juice								
Drink	1 box (4.23 oz)	70	0	0	0	17	0	10
Drink	1 box (8.5 oz)	140	0	0	0	34	0	15
Mott's								
Cherry	1 box (8 oz)	120	0	0	0	31	—	15
Ocean Spray								
Black Cherry	8 oz	140	0	0	0	33	0	35
CHERVIL								
seed	1 tsp	1	tr	tr	0	tr	—	tr
CHESTNUTS								
chinese cooked	1 oz	44	1	tr	0	10	—	1
chinese dried	1 oz	103	2	tr	0	23	—	2
chinese raw	1 oz	64	1	tr	0	14	—	1
chinese roasted	1 oz	68	1	tr	0	15	—	1
cooked	1 oz	37	1	tr	0	8	—	8
creme de marrons	1 oz	73	1	tr	0	18	1	1
dried peeled	1 oz	105	1	1	0	22	—	11
japanese cooked	1 oz	16	tr	tr	0	4	—	1
japanese dried	1 oz	102	1	tr	0	23	—	10
japanese raw	1 oz	44	1	tr	0	10	—	4
japanese roasted	1 oz	57	1	tr	0	13	—	—
raw peeled	1 oz	56	tr	tr	0	13	—	1
roasted	1 cup	350	5	3	0	76	—	3
roasted	2–3 (1 oz)	70	1	1	0	15	—	1
CHEWING GUM								
bubble gum	1 block (8 g)	27	0	0	0	8	—	0
stick	1 (3 g)	10	0	0	0	3	—	0
Aquafresh								
Peppermint	2 pieces	5	0	0	0	2	—	0

FOOD	PORTION	CALS	PROT	FAT	CHOL	CARB	FIBER	SOD
Arm & Hammer								
Dental Care Spearmint or Peppermint	2 pieces (2.5 g)	5	0	0	0	2	–	30
CareFree								
Koolerz Lemonaide	1 piece	5	0	0	0	2	0	0
Dentyne								
Ice Peppermint	2 pieces (3 g)	5	0	0	0	2	–	0
Doublemint								
Chewing Gum	1 piece	10	tr	tr	0	2	–	0
Eclipse								
Spearmint	2 pieces	5	0	0	0	2	–	0
Extra Sugar Free								
Cinnamon	1 piece	8	tr	tr	0	tr	–	0
Winter Fresh	1 piece	8	tr	tr	0	tr	–	0
Glee Gum								
Peppermint	2 pieces (2.5 g)	5	0	0	0	2	–	0
Hubba Bubba								
Bubble Gum Cola	1 piece	23	tr	tr	0	6	–	0
Bubble Gum Sugarfree Grape	1 piece	13	tr	tr	0	tr	–	0
Bubble Gum Sugarfree Original	1 piece	14	tr	tr	0	tr	–	0
Original	1 piece	23	tr	tr	0	6	–	0
Strawberry Grape Raspberry	1 piece	23	tr	tr	0	6	–	0
Speakeasy								
Natural Rainforest All Flavors	2 pieces	10	5	0	0	2	–	5
Wrigley's								
Orbit	1 piece	5	0	0	0	1	–	0
Spearmint	1 stick	10	tr	tr	0	2	–	0
Xylichew								
Licorice	2 pieces	4	0	0	0	2	0	0
CHIA SEEDS								
dried	1 oz	134	5	7	0	14	–	–

FOOD	PORTION	CALS	PROT	FAT	CHOL	CARB	FIBER	SOD

CHICKEN *(see also* CHICKEN DISHES, CHICKEN SUBSTITUTES, DINNER, HOT DOGS*)*

CANNED

FOOD	PORTION	CALS	PROT	FAT	CHOL	CARB	FIBER	SOD
chicken spread	1 tbsp	25	2	2	–	1	–	–
chicken spread	1 oz	55	4	3	–	2	–	–
chicken spread barbeque flavored	1 oz	55	4	3	–	2	–	–
w/ broth	1 can (5 oz)	234	31	11	–	0	–	714
w/ broth	½ can (2.5 oz)	117	15	6	–	0	–	357

FRESH

FOOD	PORTION	CALS	PROT	FAT	CHOL	CARB	FIBER	SOD
broiler/fryer breast w/ skin batter dipped & fried	2.9 oz	218	21	11	72	8	–	231
broiler/fryer breast w/ skin batter dipped & fried	½ breast (4.9 oz)	364	35	18	119	13	–	385
broiler/fryer breast w/ skin roasted	2 oz	115	17	5	49	0	–	41
broiler/fryer breast w/ skin roasted	½ breast (3.4 oz)	193	29	8	83	0	–	69
broiler/fryer breast w/ skin stewed	½ breast (3.9 oz)	202	30	8	83	0	–	68
broiler/fryer breast w/o skin fried	½ breast (3 oz)	161	29	4	78	tr	–	68
broiler/fryer breast w/o skin roasted	½ breast (3 oz)	142	27	3	73	0	–	63
broiler/fryer breast w/o skin stewed	2 oz	86	17	2	44	0	–	36
broiler/fryer drumstick w/ skin batter dipped & fried	1 (2.6 oz)	193	16	11	62	6	–	194
broiler/fryer drumstick w/ skin floured & fried	1 (1.7 oz)	120	13	7	44	1	–	44
broiler/fryer drumstick w/ skin roasted	1 (1.8 oz)	112	14	6	48	0	–	47

FOOD	PORTION	CALS	PROT	FAT	CHOL	CARB	FIBER	SOD
broiler/fryer drumstick w/ skin stewed	1 (2 oz)	116	14	6	48	0	—	43
broiler/fryer drumstick w/o skin fried	1 (1.5 oz)	82	12	3	40	0	—	40
broiler/fryer drumstick w/o skin roasted	1 (1.5 oz)	76	12	2	41	0	—	42
broiler/fryer drumstick w/o skin stewed	1 (1.6 oz)	78	13	3	40	0	—	37
broiler/fryer leg w/ skin batter dipped & fried	1 (5.5 oz)	431	34	26	142	14	—	442
broiler/fryer leg w/ skin floured & fried	1 (3.9 oz)	285	30	16	105	3	—	99
broiler/fryer leg w/ skin roasted	1 (4 oz)	265	30	15	105	0	—	99
broiler/fryer leg w/ skin stewed	1 (4.4 oz)	275	30	16	105	0	—	92
broiler/fryer leg w/o skin fried	1 (3.3 oz)	195	27	9	93	1	—	90
broiler/fryer leg w/o skin roasted	1 (3.3 oz)	182	26	8	89	0	—	87
broiler/fryer leg w/o skin stewed	1 (3.5 oz)	187	26	8	90	0	—	78
broiler/fryer neck w/ skin stewed	1 (1.3 oz)	94	7	7	27	0	—	20
broiler/fryer neck w/o skin stewed	1 (.6 oz)	32	4	1	14	0	—	12
broiler/fryer skin batter dipped & fried	from ½ chicken (6.7 oz)	748	20	55	140	44	—	1105
broiler/fryer skin floured & fried	from ½ chicken (2 oz)	281	24	24	41	5	—	30
broiler/fryer skin roasted	from ½ chicken (2 oz)	254	11	23	46	0	—	36

FOOD	PORTION	CALS	PROT	FAT	CHOL	CARB	FIBER	SOD
broiler/fryer skin stewed	from ½ chicken (2.5 oz)	261	11	24	45	0	–	40
broiler/fryer thigh w/ skin batter dipped & fried	1 (3 oz)	238	19	14	80	8	–	248
broiler/fryer thigh w/ skin floured & fried	1 (2.2 oz)	162	17	9	60	2	–	55
broiler/fryer thigh w/ skin roasted	1 (2.2 oz)	153	16	10	58	0	–	52
broiler/fryer thigh w/ skin stewed	1 (2.4 oz)	158	16	10	57	0	–	49
broiler/fryer thigh w/o skin fried	1 (1.8 oz)	113	15	5	53	1	–	49
broiler/fryer thigh w/o skin roasted	1 (1.8 oz)	109	13	6	49	0	–	46
broiler/fryer thigh w/o skin stewed	1 (1.9 oz)	107	14	5	49	0	–	41
broiler/fryer w/skin floured & fried	½ chicken (11 oz)	844	90	47	283	10	–	264
broiler/fryer w/ skin fried	½ chicken (16.4 oz)	1347	81	81	404	44	–	1360
broiler/fryer w/ skin roasted	½ chicken (10.5 oz)	715	82	41	263	0	–	244
broiler/fryer w/ skin stewed	½ chicken (11.7 oz)	730	82	42	262	0	–	224
broiler/fryer w/ skin neck & giblets batter dipped & fried	1 chicken (2.3 lbs)	2987	235	180	1054	93	–	2921
broiler/fryer w/ skin neck & giblets roasted	1 chicken (1.5 lbs)	1598	183	90	730	tr	–	536
broiler/fryer w/ skin neck & giblets stewed	1 chicken (1.6 lbs)	1625	184	93	726	tr	–	494
broiler/fryer w/o skin fried	1 cup	307	43	13	131	2	–	127

FOOD	PORTION	CALS	PROT	FAT	CHOL	CARB	FIBER	SOD
broiler/fryer w/o skin roasted	1 cup (5 oz)	266	41	10	125	0	–	120
broiler/fryer w/o skin stewed	1 oz	54	7	3	22	0	–	18
broiler/fryer w/o skin stewed	1 cup (5 oz)	248	38	9	116	0	–	98
broiler/fryer wing w/ skin batter dipped & fried	1 (1.7 oz)	159	10	11	39	5	–	157
broiler/fryer wing w/ skin floured & fried	1 (1.1 oz)	103	8	7	26	1	–	25
broiler/fryer wing w/ skin roasted	1 (1.2 oz)	99	9	7	29	0	–	28
broiler/fryer wing w/ skin stewed	1 (1.4 oz)	100	9	7	28	0	–	27
capon w/ skin neck & giblets roasted	1 chicken (3.1 lbs)	3211	402	165	1458	1	–	704
cornish hen w/ skin roasted	1 hen (8 oz)	595	51	42	299	0	–	146
cornish hen w/o skin & bone roasted	1 hen (3.8 oz)	144	25	4	113	0	–	67
cornish hen w/o skin & bone roasted	½ hen (2 oz)	72	13	2	57	0	–	34
cornish hen w/skin roasted	½ hen (4 oz)	296	25	21	149	0	–	73
roaster dark meat w/o skin roasted	1 cup (5 oz)	250	33	12	104	0	–	133
roaster light meat w/o skin roasted	1 cup (5 oz)	214	38	6	105	0	–	71
roaster w/ skin neck & giblets roasted	1 chicken (2.4 lbs)	2363	257	140	1003	1	–	760
roaster w/ skin roasted	½ chicken (1.1 lbs)	1071	115	64	365	0	–	349
roaster w/o skin skin roasted	1 cup (5 oz)	469	9	28	160	0	–	105

FOOD	PORTION	CALS	PROT	FAT	CHOL	CARB	FIBER	SOD
stewing dark meat w/o skin stewed	1 cup (5 oz)	361	39	21	132	0	—	133
stewing w/ skin neck & giblets stewed	1 chicken (1.3 lbs)	1636	157	107	603	tr	—	419
stewing w/ skin stewed	½ chicken (9.2 oz)	744	70	49	205	0	—	190
stewing w/ skin stewed	6.2 oz	507	34	34	140	0	—	130
Amish Select								
Boneless Skinless Breast w/ Honey Dijon Mustard	1 serv (4 oz)	130	24	2	60	4	0	390
Murray's								
Breast Boneless & Skinless	4 oz	110	26	1	70	0	0	50
Ground	3 oz	130	17	7	90	0	0	55
Whole Lean	4 oz	170	21	9	90	0	0	75
Perdue								
Boneless Skinless Breasts Cooked	3 oz	110	25	2	70	0	—	30
Boneless Breast Roasted Garlic Herb	1 piece (3 oz)	90	18	1	50	3	—	620
Breaded Breast Strips Barbecue	3 oz	120	12	1	30	16	—	720
Breaded Breast Strips Hot & Spicy	3 oz	110	12	1	30	13	—	930
Breaded Breast Strips Original	3 oz	120	14	1	35	14	—	750
Burger Cooked	1 (3 oz)	160	17	10	110	0	—	55
Chicken Breast Seasoned Italian Cooked	1 piece (3 oz)	90	18	1	50	3	—	610
Chicken Breast Seasoned Teriyaki Cooked	1 piece (3 oz)	90	18	1	50	3	—	560
Ground Cooked	3 oz	170	18	11	125	0	—	50

FOOD	PORTION	CALS	PROT	FAT	CHOL	CARB	FIBER	SOD
Ground Breast Cooked	3 oz	80	19	1	55	0	—	60
Honey Rotisserie Dark Meat	3 oz	200	12	16	80	1	—	300
Honey Rotisserie White Meat	3 oz	140	19	8	70	1	—	290
Oven Stuffer Dark Meat Roasted	3 oz	210	18	15	100	0	—	60
Oven Stuffer Drumstick Roasted	1 (3.6 oz)	190	22	11	120	0	—	100
Oven Stuffer White Meat Roasted	3 oz	170	21	9	80	0	—	50
Oven Stuffer Wingette Roasted	3 (3.4 oz)	220	21	15	120	0	—	80
Ovenables Breast Lemon Pepper Cooked	1 piece (3 oz)	90	18	1	50	2	—	380
Seasoned Roasting Chicken Toasted Garlic Dark Meat	3 oz	190	16	14	100	1	—	330
Seasoned Roasting Chicken Toasted Garlic White Meat	3 oz	160	19	9	75	1	—	320
Seasoned Strips Parmesan Garlic cooked	3 oz	100	20	2	55	2	—	710
Seasoned Strips Savory Classic cooked	3 oz	90	19	1	55	1	—	500
Seasoned Strips Spicy Fiesta cooked	3 oz	140	16	7	75	3	—	630
Split Breast Cooked	1 piece (6.8 oz)	370	48	20	180	0	—	100
Thin Sliced Breast Rosemary Garlic Thyme	1 piece (3 oz)	90	20	2	60	1	—	820
Thin Sliced Breast Tomato Herb	1 piece (3 oz)	90	20	2	60	1	—	740

FOOD	PORTION	CALS	PROT	FAT	CHOL	CARB	FIBER	SOD
Whole Dark Meat cooked	3 oz	150	17	16	110	0	—	55
Whole White Meat Cooked	3 oz	170	21	10	85	0	0	45
Wings Roasted	2 (3.2 oz)	210	19	15	115	0	—	75
Wampler								
Breast Tenders	4 oz	130	27	2	70	0	—	55
FROZEN								
Banquet								
Breast Nuggets	7	280	13	20	40	11	1	500
Breast Patties Grilled Honey BBQ	1	110	13	5	40	3	0	440
Breast Patties Grilled Honey Mustard	1	120	13	5	25	5	0	500
Breast Tenders Our Original	3	250	12	15	40	15	tr	480
Breast Tenders Southern	3 pieces	260	12	16	40	16	1	460
Country Fried	1 serv (3 oz)	270	14	18	65	13	1	620
Fat Free Baked Breast Patties	1	100	9	0	20	15	1	400
Fried Our Original	1 serv (3 oz)	280	14	18	65	15	1	830
Honey BBQ Skinless Fried	1 serv (3 oz)	230	18	13	55	9	1	480
Hot 'n Spicy Fried	1 serv (3 oz)	260	14	18	65	13	1	730
Nuggets Our Original	6	270	14	19	35	12	1	540
Nuggets Southern Fried	5	270	12	18	35	16	2	570
Patties Our Original	1	190	7	14	30	10	1	440
Patties Southern Fried	1	190	8	12	25	10	tr	430
Skinless Fried	1 serv (3 oz)	220	18	13	65	7	2	480
Smokehouse Big Wings	2	200	14	17	70	4	0	300

FOOD	PORTION	CALS	PROT	FAT	CHOL	CARB	FIBER	SOD
Southern Fried	1 serv (3 oz)	280	14	18	65	15	1	700
Wings Firehouse Big	2	190	14	14	70	1	0	650
Wings Honey BBQ	4	380	31	24	70	15	1	570
Wings Hot & Spicy	4 pieces	280	18	20	90	9	tr	450
Bell & Evans								
Breaded Breast Nuggets	1 serv (4 oz)	190	20	6	45	13	1	440
Breaded Whole Breast Tenders	1 (4 oz)	190	20	6	45	13	1	440
Burgers	1 (3 oz)	120	16	6	85	tr	0	130
Chicken Sandwich Steaks	1 serv (2 oz)	60	14	1	40	tr	0	25
Country Skillet								
Bites	5	270	12	16	20	18	1	720
Breast Tenders	3	240	11	14	25	16	1	450
Chunks	5	270	12	18	20	18	1	720
Fried	3 oz	270	14	18	65	13	1	620
Nuggets	10	280	14	17	25	16	1	610
Patties	1	190	9	12	20	12	1	490
Southern Fried Chunks	5	270	11	18	20	17	1	550
Southern Fried Patties	1	190	9	12	20	12	1	440
Health Is Wealth								
Nuggets	4 (3 oz)	150	14	6	40	9	0	180
Patties	1 (3 oz)	150	13	6	40	9	0	180
Tenders	3 (3 oz)	130	14	3	35	11	0	230
Kid Cuisine								
Dino Mite Nuggets	4 pieces	300	11	23	40	10	1	540
Radical Racin' Nuggets w/ Cheese	4 pieces	300	11	23	35	12	tr	620
Weaver								
Breast Strips	3 pieces (3.3 oz)	210	14	11	35	13	2	430
Breast Tenders	5 pieces (3 oz)	220	14	15	35	8	1	290
Croquettes	1 serv (3.5 oz)	290	11	18	45	22	2	540

FOOD	PORTION	CALS	PROT	FAT	CHOL	CARB	FIBER	SOD
Dutch Frye Nuggets	5 pieces (3.3 oz)	280	14	20	45	12	2	410
Honey Battered Tenders	5 pieces (2.9 oz)	230	12	15	35	12	1	380
Hot Wings Buffalo Style	3 pieces (2.7 oz)	190	18	13	95	0	0	370
Mini Drums Crispy	5 pieces (3.3 oz)	250	14	16	40	14	1	410
Nuggets	4 pieces (2.7 oz)	210	11	15	35	9	1	360
Patties	1 (2.6 oz)	180	10	11	30	10	1	430
Rondelet	1 (2.6 oz)	170	10	10	20	10	1	410
Rondelet Dutch Frye	1 (2.6 oz)	230	11	16	35	10	1	360
Rondelet Italian	1 (2.6 oz)	210	10	14	20	12	1	470
READY-TO-EAT								
chicken roll light meat	2 oz	90	11	4	28	1	—	331
chicken roll light meat	1 pkg (6 oz)	271	33	13	85	4	—	992
poultry salad sandwich spread	1 oz	238	3	4	9	2	—	107
poultry salad sandwich spread	1 tbsp (13 g)	109	2	2	4	1	—	49
Banquet								
Fat Free Baked Breast Tenders	3	120	13	0	30	16	2	480
Boar's Head								
Breast Hickory Smoked	2 oz	60	11	1	30	tr	0	440
Breast Oven Roasted	2 oz	50	11	1	30	tr	0	420
Breast Bar B Q Sauce Basted	2 oz	60	11	1	30	3	0	490
Butterball								
Crispy Baked Breasts Italian Style Herb	1 piece (0.5 oz)	190	17	6	55	16	1	710

FOOD	PORTION	CALS	PROT	FAT	CHOL	CARB	FIBER	SOD
Crispy Baked Breasts Lemon Pepper	1 piece (0.5 oz)	200	16	7	50	16	tr	420
Crispy Baked Breasts Original	1 piece (0.5 oz)	180	16	6	45	16	1	500
Crispy Baked Breasts Parmesan	1 piece (0.5 oz)	200	17	7	55	16	tr	650
Crispy Baked Breasts Southwestern	1 piece (0.5 oz)	170	17	6	35	13	2	590
Tenders Baked Breast	3 pieces	170	14	6	35	15	1	410
Tenders Hickory Smoked Grilled	4 pieces + sauce	160	17	5	50	12	1	570
Tenders Oriental Grilled	4 pieces + sauce	160	17	5	45	12	1	560
Carl Buddig								
Chicken Sliced	1 pkg (2.5 oz)	110	12	7	40	1	—	680
Lean Slices Honey Smoked Breast	1 pkg (2.5 oz)	70	12	1	30	3	—	630
Lean Slices Roasted Breast	1 pkg (2.5 oz)	60	13	1	30	1	—	630
Hillshire Farm								
Smoked Breast	6 slices (2 oz)	60	11	1	25	2	0	600
Perdue								
Breast Cutlets Homestyle	1 (2.9 oz)	110	14	1	35	12	—	730
Breast Cutlets Italian Style	1 (2.9 oz)	120	15	2	40	11	—	690
Breast Filets In Barbecue Sauce	1 piece + 3 tbsp sauce (5.9 oz)	200	24	1	70	24	—	1100
Breast Strips In Garlic & Herb Sauce	1 serv (5 oz)	100	18	1	50	4	2	1010
Breast Strips In Marinara Sauce	1 serv (5 oz)	120	18	3	50	5	—	1130
Breast Strips In Teriyaki Sauce	1 serv (5 oz)	190	20	1	50	26	—	1660

FOOD	PORTION	CALS	PROT	FAT	CHOL	CARB	FIBER	SOD
Carved Breast Honey Roasted	½ cup (2.5 oz)	100	18	2	45	2	—	450
Carved Breast Original Roasted	½ cup (2.5 oz)	90	19	2	50	1	—	500
Cutlets Cooked	1 (3.5 oz)	220	15	11	55	15	—	600
Nuggets	5 (3.4 oz)	210	15	11	50	15	—	580
Nuggets Chicken & Cheese	5 (3.4 oz)	230	15	13	55	15	—	670
Short Cuts Entrees In Teriyaki Sauce	5 oz	190	20	1	50	26	—	1660
Short Cuts Grilled Italian	½ cup	80	15	1	40	4	—	500
Short Cuts Lemon Pepper	½ cup (2.5 oz)	100	19	3	60	1	—	490
Short Cuts Southwestern	½ cup (2.5 oz)	100	18	3	60	1	—	410
Tyson								
Grilled Breast Strips	1 serv (3 oz)	120	21	4	60	1	0	500
Roasted Whole Chicken w/ Skin	1 serv (3 oz)	160	16	11	75	1	0	490
TAKE-OUT								
oven roasted breast of chicken	2 oz	60	11	1	25	0	—	470

CHICKEN DISHES
CANNED
Bumble Bee

FOOD	PORTION	CALS	PROT	FAT	CHOL	CARB	FIBER	SOD
Chicken Salad	1 pkg (3.5 oz)	230	10	10	25	25	0	540

MIX
Chicken Skillet Helper

FOOD	PORTION	CALS	PROT	FAT	CHOL	CARB	FIBER	SOD
Stir-Fried Chicken as prep	1 cup	270	18	9	105	30	1	760

REFRIGERATED

FOOD	PORTION	CALS	PROT	FAT	CHOL	CARB	FIBER	SOD
salad low fat	⅓ cup	90	8	2	20	9	—	440

Lloyd's

FOOD	PORTION	CALS	PROT	FAT	CHOL	CARB	FIBER	SOD
Barbecue Shredded Chicken	¼ cup (2 oz)	90	6	2	15	11	—	440

FOOD	PORTION	CALS	PROT	FAT	CHOL	CARB	FIBER	SOD
Old El Paso								
For Tacos Shredded Chicken	¼ cup	60	5	2	25	4	1	430
Oscar Mayer								
Lunchables Chicken Wraps	1 pkg	440	17	13	40	64	3	860
Tyson								
Chicken Breast Medallions In Tomato & Herb Sauce	1 serv (5 oz)	120	18	4	40	5	0	640
Wampler								
Cacciatore	1 cup	260	30	9	90	10	—	600
Fajitas	1 cup	210	23	7	70	13	—	1360
Salad	⅓ cup	200	9	14	30	9	—	420
Salad Lite	⅓ cup	130	9	7	25	9	—	370
Smokey Barbecue Chicken	1 cup	430	42	15	140	31	—	1020
Sweet-n-Sour	1 cup	250	20	4	55	35	—	510
SHELF-STABLE								
Lunch Bucket								
Chicken Fiesta	1 pkg (7.5 oz)	160	6	2	5	30	5	530
TastyBite								
Chicken Moglai	1 pkg (9.5 oz)	300	21	16	45	20	3	1080
TAKE-OUT								
boneless breaded & fried w/ barbecue sauce	6 pieces (4.6 oz)	330	17	18	61	25	—	830
boneless breaded & fried w/ honey	6 pieces (4 oz)	339	17	18	61	27	—	537
boneless breaded & fried w/ mustard sauce	6 pieces (4.6 oz)	323	17	17	62	21	—	791
boneless breaded & fried w/ sweet & sour sauce	6 pieces (4.6 oz)	346	17	18	61	29	—	791
boneless breast w/ apple stuffing	1 serv (5 oz)	260	32	9	80	10	1	250

FOOD	PORTION	CALS	PROT	FAT	CHOL	CARB	FIBER	SOD
breast & wing breaded & fried	2 pieces (5.7 oz)	494	36	30	149	20	–	975
b'stilla chicken pie	1 serv	926	–	227	64	–	–	1242
chicken & dumplings	¾ cup	256	23	12	109	12	tr	1283
chicken & noodles	1 cup	365	22	18	103	26	–	600
chicken a la king	1 cup	470	27	34	221	12	–	760
chicken cacciatore	¾ cup	394	33	24	99	9	2	671
chicken paprikash	1½ cups	296	–	10	90	–	–	–
chicken pie w/ top crust	1 slice (5.6 oz)	472	19	31	–	32	1	–
chicken cordon bleu	1 serv (5 oz)	280	29	13	70	10	0	800
drumstick breaded & fried	2 pieces (5.2 oz)	430	30	27	165	16	–	756
grilled breast strips	4 strips (3 oz)	100	20	2	50	0	0	310
groundnut stew hkatenkwan	1 serv (15.7 oz)	576	38	40	116	18	4	1009
jamaican jerk wings	4 wings (9.9 oz)	709	57	51	172	3	tr	1045
kobete turkish chicken w/ pastry	1 serv	513	–	13	71	–	–	551
sancocho de pollo dominican chicken stew	1 serv	702	71	30	195	34	1	653
souvlaki	1 serv	392	–	54	17	–	–	337
thigh breaded & fried	2 pieces (5.2 oz)	430	30	27	165	16	–	756

CHICKEN SUBSTITUTES
Health Is Wealth

FOOD	PORTION	CALS	PROT	FAT	CHOL	CARB	FIBER	SOD
Buffalo Wings	3 pieces (2.2 oz)	100	10	2	0	11	3	490
Chicken-Free Nuggets	3 pieces (2.25 oz)	90	10	1	0	11	2	330
Chicken-Free Patties	1 (3 oz)	120	14	2	0	15	2	440

FOOD	PORTION	CALS	PROT	FAT	CHOL	CARB	FIBER	SOD
Loma Linda								
Chicken Supreme Mix not prep	⅓ cup (0.9 oz)	90	15	1	0	6	4	720
Chik Nuggets	5 pieces (3 oz)	240	12	16	0	13	5	710
Fried Chik'n w/ Gravy	2 pieces (2.8 oz)	160	12	10	0	4	2	440
Morningstar Farms								
Chik Nuggets	4 pieces (3 oz)	160	13	4	0	17	5	670
Chik Patties	1 (2.5 oz)	150	9	6	0	15	2	570
Meatless Buffalo Wings	5 pieces (3 oz)	200	13	9	0	16	3	730
Quorn								
Cutlets	1 (3.5 oz)	200	10	8	0	20	4	610
Naked Cutlets	1 (2.4 oz)	80	11	3	5	5	2	420
Nuggets	3–4 pieces (3 oz)	180	8	8	0	18	3	650
Patties	1 patty (2.6 oz)	160	8	7	0	12	3	525
Tenders	1 cup (3 oz)	90	12	2	0	8	3	350
Worthington								
Chicken Sliced or Roll	2 slices (2 oz)	80	9	5	0	1	tr	370
Chic-Ketts	2 slices (1.9 oz)	120	13	7	0	2	2	390
ChikStiks	1 (1.6 oz)	110	9	7	0	3	2	360
CrispyChik Patties	1 (2.5 oz)	150	8	6	0	15	2	600
Cutlets	1 slice (2.1 oz)	70	11	1	0	3	2	340
Diced Chik	¼ cup (1.9 oz)	40	7	0	0	1	1	270
FriChik	2 pieces (3.2 oz)	120	10	8	0	1	1	430
FriChik Low Fat	2 pieces (3 oz)	80	10	3	0	2	1	430
Golden Croquettes	4 pieces (3 oz)	210	14	10	0	14	6	600
Yves								
Veggie Chicken Burgers	1 (3 oz)	120	17	3	0	6	3	390

FOOD	PORTION	CALS	PROT	FAT	CHOL	CARB	FIBER	SOD
CHICKPEAS								
CANNED								
chickpeas	1 cup	285	12	3	0	54	–	718
Progresso								
Chick Peas	½ cup (4.6 oz)	120	5	3	0	20	5	280
Garbanzo	½ cup (4.4 oz)	110	6	2	0	18	5	380
DRIED								
cooked	1 cup	269	15	4	0	45	–	11
CHICORY								
greens raw chopped	½ cup	21	2	tr	0	4	–	41
root raw	1 (2.1 oz)	44	1	tr	0	11	–	30
roots raw cut up	½ cup (1.6 oz)	33	1	tr	0	8	–	23
witloof head raw	1 (1.9 oz)	9	tr	tr	0	2	–	1
witloof raw	½ cup (1.6 oz)	8	tr	tr	0	2	–	1
CHILI								
chile pepper paste	1 tbsp	6	tr	1	–	1	1	1445
chili w/ beans	1 cup	286	15	14	43	30	–	1330
dried ancho	1 tsp	3	tr	tr	0	1	tr	0
dried casabel	1 tsp	3	tr	tr	0	1	tr	–
dried guajillo	1 tsp	3	tr	tr	0	1	tr	–
dried mulato	1 tsp	3	tr	tr	0	1	tr	–
dried pasilla	1 tsp	3	tr	tr	0	1	tr	1
dried smoked chipotle	1 tsp	3	tr	tr	0	1	tr	–
powder	1 tsp	8	tr	tr	0	1	–	26
Amy's								
Chili & Cornbread	1 pkg (10.5 oz)	320	11	6	10	59	8	680
Organic Black Bean	1 cup	200	11	2	0	31	15	680
Organic Medium	1 cup	190	8	6	0	26	7	590
Organic Medium w/ Vegetables	1 cup	190	7	6	0	29	8	590

FOOD	PORTION	CALS	PROT	FAT	CHOL	CARB	FIBER	SOD
Bush's								
Chili Beans Mild Sauce	½ cup	120	6	1	0	20	6	480
Original No Beans	1 cup	240	13	14	25	16	3	1380
Carroll Shelby's								
Original Texas Chili Kit	2 tbsp	60	2	1	0	12	0	1320
Chef Boyardee								
Chili Mac	½ can (7 oz)	260	10	11	30	30	3	1480
Chili Man								
Seasoning Mix	1 tbsp (7 g)	25	1	1	—	4	2	330
Del Monte								
Sauce	1 tbsp (0.6 oz)	20	0	0	0	5	0	480
Gebhardt								
Chili Powder	¼ tsp (0.3 g)	1	tr	tr	0	tr	tr	tr
Chili Quik Seasoning	1 tbsp (0.3 oz)	43	1	1	0	8	2	985
Plain	1 cup (9.4 oz)	232	7	19	0	11	3	737
With Beans	1 cup (9.4 oz)	322	15	15	29	32	15	673
Gringo Billy's								
Chili Mix	1 tbsp	24	0	1	0	2	2	319
Healthy Choice								
Bowls Chili & Cornbread	1 meal (9.5 oz)	350	21	8	35	49	8	600
Hunt's								
Chili Beans	½ cup (4.5 oz)	87	6	1	0	17	6	597
Family Favorites Chili Sauce	¼ cup	25	1	0	0	5	1	400
Instant India								
Chili Ginger Paste	2 tbsp (1 oz)	90	1	7	0	6	0	470
Just Rite								
With Beans	1 cup (9 oz)	379	18	27	35	31	13	51
Lean Cuisine								
Everyday Favorites Three Bean Chili w/ Rice	1 pkg (10 oz)	250	11	6	10	37	9	590

FOOD	PORTION	CALS	PROT	FAT	CHOL	CARB	FIBER	SOD
Manwich								
Homestyle Fixins	½ cup (4.6 oz)	84	6	1	0	19	6	858
Marie Callender's								
Chili & Cornbread	1 meal (16 oz)	560	27	21	60	67	7	2110
McCormick								
Mexican Style Chili Powder	¼ tsp	0	0	0	0	0	0	20
Original Chili Seasoning	1⅓ tbsp (9 g)	30	—	1	0	5	2	310
Natural Choice								
Organic Vegan Three Bean	½ cup (4.6 oz)	140	9	1	0	24	7	510
Natural Touch								
Vegetarian	1 cup (8.1 oz)	170	18	1	0	21	11	870
Nature's Entree								
Texas Chili	1 pkg (12 oz)	320	26	7	15	43	11	960
Open Range								
Plain	1 cup (8.8 oz)	353	18	26	48	19	6	1216
With Beans	1 cup (9 oz)	281	17	16	26	25	10	1291
Soy7								
Chili Mix as prep	1 cup	150	16	2	0	24	7	400
Ultimate								
No Beans Hot	1 cup (8.7 oz)	420	20	30	85	18	5	1420
Turkey w/ Beans	1 cup (8.7 oz)	260	17	9	50	28	9	930
W/ Beans	1 cup (8.7 oz)	320	18	16	50	25	9	920
W/ Beans Hot	1 cup (8.7 oz)	320	18	16	50	25	9	920
Van Camp								
Beanee Weenee Chilee	1 cup (7.7 oz)	240	14	12	35	27	9	1090
Chili With Beans	1 cup (8.9 oz)	350	19	21	45	28	7	1020

FOOD	PORTION	CALS	PROT	FAT	CHOL	CARB	FIBER	SOD
Mexican Style Chili Beans	½ cup (4.6 oz)	110	7	2	0	21	8	430
Wampler								
Turkey	1 cup	250	23	7	75	22	—	1840
Wick Fowler's								
2 Alarm Chili Kit	3 tbsp	60	2	2	0	10	0	980
False Alarm Chili Kit	2 tbsp	50	2	2	0	9	0	980
Worthington								
Chili	1 cup (8.1 oz)	290	19	15	0	21	9	1130
Low Fat	1 cup (8.1 oz)	170	18	1	0	21	11	870
Yves								
Veggie Chili	1 pkg (10.5 oz)	230	21	1	0	37	14	850
TAKE-OUT								
con carne w/ beans	8.9 oz	254	25	8	133	22	—	1008

CHILI PEPPER (see PEPPERS)

CHINESE FOOD (see ASIAN FOOD)

CHINESE PRESERVING MELON

FOOD	PORTION	CALS	PROT	FAT	CHOL	CARB	FIBER	SOD
cooked	½ cup	11	tr	tr	0	3	—	93

CHIPS

FOOD	PORTION	CALS	PROT	FAT	CHOL	CARB	FIBER	SOD
barbecue	1 oz	139	2	9	0	15	—	213
barbecue	1 bag (7 oz)	971	15	64	0	105	—	1486
corn	1 oz	153	2	10	0	16	1	179
corn	1 bag (7 oz)	1067	13	66	0	113	9	1248
corn barbecue	1 oz	148	2	9	0	16	1	216
corn barbecue	1 bag (7 oz)	1036	14	65	0	111	10	1511
corn cones	1 oz	145	2	8	0	18	—	290
corn cones nacho	1 oz	152	2	9	—	17	—	270
corn onion	1 oz	142	2	6	0	19	—	278
potato	1 oz	152	2	10	0	15	—	168
potato	1 bag (8 oz)	1217	16	79	0	120	—	1347
potato cheese	1 oz	140	2	8	—	16	—	225
potato cheese	1 bag (6 oz)	842	14	46	—	98	—	1348
potato light	1 oz	134	2	6	0	19	—	139
potato light	1 bag (6 oz)	801	12	35	0	114	—	836

FOOD	PORTION	CALS	PROT	FAT	CHOL	CARB	FIBER	SOD
potato sour cream & onion	1 oz	150	2	10	2	15	—	177
potato sour cream & onion	1 bag (7 oz)	1051	16	67	14	102	—	1237
potato sticks	½ cup (0.6 oz)	94	1	6	0	10	1	45
potato sticks	1 pkg (1 oz)	148	2	10	0	15	—	71
potato sticks	1 oz	148	2	10	0	15	1	71
taco	1 oz	136	2	7	—	18	—	223
taco	1 bag (8 oz)	1089	18	55	—	143	—	1788
taro	10 (0.8 oz)	115	1	6	0	16	—	79
taro	1 oz	141	1	7	0	19	—	97
tortilla	1 oz	142	2	7	0	18	2	150
tortilla	1 bag (7.5 oz)	1067	15	56	0	134	14	1124
tortilla nacho	1 oz	141	2	7	0	18	2	201
tortilla nacho	1 bag (8 oz)	1131	18	58	0	142	12	1606
tortilla nacho light	1 oz	126	3	4	0	20	—	284
tortilla nacho light	1 bag (6 oz)	757	15	26	0	122	—	1705
tortilla ranch	1 oz	139	2	7	0	18	—	174
tortilla ranch	1 bag (7 oz)	969	15	47	1	128	—	1212
Atkins								
Crunchers Barbeque	1 pkg (1 oz)	100	13	3	0	8	4	430
Crunchers Nacho Cheese	1 pkg (1 oz)	100	13	3	0	8	3	400
Crunchers Original	1 pkg (1 oz)	90	13	3	0	8	4	440
Crunchers Sour Cream & Onion	1 pkg (1 oz)	100	12	4	5	8	3	410
Barbara's Bakery								
Potato	1¼ cup (1 oz)	150	2	10	0	15	1	180
Potato No Salt Added	1¼ cups (1 oz)	150	2	10	0	15	1	20
Potato Ripple	1¼ cup (1 oz)	150	2	10	0	15	1	180
Potato Yogurt & Green Onion	1¼ cup (1 oz)	150	2	9	0	15	1	240

FOOD	PORTION	CALS	PROT	FAT	CHOL	CARB	FIBER	SOD
Tortilla Blue Corn	15 chips (1 oz)	140	3	7	0	16	1	40
Tortilla Blue Corn No Salt	15 chips (1 oz)	140	3	7	0	16	1	0
Tortilla Pinta Salsa	15 chips (1 oz)	130	2	6	0	19	2	210
Bruno & Luigi's								
Pasta Chips Garlic & Herb	1 oz	117	4	1	0	23	1	25
Cape Cod								
Potato Golden Russet	1 pkg (0.5 oz)	70	1	4	0	8	tr	75
Chester's								
Flamin'Hot	1 oz	140	2	8	0	17	tr	250
Salsa	1 oz	140	2	7	0	18	tr	290
Deliciously Slim								
Tortilla Black Bean & Sour Cream	1 oz	140	5	9	0	13	5	125
Tortilla Lightly Salted	1 oz	140	4	8	0	13	5	150
Tortilla Ranch	1 oz	140	5	9	0	13	5	140
Doritos								
3D's Cooler Ranch	27 (1 oz)	140	2	6	<5	18	1	350
3D's Nacho Cheesier	27 (1 oz)	140	2	7	<5	17	1	360
Cooler Ranch	12 (1 oz)	140	2	7	0	18	1	170
Flamin' Hot	11 (1 oz)	140	2	7	0	17	1	210
Nacho Cheesier	11 (1 oz)	140	2	7	0	17	1	200
Salsa Verde	12 (1 oz)	150	2	7	0	20	1	210
Smokey Red	12 (1 oz)	150	2	7	0	21	1	210
Spicy Nacho	12 (1 oz)	140	2	6	0	18	1	210
Toasted Corn	13 (1 oz)	140	2	7	0	18	1	120
Durangos								
Tortilla	15 (1 oz)	150	2	7	0	20	2	105
Eden								
Brown Rice Chips	1 oz	150	2	7	0	19	0	100
Sea Vegetable Chips	1 oz	140	1	5	0	23	0	220
Fritos								
Chili Cheese	31 (1 oz)	160	2	10	0	16	1	240
Corn Chips BBQ	29 (1 oz)	150	2	9	0	16	1	290

FOOD	PORTION	CALS	PROT	FAT	CHOL	CARB	FIBER	SOD
Corn Chips King Size	12 (1 oz)	150	2	10	0	16	1	150
Corn Chips Sabrositas Flamin' Hot	30 (1 oz)	150	2	9	0	16	1	180
Corn Chips Sabrositas Lime 'N Chile	28 (1 oz)	150	2	9	0	17	1	240
Corn Chips Wild N' Mild Ranch	28 (1 oz)	160	2	10	0	15	1	160
Original	32 (1 oz)	160	2	10	0	15	1	170
Scoops	11 (1 oz)	160	2	10	0	17	1	105
Texas Grill Honey BBQ	15 (1 oz)	150	2	9	0	16	1	200
GeniSoy								
Soy Crisps	1 oz	110	7	2	0	14	2	290
Soy Crisps Apple Cinnamon Crunch	1 oz	120	7	2	0	17	2	160
Soy Crisps Creamy Ranch	1 oz	110	7	2	0	15	2	330
Soy Crisps Deep Sea Salt	1 oz	110	7	2	0	14	2	260
Soy Crisps Rich Cheddar Cheese	1 oz	110	7	2	0	14	2	320
Soy Crisps Roasted Garlic & Onion	1 oz	100	7	2	0	14	2	280
Soy Crisps Zesty Barbeque	1 oz	110	7	2	0	17	2	160
Guiltless Gourmet								
Guiltless Carbs Salsa Verde	1 oz	110	14	3	0	9	3	460
Guiltless Carbs Southwestern Ranch	1 oz	110	14	3	0	9	3	420
Guiltless Carbs Three Pepper	1 oz	110	14	3	0	9	3	300
Tortilla Blue Corn	18 (1 oz)	110	3	2	0	22	2	140

FOOD	PORTION	CALS	PROT	FAT	CHOL	CARB	FIBER	SOD
Tortilla Chili Lime	18 (1 oz)	110	2	2	0	22	2	200
Tortilla Chili Verde	18 (1 oz)	120	2	2	0	22	2	200
Tortilla Chipotle	18 (1 oz)	120	2	2	0	22	2	200
Tortilla Mucho Nacho	18 (1 oz)	110	2	2	0	20	3	200
Tortilla Organic Red Corn	18 (1 oz)	110	3	2	0	22	2	160
Tortilla Spicy Black Bean	18 (1 oz)	110	3	2	0	22	2	200
Tortilla Sweet White Corn	18 (1 oz)	110	3	2	0	22	2	160
Tortilla Yellow Corn	18 (1 oz)	110	3	2	0	22	2	160
Tortilla Yellow Corn Unsalted	18 (1 oz)	110	2	1	0	22	2	26
Herr's								
Potato	1 oz	140	2	8	0	16	1	180
Husman's								
Deli Style Tortilla	11 chips	150	3	7	0	19	1	200
Potato	18 (1 oz)	160	2	11	0	14	1	75
Potato Sour Cream & Onion	18 (1 oz)	150	2	9	0	14	1	200
Potato Sweet N'Sassy	18 (1 oz)	155	1	10	0	15	1	110
Keto								
Low Carb Tortilla All Flavors	1 oz	150	12	8	0	8	4	240
Lay's								
Adobadas	16 (1 oz)	170	2	10	0	18	1	240
Baked KC Masterpiece BBQ	11 (1 oz)	120	2	3	0	22	2	210
Baked Original	11 (1 oz)	110	2	2	0	23	2	150
Baked Roasted Herb	12 (1 oz)	130	2	3	0	25	2	190
Baked Sour Cream & Onion	12 (1 oz)	120	2	2	0	21	2	210
Classic	20 (1 oz)	150	2	10	0	15	1	180
Deli Style Hot N'Tangy BBQ	18 (1 oz)	150	2	10	0	16	1	220
Deli Style Jalapeno	17 (1 oz)	150	2	10	0	16	1	230

FOOD	PORTION	CALS	PROT	FAT	CHOL	CARB	FIBER	SOD
Deli Style Original	17 (1 oz)	140	1	10	0	16	1	180
Deli Style Salt & Vinegar	16 (1 oz)	90	1	10	0	16	1	380
Flamin' Hot	17 pieces (1 oz)	150	2	10	0	16	1	180
KC Masterpiece BBQ	15 (1 oz)	150	2	10	0	15	1	200
Onion & Garlic	19 (1 oz)	150	2	9	0	16	1	200
Original Baked	1 pkg (1⅛ oz)	130	2	2	0	26	2	170
Salt & Vinegar	17 pieces (1 oz)	150	2	10	0	15	1	300
Sour Cream & Onion	17 pieces (1 oz)	160	2	11	<5	12	1	200
Toasted Onion & Cheese	17 pieces (1 oz)	160	2	10	0	14	1	240
Wavy	11 pieces (1 oz)	150	2	10	0	15	1	180
Wavy Au Gratin	13 (1 oz)	150	2	10	<5	14	1	200
Wavy Ranch	11 (1 oz)	160	2	11	0	14	1	150
Wow Mesquite BBQ	20 (1 oz)	75	2	0	0	17	1	250
Wow Original	20 (1 oz)	75	2	0	0	18	1	200
Wow Sour Cream & Chive	19 (1 oz)	80	2	0	0	17	1	230
Wow Sour Cream & Chive	19 (1 oz)	80	2	0	0	17	1	230
Met-Rx								
Pro Chips Bar-B-Que	1 pkg (2 oz)	260	38	9	0	8	0	440
Pro Chips Nacho	1 pkg (2 oz)	260	38	10	0	6	0	500
Old Dutch Foods								
Potato	12–15 chips (1 oz)	150	2	8	0	16	1	130
Potato BBQ	12–15 chips (1 oz)	150	2	9	0	15	1	300
Potato BBQ Ripple	12–15 chips (1 oz)	150	2	9	0	16	tr	180
Potato Cajun Ripple	12–15 chips (1 oz)	150	2	10	0	15	1	160

FOOD	PORTION	CALS	PROT	FAT	CHOL	CARB	FIBER	SOD
Potato Cheddar & Sour Cream Ripple	12–15 chips (1 oz)	160	2	9	0	16	1	190
Potato Cheddar & Sour Cream Ripples	12–15 chips (1 oz)	150	2	9	0	15	1	190
Potato Dill	12–15 chips (1 oz)	140	2	8	0	16	1	310
Potato Dutch Crunch	15–20 chips (1 oz)	130	2	6	0	18	2	140
Potato French Onion Ripple	12–15 chips (1 oz)	150	2	10	0	15	1	180
Potato Jalapeno & Cheddar Dutch Crunch	15–20 chips (1 oz)	130	2	6	0	17	1	190
Potato Jalapeno Cheese	12–15 chips (1 oz)	150	2	9	0	16	1	170
Potato Mesquite BBQ Dutch Crunch	15–20 chips (1 oz)	130	2	6	0	19	2	230
Potato Onion & Garlic	12–15 chips (1 oz)	140	2	8	0	16	1	210
Potato Outback Spicy BBQ	12–15 chips (1 oz)	150	2	10	0	15	1	170
Potato Ripples	12–15 chips (1 oz)	150	2	9	0	15	1	115
Potato Salt & Vinegar Dutch Crunch	15–20 chips (1 oz)	130	0	6	0	18	1	360
Potato Sour Cream & Onion	12–15 chips (1 oz)	150	2	9	0	15	1	230
Tortilla Bite Size White Corn	20 chips (1 oz)	150	2	8	0	18	1	105
Tortilla Nacho Cheese	15 chips (1 oz)	150	2	7	0	19	1	150
Tortilla Restaurant Style White	9 chips (1 oz)	140	2	7	0	20	2	95
Tostados White Corn	11 chips (1 oz)	140	2	7	0	20	2	115

FOOD	PORTION	CALS	PROT	FAT	CHOL	CARB	FIBER	SOD
Tostados Yellow	11 chips (1 oz)	140	2	6	0	21	1	90
Pita-Snax								
Cheddar Cheese	34 (1 oz)	110	3	2	0	21	tr	240
Chili & Lime	34 (1 oz)	120	3	2	0	20	tr	210
Cinnamon	34 (1 oz)	120	3	2	0	22	tr	60
Dill Ranch	34 (1 oz)	120	3	2	0	21	tr	170
Garlic	34 (1 oz)	120	3	2	0	22	tr	120
Lightly Salted	34 (1 oz)	110	3	1	0	22	tr	170
Pringles								
BBQ	14 chips (1 oz)	150	2	10	0	15	1	200
Cheese & Onion	14 chips (1 oz)	160	1	11	0	15	1	220
Cheez-ums	14 chips (1 oz)	150	2	10	0	14	1	190
Original	14 chips (1 oz)	160	2	11	0	15	1	170
Pizzalicious	14 chips (1 oz)	160	1	11	0	14	1	200
Ranch	14 chips (1 oz)	150	2	10	0	15	1	130
Salt & Vinegar	14 chips (1 oz)	160	1	11	0	15	1	200
Sour Cream & Onion	14 chips (1 oz)	160	2	10	0	15	1	135
Racquet								
Wheat Chips All Flavors	6 chips	30	1	1	0	4	0	30
Revival								
Baked Soy Pasta Chips Lightly Salted Sunshine	1 bag (0.9 oz)	100	7	2	0	13	0	180
Baked Soy Pasta Chips Naturally Nice	1 bag (0.9 oz)	80	7	1	0	12	0	120
Baked Soy Pasta Chips Rev It Up Ranch	1 bag (0.9 oz)	105	7	3	0	12	0	190

FOOD	PORTION	CALS	PROT	FAT	CHOL	CARB	FIBER	SOD
Ruffles								
Baked	10 (1 oz)	110	2	2	0	23	2	180
Baked Cheddar & Sour Cream	9 (1 oz)	120	2	3	0	21	2	270
Buffalo Style	11 chips (1 oz)	160	2	10	0	16	1	230
Cheddar & Sour Cream	11 chips (1 oz)	160	2	10	0	14	1	190
French Onion	11 (1 oz)	150	2	10	0	15	1	190
MC Masterpiece Mesquite BBQ	11 (1 oz)	150	1	10	0	15	1	190
Original	1 pkg (1.5 oz)	240	3	16	0	22	2	250
Original	12 chips (1 oz)	150	2	10	0	14	1	180
Ranch	13 (1 oz)	150	2	9	0	15	1	280
Reduced Fat	16 (1 oz)	130	2	7	0	18	1	130
The Works	12 (1 oz)	160	2	11	0	14	1	210
Wow Cheddar & Sour Cream	15 (1 oz)	75	3	0	0	16	1	230
Wow Original	17 (1 oz)	75	2	0	0	17	1	200
Santitas								
100% White Corn	6 (1 oz)	130	2	6	0	19	1	110
Restaurant Style Chips	7 (1 oz)	130	2	6	0	19	1	110
Restaurant Style Strips	10 (1 oz)	130	2	6	0	19	1	110
Skinny								
BBQ	1½ cups	90	2	2	0	17	1	210
Corn	1½ cups	90	2	2	0	17	1	90
Nacho Cheese	1½ cups	90	2	3	0	15	1	200
Sour Cream & Onion	1½ cups	90	2	2	0	17	1	110
Sticks Garden Veggie	1 oz	140	1	6	0	17	1	280
Sticks Island Lime Chili	1 oz	140	1	6	0	17	1	280
Sticks Maui Wowie	1 oz	140	1	6	0	17	1	280

FOOD	PORTION	CALS	PROT	FAT	CHOL	CARB	FIBER	SOD
Sticks Original Spud	1 oz	140	1	6	0	17	1	280
Snyder's Of Hanover								
Barbeque Corn	1.5 oz	230	3	14	0	22	2	350
BBQ Rib	1 oz	140	2	7	0	17	tr	290
Cheddar Bacon	1 oz	150	2	6	0	20	3	270
Corn Chips	1.5 oz	230	3	15	0	22	2	220
Grilled Steak & Onion	1 oz	140	2	6	0	20	4	140
Hot Buffalo	1 oz	150	2	7	0	20	4	330
Kosher Dill	1 oz	140	2	6	0	20	3	360
No Salt	1 oz	140	2	6	0	19	3	0
Potato	1 oz	140	2	6	0	19	3	90
Ripple	1 oz	140	2	6	0	18	4	100
Salt & Vinegar	1 oz	140	2	6	0	19	4	150
Sausage Pizza	1 oz	150	2	6	0	20	4	250
Sour Cream & Onion	1 oz	150	2	7	0	19	4	150
Tasty Veggie Potato Chips	1 oz	150	3	6	0	20	4	260
Tortilla Nacho	1 oz	140	2	7	0	19	1	130
Tortilla No Salt Yellow Corn	1 oz	140	2	6	0	19	1	0
Tortilla White Corn	1 oz	140	2	6	0	20	1	130
Tortilla Yellow Corn	1 oz	140	2	6	0	19	1	130
Tortilla Yellow Corn Mini	1 oz	160	2	8	0	20	1	130
Veggie Crisps	1 pkg (1.5 oz)	190	1	9	0	26	2	470
Soya King								
Soy Mongolian BBQ	23 chips (1 oz)	140	1	7	0	19	3	115
Soy Original	23 chips (1 oz)	140	1	7	0	19	3	115
Soy Sour Cream & Onion	23 chips (1 oz)	140	1	7	0	19	3	115
Soy Taco	23 chips (1 oz)	140	1	7	0	19	3	115

FOOD	PORTION	CALS	PROT	FAT	CHOL	CARB	FIBER	SOD
Stacy's								
Pita Chips Cinnamon Sugar	1 oz	130	3	4	0	18	3	130
Pita Chips Parmesan Garlic & Herb	1 oz	130	3	4	0	18	3	200
Pita Chips Simply Naked	1 oz	130	3	4	0	18	3	140
Twisted Pasta Low Fat	1 oz	110	3	2	0	21	1	135
Sunchips								
French Onion	13 (1 oz)	140	2	7	0	18	2	115
Harvest Cheddar	13 (1 oz)	140	2	6	0	19	2	115
Original	14 (1 oz)	140	2	6	0	19	2	115
Terra Chips								
Spiced Sweet Potato	1 pkg (½ oz)	190	1	13	0	17	3	180
Torengos								
Chips	13 chips (1 oz)	140	2	9	0	15	1	150
Tostitos								
Baked Bite Size	20 (1 oz)	110	3	1	0	24	2	200
Baked Bite Size Salsa & Cream Cheese	16 (1 oz)	120	2	3	0	21	1	190
Baked Original	13 (1 oz)	110	3	1	3	21	1	200
Bite Size	15 (1 oz)	140	2	8	0	17	1	110
Crispy Rounds	13 (1 oz)	150	2	8	0	17	1	85
Nacho Style	6 (1 oz)	140	2	6	0	19	1	100
Restaurant Style	7 (1 oz)	140	2	6	0	19	1	110
Restaurant Style Hint Of Lime	6 (1 oz)	140	2	6	0	19	1	160
Santa Fe Gold	7 (1 oz)	140	2	6	0	19	1	80
Wow Original	6 (1 oz)	90	2	1	0	20	1	105
Utz								
Baked Crisps	12 (1 oz)	110	2	2	0	23	2	180
Carolina Barbeque	20 (1 oz)	150	2	9	0	14	1	270
Cheddar & Sour Cream	20 (1 oz)	160	2	10	0	14	1	200

FOOD	PORTION	CALS	PROT	FAT	CHOL	CARB	FIBER	SOD
Corn Chips	24 (1 oz)	160	2	10	0	16	1	160
Corn Chips Barbecue	24 (1 oz)	160	2	10	0	16	1	180
Grandma	20 (1 oz)	140	2	8	5	14	1	120
Grandma BBQ	20 (1 oz)	140	2	8	5	15	1	240
Home Style Kettle	20 (1 oz)	140	2	8	0	14	1	120
Home Style Kettle BBQ	20 (1 oz)	140	2	8	0	15	1	240
Kettle Classics Crunchy	20 (1 oz)	150	2	9	0	15	1	95
Kettle Classics Crunchy Mesquite BBQ	20 (1 oz)	150	2	9	0	15	1	200
No Salt Added	20 (1 oz)	150	2	9	0	14	1	5
Onion & Garlic	20 (1 oz)	150	2	9	0	14	1	180
Potato	20 (1 oz)	150	2	9	0	14	1	95
Reduced Fat BBQ	22 (1 oz)	140	2	6	0	19	1	190
Reducted Fat Ripple	24 (1 oz)	140	2	7	0	18	1	120
Ripple	20 (1 oz)	150	2	10	0	14	1	95
Ripple Sour Cream & Onion	20 (1 oz)	160	2	10	0	14	1	140
Ripple Barbeque	20 (1 oz)	150	2	10	0	14	1	200
Salt'N Vinegar	20 (1 oz)	150	2	9	0	14	1	270
The Crab Chip	20 (1 oz)	150	2	9	0	14	1	300
Tortilla Black Bean & Salsa	13 (1 oz)	150	2	7	0	19	1	230
Tortilla Low Fat Baked	10 (1 oz)	120	2	2	0	24	2	200
Tortilla Nacho	13 (1 oz)	150	2	8	0	19	1	200
Tortilla Restaurant Style	6 (1 oz)	140	2	7	0	18	1	120
Tortilla Spicy Nacho	13 (1 oz)	150	2	8	0	19	1	220
Tortilla White Corn	12 (1 oz)	140	2	7	0	18	1	120
Yes! Fat Free	20 (1 oz)	75	2	0	0	17	1	180
Yes! Fat Free Barbeque	20 (1 oz)	75	2	0	0	16	1	210
Yes! Fat Free Ripple	20 (1 oz)	75	2	0	0	17	1	180

CHITTERLINGS

FOOD	PORTION	CALS	PROT	FAT	CHOL	CARB	FIBER	SOD
pork cooked	3 oz	258	9	24	122	0	0	33

FOOD	PORTION	CALS	PROT	FAT	CHOL	CARB	FIBER	SOD
CHIVES								
freeze-dried	1 tbsp	1	tr	tr	0	tr	–	–
fresh chopped	1 tsp	0	tr	tr	0	tr	–	0
fresh chopped	1 tbsp	1	tr	tr	0	tr	–	0

CHOCOLATE (see also CANDY, CHOCOLATE SPREAD, CHOCOLATE SYRUP, COCOA, HOT CHOCOLATE, ICE CREAM TOPPINGS, MILK DRINKS)

FOOD	PORTION	CALS	PROT	FAT	CHOL	CARB	FIBER	SOD
BAKING								
baking	1 oz	145	3	15	0	8	–	1
grated unsweetened	1 cup	689	14	73	0	37	20	18
liquid unsweetened	1 oz	134	3	14	0	10	5	3
squares unsweetened	1 square (1 oz)	146	3	16	0	8	4	4
Nestle								
Choco Bake	½ oz	80	1	8	0	5	2	0
Premier White Bar	½ oz	80	1	5	<5	8	0	15
Premier White Morsels	1 tbsp	80	tr	4	0	9	0	20
Semi-Sweet Bar	½ oz	70	<1	4	0	9	tr	0
Unsweetened Bar	½ oz	80	2	7	0	4	2	0
CHIPS								
milk chocolate	1 cup (6 oz)	862	12	52	38	100	–	138
semisweet	60 pieces (1 oz)	136	1	9	0	18	–	3
semisweet	1 cup (6 oz)	804	7	50	0	106	–	19
Cloud Nine								
Double Dark Chocolate	13 pieces (0.5 oz)	80	1	4	5	9	0	0
Ghirardelli								
Semi-Sweet	33 pieces (0.5 oz)	70	1	4	0	9	tr	0
Hershey's								
Holiday Baking Bits	1 tbsp	70	tr	3	0	11	–	0
Milk Chocolate	1 tbsp	80	1	5	<5	9	–	10
Mini Milk Chocolate	1 tbsp	80	tr	4	0	10	–	0
Mini Kisses For Baking	11 pieces	80	1	5	<5	9	–	15
Premier White Milk Chips	1 tbsp	80	1	4	0	9	–	30
Raspberry Chips	1 tbsp	80	tr	4	0	10	–	0

FOOD	PORTION	CALS	PROT	FAT	CHOL	CARB	FIBER	SOD
Semi-Sweet	1 tbsp	80	tr	4	0	10	—	0
Semi-Sweet Mini	1 tbsp	80	tr	4	0	10	—	0
Skor English Toffee Baking Bits	1 tbsp	70	0	5	10	7	—	60
Nestle								
Crunch Baking Pieces	1½ tbsp	80	tr	4	0	10	0	25
Milk Chocolate Morsels	1 tbsp	70	tr	4	<5	9	0	0
Mint Chocolate Morsels	1 tbsp	70	tr	4	0	9	tr	0
Morsels Semi-Sweet	1 tbsp	70	tr	4	0	9	tr	0
Semi-Sweet Mega Morsels	1 tbsp	70	tr	4	0	9	tr	0
Semi-Sweet Mini Morsels	1 tbsp	70	tr	4	0	9	tr	0
Sunspire								
Chocolate Sundrops	47 pieces (1.4 oz)	190	2	5	0	27	1	50
Dark Chocolate Grain Sweetened	13 pieces (0.5 oz)	70	0	4	0	10	1	1
Organic	13 pieces (0.5 oz)	70	1	5	0	9	0	0
Tropical Source								
Espresso Roast Dairy Free	13 pieces (1.5 oz)	70	1	4	0	9	1	1
Semi-Sweet Dairy Free	13 pieces (1.5 oz)	80	1	4	5	9	0	0
MIX								
powder	2–3 heaping tsp	75	1	1	0	20	—	45
powder as prep w/ whole milk	9 oz	226	9	9	33	31	—	165
Quik								
Chocolate Powder	2 tbsp (0.8 oz)	90	1	1	0	19	1	30
Chocolate Powder No Sugar	2 tbsp (0.4 oz)	40	1	1	0	7	2	45

CHOCOLATE MILK *(see MILK DRINKS)*

FOOD	PORTION	CALS	PROT	FAT	CHOL	CARB	FIBER	SOD
CHOCOLATE SPREAD								
Twist								
Sugar Free Chocolate Spread	2 tbsp	170	2	12	0	2	0	55
CHOCOLATE SYRUP								
chocolate fudge	1 tbsp (0.7 oz)	73	1	3	–	12	–	27
chocolate fudge	1 cup (11.9 oz)	1176	15	46	–	200	–	442
syrup	2 tbsp	82	1	tr	0	22	–	36
syrup	1 cup	653	6	3	0	177	–	287
syrup as prep w/ whole milk	9 oz	232	9	9	33	34	–	156
Ah!Laska								
Organic	2 tbsp	85	2	0	0	20	–	5
Colac								
Chocolate Topping	1 tbsp	37	0	1	0	15	0	5
DaVinci Gourmet								
Sugar Free	2 tbsp	15	1	0	0	5	1	0
Hershey's								
Chocolate Fudge	1 tbsp	70	tr	3	<5	10	–	25
Double Chocolate	1 tbsp	50	0	0	0	13	–	15
Lite	2 tbsp	50	0	0	0	12	–	35
Syrup	2 tbsp	100	1	0	0	24	–	25
Quik								
Chocolate	2 tbsp (1.3 oz)	100	1	1	0	23	tr	30
Smucker's								
Plate Scapers Chocolate	2 tbsp	100	1	5	–	23	1	20
Toll House								
Mint Chocolate	2 tbsp (1.5 oz)	130	1	3	0	25	1	30
Semi-Sweet	2 tbsp (1.5 oz)	130	1	4	0	24	1	30
Walden Farms								
Sugar Free	2 tbsp	0	0	0	0	0	0	35
Whoppers								
Chocolate Malt	2 tbsp	100	tr	0	0	25	–	55

FOOD	PORTION	CALS	PROT	FAT	CHOL	CARB	FIBER	SOD
CHUTNEY								
apple	1.2 oz	68	tr	0	–	18	1	–
apple cranberry	1 tbsp	16	tr	0	0	4	–	1
coconut	¼ cup	74	1	7	0	4	2	5
mango	1 tbsp	54	tr	2	0	10	tr	207
tomato	1 tbsp	32	tr	tr	0	8	tr	26
Wild Thyme Farms								
Apricot Cranberry Walnut	1 tbsp	15	0	0	0	3	–	0
Pineapple Peach Lime	1 tbsp	14	0	0	0	6	–	0
CILANTRO								
fresh	1 cup (1.6 oz)	11	1	tr	0	2	1	25
fresh	1 tsp (2 g)	tr	tr	tr	0	tr	tr	1
CINNAMON								
ground	1 tsp	6	tr	tr	0	2	–	1
sticks	0.5 oz	39	1	tr	–	8	3	4
Gringo Billy's								
Cinnamon Sweetener	½ tsp	0	0	0	0	0	0	57
CISCO								
raw	3 oz	84	16	2	–	0	–	47
smoked	1 oz	50	5	3	9	0	–	135
smoked	3 oz	151	14	10	27	0	–	409
CLAMS								
CANNED								
liquid only	1 cup	6	1	tr	–	tr	–	516
liquid only	3 oz	2	tr	tr	–	tr	–	183
meat only	1 cup	236	41	3	107	8	–	179
meat only	3 oz	126	22	2	57	4	–	95
Bumble Bee								
Baby	2 oz	50	9	1	40	2	0	270
Progresso								
Creamy Clam Sauce	½ cup (4.2 oz)	110	5	6	10	8	0	440
Minced	¼ cup (2.1 oz)	25	4	0	10	2	0	250

FOOD	PORTION	CALS	PROT	FAT	CHOL	CARB	FIBER	SOD
Red Clam Sauce	½ cup (4.4 oz)	60	4	1	10	8	1	350
White Clam Sauce	½ cup (4.4 oz)	150	9	10	20	5	0	710
FRESH								
cooked	3 oz	126	22	2	57	4	—	95
cooked	20 sm	133	23	2	60	5	—	100
raw	20 sm (6.3 oz)	133	23	2	60	5	—	100
raw	3 oz	63	11	1	29	2	—	47
raw	9 lg (6.3 oz)	133	23	2	60	5	—	100
TAKE-OUT								
breaded & fried	20 sm	379	27	21	115	19	—	684
CLEMENTINES								
Haddon House								
In Light Syrup	½ cup	80	0	0	0	19	1	10
Tina								
Fresh	1	50	1	1	0	15	3	0
CLOVES								
ground	1 tsp	7	tr	tr	0	1	—	5
COCOA (see also HOT CHOCOLATE)								
powder unsweetened	1 tbsp (5 g)	11	1	1	0	3	2	1
powder unsweetened	1 cup (3 oz)	197	17	12	0	47	29	18
Ah!Laska								
Organic	2 tbsp	100	2	0	0	23	5	35
Organic Bakers Cocoa	1 tbsp	20	1	0	0	3	1	0
Hershey's								
Cocoa	1 tbsp	20	1	1	0	3	—	0
European Cocoa	1 tbsp	20	1	1	0	3	—	0
Nestle								
Cocoa	1 tbsp	15	1	1	0	3	1	0
COCONUT								
dried sweetened flaked	7 oz pkg	944	7	64	0	95	—	509

FOOD	PORTION	CALS	PROT	FAT	CHOL	CARB	FIBER	SOD
dried sweetened flaked	1 cup	351	2	24	0	35	–	189
dried sweetened flaked canned	1 cup	341	3	24	0	32	–	15
dried sweetened shredded	1 cup	466	2	33	0	44	–	244
dried sweetened shredded	7 oz pkg	997	6	71	0	95	–	522
dried toasted	1 oz	168	2	13	0	13	–	11
dried unsweetened	1 oz	187	2	18	0	7	–	11
fresh	1 piece (1.5 oz)	159	2	15	0	7	4	9
fresh shredded	1 cup	283	3	27	0	12	7	16

COCONUT JUICE

FOOD	PORTION	CALS	PROT	FAT	CHOL	CARB	FIBER	SOD
coconut water	1 tbsp	3	tr	tr	0	1	–	16
coconut water	1 cup	46	2	tr	0	9	–	252
cream canned	1 tbsp	36	1	3	0	2	–	10
cream canned	1 cup	568	8	52	0	25	–	149
milk canned	1 tbsp	30	tr	3	0	tr	–	2
milk canned	1 cup	445	5	48	0	6	–	29
milk frozen	1 tbsp	30	tr	3	0	1	–	2
milk frozen	1 cup	486	4	50	0	13	–	29
Amy & Brian								
Juice	8 oz	76	0	0	0	19	–	42
Thai Kitchen								
Milk	2 oz	124	1	12	0	3	0	13
Vita Coco								
Coconut Water	1 box	65	0	0	0	17	–	65
Zico								
Coconut Water Mango	11 oz	60	1	0	0	15	0	60
Coconut Water Natural	11 oz	60	1	0	0	15	0	60

COD

FOOD	PORTION	CALS	PROT	FAT	CHOL	CARB	FIBER	SOD
atlantic canned	1 can (11 oz)	327	71	3	171	0	–	680
atlantic canned	3 oz	89	19	1	47	0	–	185
atlantic dried	3 oz	246	53	2	129	0	–	5973

FOOD	PORTION	CALS	PROT	FAT	CHOL	CARB	FIBER	SOD
atlantic fresh cooked	3 oz	89	19	1	47	0	–	66
atlantic fresh cooked	1 fillet (6.3 oz)	189	41	2	99	0	–	141
atlantic fresh raw	3 oz	70	15	1	37	0	–	46
pacific fresh baked	3 oz	95	21	1	43	0	–	82
roe canned	1 oz	34	6	1	–	tr	–	–
roe raw	1 oz	37	7	tr	103	tr	–	–
roe tarama	3.5 oz	547	8	55	–	6	–	600
TAKE-OUT								
roe baked w/ butter & lemon juice	1 oz	36	6	1	–	tr	–	21

COFFEE (see also COFFEE BEVERAGES, COFFEE SUBSTITUTES)

FOOD	PORTION	CALS	PROT	FAT	CHOL	CARB	FIBER	SOD
INSTANT								
decaffeinated	1 rounded tsp	4	tr	0	0	1	–	0
decaffeinated as prep	6 oz	4	tr	0	0	1	–	6
regular as prep	1 cup (6 oz)	4	tr	0	0	1	0	5
regular w/ chicory	1 rounded tsp	6	tr	0	0	1	–	5
regular w/ chicory as prep	6 oz	6	tr	0	0	1	–	10
Nescafe								
Decafe	1 tsp (2 g)	0	tr	0	0	tr	0	0
Decafe w/ Chicory	1 tsp (2 g)	0	tr	0	0	tr	0	0
French Vanilla	1 tsp (2 g)	5	0	0	0	1	0	0
French Vanilla Decaf	1 tsp (2 g)	5	0	0	0	1	0	0
Hazelnut	1 tsp (2 g)	5	0	0	0	1	0	0
Irish Creme	1 tsp (2 g)	5	0	0	0	1	0	0
Regular	1 tsp (2 g)	0	tr	0	0	tr	0	0
With Chicory	1 tsp (2 g)	5	0	0	0	1	0	0
REGULAR								
brewed	8 oz	2	tr	0	0	tr	–	1
roasted beans	1 oz	64	4	4	–	18	2	–
Nescafe								
Cafe Mocha	1 can (10 oz)	140	3	3	10	27	1	115
Caffe Latte	1 can (10 oz)	130	3	3	15	22	1	130
Caffe Latte Decaffeinated	1 can (10 oz)	130	3	3	15	22	0	100
Espresso	1 tsp (2 g)	0	tr	0	0	tr	0	0

FOOD	PORTION	CALS	PROT	FAT	CHOL	CARB	FIBER	SOD
Espresso Cafe Latte	1 pkg (0.6 oz)	70	3	2	10	10	0	50
Espresso Cafe Mocha	1 pkg (1 oz)	110	3	3	10	20	1	35
Espresso Cappuccino	1 pkg (0.6 oz)	80	3	3	10	11	0	40
Espresso Roast	1 can (10 oz)	90	1	1	<5	21	0	75
French Vanilla	1 can (10 oz)	150	4	4	15	25	2	140
Hazelnut	1 can (10 oz)	130	3	3	15	22	0	100
Roasted Ground as prep	1 cup (6 oz)	0	tr	0	0	tr	0	0
Roasted Ground Decaffeinated as prep	1 cup (6 oz)	0	tr	0	0	tr	0	0
Revival								
Soy Caramel Corn	1 cup (8 oz)	0	0	0	0	0	0	0
Soy Hazelnut	1 cup (8 oz)	0	0	0	0	0	0	0
Soy Original Roast	1 cup (8 oz)	0	0	0	0	0	0	0
COFFEE BEVERAGES								
cappuccino mix as prep	7 oz	62	tr	2	–	11	–	104
french mix as prep	7 oz	57	1	3	–	7	–	–
mocha mix as prep	7 oz	51	1	2	–	8	–	36
AchievONE								
All Flavors	1 bottle (9.5 oz)	120	20	0	20	5	–	200
America's Best Brew								
Iced Coffee All Flavors	8 oz	110	3	2	0	25	–	15
Arizona								
Iced Latte Supreme	8 oz	110	3	2	6	21	1	95
Iced Mocha Latte	8 oz	110	4	2	5	21	1	98
Big Train								
Low Carb Blended Ice Mocha as prep	1 serv (16 oz)	90	6	5	0	14	1	190
Chock full o'Nuts								
New York Cappuccino French Vanilla	1 pkg (0.9 oz)	90	2	2	0	19	0	115

FOOD	PORTION	CALS	PROT	FAT	CHOL	CARB	FIBER	SOD
New York Cappuccino Hazelnut	1 pkg. (0.9 oz)	90	2	2	0	19	0	115
Coffee House USA								
All Flavors	1 bottle (9.5 oz)	100	4	4	15	29	tr	160
Flavour Creations								
Coffee Flavoring Tablets All Flavors	1 tablet	0	0	0	0	tr	0	0
Gehl's								
Iced Cappuccino	1 can (11 oz)	190	11	2	13	33	0	330
Jakada								
Latte Mocha	1 bottle (10.5 oz)	180	5	3.5	10	33	0	70
Latte Vanilla	1 bottle (10.5 oz)	180	4	4	10	32	0	70
Low Carb Creations								
Cappuccino	1 cup	30	0	2	0	3	0	39
Silk								
Coffee Soylatte	1 bottle (11 oz)	220	7	5	0	38	0	70
Sipper Sweets								
Sugar Free Low Carb Cappuccino	1 serv	50	1	3	0	3	0	80
Starbucks								
Frappuccino	1 bottle (9.5 oz)	190	6	3	12	39	0	110
Frappuccino Mocha	1 bottle (9.5 oz)	190	6	3	12	39	0	110
Frappuccino Vanilla	1 bottle (9.5 oz)	190	6	3	12	39	0	110
TAKE-OUT								
cafe amaretto w/ alcohol	1 serv	192	1	9	33	15	0	14
cafe au lait	1 cup (8 fl oz)	77	4	4	17	6	–	62
cafe brulot	1 cup	48	tr	0	0	3	–	2
cafe brulot w/ alcohol	1 serv	130	1	tr	0	16	3	4

FOOD	PORTION	CALS	PROT	FAT	CHOL	CARB	FIBER	SOD
cappuccino	1 cup (8 fl oz)	77	4	4	17	6	—	62
coffee con leche	1 cup (8 fl oz)	77	4	4	17	6	—	62
espresso	1 cup (3 fl oz)	2	tr	0	0	tr	—	2
irish coffee	1 serv	226	1	11	41	6	0	15
latte w/ skim milk	13 oz	88	8	tr	4	12	0	128
latte w/ whole milk	13 oz	152	8	8	33	12	0	122
mocha	1 mug (9.6 fl oz)	202	3	15	40	17	—	28

COFFEE SUBSTITUTES

FOOD	PORTION	CALS	PROT	FAT	CHOL	CARB	FIBER	SOD
powder	1 tsp	9	tr	tr	0	2	—	2
powder as prep	6 oz	9	tr	tr	0	2	—	7
powder as prep w/ milk	6 oz	121	6	6	25	10	—	91
Natural Touch								
Kaffree Roma	1 tsp (2 g)	10	0	0	0	2	0	0
Roma Cappuccino	3 tbsp (0.4 oz)	50	1	3	0	5	0	15

COFFEE WHITENERS

FOOD	PORTION	CALS	PROT	FAT	CHOL	CARB	FIBER	SOD
liquid nondairy frzn	1 tbsp (0.5 oz)	20	tr	2	0	2	—	12
powder nondairy	1 tsp	11	tr	tr	0	1	—	4
N-Rich								
Coffee Creamer	1 tsp (2 g)	10	tr	1	0	1	0	4
Silk								
Creamer	1 tbsp	15	0	1	0	1	0	5
Creamer French Vanilla	1 tbsp	20	0	1	0	3	0	5
Creamer Hazelnut	1 tbsp	15	0	1	0	1	0	5

COLESLAW

FOOD	PORTION	CALS	PROT	FAT	CHOL	CARB	FIBER	SOD
Fresh Express								
Cole Slaw Kit as prep	2 cups	120	1	8	5	12	2	135
TAKE-OUT								
coleslaw w/ dressing	½ cup	42	1	2	5	7	—	14

FOOD	PORTION	CALS	PROT	FAT	CHOL	CARB	FIBER	SOD
vinegar & oil coleslaw	3.5 oz	150	1	9	0	16	–	480

COLLARDS
fresh cooked	½ cup	17	1	tr	0	4	–	10
frzn chopped cooked	½ cup	31	3	tr	0	6	–	42
raw chopped	½ cup	6	tr	tr	0	1	–	4
Birds Eye								
Chopped Greens frzn	1 cup	30	2	0	0	2	2	20

COOKIES
MIX

FOOD	PORTION	CALS	PROT	FAT	CHOL	CARB	FIBER	SOD
chocolate chip	1 (0.56 oz)	79	1	4	7	10	–	47
oatmeal	1 (0.6 oz)	74	1	3	7	10	tr	75
oatmeal raisin	1 (0.6 oz)	74	1	3	7	10	tr	75
Aunt Paula's								
Low Carb Chef Chocolate Chip as prep	1	66	9	4	2	4	1	–
Low Carb Chef Peanut Butter as prep	1	66	9	4	2	4	1	–
Betty Crocker								
Chocolate Peanut Butter as prep	1 bar	180	2	9	18	25	–	150
Date Bar as prep	1 bar	150	1	6	0	23	1	30
Oatmeal as prep	2	150	2	6	12	22	1	100
Big Train								
Low Carb Chocolate Chip as prep	2	140	2	9	42	11	4	45
Low Carb Peanut Butter as prep	2	140	2	9	24	9	4	120
GoldnBrown								
Fat Free	1 (1.1 oz)	120	2	0	0	27	0	135
Keto								
Chocolate Chip as prep	1	47	3	2	–	2	1	25

FOOD	PORTION	CALS	PROT	FAT	CHOL	CARB	FIBER	SOD
Oatmeal Raisin as prep	2	59	6	3	–	2	1	50
MiniCarb								
All Flavors as prep	1	110	4	2	5	7	5	45
READY-TO-EAT								
animal	11 crackers (1 oz)	126	2	4	–	21	–	112
animal crackers	1 (2.5 g)	11	tr	tr	–	2	–	10
animal crackers	1 box (2.4 oz)	299	4	9	11	51	–	274
australian anzac biscuit	1	98	1	3	0	17	1	59
butter	1 (5 g)	23	tr	1	–	3	tr	18
chocolate chip	1 box (1.9 oz)	233	3	12	12	36	–	188
chocolate chip	1 (0.4 oz)	48	1	2	–	7	tr	32
chocolate chip low fat	1 (0.25 oz)	45	1	2	0	7	–	38
chocolate chip low sugar low sodium	1 (0.24 oz)	31	tr	1	0	5	–	1
chocolate chip soft-type	1 (0.5 oz)	69	1	4	0	9	tr	49
chocolate w/ creme filling	1 (0.35 oz)	47	1	2	–	7	tr	36
chocolate w/ creme filling chocolate coated	1 (0.60 oz)	82	1	5	–	11	–	55
chocolate w/ creme filling sugar free low sodium	1 (0.35 oz)	46	1	2	–	7	–	24
chocolate w/ extra creme filling	1 (0.46 oz)	65	1	3	–	9	–	64
chocolate wafer	1 (0.2 oz)	26	tr	1	0	4	–	35
cream cheese	1 (1.1 oz)	141	2	9	25	14	tr	53
digestive biscuits plain	2	141	2	7	–	21	1	–
fig bars	1 (0.56 oz)	56	1	1	–	11	1	56
fortune	1 (0.28 oz)	30	tr	tr	–	7	tr	22

FOOD	PORTION	CALS	PROT	FAT	CHOL	CARB	FIBER	SOD
fudge	1 (0.73 oz)	73	1	1	–	17	tr	40
gingersnaps	1 (0.24 oz)	29	tr	1	0	5	–	48
graham	1 square (0.24 oz)	30	1	1	0	5	–	42
graham chocolate covered	1 (0.49 oz)	68	1	3	0	9	–	41
graham honey	1 (0.24 oz)	30	1	1	0	5	tr	42
hermits	1 (1 oz)	117	2	5	23	18	1	54
jumbles coconut	1 (1 oz)	121	1	7	26	13	1	19
ladyfingers	1 (0.38 oz)	40	1	1	40	7	–	16
macaroons	1 (0.8 oz)	97	1	3	0	17	–	59
madeleines	1 (0.8 oz)	86	2	5	46	10	tr	34
marshmallow chocolate coated	1 (0.46 oz)	55	1	2	–	9	–	22
marshmallow pie chocolate coated	1 (1.4 oz)	165	2	7	–	26	–	66
meringue	1 (0.3 oz)	20	tr	0	0	5	0	20
molasses	1 (0.5 oz)	65	1	2	0	11	–	69
neapolitan tri-color cookie	1 (0.6 oz)	79	1	5	17	8	tr	10
oatmeal	1 (0.6 oz)	81	1	3	0	12	1	69
oatmeal soft-type	1 (0.5 oz)	61	1	2	–	10	tr	52
oatmeal raisin	1 (0.6 oz)	81	1	3	0	12	1	69
oatmeal raisin low sugar no sodium	1 (0.24 oz)	31	tr	1	0	5	–	1
oatmeal raisin soft-type	1 (0.5 oz)	61	1	2	–	10	tr	52
peanut butter sandwich	1 (0.5 oz)	67	1	3	0	9	–	52
peanut butter sandwich sugar free low sodium	1 (0.35 oz)	54	1	3	–	5	–	41
peanut butter soft-type	1 (0.5 oz)	69	1	4	0	9	tr	50
pinenut cookies	1 (1.1 oz)	134	4	9	0	11	1	11
raisin soft-type	1 (0.5 oz)	60	1	2	0	10	–	51
reginette queen'a biscuit	1 (0.8 oz)	86	2	3	tr	13	tr	83

FOOD	PORTION	CALS	PROT	FAT	CHOL	CARB	FIBER	SOD
shortbread	1 (0.28 oz)	40	1	2	2	5	—	36
shortbread pecan	1 (0.49 oz)	79	1	5	5	8	tr	39
spritz	1 (0.4 oz)	42	1	2	6	6	tr	9
sugar	1 (0.52 oz)	72	1	3	8	10	—	53
sugar low sugar sodium free	1 (0.24 oz)	30	1	1	0	5	—	0
sugar wafers w/ creme filling	1 (0.12 oz)	18	tr	1	0	3	—	5
sugar wafers w/ creme filling sugar free sodium free	1 (0.14 oz)	20	tr	1	0	3	—	0
toll house original	1 (0.8 oz)	105	2	6	15	13	tr	57
vanilla sandwich	1 (0.35 oz)	48	tr	2	0	7	tr	35
vanilla wafers	1 (0.21 oz)	28	tr	1	—	4	—	18
zeppole	1 (0.8 oz)	78	1	6	24	6	tr	14
Alternative Baking								
Vegan Chocolate Chip	1 serv (2.5 oz)	280	3	10	0	46	1	150
Vegan Expresso Chocolate Chip	1 serv (2 oz)	230	3	9	0	35	1	125
Vegan Lemon	1 serv (2.25 oz)	250	3	7	0	42	1	170
Vegan Oatmeal	1 serv (2.25 oz)	250	5	10	0	35	2	105
Vegan Peanut Butter	1 serv (2.25 oz)	270	5	10	0	40	1	115
Vegan Pumpkin	1 serv (2 oz)	200	2	6	0	35	1	120
Vegan Wheat Free Choco Cherry Chunk	1 serv (1.75 oz)	190	3	6	0	32	1	30
Vegan Wheat Free Hula Nut	1 serv (1.75 oz)	190	6	6	0	29	2	65
Vegan Wheat Free P-nut Fudge Fusion	1 serv (1.75 oz)	190	4	7	0	29	1	75
Vegan Wheat Free Snickerdoodle	1 serv (1.75 oz)	170	3	3	0	35	1	70

FOOD	PORTION	CALS	PROT	FAT	CHOL	CARB	FIBER	SOD
Amay's								
Chinese Style Almond	1 (0.5 oz)	80	1	4	4	10	0	13
Archway								
Alpine Fudge	1 (1.3 oz)	160	1	6	<5	24	tr	80
Devils Food Chocolate Drop Fat Free	1 (0.7 oz)	60	1	0	0	15	0	70
Dutch Cocoa	1 (0.9 oz)	100	1	4	0	18	0	65
Frosty Lemon	1 (0.9 oz)	100	tr	4	0	16	0	100
Fruit & Honey Bar	1 (0.9 oz)	110	1	3	5	19	0	100
Fruit Bar Fat Free	1 (0.9 oz)	90	tr	0	0	21	0	90
Fruit Filled Apricot	1 (0.8 oz)	90	1	3	<5	15	0	75
Fruit Filled Raspberry	1 (0.8 oz)	90	1	3	<5	15	0	80
Ginger Snaps	5 (1 oz)	120	1	5	0	20	0	150
Homestyle Chocolate Chip	3 (1 oz)	130	1	7	5	17	1	60
Oatmeal	1 (0.9 oz)	100	1	4	5	16	0	100
Oatmeal Apple Filled	1 (0.9 oz)	90	1	3	<5	16	0	70
Oatmeal Pecan	1 (0.9 oz)	110	1	4	5	16	1	120
Oatmeal Raisin	1	120	2	4	<5	20	tr	100
Oatmeal Raspberry Fat Free	1 (1.1 oz)	100	1	0	0	23	1	170
Oatmeal Sugar Free	1 (0.8 oz)	110	1	5	0	16	0	75
Oatmeal Raisin Fat Free	1 (1.1 oz)	100	1	0	0	24	1	60
Old Dutch Apple	1 (0.9 oz)	110	1	4	5	18	0	115
Peanut Butter	1 (1 oz)	150	2	9	5	16	0	110
Peanut Butter Fudge	1 (1.3 oz)	220	3	13	<5	23	1	135
Pecan Crunch	3 (1.2 oz)	180	2	10	5	20	0	140
Rocky Road	1 (0.8 oz)	110	1	5	10	16	0	70
Shortbread Sugar Free	1 (0.8 oz)	110	1	5	0	16	0	45
Windmill	1	90	1	4	0	14	0	95
Arnott's								
Raspberry Tartlets	2	100	1	4	0	17	tr	70

FOOD	PORTION	CALS	PROT	FAT	CHOL	CARB	FIBER	SOD
Atkins								
Endulge Wafer Bars Chocolate Creme	2 bars (1 oz)	120	4	9	0	15	3	115
Endulge Wafer Bars Mint	2 bars (1 oz)	120	4	9	0	15	3	115
Endulge Wafer Bars Peanut Butter	2 bars (1 oz)	120	4	9	0	14	3	125
Bahlsen								
Afrika	8 (1.1 oz)	170	2	10	5	17	2	20
Butter Leaves	7 (1 oz)	140	2	7	15	19	tr	50
Choco Leibniz	2 (1 oz)	140	2	7	5	18	tr	50
Choco Star Dark Chocolate	3 (1.1 oz)	170	2	12	0	16	1	10
Choco Star Milk Chocolate	3 (1.1 oz)	180	2	12	<5	16	1	25
Chocolate Hearts	4 (1 oz)	160	2	9	5	18	1	25
Delice	6 (1 oz)	140	2	6	0	19	tr	100
Deloba	4 (0.9 oz)	130	2	5	0	19	tr	80
Hanover Waffelin	5 (1 oz)	160	1	10	0	16	0	35
Hit Chocolate Vanilla Filled	2 (1 oz)	140	2	8	0	18	tr	75
Hit Vanilla Chocolate Filled	2 (1 oz)	140	2	7	0	19	tr	65
Kipferl	4 (1 oz)	150	2	9	5	16	0	10
Leibniz	6 (1 oz)	130	2	4	10	23	1	125
Nuss Dessert	3 (1.1 oz)	180	2	11	10	19	tr	60
Probiers	6 (1.1 oz)	150	2	6	0	21	tr	60
Twingo	6 (1.1 oz)	170	2	11	0	18	1	15
Waffeletten	4 (1 oz)	160	2	9	<5	18	1	40
Baker's Breakfast Cookie								
Apple Pie	1 (3 oz)	204	8	2	0	44	6	220
Banana Walnut	1 (3 oz)	274	8	8	0	52	5	200
Chocolate Chunk Raisin	1 (3 oz)	260	8	5	0	54	5	200
Double Chocolate Chunk	1 (3 oz)	250	8	5	0	50	5	200
Fruit & Nut	1 (3 oz)	270	8	5	0	54	5	210
Lemon Poppy Seed	1 (3 oz)	230	8	3	0	52	5	200
Mocha Chocolate Chunk	1 (3 oz)	250	8	5	0	50	5	230

FOOD	PORTION	CALS	PROT	FAT	CHOL	CARB	FIBER	SOD
Oatmeal Raisin	1 (3 oz)	250	8	4	0	54	5	200
Peanut Butter	1 (3 oz)	290	10	8	0	48	6	230
Peanut Butter & Jelly	1 (3 oz)	320	10	9	0	64	6	340
Pumpkin Spice	1 (3 oz)	230	8	3	0	52	5	200
Vegan Chocolate Chunk	1 (3 oz)	260	8	6	0	52	5	200
Vegan Peanut Butter Chocolate Chunk	1 (3 oz)	310	10	10	0	58	6	240
Baker's Harvest								
Animal	12 (0.9 oz)	130	2	3	—	22	—	80
Chocolate Graham	2 (0.9 oz)	130	2	3	—	24	1	120
Cinnamon Grahams	2 (0.9 oz)	130	1	5	—	19	tr	85
Cinnamon Grahams Low Fat	2 (0.9 oz)	110	2	2	0	22	1	120
Fig Bars	2 (1.2 oz)	120	tr	3	—	23	1	55
Graham	2 (0.9 oz)	120	1	4	—	21	tr	95
Graham Low Fat	2 (0.9 oz)	110	2	2	0	22	1	120
Iced Oatmeal	1 (0.6 oz)	70	1	3	0	11	0	65
Pecan Shortbread	1 (0.5 oz)	80	1	5	<5	10	0	55
Vanilla Wafers	7 (1.1 oz)	150	1	6	—	22	1	115
Barbara's Bakery								
Apple Cinnamon Bars Fat Free Whole Wheat	1 (0.7 oz)	60	1	0	0	14	2	20
Chocolate Chip	1 (0.6 oz)	80	1	4	5	10	1	60
Double Dutch Chocolate	1 (0.6 oz)	80	1	4	5	10	1	60
Fig Bars Fat Free Wheat Free	1 (0.7 oz)	60	tr	0	0	15	1	20
Fig Bars Fat Free Whole Wheat	1 (0.7 oz)	60	tr	0	0	16	2	20
Nature's Choice Coconut Almond	1 bar (1 oz)	120	2	5	0	20	1	10
Nature's Choice Expresso Bean	1 bar (1 oz)	120	2	3	0	22	1	10
Nature's Choice Lemon Yogurt	1 bar (1 oz)	120	2	4	0	22	1	10

FOOD	PORTION	CALS	PROT	FAT	CHOL	CARB	FIBER	SOD
Nature's Choice Roasted Peanut	1 bar (1 oz)	130	3	5	0	20	1	50
Old Fashioned Oatmeal	1 (0.6 oz)	70	1	3	5	11	1	65
Raspberry Bars Fat Free Wheat Free Raspberry	1 (0.7 oz)	60	1	0	0	15	1	25
Snackimals Chocolate Chip	8 (1 oz)	120	2	5	0	18	1	85
Snackimals Oatmeal Wheat Free	8 (1 oz)	120	2	5	0	19	2	75
Snackimals Vanilla	8 (1 oz)	120	2	5	0	19	1	55
Traditional Blueberry Low Fat	1 (0.7 oz)	60	1	1	0	14	1	25
Traditional Fig Low Fat	1 (0.7 oz)	60	1	1	0	14	1	25
Traditional Shortbread	1 (0.6 oz)	80	1	4	10	10	1	40
Bed & Breakfast								
Cranberry Orange Oatmeal	1 (0.8 oz)	110	1	5	10	17	1	75
Enrobed Shortbread	2 (1.4 oz)	190	2	9	15	24	1	125
Fruit Center Key Lime	2 (1.1 oz)	140	1	6	<5	22	0	55
Fruit Center Raspberry	2 (1.1 oz)	140	1	6	<5	22	0	55
Beigel's								
Black & White	1 (1 oz)	100	1	3	0	18	0	20
BP Gourmet								
Biscotti Fat Free Cinnamon Crunch	6 (1 oz)	110	2	0	0	24	0	75
Biscotti Fat Free Vanilla Crunch	4 (1 oz)	80	2	0	0	18	0	25
Chocolate Fudge Chip Sugar Free	5 (1 oz)	100	1	6	0	13	0	80
Dreams Chocolate	7 (1 oz)	120	2	3	0	21	0	35

FOOD	PORTION	CALS	PROT	FAT	CHOL	CARB	FIBER	SOD
Dreams Fat Free Chocolate Fudge	13 (1 oz)	100	2	0	0	25	0	35
Dreams Fat Free Vanilla	19 (1 oz)	100	2	0	0	25	0	35
Tangos Fat Free Chocolate Fudge Chip	4 (1 oz)	100	2	0	0	23	0	95
Breaktime								
Chocolate Chip	1 (0.3 oz)	37	tr	2	0	5	tr	37
Coconut	1 (0.3 oz)	35	1	1	0	5	tr	15
Ginger	1 (0.3 oz)	34	tr	1	0	6	—	<15
Oatmeal	1 (0.3 oz)	35	1	1	0	5	tr	27
Sprinkles	1 (0.3 oz)	36	tr	2	0	5	—	46
Brent & Sam's								
Chocolate Chip Pecan	2 (0.5 oz)	80	1	5	<5	9	0	60
Chocolate Chip Raspberry	2 (0.5 oz)	70	tr	4	<5	10	0	60
Chocolate Chips	2 (0.5 oz)	70	1	4	<5	10	0	65
Key Lime White Chocolate	2 (0.5 oz)	70	tr	4	<5	10	0	65
Oatmeal Raisin Pecan	2 (0.5 oz)	70	tr	7	<5	9	1	70
Toffee Pecan	2 (0.5 oz)	80	tr	5	5	9	0	75
White Chocolate Macadamia	2 (0.5 oz)	80	tr	5	<5	9	0	65
Bud's Best								
Caco Creme	7 (1 oz)	140	2	6	0	21	2	110
Chocolate Chip	6 (1 oz)	140	2	6	0	19	1	65
French Vanilla	7 (1 oz)	150	2	6	0	20	2	70
Oatmeal	6 (1 oz)	130	2	5	0	20	tr	65
Cafe								
Cinnamony Twists Chocolate Chip	1 (0.5 oz)	40	0	2	0	7	0	25
Sugar Free California Almond	4 (1 oz)	110	2	4	0	17	0	60
Twists Cinnamony	1 (0.3 oz)	40	0	2	0	7	0	25
Carbolite								
Chocolate Chip	1 (1 oz)	120	4	9	11	12	4	71
Peanut Butter	1 (1 oz)	120	4	9	11	12	4	71

FOOD	PORTION	CALS	PROT	FAT	CHOL	CARB	FIBER	SOD
Shortbread	1 (1 oz)	180	4	9	2	14	5	100
Carriage Trade								
Finnish Ginger Snaps	3	60	2	7	—	21	tr	135
Carr's								
Ginger Lemon Cremes	2 (1 oz)	140	1	7	<5	19	tr	105
Cookie Lover's								
Chocolate Chip	1 (0.8 oz)	90	1	4	10	16	0	90
Creme Supremes	2 (0.9 oz)	120	1	5	0	18	1	90
Creme Supremes Mint	2 (0.9 oz)	120	1	5	0	18	1	90
Grahams	2 (1 oz)	100	2	1	0	22	1	130
Grahams Cinnamon	2 (1 oz)	110	2	1	0	24	1	130
Peanut Butter	1 (0.8 oz)	100	2	4	15	16	0	55
Shortbread	1 (0.8 oz)	120	2	7	15	13	0	70
Country Choice								
Chocolate Chip Walnut	1	100	1	4	5	16	tr	65
Double Fugde Brownie	1	90	1	3	5	16	tr	85
Ginger	1	90	1	2	5	17	tr	75
Ginger Snaps	5	120	1	5	0	19	2	85
Lemon	1	90	1	3	5	17	tr	75
Oatmeal Chocolate Chip	1	100	2	4	5	15	1	70
Oatmeal Raisin	1	100	1	3	5	16	1	70
Old Fashioned Oatmeal	1	100	2	3	5	16	1	90
Peanut Butter	1	100	2	5	5	13	tr	75
Sandwich Cremes Chocolate	1	130	1	5	0	19	0	100
Sandwich Cremes Duplex	2	130	1	5	0	19	0	115
Sandwich Cremes Ginger Lemon	2	130	1	5	0	19	0	130
Sandwich Cremes Mint Creme	2	130	1	5	0	19	0	100
Vanilla Wafers	7	120	1	5	5	19	2	100

FOOD	PORTION	CALS	PROT	FAT	CHOL	CARB	FIBER	SOD
Country Naturals								
Sandwich Cremes Vanilla	2	130	1	5	0	19	0	125
Dare								
Blueberry Cheesecake	1 (0.6 oz)	90	1	5	4	11	tr	56
Butter Shortbread	1 (0.5 oz)	63	1	4	6	7	tr	45
Butter Creme	1 (0.6 oz)	85	1	4	2	11	1	96
Carrot Cake	1 (0.6 oz)	92	1	5	3	11	tr	61
Chocolate Chip	1 (0.5 oz)	77	1	4	2	9	tr	42
Chocolate Fudge	1 (0.7 oz)	97	1	5	1	13	1	36
Cinnamon Danish	1 (0.4 oz)	47	1	2	2	7	tr	25
Coconut Creme	1 (0.7 oz)	99	1	5	1	12	tr	42
French Creme	1 (0.5 oz)	80	1	5	1	8	tr	21
Harvest From The Rain Forest	1 (0.5 oz)	70	1	4	2	7	tr	39
Key Lime Creme	1 (0.6 oz)	86	1	4	0	12	tr	69
Lemon Creme	1 (0.7 oz)	95	1	5	1	13	tr	66
Maple Leaf Creme	1 (0.6 oz)	83	1	4	0	12	tr	53
Maple Walnut Fudge	1 (0.7 oz)	99	1	5	0	13	tr	36
Milk Chocolate Fudge	1 (0.7 oz)	99	1	5	1	12	tr	32
Oatmeal Raisin	1 (0.4 oz)	59	1	3	4	8	tr	22
Social Tea	1 (0.2 oz)	26	tr	1	0	4	tr	25
Sun Maid Raisin Oatmeal	1 (0.5 oz)	52	1	3	5	8	tr	30
De Beukelaer								
Pirouline	8 (1 oz)	130	3	4	15	23	tr	50
Pirouline Viennese Wafers	1 (1 oz)	150	1	7	30	20	tr	25
Delacre								
Chocosprits	1 (0.6 oz)	90	1	5	9	11	tr	50
Marquisettes	3 (0.9 oz)	140	2	7	5	17	1	45
Roules d'Or	4 (1 oz)	180	1	8	0	19	0	35
Dunkaroos								
Chocolate Graham	1 pkg	120	1	5	0	20	–	120
Cinnamon Graham	1 pkg	130	1	5	0	21	–	75
Honey Graham	1 pkg	120	1	5	0	20	tr	100

FOOD	PORTION	CALS	PROT	FAT	CHOL	CARB	FIBER	SOD
Eddyleon								
Jelly Graham Raspberry	1 (0.9 oz)	134	1	8	2	15	tr	44
Pudding Cookies	1 (0.9 oz)	134	1	6	2	15	tr	44
Elite								
Tea Biscuits Chocolate	4	80	1	2	0	14	0	55
English Bay								
Strawberry Fruit Bar	1 (1.2 oz)	120	1	3	5	22	1	100
Falcone's								
Sorrentini	1 (1 oz)	100	2	4	10	16	2	55
Famous Amos								
Butter Shortie	1 (0.5 oz)	80	1	5	10	9	tr	65
Chocolate Chip & Pecan	4 (1 oz)	140	1	8	0	18	tr	100
Chocolate Chip Toffee	4 (1 oz)	130	1	6	0	18	0	115
Chocolate Creme Sandwich	3 (1.2 oz)	140	2	6	0	22	tr	90
Chunky Chocolate Chip	1 (0.5 oz)	70	1	4	0	9	0	80
Fat Free Fig Bar	2 (1 oz)	90	1	0	0	21	1	60
Fat Free Strawberry Fruit Bar	2 (1 oz)	90	1	0	0	22	0	50
Fig Bar	2 (1.1 oz)	120	1	3	0	22	tr	150
Oatmeal Chocolate Chip Walnut	4 (1 oz)	140	2	7	0	16	tr	120
Oatmeal Raisin	4 (1 oz)	130	2	6	5	20	tr	135
Oatmeal Macaroon Creme Sandwich	3 (1.2 oz)	160	2	7	0	23	1	—
Peanut Butter Chocolate Chunk	1 (0.5 oz)	80	1	5	0	9	tr	70
Peanut Butter Creme Sandwich	3 (1.2 oz)	160	4	8	0	19	1	115
Pecan Shortie	1 (0.5 oz)	80	1	5	0	9	tr	55
Vanilla Creme Sandwich	3 (1.2 oz)	160	2	7	0	24	0	85
Frookie								
Animal Frackers	14 (1 oz)	130	2	5	0	18	1	90

FOOD	PORTION	CALS	PROT	FAT	CHOL	CARB	FIBER	SOD
Chocolate Chip Wheat & Gluten Free	3 (1.1 oz)	140	1	5	0	23	1	100
Double Chocolate Wheat & Gluten Free	3 (1.1 oz)	130	1	4	0	23	1	105
Dream Creams Strawberry	4 (1 oz)	140	2	8	0	18	4	55
Dream Creams Vanilla	4 (1 oz)	140	2	8	0	18	4	55
Funky Monkeys Chocolate	16 (1 oz)	120	2	4	0	20	1	120
Funky Monkeys Vanilla	16 (1 oz)	120	2	4	0	20	1	120
Graham Cinnamon	2 (1 oz)	100	2	3	0	17	1	105
Graham Honey	2 (1 oz)	110	2	3	0	18	1	120
Lemon Wafers	8 (1 oz)	110	2	0	0	26	tr	130
Old Fashioned Ginger Snaps	8 (1 oz)	120	1	2	0	24	tr	110
Organic Chocolate Chip	3 (1.1 oz)	150	2	7	0	20	1	115
Organic Double Chocolate Chip	3 (1.1 oz)	140	2	6	0	20	1	95
Organic Iced Lemon	3 (1.3 oz)	165	2	6	0	27	0	115
Organic Oatmeal Raisin	3 (1.1 oz)	140	2	5	0	22	1	110
Peanut Butter Chunk Wheat & Gluten Free	3 (1.1 oz)	140	3	5	0	21	0	140
Sandwich Chocolate	2 (0.7 oz)	100	1	4	0	14	1	60
Sandwich Lemon	2 (0.7 oz)	100	1	4	0	14	1	60
Sandwich Peanut Butter	2 (0.7 oz)	100	1	4	0	14	1	60
Sandwich Vanilla	2 (0.7 oz)	100	1	4	0	14	1	60
Shortbread	5 (1 oz)	130	2	5	15	20	tr	95
Vanilla Wafers	8 (1 oz)	110	2	0	0	26	0	120
General Henry								
Fruit Bars Apple	1 (0.6 oz)	60	1	1	0	13	tr	70

FOOD	PORTION	CALS	PROT	FAT	CHOL	CARB	FIBER	SOD
Fruit Bars Blueberry	1 (0.6 oz)	60	1	1	0	12	tr	75
Fruit Bars Fig	1 (0.6 oz)	60	1	1	0	12	tr	70
Girl Scout								
Apple Cinnamon Reduced Fat	3 (1 oz)	120	2	5	0	18	tr	140
Lemon Drops	3 (1.2 oz)	160	2	8	0	20	0	150
Samoas	2 (1 oz)	160	2	9	0	17	2	45
Striped Chocolate Chip	3 (1.2 oz)	180	2	10	0	20	tr	100
Tagalongs	2 (0.9 oz)	150	3	10	0	13	2	85
Thin Mints	4 (1 oz)	140	1	8	0	18	tr	80
Trefoils	5 (1.1 oz)	160	2	8	0	20	1	90
Glenny's								
Soy Fudgies All Flavors	3	70	3	2	0	14	1	10
Godiva								
Biscotti Dipped In Milk Chocolate	1 (0.9 oz)	120	2	6	20	15	0	45
Gol D Lite								
Low Carb Pizzelle	1 (0.3 oz)	46	1	2	0	6	1	0
Golden Grahams Treats								
Chocolate Chunk	1 bar (0.8 oz)	90	1	3	0	17	0	110
Honey Graham	1 bar (0.8 oz)	90	1	2	0	17	0	120
King Size Chocolate Chunk	1 bar (1.6 oz)	190	2	5	0	35	1	220
King Size Honey Graham	1 bar (1.6 oz)	180	1	4	0	36	1	240
Golightly								
Fabulous Tastes Caramel Dulce De Leche	4	100	2	6	0	14	5	65
Goody Man								
Marshmallow Crispy Squares	1 (1.17 oz)	130	1	3	0	24	0	170
Gourmet								
Chocolate Chip	2 (1.1 oz)	160	2	9	15	19	1	85
Lemon Creme	2 (1.4 oz)	210	1	10	0	27	0	60
Oatmeal Raisin	2 (0.9 oz)	120	2	6	15	15	1	105
Peanut Butter Chip	2 (1 oz)	150	3	8	10	17	tr	135
Raspberry Center	2 (1.1 oz)	140	1	5	10	21	tr	60

FOOD	PORTION	CALS	PROT	FAT	CHOL	CARB	FIBER	SOD
Grandma's								
Chocolate Chip	1 (1.4 oz)	190	2	9	0	25	tr	135
Fudge Chocolate Chip	1 (1.4 oz)	170	1	7	<5	26	1	160
Fudge Sandwich	3	180	2	5	0	31	tr	200
Fudge Vanilla Sandwich	3	120	1	4	0	21	tr	130
Mini Fudge	9	150	2	7	0	21	1	180
Mini Peanut Butter	9	150	2	7	0	21	1	140
Mini Vanilla	9	150	2	7	<5	22	tr	85
Oatmeal Raisin	1 (1.4 oz)	160	1	6	5	26	1	250
Old Time Molasses	1 (1.4 oz)	160	2	4	<5	29	tr	230
Peanut Butter	1 (1.4 oz)	190	2	9	5	22	1	200
Peanut Butter Chocolate Chip	1 (1.4 oz)	190	4	9	<5	23	1	170
Peanut Butter Sandwich	5	210	3	10	0	28	1	200
Rich N'Chewy	1 pkg	270	2	12	10	39	1	130
Vanilla Sandwich	3	180	2	5	0	32	tr	160
Vanilla Sandwich	5	210	2	10	5	30	tr	125
Granny Oats								
Low Carb Oatmeal	4	98	1	6	25	10	3	140
Heavenly								
Meringues All Flavors Sugar Free Fat Free	1	0	2	0	0	1	0	0
Hellema								
Almond	1 pkg (0.6 oz)	90	1	5	0	9	tr	35
Hershey's								
Cripsy Rice Snacks Peanut Butter	1 (0.6 oz)	70	1	3	0	10	tr	130
Jacques Gourmet								
Palmier Cinnamon	3 (1 oz)	140	1	9	0	15	0	65
Palmier Vanilla	3 (1 oz)	140	1	9	0	15	0	65
Joseph's								
Almond Sugar Free	2 (0.9 oz)	100	1	5	0	14	0	20

FOOD	PORTION	CALS	PROT	FAT	CHOL	CARB	FIBER	SOD
Chocolate Chip Sugar Free	2 (0.9 oz)	100	1	5	0	15	0	40
Chocolate Walnut Sugar Free	2 (0.9 oz)	100	1	6	0	14	1	40
Coconut Sugar Free	2 (0.9 oz)	105	1	5	0	14	0	40
Lemon Sugar Free	2 (0.9 oz)	95	1	4	0	15	0	30
Oatmeal Raisin Sugar Free	2 (0.9 oz)	100	2	5	0	15	0	40
Peanut Butter Sugar Free	2 (0.9 oz)	95	2	5	0	13	1	40
Pecan Shortbread Sugar Free	2 (0.9 oz)	100	1	5	0	14	0	40
Karen's								
Fabulous Tastes Heavenly Chocolate Chip	4	90	2	5	0	16	5	65
Fabulous Tastes Luscious Raspberry Almond	4	110	3	6	0	15	5	65
Fabulous Tastes Pecan Vanilla Pralines	4	120	2	8	0	15	6	75
Kedem								
Tea Biscuits Chocolate	2	32	1	1	0	6	tr	29
Tea Biscuits Orange	2	32	1	1	0	6	tr	29
Keebler								
Animal Crackers Chocolate Chip	7 (1 oz)	130	2	5	0	22	0	120
Animal Crackers Ernie's	1 box	250	<4	9	0	41	1	290
Animal Crackers Iced	6 (1.1 oz)	150	2	5	0	24	0	110
Animal Crackers Sprinkled	6 (1.1 oz)	150	<2	5	0	24	0	105
Butter	5 (1.1 oz)	150	<2	6	10	22	tr	170
Chips Deluxe	1 (0.5 oz)	80	tr	5	0	9	tr	50
Chips Deluxe Chocolate Lovers	1 (0.6 oz)	90	tr	5	5	11	0	80

FOOD	PORTION	CALS	PROT	FAT	CHOL	CARB	FIBER	SOD
Chips Deluxe Coconut	1 (0.5 oz)	80	tr	5	0	10	tr	50
Chips Deluxe Rainbow	1 (0.6 oz)	80	tr	4	<5	10	tr	45
Chips Deluxe Soft 'n Chewy	1 (0.6 oz)	80	tr	4	5	11	0	60
Chips Deluxe w/ Peanut Butter Cups	1 (0.6 oz)	90	tr	5	0	9	0	45
Classic Collection Chocolate Fudge Creme	1 (0.6 oz)	80	tr	4	0	12	0	75
Classic Collection French Vanilla Creme	1 (0.6 oz)	80	tr	4	0	12	0	65
Cookie Stix Butter	5 (1.2 oz)	160	<2	6	10	22	1	150
Cookie Stix Chocolate Chip	4 (0.9 oz)	130	<2	5	5	19	tr	100
Cookie Stix Rainbow	5 (1.2 oz)	150	<2	6	5	23	tr	110
Danish Wedding	4 (0.9 oz)	120	tr	5	0	20	tr	80
Droxies	3 (1.1 oz)	140	<2	6	0	21	tr	95
Droxies Reduced Fat	3 (1.1 oz)	140	<2	5	0	23	1	150
E.L. Fudge Butter w/ Fudge Filling	2 (0.9 oz)	120	tr	6	<5	17	tr	70
E.L. Fudge Fudge w/ Fudge Filling	2 (0.9 oz)	120	<2	6	0	17	tr	70
E.L. Fudge w/ Peanut Butter Filling	2 (0.9 oz)	120	<2	6	0	16	tr	150
Fudge Shoppe Deluxe Grahams	3 (1 oz)	140	tr	7	0	19	tr	105
Fudge Shoppe Double Fudge 'n Caramel	2 (1 oz)	140	tr	7	0	20	tr	65
Fudge Shoppe Fudge Sticks	3 (1 oz)	150	tr	8	0	20	tr	55

FOOD	PORTION	CALS	PROT	FAT	CHOL	CARB	FIBER	SOD
Fudge Shoppe Fudge Sticks Peanut Butter	3 (1 oz)	150	<2	8	0	18	tr	45
Fudge Shoppe Fudge Stripes	3 (1.1 oz)	160	tr	8	0	21	tr	140
Fudge Shoppe Fudge Stripes Reduced Fat	3 (1 oz)	140	tr	5	0	21	0	120
Fudge Shoppe Grasshoppers	4 (1 oz)	150	tr	7	0	20	tr	70
Fudge Shoppe S'mores	3 (1.2 oz)	160	tr	8	0	22	tr	95
Ginger Snaps	5 (1.1 oz)	150	<2	6	0	24	0	120
Golden Fruit Cranberry	1 (0.7 oz)	80	tr	2	0	14	tr	55
Golden Fruit Raisin	1 (0.7 oz)	80	tr	2	0	15	tr	50
Graham Cinnamon Crisp	8 (1 oz)	140	2	5	0	22	1	170
Graham Cinnamon Crisp Low Fat	8 (1 oz)	110	2	2	0	24	1	190
Graham Honey	8 (1.1 oz)	140	2	4	0	23	0	140
Graham Honey Low Fat	8 (1.1 oz)	120	2	2	0	26	1	210
Graham Original	8 (1 oz)	130	2	3	0	23	tr	135
Lemon Coolers	5 (1 oz)	140	tr	6	0	21	tr	100
Oatmeal Country Style	2 (0.8 oz)	120	<2	5	0	17	tr	115
Sandies Almond Shortbread	1 (0.5 oz)	80	tr	5	5	9	0	50
Sandies Pecan Shortbread	1 (0.5 oz)	80	tr	5	<5	9	tr	75
Sandies Simply Shortbread	1 (0.5 oz)	80	tr	5	10	9	0	70
Snack Size Chips Deluxe	1 pkg (2 oz)	300	3	16	5	36	tr	170
Snack Size Chips Deluxe Chocolate Lovers	1 pkg (2 oz)	280	3	15	20	36	1	170
Snack Size Mini Fudge Stripes	1 pkg (2 oz)	280	3	14	0	38	2	150

FOOD	PORTION	CALS	PROT	FAT	CHOL	CARB	FIBER	SOD
Snack Size Rainbow Chips Deluxe	1 pkg (2 oz)	290	3	16	5	36	1	170
Snack Size Sandies w/ Pecans	1 pkg (2 oz)	300	3	17	10	33	1	190
Snackin' Grahams Cinnamon	21 (1 oz)	130	<2	3	0	23	1	210
Snackin' Grahams Honey	23 (1 oz)	130	<2	4	0	22	tr	120
Soft Batch Chocolate Chip	1 (0.6 oz)	80	tr	4	0	10	tr	70
Soft Batch Homestyle Chocolate Chunk	1 (0.9 oz)	130	1	7	0	17	1	80
Soft Batch Homestyle Double Chocolate	1 (0.9 oz)	130	1	7	0	17	1	90
Soft Batch Homestyle Oatmeal Raisin	1 (0.9 oz)	130	1	5	0	20	tr	150
Soft Batch Oatmeal Raisin	1 (0.5 oz)	70	tr	3	0	10	tr	65
Sugar Wafers Creme	3 (0.9 oz)	130	tr	6	0	18	tr	20
Sugar Wafers Lemon	3 (0.9 oz)	130	tr	6	0	19	0	20
Sugar Wafers Peanut Butter	4 (1.1 oz)	170	<3	9	0	19	1	75
Vanilla Wafers	8 (1.1 oz)	150	tr	7	0	20	tr	120
Vanilla Wafers Reduced Fat	8 (1.1 oz)	130	<2	4	0	25	tr	140
Vienna Fingers	2 (1 oz)	140	2	6	0	21	tr	105
Vienna Fingers Lemon	2 (1 oz)	140	2	6	0	21	0	90
Keto								
Low Carb Biscotti Chocolate	1 (1.2 oz)	157	13	9	200	6	3	80
Low Carb Biscotti Lemon Nut	1 (1.2 oz)	157	13	9	200	6	3	80
Low Carb Biscotti Vanilla Almond	1 (1.2 oz)	157	13	9	200	6	3	80

FOOD	PORTION	CALS	PROT	FAT	CHOL	CARB	FIBER	SOD
Knott's Berry Farm								
Shortbread Apricot	3 (1 oz)	120	2	5	4	17	0	70
Shortbread Boysenberry	3 (1 oz)	120	2	5	4	17	0	60
Shortbread Raspberry	3 (1 oz)	120	2	5	4	17	0	60
La Choy								
Fortune	4 (1 oz)	112	2	tr	0	26	1	11
La Dolce Vita								
Biscotti Chocolate Passion	1 (1.2 oz)	130	2	8	45	11	1	135
Landies Candies								
Sugar Free Dark Royal Pecan Shortbread	2	167	1	9	0	16	1	27
Sugar Free Milk Chocolate Chip	2	173	4	11	<5	17	tr	91
Sugar Free Milk Chocolate Peanut Butter	2	171	4	8	<5	17	tr	91
Sugar Free White Chocolate Lemon	2	177	3	11	<5	20	0	67
Larzaroni								
Arancelli	8 (1 oz)	160	3	8	8	19	tr	36
Calypso	3 (1 oz)	150	2	8	0	18	1	30
Limonelli	5 (1 oz)	140	2	8	5	16	2	30
Malaika	5 (1 oz)	158	3	9	17	17	1	36
Nanette	4 (1.2 oz)	170	3	9	<5	20	tr	30
Okla	3 (1 oz)	186	3	10	6	21	1	43
Oskar	10 (1 oz)	150	2	9	0	18	tr	10
Samba	5 (1 oz)	160	3	10	0	14	2	150
Velieri	3 (0.9 oz)	120	2	5	10	17	tr	60
Linden's								
Lemon	1 (1 oz)	120	–	5	10	–	–	135
Little Debbie								
Apple Flips	1 (1.2 oz)	150	1	5	5	24	tr	115
Marshmallow Crispy Bar	1 (1.3 oz)	140	1	4	0	26	0	170
Low Carb Creations								
Chocolate Chip	1 (1 oz)	140	4	10	25	11	1	40

FOOD	PORTION	CALS	PROT	FAT	CHOL	CARB	FIBER	SOD
Coconut	1 (1 oz)	140	5	10	30	9	1	50
Lemon	1 (1 oz)	140	5	11	30	9	1	50
Snickerdoodle	1 (1 oz)	140	5	11	30	9	1	50
LU								
Chocolatier	3 (1 oz)	150	1	9	0	17	1	5
Le Bastogne	2 (0.8 oz)	120	1	5	0	18	0	50
Le Dore	4 (1 oz)	140	2	6	<5	21	0	55
Le Fondant	4 (1.1 oz)	170	1	10	0	19	1	5
Le Palmier	4 (1.2 oz)	180	2	10	0	20	tr	140
Le Petit Beurre	4 (1.2 oz)	150	3	4	10	26	tr	160
Le Petit Ecolier Dark Chocolate	2 (0.9 oz)	130	2	6	<5	17	1	50
Le Petit Ecolier Extra Dark Chocolate	2	120	2	7	<5	15	2	50
Le Petit Ecolier Hazelnut Milk Chocolate	2 (0.9 oz)	130	2	7	5	16	0	55
Le Petit Ecolier Milk Chocolate	2 (0.9 oz)	130	1	6	5	17	tr	55
Le Petit Fruit Strawberry	5 (1.2 oz)	110	1	1	30	26	0	10
Le Raisin Dore	4 (1.2 oz)	160	2	7	20	23	tr	130
Le Truffe Coconut	4 (1.2 oz)	190	1	12	0	17	1	15
Le Truffe Praline Chocolate	4 (1.2 oz)	170	2	9	0	20	2	15
Pim's Orange	2 (0.9 oz)	90	1	3	10	16	tr	25
Pim's Raspberry	2 (0.9 oz)	90	1	3	5	17	tr	25
Pim's Sensation Bar Chocolate	1	110	1	6	0	13	tr	30
Pim's Sensation Bar Hazelnut	1	110	1	6	0	13	tr	30
M&M's								
Cookies & Milky Way	1 bar (1.20 oz)	180	2	11	0	21	1	95
Mamma Says'								
Biscotti Almond Pistachio	1 (0.5 oz)	50	1	3	7	7	1	26
Biscotti Chocolate Macadamia	1 (0.5 oz)	45	1	3	10	5	1	23

FOOD	PORTION	CALS	PROT	FAT	CHOL	CARB	FIBER	SOD
Biscotti Orange Citrine	1 (0.5 oz)	60	2	2	10	8	1	40
Mauna Loa								
Macadamia Nut Chocolate Chip	2	130	2	6	5	18	1	55
Macadamia Nut Hawaiian Crunch	2	150	2	8	10	15	1	30
Macadamia Nut White Chocolate Chip	2	130	2	6	6	18	1	55
Milk Lunch Brand								
New England Biscuits	4 (1.1 oz)	140	2	5	<5	24	1	220
Miss Meringue								
Minis Chocolate Raspberry	13 (1 oz)	80	1	0	0	20	0	15
Minis Chocolate Chip	13 (1 oz)	120	2	2	0	27	1	20
Minis Mint Chocolate Chip	13 (1 oz)	120	2	2	0	26	1	20
Minis Mochaccino	13 (1 oz)	80	1	0	0	20	0	15
Minis Orange	13 (1 oz)	80	1	0	0	20	0	15
Minis Rainbow Vanilla	13 (1 oz)	110	1	0	0	27	0	25
Minis Toasted Coconut	13 (1 oz)	90	1	2	0	19	0	15
Minis Very Chocolate	13 (1 oz)	80	1	0	0	20	0	15
Minis Very Minty	13 (1 oz)	80	1	0	0	20	0	15
Minis Very Vanilla	13 (1 oz)	80	1	0	0	20	0	15
MoonPie								
Chocolate	1 (2.75 oz)	330	4	10	0	56	0	256
Mini Banana	1 (1.2 oz)	152	3	5	0	26	0	120
Mini Chocolate	1 (1.2 oz)	152	3	5	0	26	0	120
Mini Vanilla	1 (1.2 oz)	152	3	5	0	26	0	120
Mother's								
Almond Shortbread	3	180	2	11	0	19	1	115
Checkerboard Wafers	8	150	1	8	0	20	1	40
Chocolate Chip	2	160	2	8	10	20	0	105

FOOD	PORTION	CALS	PROT	FAT	CHOL	CARB	FIBER	SOD
Chocolate Chip Angel	3	180	2	9	0	21	1	70
Chocolate Chip Parade	4	130	1	5	0	19	1	100
Circus Animals	6	140	1	6	0	20	0	55
Classic Assortments	2	140	1	7	0	18	1	105
Cocadas	5	150	2	7	5	20	2	140
Cookie Parade	4	140	1	7	0	18	2	95
Dinosaur Grrrahams	2	130	2	3	0	24	2	130
Double Fudge	2	180	2	9	0	24	2	110
English Tea	2	180	2	7	0	26	1	100
Flaky Flix Fudge	2	140	1	7	0	17	2	50
Flaky Flix Vanilla	2	140	1	8	0	17	1	40
Gaucho Peanut Butter	2	190	3	10	0	22	2	200
Iced Oatmeal	2	130	2	4	0	22	1	160
Iced Raisin	2	180	1	8	0	24	1	110
Macaroon	2	150	1	8	0	18	2	80
Marias	3	170	2	6	5	28	1	150
MLB Double Header Duplex	3	170	2	8	5	23	1	130
Oatmeal	2	110	1	5	0	17	1	150
Oatmeal Chocolate Chip	2	120	2	5	0	19	1	140
Oatmeal Raisin	5	150	2	7	5	20	2	125
Oatmeal Walnut Chocolate Chip	2	130	2	6	0	17	1	135
Rainbow Wafers	8	150	1	8	0	20	1	40
Striped Shortbread	3	170	2	8	0	22	1	75
Sugar	2	140	1	6	0	19	1	75
Taffy	2	180	2	8	0	25	2	160
Triplet Assortment	2	140	1	7	0	18	1	112
Vanilla Wafers	6	150	2	6	4	24	1	85
Wallops Boysenberry	1	80	1	2	0	15	1	40
Wallops Honey Crust Fig	1	80	1	2	0	15	0	55

FOOD	PORTION	CALS	PROT	FAT	CHOL	CARB	FIBER	SOD
Wallops Honey Graham Fig	1	80	1	2	0	15	1	55
Wallops Mixed Berry	1	80	1	2	0	15	1	40
Wallops Peach Apricot	1	80	1	2	0	15	1	40
Wallops Raspberry	1	80	1	2	0	15	1	40
Wallops Strawberry	1	80	1	2	0	15	1	40
Walnut Fudge	2	130	1	7	0	16	1	90
Zoo Pals	14	140	2	5	0	23	1	120
Mrs. Alison's								
Coconut Bar	2 (1 oz)	130	2	6	0	19	0	85
Creme Wafers	5 (1.1 oz)	170	1	10	0	21	tr	35
Duplex Sandwich	3 (1 oz)	130	1	5	0	20	0	105
Fudge Fingers	3 (1 oz)	160	tr	10	0	19	0	20
Ginger Snaps	4 (1 oz)	130	2	3	<2	23	tr	170
Jelly Tops	5 (1 oz)	140	2	7	0	18	0	45
Lemon Creme	3 (1 oz)	130	1	5	0	21	0	115
Macaroons	2 (1 oz)	140	2	7	0	18	tr	95
Pecan	2 (1 oz)	140	2	7	0	19	0	75
Shortbread	5 (1 oz)	120	2	5	0	19	0	100
Vanilla Sandwich	3 (1 oz)	130	1	5	0	21	0	115
Murray's								
Sugar Free Double Fudge	3 (1.2 oz)	140	2	6	0	23	3	110
Sugar Free Ginger Snap	6 (1 oz)	110	2	4	0	21	tr	100
Sugar Free Oatmeal	6 (1.1 oz)	120	2	4	0	23	1	130
Sugar Free Peanut Butter	6 (1 oz)	130	3	7	0	17	1	85
Sugar Free Vanilla Sandwich Creme	3 (1 oz)	120	1	5	0	21	2	65
Sugar Free Vanilla Wafers	9 (1.1 oz)	120	2	4	0	23	tr	85
Nabisco								
Barnum's Animal Crackers	10 (1 oz)	130	2	4	0	23	tr	150

FOOD	PORTION	CALS	PROT	FAT	CHOL	CARB	FIBER	SOD
Barnum's Animal Crackers Chocolate	10 (1 oz)	130	2	4	0	23	1	160
Biscos Sugar Wafers	8 (1 oz)	140	tr	6	0	21	0	40
Cafe Cremes Cappuccino	2 (1.1 oz)	160	1	8	0	22	0	130
Cafe Cremes Vanilla	2 (1.1 oz)	160	1	7	0	22	0	130
Cafe Cremes Vanilla Fudge	2 (1.1 oz)	200	2	10	0	27	tr	140
Cameo	2 (1 oz)	130	1	5	0	21	0	105
Chips Ahoy!	3 (1.1 oz)	160	2	8	0	21	1	105
Chips Ahoy! Chewy	3 (1.3 oz)	170	1	8	0	24	tr	125
Chips Ahoy! Chunky	1 (0.5 oz)	80	tr	4	5	10	0	35
Chips Ahoy! Munch Size	6 (1.1 oz)	160	2	8	0	21	1	150
Chips Ahoy! Reduced Fat	3 (1.1 oz)	140	2	5	0	22	tr	150
Family Favorites Iced Oatmeal	1 (0.6 oz)	80	1	3	0	12	0	55
Family Favorites Oatmeal	1 (0.6 oz)	80	1	3	0	12	0	65
Famous Chocolate Wafers	5 (1.1 oz)	140	2	4	<5	24	1	230
Grahams	4 (1 oz)	120	2	3	0	22	1	180
Honey Maid Chocolate	8 (1 oz)	120	2	3	0	22	1	170
Honey Maid Cinnamon Grahams	8 (1 oz)	120	2	3	0	23	tr	180
Honey Maid Honey Grahams	8 (1 oz)	120	2	3	0	22	1	180
Honey Maid Low Fat Cinnamon Grahams	8 (1 oz)	110	2	2	0	23	tr	170
Honey Maid Low Fat Grahams	8 (1 oz)	110	2	2	0	23	tr	200

FOOD	PORTION	CALS	PROT	FAT	CHOL	CARB	FIBER	SOD
Honey Maid Oatmeal Crunch	8 (1 oz)	120	2	3	0	22	1	140
Lorna Doone	4 (1 oz)	140	2	7	5	19	tr	130
Mallomars	2	120	1	5	0	17	tr	35
Marshmallow Twirls	1 (1 oz)	130	1	6	0	20	0	75
Mystic Mint	1 (0.5 oz)	90	1	5	0	11	0	65
National Arrowroot	1 (5 g)	20	0	1	–	4	0	15
Newton Fat Free Fig	2 (1 oz)	90	1	0	0	22	1	115
Newtons Fig	2 (1.1 oz)	110	1	3	0	22	1	125
Newtons Fat Free Apple	2 (1 oz)	90	1	0	0	21	tr	65
Newtons Fat Free Cobblers Apple Cinnamon	1 (0.8 oz)	70	1	0	0	17	tr	40
Newtons Fat Free Cobblers Peach Apricot	1 (0.8 oz)	70	1	0	0	17	0	55
Newtons Fat Free Cranberry	2 (1 oz)	100	1	0	0	22	tr	95
Newtons Fat Free Raspberry	2 (1 oz)	100	1	0	0	23	tr	115
Newtons Fat Free Strawberry	2 (1 oz)	90	1	0	0	21	0	95
Nilla Wafers	8 (1.1 oz)	140	1	5	<5	24	0	100
Nilla Wafers Chocolate Reduced Fat	8 (1 oz)	110	2	2	0	23	tr	120
Nilla Wafers Reduced Fat	8 (1 oz)	120	1	2	0	24	0	105
Nutter Butter Bites	10 (1 oz)	150	3	7	<5	20	1	125
Nutter Butter Chocolate Peanut Butter Sandwich	2 (1 oz)	130	2	5	0	19	1	140
Nutter Butter Peanut Butter Sandwich	2 (1 oz)	130	2	6	<5	19	tr	110

FOOD	PORTION	CALS	PROT	FAT	CHOL	CARB	FIBER	SOD
Old Fashioned Ginger Snaps	4 (1 oz)	120	1	3	0	22	tr	230
Oreo	3 (1.2 oz)	160	1	7	0	23	1	220
Oreo Double Stuff	2 (1 oz)	140	1	7	0	19	tr	150
Oreo Mini	1 pkg (0.5 oz)	65	tr	3	0	10	1	75
Oreo Reduced Fat	3 (1.1 oz)	130	–	4	0	25	1	190
Oreo Halloween	2 (1 oz)	140	1	7	0	19	tr	115
Pecanz	1 (0.5 oz)	90	1	5	<5	9	0	50
Pinwheels Chocolate Marshmallow	1 (1 oz)	130	1	5	0	21	tr	35
Rugrats Chocolate Frosted	8 (1.1 oz)	150	1	5	0	24	tr	110
Rugrats Vanilla Frosted	8 (1.1 oz)	150	1	6	0	24	tr	105
Social Tea	6 (1 oz)	120	2	4	5	20	tr	115
Sweet Crispers Chocolate	18 (1.1 oz)	130	2	3	0	25	1	190
Sweet Crispers Chocolate Chip	18 (1.1 oz)	130	2	3	0	23	tr	160
Teddy Grahams Chocolate	24 (1 oz)	130	2	5	0	22	1	170
Teddy Grahams Chocolately Chip	24 (1 oz)	130	2	5	0	23	tr	135
Teddy Grahams Cinnamon	24 (1 oz)	130	2	4	0	23	1	150
Teddy Grahams Honey	24 (1 oz)	130	2	4	0	23	tr	150
Natural Ovens								
Carob Chip	1	90	2	4	0	16	3	15
Chocolate Raspberry	1	120	2	5	0	19	3	70
Oatmeal Raisin	1	90	3	3	0	15	3	15
Nestle								
Flipz Crunchy Graham White Fudge Chocolate	8 (1 oz)	140	2	6	0	19	0	85
Nonni's								
Biscotti Cioccalati	1 (1 oz)	130	2	5	5	19	1	50

FOOD	PORTION	CALS	PROT	FAT	CHOL	CARB	FIBER	SOD
Biscotti Decadence	1 (1.1 oz)	130	2	5	25	19	1	65
Biscotti Original	1 (1 oz)	100	2	4	25	15	1	65
Biscotti Paradiso	1 (1.1 oz)	130	2	6	5	19	0	60
Old Brussels								
Ginger Crisps	2 (0.9 oz)	140	2	4	0	23	2	115
Olde World								
Pizzelle Almond	3 (1 oz)	90	2	4	45	12	0	15
Pizzelle Anise	3 (1 oz)	90	2	4	45	12	0	15
Pizzelle Chocolate	3 (1 oz)	100	2	5	45	11	0	15
Pizzelle Lemon	3 (1 oz)	90	2	4	45	12	0	15
Pizzelle Vanilla	3 (1 oz)	90	2	4	45	12	0	15
Pally								
Butter	5 (1 oz)	140	3	3	1	23	1	170
Carnival	5 (1 oz)	130	2	3	0	24	1	130
Cinnamon Biscuit	5 (1 oz)	130	2	3	0	23	0	130
Mariel Biscuit	6 (1 oz)	150	3	4	0	23	1	140
Tea Biscuits	5 (1 oz)	150	2	4	0	23	1	170
Pamela's								
Pecan Shortbread Rice Flour	1 (0.8 oz)	130	tr	8	20	15	tr	65
Parmalat								
Grisbi Lemon	1 (0.6 oz)	90	1	6	5	9	1	0
Peek Freans								
Arrowroot	4 (1.2 oz)	150	2	5	0	26	1	80
Assorted Creme	1 (1 oz)	130	1	6	<5	19	0	50
Dream Puffs	2 (0.9 oz)	110	tr	4	0	18	0	50
Fruit Creme	2 (0.9 oz)	130	1	5	0	20	0	35
Ginger Crisp	4 (1.2 oz)	150	2	4	0	28	tr	65
Nice	4 (1.2 oz)	160	2	6	0	25	1	100
Petit Beret Creme Caramel	2 (0.8 oz)	110	tr	5	0	15	tr	120
Petit Beret Fudge Truffle	2 (0.8 oz)	110	tr	5	0	15	tr	100
Petit Beurre	4 (1 oz)	130	2	4	tr	22	tr	115
Rich Tea	4 (1.2 oz)	160	2	5	0	25	tr	150
Shortcake	2 (0.9 oz)	140	1	7	20	18	0	70
Traditional Oatmeal	1 (0.7 oz)	90	1	3	0	15	tr	100
Tropical Cremes Calypso Lime	2 (0.9 oz)	130	1	5	0	20	0	15

FOOD	PORTION	CALS	PROT	FAT	CHOL	CARB	FIBER	SOD
Pepperidge Farm								
Brussels	2	100	1	5	<5	13	tr	55
Chocolate Chunk Minis Nantucket	1 pkg (1.75 oz)	260	tr	13	10	34	0	115
Chocolate Chunk Soft Baked	1	140	1	5	<5	22	1	65
Goldfish Grahams Cinnamon	1 pkg (1.75 oz)	240	2	10	5	37	2	220
Spritzers Cool Key Lime	6 (1.1 oz)	140	1	7	<5	21	0	60
Spritzers Ripe Red Raspberry	5 (1.1 oz)	140	1	7	<5	21	0	60
Spritzers Zesty Lemon	5 (1.1 oz)	140	1	7	<5	21	0	60
Pure De-Lite								
High Protein Chocolate Fudge	1 (2.2 oz)	210	18	8	10	29	5	260
High Protein Peanut Butter Crunch	1 (2.2 oz)	210	18	8	5	28	5	300
Ralston								
Animal	12 (0.9 oz)	130	2	3	—	22	—	80
Chocolate Graham	2 (0.9 oz)	130	2	3	—	24	1	120
Cinnamon Grahams	2 (0.9 oz)	130	1	5	—	19	tr	85
Cinnamon Grahams Low Fat	2 (0.9 oz)	110	2	2	0	22	1	120
Fig Bars	2 (1.2 oz)	120	tr	3	—	23	1	55
Vanilla Wafers	7 (1.1 oz)	150	1	6	—	22	1	115
Real Torino								
Lady Fingers	3 (1 oz)	110	2	1	5	23	0	70
Reko								
Pizzelle Maple	5 (1 oz)	150	3	6	15	20	0	20
Pizzelle Vanilla	1 (6 g)	30	1	1	3	4	0	4
Royal								
Apple Bars	1 (1.1 oz)	100	1	2	0	21	1	65
Apple Cake	1 (1.1 oz)	110	1	3	0	19	1	50
Brownie Rounds	1 (1.1 oz)	130	1	6	0	19	0	135
Chocolate Chip	1 (1.1 oz)	140	1	6	0	20	1	120
Devilfood	1 (1 oz)	110	1	5	0	17	0	110
Fig Bars	1 (1.1 oz)	100	1	2	0	20	1	65
Oatmeal	1 (1.1 oz)	130	2	6	0	19	1	140

FOOD	PORTION	CALS	PROT	FAT	CHOL	CARB	FIBER	SOD
Raisin	1 (1 oz)	110	1	5	0	17	0	115
Strawberry Bars	1 (1.1 oz)	100	1	2	0	20	1	65
Salerno								
Mini Butter	25 (1 oz)	180	2	6	15	20	tr	125
Mini Dinosaur Chocolate Graham	16 (1.1 oz)	140	2	5	0	22	1	125
Scotter Pie	1 (1.2 oz)	140	1	5	0	23	0	80
Santa Fe Farms								
Chocolate Chocolate Chip Fat Free	2 (1 oz)	60	2	0	0	16	3	90
Chocolate Mint Fat Free	2 (1 oz)	60	2	0	0	16	3	90
Ginger Fat Free	2 (1 oz)	70	2	0	0	17	2	95
Sargento								
MooTown Snackers Honey Graham Sticks & Vanilla Creme w/ Sprinkles	1 pkg (1 oz)	140	2	7	0	17	0	50
MooTown Snackers Vanilla Sticks & Chocolate Fudge Creme	1 pkg (1 oz)	130	1	6	0	18	tr	50
Savion								
Chocolate Biscuits	5 (1 oz)	120	2	3	0	22	0	45
Tea Biscuits	5 (1 oz)	120	2	3	0	22	0	80
Tea Biscuits Vanilla	5 (1 oz)	120	2	3	0	22	0	80
Scotto's								
Biscotti Fat Free French Vanilla	4 (1 oz)	80	2	0	0	18	0	25
Season								
Hamantashen Poppy	1 (1 oz)	150	1	7	7	20	1	60
Simple Pleasures								
Almond	1 (0.3 oz)	37	1	2	0	5	tr	9
Cinnamon Snaps	1 (0.2 oz)	31	1	1	0	6	tr	27
Digestive	1 (0.3 oz)	46	1	2	0	6	tr	34
Encore Tea Cookie	1 (0.2 oz)	29	tr	1	0	6	tr	32
Lemon Social Tea	1 (0.2 oz)	29	tr	1	0	6	tr	32
Oatmeal	1 (0.5 oz)	74	1	3	0	5	1	–

FOOD	PORTION	CALS	PROT	FAT	CHOL	CARB	FIBER	SOD
Spice Snaps	1 (0.3 oz)	34	1	1	0	6	tr	56
Sugar	1 (0.4 oz)	45	1	2	3	7	tr	–
SnackWell's								
Creme Sandwich	1 pkg (1.7 oz)	210	2	5	0	38	tr	230
Mint Creme	2	110	1	4	0	19	tr	70
Sugar Free Chocolate Chip	3 (1.2 oz)	150	2	8	<5	23	tr	160
Sugar Free Oatmeal	1 (0.8 oz)	90	1	3	0	17	tr	80
Soybite								
All Flavors	1	79	5	5	0	7	1	3
Stella D'Oro								
Lady Stella	3	130	1	5	5	20	tr	55
Stieffenhofer								
Choco Minis	4 (1 oz)	160	1	8	15	19	1	40
Snaky	3 (1 oz)	160	2	8	0	19	0	20
Streit's								
Wafers	3 (1 oz)	160	1	9	0	19	1	35
Suissette								
Swiss Chocolate Hearts	4 (1 oz)	170	2	10	5	17	–	40
Swiss Delight	4 (1 oz)	160	2	9	5	19	–	35
Swiss Praline	4 (1 oz)	150	1	9	15	17	1	15
Sunshine								
Vienna Fingers Reduced Fat	2 (1 oz)	130	1	5	0	22	tr	105
Super Chip								
Chocolate Chip	2 (0.9 oz)	100	1	7	–	10	3	170
Sweet'N Low								
Sugar Free Amaretto Biscotti	4 (1 oz)	120	2	6	10	17	tr	180
Sugar Free Chocolate Chip	4 (1 oz)	135	2	8	10	17	tr	35
Sugar Free Cinnamon Graham	7 (1 oz)	120	2	6	15	19	tr	90
Sugar Free Morning Crunch Bars	2 (1 oz)	120	2	6	10	19	tr	150
Sugar Free Vanilla Wafers	7 (1 oz)	120	2	6	15	19	tr	80

FOOD	PORTION	CALS	PROT	FAT	CHOL	CARB	FIBER	SOD
Sweetzels								
Chocolate Chip	7 (1 oz)	160	1	9	5	18	0	70
Ginger Snaps	4 (1.2 oz)	140	2	3	0	25	tr	120
Vanilla Wafers	7 (1.1 oz)	137	2	5	0	22	0	94
The Source								
Barry's Raspberry Palmiers	1 (0.7 oz)	80	1	3	0	14	0	50
Tree Of Life								
Fat Free Almond Butter	1 (0.8 oz)	60	1	0	0	14	1	50
Fat Free Carrot Cake	1 (0.8 oz)	60	1	0	0	14	1	50
Fat Free Devil's Food Chocolate	1 (0.8 oz)	70	2	0	0	15	1	80
Fat Free Oatmeal Raisin	1 (0.8 oz)	70	2	0	0	16	1	40
Fruit Bars Fat Free Fig	1 (0.8 oz)	70	1	0	0	16	2	100
Fruit Bars Fat Free Peach Apricot	1 (0.8 oz)	70	1	0	0	17	1	110
Fruit Bars Fat Free Wildberry	1 (0.8 oz)	70	1	0	0	16	2	170
Monster Carob Chip	1 (4.7 oz)	700	10	35	10	95	5	375
Monster Granola	1 (4.7 oz)	700	10	30	10	95	5	475
Monster Macaroon	1 (4.7 oz)	750	5	45	10	85	5	375
Monster Peanut Butter	1 (4.7 oz)	700	15	35	20	85	5	525
Monster Fat Free Carrot Cake	1 cookie (3.8 oz)	240	4	0	0	60	4	120
Monster Fat Free Devil's Food Chocolate	1 cookie (3.8 oz)	320	8	0	0	80	8	180
Monster Fat Free Gingerbread	1 cookie (3.8 oz)	320	8	0	0	76	8	200
Monster Fat Free Maple Pecan	1 cookie (3.8 oz)	360	8	0	0	80	8	200
Oatmeal	1 (0.8 oz)	100	2	4	15	16	0	55
Sandwich Royal Vanilla	2 (0.9 oz)	120	1	5	0	17	1	115

FOOD	PORTION	CALS	PROT	FAT	CHOL	CARB	FIBER	SOD
Wheat Free Carob	1 (0.8 oz)	100	1	5	0	14	6	75
Wheat Free Maple Walnut	1 (0.8 oz)	100	2	6	0	13	6	50
Wheat Free Oatmeal	1 (0.8 oz)	90	1	5	0	11	1	25
Wheat Free Peanut Butter	1 (0.8 oz)	109	2	6	0	8	1	100
Twix								
Bars Chocolate Caramel	1 (0.9 oz)	140	1	7	0	18	0	55
Voortman								
Almonette	2 (1 oz)	150	1	8	0	17	tr	65
Chocolate Chip	1 (0.7 oz)	100	tr	5	0	13	0	45
Chocolate Wafers Sugar Free	3 (1 oz)	160	tr	11	0	18	0	30
Coconut Delight	1 (0.6 oz)	90	tr	5	0	10	0	25
Peanut Delight	1 (0.9 oz)	130	2	7	<5	15	tr	90
Strawberry Wafers Sugar Free	3 (1 oz)	160	tr	11	0	18	0	30
Sugar	1 (0.6 oz)	80	tr	4	0	11	0	45
Turnovers Blueberry	1 (0.9 oz)	100	1	3	<5	16	0	50
Turnovers Cherry	1 (0.9 oz)	100	1	3	<5	16	0	50
Turnovers Strawberry	1 (0.9 oz)	100	1	3	<5	16	0	50
Vanilla Wafers Sugar Free	3 (1 oz)	160	tr	11	0	18	0	30
Windmill	1 (0.7 oz)	90	tr	4	0	13	0	100
White Eagle Bakery								
Chruscik	2 (1 oz)	140	2	8	45	16	0	95
Wortz								
Animal	9 (1.1 oz)	140	2	5	—	22	1	140
Chocolate Graham	2 (0.9 oz)	130	2	3	—	24	1	120
Cinnamon Grahams	2 (0.9 oz)	130	1	5	—	19	tr	85
Vanilla Wafers	7 (1.1 oz)	150	1	6	—	22	1	115
REFRIGERATED								
chocolate chip	1 (0.42 oz)	59	1	3	3	8	—	28
chocolate chip unbaked	1 oz	126	1	6	7	17	—	59
oatmeal	1 (0.4 oz)	56	1	3	3	8	—	39

FOOD	PORTION	CALS	PROT	FAT	CHOL	CARB	FIBER	SOD
oatmeal raisin	1 (0.4 oz)	56	1	3	3	8	−	39
peanut butter	1 (0.4 oz)	60	1	3	4	7	−	52
peanut butter dough	1 oz	130	2	7	8	15	−	112
sugar	1 (0.42 oz)	58	1	3	4	8	−	56
sugar dough	1 oz	124	1	6	8	17	−	120
TAKE-OUT								
biscotti with nuts chocolate dipped	1 (1.3 oz)	117	2	6	18	16	1	33
black & white	1 lg (3 oz)	302	4	9	58	52	1	72
finikia	1 (1.2 oz)	171	2	5	27	16	1	26
koulourakia butter cookie twist	1 (0.9 oz)	113	2	6	32	14	tr	59
linzer tart	1 (2.4 oz)	280	2	14	40	34	0	130

CORIANDER

FOOD	PORTION	CALS	PROT	FAT	CHOL	CARB	FIBER	SOD
leaf dried	1 tsp	2	tr	tr	0	tr	−	1
leaf fresh	¼ cup	1	tr	tr	0	tr	−	1
seed	1 tsp	5	tr	tr	0	1	−	1
Instant India								
Tomato Coriander Paste	2 tbsp (1 oz)	90	1	6	0	8	0	570

CORN
CANNED

FOOD	PORTION	CALS	PROT	FAT	CHOL	CARB	FIBER	SOD
cream style	½ cup	93	2	1	0	23	−	365
w/ red & green peppers	½ cup	86	3	1	0	21	−	396
white	½ cup	66	2	1	0	15	−	−
yellow	½ cup	66	2	1	0	15	1	−
Del Monte								
Cream Style Golden	½ cup (4.4 oz)	90	2	1	0	20	2	360
Cream Style Golden No Salt Added	½ cup (4.4 oz)	60	1	1	0	14	2	10
Cream Style White	½ cup (4.4 oz)	100	2	1	0	21	2	360
Fiesta	½ cup (4.4 oz)	50	2	1	0	12	2	310

FOOD	PORTION	CALS	PROT	FAT	CHOL	CARB	FIBER	SOD
Gold & White Supersweet	½ cup (4.4 oz)	80	2	1	0	18	2	360
Whole Kernel Golden	½ cup (4.4 oz)	90	2	1	0	18	3	360
Whole Kernel Golden Supersweet No Salt Added	½ cup (4.4 oz)	60	2	1	0	11	3	10
Whole Kernel Golden Supersweet No Sugar	½ cup (4.4 oz)	60	2	1	0	11	3	360
Whole Kernel Golden Supersweet Vacuum Packed	½ cup (3.7 oz)	70	2	1	0	13	3	270
Whole Kernel White Sweet	½ cup (4.4 oz)	60	2	1	0	11	3	360
Green Giant								
Mexicorn	⅓ cup	60	2	0	0	14	1	250
S&W								
Cream Style	½ cup (4.4 oz)	60	1	1	0	14	2	360
Whole Kernel	⅓ cup (3 oz)	70	2	2	0	12	2	170
Veg-All								
Whole Kernel	½ cup	80	2	1	0	16	2	340
FRESH								
on-the-cob w/ butter cooked	1 ear	155	4	3	6	32	—	30
white cooked	½ cup	89	3	1	0	21	—	14
white raw	½ cup	66	2	1	0	15	—	12
yellow cooked	½ cup	89	3	1	0	21	—	14
yellow cooked	1 ear (2.7 oz)	83	3	1	0	19	—	13
yellow raw	1 ear (3 oz)	77	3	1	0	17	—	14
yellow raw	½ cup	66	2	1	0	15	—	12

FOOD	PORTION	CALS	PROT	FAT	CHOL	CARB	FIBER	SOD
FROZEN								
cooked	½ cup	67	2	tr	0	17	—	4
on-the-cob cooked	1 ear (2.2 oz)	59	2	tr	0	14	—	3
Birds Eye								
Baby Gold & White	⅔ cup	100	3	1	0	21	3	0
Cob Big Ear	1 ear	120	—	1	0	—	3	0
Cut	⅓ cup	70	—	1	0	—	2	0
Fresh Like								
Cut	3.5 oz	85	3	1	—	21	1	5
On The Cob	1 ear (3 in)	96	3	1	—	24	1	4
Tree Of Life								
Corn	⅔ cup (3.2 oz)	80	3	1	0	19	1	10
TAKE-OUT								
fritters	1 (1 oz)	62	2	2	12	9	1	126
scalloped	½ cup	258	7	7	47	43	—	246

CORN CHIPS (see CHIPS)

CORNISH HEN (see CHICKEN)

CORNMEAL

FOOD	PORTION	CALS	PROT	FAT	CHOL	CARB	FIBER	SOD
corn grits cooked	1 cup	146	4	tr	0	31	—	0
corn grits uncooked	1 cup	579	14	2	0	124	—	1
white	1 cup (4.8 oz)	505	12	2	0	107	10	4
whole grain	1 cup (4.3 oz)	442	10	4	0	94	9	43
yellow	1 cup (4.8 oz)	505	12	2	0	107	10	4
yellow self-rising	1 cup (4.3 oz)	407	10	4	0	86	8	1521
Albers								
White	3 tbsp	110	2	0	0	24	tr	0
Yellow	3 tbsp	110	2	0	0	24	tr	0
Expert Foods								
Low Carb Grits Mix	1½ tsp	15	2	0	0	2	2	34

FOOD	PORTION	CALS	PROT	FAT	CHOL	CARB	FIBER	SOD
Hodgson Mill								
Cornbread Mix Jalapeno Mexican	¼ cup (1 oz)	100	4	1	0	21	1	310
Yellow Organic	¼ cup (1 oz)	100	3	1	0	22	3	0
Yellow Self Rising	¼ cup (1 oz)	90	3	1	0	21	3	260
Indian Head								
Stone Ground	¼ cup	100	3	1	0	20	2	0
Kentucky Kernal								
Sweet Cornbread Mix	¼ cup (1 oz)	120	2	2	0	24	0	310
McKenzie's								
Hush Puppies	1 serv (1.9 oz)	190	2	10	0	23	2	470
Quaker								
Old Fashioned Grits not prep	¼ cup	140	3	1	—	32	2	0
Yellow	3 tbsp (1 oz)	90	2	1	0	21	2	0
TAKE-OUT								
hush puppies	1 (0.75 oz)	74	3	3	10	10	1	147
CORNSTARCH								
cornstarch	1 cup (4.5 oz)	488	tr	tr	0	117	1	12
Argo								
Cornstarch	1 cup (128 g)	460	tr	tr	0	115	—	tr
Cornstarch	1 tbsp (8 g)	30	tr	0	0	7	—	0
COTTAGE CHEESE								
creamed	4 oz	117	14	5	17	3	—	457
creamed	1 cup (7.4 oz)	217	26	9	31	6	—	850
creamed w/ fruit	4 oz	140	11	4	13	15	—	457
dry curd	4 oz	96	20	tr	8	2	—	14
dry curd	1 cup (5.1 oz)	123	25	1	10	3	—	19
low fat 1%	1 cup (7.9 oz)	164	28	2	10	6	—	918
low fat 1%	4 oz	82	14	1	5	3	—	459
low fat 2%	1 cup (7.9 oz)	203	31	4	19	8	—	918
low fat 2%	4 oz	101	16	2	9	4	—	459

FOOD	PORTION	CALS	PROT	FAT	CHOL	CARB	FIBER	SOD
Breakstone's								
Cottage Doubles Peach	1 pkg (5.5 oz)	140	12	3	15	16	tr	390
Fat Free	½ cup	90	12	0	10	8	0	450
Cabot								
Cottage Cheese	½ cup	100	13	5	15	4	0	400
No Fat	½ cup	70	13	0	5	5	0	410
Horizon Organic								
Cottage Cheese	½ cup (3.9 oz)	110	13	5	15	4	0	340
Light N'Lively								
Low fat	½ cup	80	12	2	10	6	0	420
COTTONSEED								
kernels roasted	1 tbsp	51	3	4	0	2	–	3
COUSCOUS								
cooked	1 cup (5.5 oz)	176	6	tr	0	36	2	8
dry	1 cup (6.1 oz)	650	22	1	0	134	9	17
Near East								
Broccoli & Cheese as prep	1 cup	230	7	3	9	41	3	670
Curry as prep	1 cup	220	7	4	0	42	3	550
Herbed Chicken as prep	1 cup	220	7	3	0	42	3	510
Original as prep	1 cup	230	8	5	0	46	2	5
Parmesan as prep	1 cup	220	8	5	9	41	2	580
Roasted Garlic Olive Oil as prep	1 cup	230	7	5	0	41	2	570
Toasted Pine Nut as prep	1 cup	230	7	6	27	40	2	510
Tomato Lentil as prep	1 cup	220	8	3	0	42	3	670
Wild Mushroom Herb as prep	1 cup	230	8	4	9	42	3	590
COWPEAS								
catjang dried cooked	1 cup (2.9 oz)	200	14	1	0	35	–	32

FOOD	PORTION	CALS	PROT	FAT	CHOL	CARB	FIBER	SOD
common canned	1 cup	184	11	1	0	33	—	718
frozen cooked	½ cup	112	7	tr	0	20	—	5
leafy tips chopped cooked	1 cup	12	2	tr	0	1	—	3
leafy tips raw chopped	1 cup	10	1	tr	0	2	—	2

CRAB
CANNED
blue	3 oz	84	17	1	76	0	—	283
blue	1 cup	133	28	2	120	0	—	450
Bumble Bee								
Fancy Lump Meat	½ can (1.9 oz)	40	8	1	50	0	0	300
Fancy White Meat	½ can (1.9 oz)	28	6	0	43	1	0	403
FRESH								
alaska king cooked	1 leg (4.7 oz)	129	26	2	72	0	—	1436
alaska king cooked	3 oz	82	16	1	45	0	—	911
alaska king raw	3 oz	71	16	1	35	0	—	711
alaska king raw	1 leg (6 oz)	144	32	1	72	0	—	1438
blue cooked	3 oz	87	17	2	85	0	—	237
blue cooked	1 cup	138	27	2	135	0	—	376
blue raw	3 oz	74	15	1	66	tr	—	249
blue raw	1 crab (7 oz)	18	4	tr	16	tr	—	62
dungeness raw	1 crab (5.7 oz)	140	28	2	97	1	—	481
dungeness raw	3 oz	73	15	1	50	1	—	251
queen steamed	3 oz	98	20	1	60	0	—	587
TAKE-OUT								
baked	1 (3.8 oz)	160	29	2	184	4	—	550
cake	1 (2 oz)	160	11	10	82	5	—	492
kenagi korean crab cooked	1 serv (3 oz)	71	16	tr	—	0	0	204
mousse	¼ cup	364	—	20	136	—	—	—
soft-shell fried	1 (4.4 oz)	334	11	18	45	31	—	1118

CRACKER CRUMBS
chocolate wafer cookie crumbs	½ cup (5.9 oz)	728	11	25	0	120	—	980
cracker meal	1 cup (4 oz)	440	11	2	0	93	—	32

FOOD	PORTION	CALS	PROT	FAT	CHOL	CARB	FIBER	SOD
graham cracker crumbs	½ cup (4.4 oz)	540	9	13	0	97	3	756
Baker's Harvest								
Graham	⅓ cup (1 oz)	130	2	4	0	23	1	110

CRACKERS

FOOD	PORTION	CALS	PROT	FAT	CHOL	CARB	FIBER	SOD
cheese	1 (1 in sq) (1 g)	5	tr	tr	0	1	–	10
cheese	14 (½ oz)	71	1	4	2	8	–	141
cheese low sodium	14 (½ oz)	71	1	4	2	8	–	68
cheese low sodium	1 (1 in sq) (1 g)	5	tr	tr	0	1	–	5
cheese w/ peanut butter filling	1 (0.24 oz)	34	1	2	0	4	tr	69
crispbread	3	61	1	2	–	9	1	–
crispbread rye	1 (0.35 oz)	37	1	tr	0	8	2	26
crispbread rye	3	77	2	1	–	17	3	–
melba toast plain	1 (5 g)	19	1	tr	0	4	tr	41
melba toast pumpernickel	1 (5 g)	19	1	tr	0	4	tr	45
melba toast rye	1 (5 g)	19	1	tr	0	4	tr	45
melba toast wheat	1 (5 g)	19	1	tr	0	4	tr	42
milk	1 (0.42 oz)	55	1	2	–	8	–	71
oyster cracker	1 (1 g)	4	tr	tr	0	1	tr	13
peanut butter sandwich	1 (7 g)	34	1	2	–	4	–	66
rusk toast	1 (0.35 oz)	41	1	1	–	7	–	25
rye w/ cheese filling	1 (0.24 oz)	34	1	2	1	4	–	73
rye wafers plain	1 (0.9 oz)	84	2	tr	0	20	–	199
rye wafers seasoned	1 (0.8 oz)	84	2	2	0	16	–	195
saltines	1 (3 g)	13	tr	tr	0	2	tr	38
saltines fat free low sodium	6 (1 oz)	118	3	tr	0	25	–	191
saltines fat free low sodium	3 (0.5 oz)	59	2	tr	0	12	–	95
saltines low salt	1 (3 g)	13	tr	tr	0	2	tr	19
snack cracker	1 (3 g)	15	tr	1	0	2	tr	25

FOOD	PORTION	CALS	PROT	FAT	CHOL	CARB	FIBER	SOD
snack cracker low salt	1 (3 g)	15	tr	1	0	2	tr	11
snack cracker w/ cheese filling	1 (7 g)	33	1	2	0	4	–	98
soup cracker	1 (1 g)	4	tr	tr	0	1	tr	13
water biscuits	3	92	2	3	–	16	1	–
wheat w/ cheese filling	1 (0.24 oz)	35	1	2	1	4	–	64
wheat w/ peanut butter filling	1 (0.24 oz)	35	1	2	0	4	–	57
wheat thins	7 (0.5 oz)	67	1	3	0	9	1	113
wheat thins	1 (2 g)	9	tr	tr	0	1	–	16
wheat thins low salt	7 (0.5 oz)	67	1	3	0	9	1	40
whole wheat	1 (4 g)	18	tr	1	0	3	–	26
whole wheat low salt	1 (4 g)	18	tr	1	0	3	–	10
zwieback	1 oz	107	3	1	–	21	1	75
American Vintage								
Wine Biscuits All Flavors	5	140	1	7	1	17	tr	190
Andre's								
CarboSave Crackerbread All Flavors	1 oz	140	10	8	0	8	4	120
Austin								
Cracker Sandwich Cheese On Cheese	6 (1.3 oz)	170	3	7	0	25	tr	310
Cracker Sandwich Cheese Peanut Butter	6 (1.3 oz)	170	5	7	0	24	1	320
Cracker Sandwich Toasty Peanut Butter	6 (1.3 oz)	170	5	7	0	24	1	340
Cracker Sandwich Whole Wheat Cheese	6 (1.3 oz)	170	3	7	0	25	tr	280
Baker's Harvest								
Cheese	23 (1 oz)	150	3	6	0	18	tr	370
Cheese Reduced Fat	29 (1 oz)	130	3	4	0	21	tr	310
Oyster	35 (0.5 oz)	70	1	2	–	11	1	150

FOOD	PORTION	CALS	PROT	FAT	CHOL	CARB	FIBER	SOD
Saltines Unsalted	5 (0.5 oz)	70	1	2	–	11	–	110
Saltines Deluxe	5 (0.5 oz)	60	1	2	–	10	–	130
Snackers	9 (1.1 oz)	160	2	8	–	19	tr	250
Snackers Reduced Fat	10 (1.1 oz)	140	3	4	0	23	tr	260
Snackers Unsalted	9 (1.1 oz)	160	2	8	–	19	tr	80
Wheat Snacks	16 (1 oz)	140	3	6	–	20	2	120
Wheat Snacks Reduced Fat	16 (1.1 oz)	140	2	4	0	23	1	220
Woven Wheats	7 (1.1 oz)	140	3	5	0	21	4	170
Woven Wheats Reduced Fat	8 (1.1 oz)	130	3	3	0	24	4	180
Barbara's Bakery								
Cheese Bites	26 (1 oz)	120	3	2	0	24	1	290
Right Lite Rounds Original	5 (0.5 oz)	55	1	5	0	12	0	150
Rite Lite Rounds Savory Poppy	5 (0.5 oz)	70	tr	2	0	11	0	135
Rite Lite Rounds Tamari Sesame	5 (0.5 oz)	70	1	2	0	12	0	160
Wheatines All Flavors	1 lg sq (0.5 oz)	50	1	2	0	10	1	110
Blue Diamond								
Nut Thins Almond	16 (1 oz)	130	3	5	0	19	tr	75
Nut Thins Hazelnut	16 (1 oz)	120	2	4	0	20	1	75
Nut Thins Pecans	16 (1 oz)	130	2	5	0	20	tr	75
Bran-A-Crisp								
Low Carb Wheat Bran	1	20	1	0	0	6	2	0
Breton								
Cabaret	3 (5 g)	70	1	4	0	9	0	160
Garden Vegetable	3	60	1	3	0	8	1	190
Light	1 (5 g)	20	1	1	0	3	tr	39
Minis	20 (0.6 oz)	89	2	4	0	11	tr	169
Minis Cheddar Cheese	20 (0.6 oz)	87	3	4	3	11	–	211
Minis Garden Vegetable	20 (0.6 oz)	87	2	4	0	12	1	144
Multi Grain	3	70	2	4	0	8	1	170
Original	3	60	2	3	0	8	0	140

FOOD	PORTION	CALS	PROT	FAT	CHOL	CARB	FIBER	SOD
Reduced Fat & Sodium	3	60	2	2	0	9	tr	75
Sesame	3	60	2	3	0	7	tr	100
Cheeters								
Low Carb All Flavors	1 pkg (1 oz)	104	4	8	0	4	2	110
Cheetos								
Bacon Cheddar	1 pkg	190	3	9	<5	25	1	410
Cheddar Cheese	1 pkg	210	3	11	<5	23	1	340
Golden Toast	1 pkg	240	4	14	5	25	1	440
Cheez It								
Hot & Spicy	26 (1 oz)	150	4	8	0	17	tr	300
Party Mix	½ cup (1 oz)	140	4	5	0	19	1	270
Reduced Fat	29 (1 oz)	140	4	5	0	20	tr	280
White Cheddar	26 (1 oz)	150	3	7	<5	18	tr	280
Courtney's								
Sun-Dried Tomato Organic	4 (0.5 oz)	60	1	1	0	10	0	130
Dare								
Cabaret	3	70	1	4	0	9	0	160
Vinta	1 (6 g)	30	1	1	0	4	1	–
Doritos								
Jalapeno Cheese	1 pkg	230	3	14	<5	26	1	450
Nacho Cheddar	1 pkg	240	4	14	<5	25	1	340
Eden								
Nori Nori Rice	15 (1 oz)	110	3	0	0	24	2	160
Frito Lay								
Cheddar Snacks	1 pkg	200	5	10	<5	27	1	530
Frookie								
Cheddar	17 (1 oz)	140	4	4	0	23	1	420
Cracked Pepper	8 (0.7 oz)	70	2	0	0	15	1	85
Garden Vegetable	13 (1 oz)	130	3	4	0	19	2	380
Garlic & Herb	8 (0.7 oz)	70	2	0	0	16	1	170
Pizza	17 (1 oz)	130	3	3	0	24	1	420
Snack & Party	10 (1 oz)	140	2	5	0	20	1	260
Water Crackers	8 (0.7 oz)	70	2	0	0	16	1	135
Wheat & Onion	12 (1 oz)	120	3	4	0	18	2	400
Wheat & Rye	13 (1 oz)	120	3	4	0	18	3	380
Gold'n Krackle								
Cheese	½ oz	65	2	2	2	9	0	85

FOOD	PORTION	CALS	PROT	FAT	CHOL	CARB	FIBER	SOD
Cheese & Oregano	½ oz	65	2	2	2	9	0	85
Hot & Spicy	½ oz	58	2	1	0	11	0	15
Onion & Garlic	½ oz	58	2	1	0	11	0	15
Plain	½ oz	58	2	1	0	11	0	15
Heavenly								
All Flavors	1	16	1	4	0	3	0	19
Cholesterol Free								
Sugar Free								
Kashi								
TLC Country	15	130	3	3	0	21	0	220
Cheddar	(1 oz)							
TLC Honey Sesame	15 (1 oz)	130	3	3	0	22	2	190
TLC Natural Ranch	15 (1 oz)	130	3	3	0	22	2	200
TLC Original 7 Grain	15 (1 oz)	130	3	3	0	22	2	200
Keebler								
Club	5	70	1	2	0	12	0	200
33% Reduced Fat	(0.6 oz)							
Club 50% Reduced	4	70	1	3	0	9	tr	80
Sodium	(0.5 oz)							
Club Original	4 (0.5 oz)	70	1	3	0	9	tr	160
Elfin	23 (1 oz)	130	2	2	0	24	tr	140
Export Soda	3 (0.5 oz)	60	1	2	0	10	tr	80
Harvest Bakery	2	70	1	3	0	10	tr	80
Multigrain	(0.6 oz)							
Munch'ems	39	140	3	5	0	20	1	320
Cheddar	(1 oz)							
Munch'ems	30	130	3	4	0	21	tr	320
Cheddar	(1 oz)							
55% Reduced Fat								
Munch'ems	28	130	2	4	0	23	1	470
Chili Cheese	(1.1 oz)							
Munch'ems	40	140	2	5	0	22	1	290
Mexquite BBQ	(1 oz)							
Munch'ems Ranch	40 (1 oz)	140	3	5	0	20	1	260
Munch'ems Ranch								
55% Reduced Fat	33 (1 oz)	130	3	4	0	21	tr	310
Munch'ems Salsa	28 (1.1 oz)	130	2	4	0	23	1	260
Munch'ems	30	130	3	5	0	20	tr	350
Seasoned Original	(1 oz)							

FOOD	PORTION	CALS	PROT	FAT	CHOL	CARB	FIBER	SOD
Munch'ems Sour Cream & Onion	39 (1 oz)	140	3	5	0	20	1	280
Munch'ems Sour Cream & Onion 55% Reduced Fat	33 (1 oz)	130	2	4	0	22	0	390
Paks Cheese & Peanut Butter	1 pkg	190	6	9	<5	22	tr	420
Paks Club & Cheddar	1 pkg	190	3	11	10	20	tr	320
Paks Toast & Peanut Butter	1 pkg	190	5	9	0	23	1	300
Sandwich Cracker Wheat & Cheddar	1 pkg	200	3	10	<5	23	tr	310
Toasteds Buttercrisp	5 (0.6 oz)	80	1	4	0	10	0	150
Toasteds Buttercrisp	9 (1 oz)	140	2	7	<5	19	tr	280
Toasteds Onion	9 (1 oz)	140	2	6	0	19	tr	310
Toasteds Sesame	5 (0.6 oz)	80	1	4	0	10	tr	135
Toasteds Sesame	9 (1 oz)	140	3	6	0	19	tr	320
Toasteds Sesame Reduced Fat	10 (1 oz)	120	3	3	0	21	2	310
Toasteds Wheat	5 (0.6 oz)	80	1	4	0	10	tr	150
Toasteds Wheat	9 (1 oz)	140	2	6	0	19	tr	270
Toasteds Wheat Reduced Fat	5 (0.5 oz)	60	1	2	0	10	tr	160
Toasteds Wheat Reduced Fat	10 (1 oz)	120	3	3	0	22	1	300
Town House	5 (0.6 oz)	80	1	5	0	9	tr	150
Town House 50% Reduced Sodium	5 (0.6 oz)	80	1	5	0	10	tr	75
Town House Reduced Fat	6 (0.6 oz)	70	1	2	0	11	tr	180
Town House Wheat	5 (0.6 oz)	80	1	4	0	10	tr	140
Wheatables Honey Wheat	12 (1 oz)	140	2	6	0	20	1	200
Wheatables Original	12 (1 oz)	140	2	6	0	10	1	210
Wheatables Seven Grain	12 (1 oz)	140	2	6	0	20	1	250

FOOD	PORTION	CALS	PROT	FAT	CHOL	CARB	FIBER	SOD
Zesta Saltine 50% Reduced Sodium	5 (0.5 oz)	60	1	2	0	11	tr	95
Zesta Saltine Fat Free	5 (0.5 oz)	50	1	0	0	11	0	150
Zesta Saltine Original	5 (0.5 oz)	60	1	2	0	10	tr	190
Zesta Saltine Unsalted Top	5 (0.5 oz)	70	1	2	0	10	tr	90
Zesta Soup & Oyster	42 (0.5 oz)	80	1	3	0	10	tr	160
Nabisco								
Royal Lunch	1 (0.4 oz)	60	tr	2	0	8	0	70
Zwieback	1 (8 g)	35	1	1	0	6	0	10
No-Carb Kitchen								
Cheese	1	25	3	3	5	0	0	90
No-No								
Flatbreads Tortilla Corn Low Fat Sugar Free Everything	3 (1 oz)	95	3	1	0	18	1	140
Old London								
Mediterranean Toast	3	60	2	2	0	9	0	190
Pepperidge Farm								
Giant Goldfish Peanut Butter Sandwich	1 pkg (1.4 oz)	190	5	9	<5	22	1	310
Giant Goldfish Wheat	14	140	2	5	0	21	1	260
Goldfish Colors On The Go	1 pkg	170	4	7	5	24	1	320
Peter Pan								
Cheese Peanut Butter	1 pkg	210	5	10	0	23	1	350
Toast Peanut Butter	1 pkg	210	5	11	0	23	tr	280
Premium								
Saltine Fat Free	5	60	1	0	0	12	0	170
Saltine Multigrain	5 (0.5 oz)	60	1	2	0	10	tr	150
Saltine Unsalted Tops	5	70	1	2	0	11	0	115

FOOD	PORTION	CALS	PROT	FAT	CHOL	CARB	FIBER	SOD
Ralston								
Cheese	23 (1 oz)	150	3	6	0	18	tr	370
Cheese Reduced Fat	29 (1 oz)	130	3	4	0	21	tr	310
Oyster	35 (0.5 oz)	70	1	2	–	11	1	150
Rich & Crisp	1 (0.5 oz)	70	1	3	–	9	0	105
Saltines Fat Free	5 (0.5 oz)	60	1	0	0	13	–	135
Saltines Deluxe	5 (0.5 oz)	60	1	2	–	10	–	130
Snackers	9 (1.1 oz)	160	2	8	–	19	tr	250
Snackers Reduced Fat	10 (1.1 oz)	140	2	4	0	23	tr	260
Snackers Unsalted	9 (1.1 oz)	160	2	8	–	19	tr	80
Wheat Snacks	16 (1 oz)	140	3	6	–	20	2	120
Wheat Snacks Reduced Fat	16 (1.1 oz)	140	2	4	0	23	1	220
Woven Wheats	7 (1.1 oz)	140	3	5	0	21	4	170
Woven Wheats Reduced Fat	8 (1.1 oz)	130	3	3	0	24	4	180
RedOval Farms								
Stoned Wheat Thins Cracked Pepper	4 (0.6 oz)	70	1	3	0	10	tr	190
Ritz								
Reduced Fat	5	70	1	2	0	11	0	150
Rykrisp								
Seasoned	2	60	1	2	0	10	3	90
Smucker's								
Snackers Grape	1 pkg (3.3 oz)	410	11	20	0	47	3	480
Snackers Strawberry	1 pkg (3.3 oz)	410	11	20	0	47	3	480
SnackWell's								
Cracked Pepper	5	60	1	2	0	10	0	115
Sunshine								
Hi Ho Reduced Fat	5 (0.5 oz)	70	1	3	0	10	tr	140
Krispy	5 (0.5 oz)	60	2	2	0	10	tr	180
Krispy Fat Free	5 (0.5 oz)	50	1	0	0	11	0	150
Krispy Mild Cheddar	5 (0.5 oz)	60	2	2	0	10	tr	180
Krispy Soup & Oyster	17 (0.5 oz)	60	2	2	0	11	tr	200

FOOD	PORTION	CALS	PROT	FAT	CHOL	CARB	FIBER	SOD
Krispy Whole Wheat	5 (0.5 oz)	60	2	2	0	10	tr	130
Tree Of Life								
Bite Size Fat Free Cracked Pepper	12 (0.5)	55	1	0	0	12	0	80
Bite Size Fat Free Garden Vegetable	12 (0.5 oz)	55	2	0	0	12	0	80
Bite Size Fat Free Garlic & Herb	12 (0.5 oz)	55	2	0	0	12	0	80
Bite Size Fat Free Toasted Onion	12 (0.5 oz)	55	2	0	0	12	0	80
Oyster	40 (0.5 oz)	60	2	0	0	13	0	130
Saltine Cracked Pepper Fat Free	4 (0.5 oz)	60	2	0	0	13	1	130
Saltine Fat Free	4 (0.5 oz)	50	2	0	0	11	0	140
Venus								
Fat Free Cracked Pepper	11 (0.5 oz)	60	1	0	0	12	0	80
Fat Free Garden Vegetable	5 (0.5 oz)	60	2	0	0	12	0	80
Fat Free Garlic & Herb	11 (0.5 oz)	60	2	0	0	12	0	90
Fat Free Multi-Grain	5 (0.5 oz)	60	1	0	0	12	tr	100
Fat Free Spicy Chili	10 (0.5 oz)	60	1	0	0	12	tr	100
Fat Free Toasted Onion	5 (0.5 oz)	60	1	0	0	12	tr	120
Fat Free Toasted Wheat	5 (0.5 oz)	60	2	0	0	12	tr	140
Fat Free Tomato & Basil	10 (0.5 oz)	60	1	0	0	12	tr	100
Fat Free Zesty Italian	10 (0.5 oz)	60	1	0	0	12	tr	120
Garden Vegetable	6 (1 oz)	150	2	8	0	20	1	230
Honey Wheat	1 oz	140	2	5	0	21	1	200
Low Fat Cracker Bread	5 (0.5 oz)	60	1	2	0	10	tr	105
Low Fat Water Crackers	4 (0.5 oz)	60	1	1	0	12	0	75

FOOD	PORTION	CALS	PROT	FAT	CHOL	CARB	FIBER	SOD
Sesame & Flaxseed	1 oz	130	3	3	0	23	1	240
Soup Original	0.5 oz	60	1	2	0	11	0	90
Wine Cheese Caviar Original	0.5 oz	60	1	2	0	11	0	90
Wine Cheese Caviar Pepper & Poppy	0.5 oz	60	1	2	0	11	0	90
Wasa								
Crispbread Fiber Rye	1 (0.4 oz)	30	1	1	0	7	2	60
Wheat Thins								
Harvest Crisps Five-Grain	13	140	3	4	0	23	1	240
Wheatsworth								
Crackers	5	80	2	4	0	10	tr	170
Wisecrackers								
Low Fat Poblano Chili & Sweet Onion	4 (0.5 oz)	45	1	1	0	8	tr	89
Wortz								
Cheese	23 (1 oz)	150	3	6	0	18	tr	370
Oyster	35 (0.5 oz)	70	1	2	–	11	1	150
Rich & Crisp	1 (0.5 oz)	70	1	3	–	9	0	105
Saltines Fat Free	5 (0.5 oz)	60	1	0	0	13	–	135
Saltines Deluxe	5 (0.5 oz)	60	1	2	–	10	–	130
Wheat Snacks	16 (1 oz)	140	3	6	–	20	2	120
Wheat Snacks Reduced Fat	16 (1.1 oz)	140	2	4	0	23	1	220
Woven Wheats	7 (1.1 oz)	140	3	5	0	21	4	170
CRANBERRIES								
cranberry sauce sweetened	½ cup	209	tr	tr	0	54	–	40
fresh chopped	1 cup	54	tr	tr	0	14	–	1
Jok'n'Al								
Cranberry Sauce	1 tbsp	8	0	0	0	2	–	0
Ocean Spray								
Craisins	⅓ cup	130	0	0	0	33	2	2
Cranberry Sauce Jellied	¼ cup	110	0	0	0	27	tr	35

FOOD	PORTION	CALS	PROT	FAT	CHOL	CARB	FIBER	SOD
Cranorange	¼ cup	120	0	0	0	30	1	35
Whole Berry Sauce	¼ cup	110	0	0	0	28	1	35
Steel's								
Spiced Cranberry Sauce	⅓ cup	20	0	0	0	5	1	0
Wild Thyme Farms								
Cranberry Sauce	1 tbsp	19	0	0	0	5	—	0

CRANBERRY BEANS

canned	1 cup	216	14	1	0	39	16	863
dried cooked	1 cup	241	17	1	0	43	18	1

CRANBERRY JUICE

cocktail	1 cup	147	tr	tr	0	38	—	10
cranberry juice cocktail	6 oz	108	0	tr	0	27	—	4
cranberry juice cocktail low calorie	6 oz	33	0	0	0	9	—	6
cranberry juice cocktail frzn	12 oz can	821	tr	0	0	210	—	13
cranberry juice cocktail frzn as prep	6 oz	102	0	0	0	26	—	6
Keto								
Kooler	½ tsp	0	0	0	0	0	0	0
Langers								
Cocktail	8 oz	140	0	0	0	35	—	10
Diet	8 oz	30	0	0	0	9	—	10
White	8 oz	120	0	0	0	28	—	10
Mott's								
Cocktail	8 fl oz	150	0	0	0	37	—	5
Nantucket Nectars								
Big Cran	8 oz	140	0	0	0	34	0	5
Ocean Spray								
Cocktail	8 oz	140	0	0	0	34	0	35
Cocktail Reduced Calorie	8 oz	50	0	0	0	13	0	35
Cocktail Light Low Calorie	8 oz	40	0	0	0	10	0	35
Cranberry Spritzer	8 oz	160	0	0	0	41	—	50

FOOD	PORTION	CALS	PROT	FAT	CHOL	CARB	FIBER	SOD
Cranberry Drink	8 oz	130	–	0	0	32	–	35
Crantastic	8 oz	100	0	0	0	32	0	35
White Cranberry	8 oz	120	0	0	0	29	–	35
White Cranberry Peach	8 oz	120	0	0	0	30	–	35
White Cranberry Strawberry	8 oz	120	0	0	0	31	–	35
CRAYFISH								
cooked	3 oz	97	20	1	151	0	–	58
raw	3 oz	76	16	1	118	0	–	45
raw	8	24	5	tr	37	0	–	14
CREAM (see also WHIPPED TOPPINGS)								
clotted cream	2 tbsp (1 oz)	164	tr	18	48	1	0	18
creme fraiche	2 tbsp (1 oz)	100	1	11	40	1	0	10
half & half	1 cup (8.5 oz)	315	7	28	89	10	–	98
half & half	1 tbsp (0.5 oz)	20	tr	2	6	1	–	6
heavy whipping	1 tbsp (0.5 oz)	52	tr	6	21	tr	–	6
heavy whipping whipped	1 cup (4.1 oz)	411	5	44	163	7	–	89
light coffee	1 cup (8.4 oz)	496	6	46	159	9	–	95
light coffee	1 tbsp (0.5 oz)	29	tr	3	10	1	–	6
light whipping	1 tbsp (0.5 oz)	44	tr	5	17	tr	–	5
light whipping cream whipped	1 cup (4.2 oz)	345	5	37	132	7	–	82
Cabot								
Whipped	2 tbsp	30	0	2	10	2	0	0
Land O Lakes								
Fat Free Half & Half	2 tbsp (1 oz)	20	tr	0	0	3	0	30
Half & Half	2 tbsp (1 oz)	40	1	4	15	1	0	20
Heavy Whipping	1 tbsp (0.5 oz)	50	0	6	20	0	0	10

FOOD	PORTION	CALS	PROT	FAT	CHOL	CARB	FIBER	SOD
CREAM CHEESE								
cream cheese	1 pkg (3 oz)	297	6	30	93	2	–	251
cream cheese	1 oz	99	2	10	31	1	–	84
Alpine Lace								
Reduced Fat Roasted Garlic & Herbs	1 tsp (1 oz)	60	4	4	10	2	0	190
Reduced Fat Sundried Tomato & Basil	2 tsp (1 oz)	70	4	5	15	2	0	300
Boar's Head								
Cream Cheese	2 tbsp (1 oz)	100	2	10	30	2	0	100
Galaxy								
Slices	1 slice (1 oz)	50	4	3	10	2	0	190
Horizon Organic								
Spreadable	2 tbsp	100	2	10	30	1	0	100
Philadelphia								
½ Less Fat	1 oz	70	3	6	20	tr	0	120
Fat Free	1 oz	30	4	0	5	2	0	200
CREAM OF TARTAR								
cream of tartar	1 tsp	8	0	0	0	2	–	2
CREAM SUBSTITUTES								
ExpertExtras								
RealCream	1 tsp	14	tr	1	6	tr	–	3
CREPES								
basic crepe unfilled	1	75	–	2	55	–	–	–
Frieda's								
Ready-To-Use	2 (0.8 oz)	50	1	1	5	9	0	90
CROAKER								
atlantic breaded & fried	3 oz	188	15	11	71	6	–	296
atlantic raw	3 oz	89	15	3	52	0	–	47
CROCODILE								
cooked	3 oz	78	17	1	–	0	0	–
CROISSANT								
apple	1 (2 oz)	145	4	5	–	21	1	156
cheese	1 (2 oz)	236	5	12	–	27	2	316

FOOD	PORTION	CALS	PROT	FAT	CHOL	CARB	FIBER	SOD
plain	1 mini (1 oz)	115	2	6	–	13	1	211
plain	1 (2 oz)	232	5	12	–	26	2	424
Sara Lee								
Broccoli & Cheese	1 (3.7 oz)	280	11	13	30	30	2	430
French Style	1 (1.5 oz)	170	4	8	<5	20	1	200
Ham & Swiss	1 (3.7 oz)	300	12	16	45	27	2	570
Petite	2 (2 oz)	230	6	11	<5	26	1	260
TAKE-OUT								
w/ egg & cheese	1 (4.5 oz)	368	13	25	216	24	–	551
w/ egg cheese & bacon	1 (4.5 oz)	413	16	28	215	24	–	889
w/ egg cheese & ham	1 (5.3 oz)	474	19	34	213	24	–	1081
w/ egg cheese & sausage	1 (5.6 oz)	523	20	38	216	25	–	1115

CROUTONS

FOOD	PORTION	CALS	PROT	FAT	CHOL	CARB	FIBER	SOD
plain	1 cup (1 oz)	122	4	2	0	22	2	209
seasoned	1 cup (1.4 oz)	186	4	7	–	25	2	495
Up Country Naturals								
Organic Whole Wheat Garlic & Herb	¼ cup (0.3 oz)	35	1	2	0	5	tr	110

CUCUMBER

FOOD	PORTION	CALS	PROT	FAT	CHOL	CARB	FIBER	SOD
fresh raw	1 (11 oz)	38	2	tr	0	8	3	6
fresh raw sliced	½ cup (1.8 oz)	7	tr	tr	0	1	1	1
Chiquita								
Cucumber	⅓ med (3.5 oz)	15	1	0	0	3	1	0
TAKE-OUT								
cucumber salad	3.5 oz	50	1	tr	0	11	–	480
kimchee	½ cup (1.8 oz)	36	tr	2	0	4	tr	173
tzatziki	½ cup (3.4 oz)	72	2	6	5	4	1	197

CUMIN

FOOD	PORTION	CALS	PROT	FAT	CHOL	CARB	FIBER	SOD
seed	1 tsp	8	tr	tr	0	1	–	4

CURRANT JUICE

FOOD	PORTION	CALS	PROT	FAT	CHOL	CARB	FIBER	SOD
black currant nectar	7 oz	110	tr	0	–	26	–	10
red currant nectar	7 oz	108	tr	tr	–	26	–	tr

FOOD	PORTION	CALS	PROT	FAT	CHOL	CARB	FIBER	SOD
CURRANTS								
black fresh	½ cup	36	1	tr	0	9	–	1
zante dried	½ cup	204	3	tr	0	53	–	6
Sun-Maid								
Zante	¼ cup	130	1	0	0	31	2	10
CUSK								
fillet baked	3 oz	106	23	1	50	0	–	38
CUSTARD								
MIX								
as prep w/ 2% milk	½ cup (4.7 oz)	148	7	4	74	24	–	200
as prep w/ whole milk	½ cup (4.7 oz)	163	6	5	–	23	–	–
flan as prep w/ 2% milk	½ cup (4.7 oz)	135	4	2	9	26	–	68
flan as prep w/ whole milk	½ cup (4.7 oz)	150	4	4	17	25	–	65
Betty Crocker								
Flan w/ Caramel Sauce as prep	1 serv	330	0	7	24	60	–	25
READY-TO-EAT								
Swiss Miss								
Egg Custard	1 pkg (4 oz)	153	5	5	4	22	0	138
TAKE-OUT								
baked	½ cup (5 oz)	148	7	7	123	15	–	109
flan	½ cup (5.4 oz)	220	7	6	140	35	–	86
zabaione	½ cup (57.2 g)	135	3	5	213	13	0	9
CUTTLEFISH								
steamed	3 oz	134	28	1	190	1	–	632
DANDELION GREENS								
fresh cooked	½ cup	17	1	tr	0	3	–	23
raw chopped	½ cup	13	1	tr	0	3	–	21

FOOD	PORTION	CALS	PROT	FAT	CHOL	CARB	FIBER	SOD
DANISH PASTRY								
FROZEN								
Morton								
Honey Buns	1 (2.28 oz)	270	3	13	0	35	1	160
Honey Buns Mini	1 (1.3 oz)	160	2	8	0	19	1	100
READY-TO-EAT								
plain ring	1 (12 oz)	1305	21	71	292	152	–	1302
TAKE-OUT								
almond	1 (4¼ in) (2.3 oz)	280	5	16	30	30	2	236
apple	1 (4¼ in) (2.5 oz)	264	4	13	–	34	1	251
cheese	1 (4¼ in) (2.5 oz)	266	6	16	–	26	–	319
cinnamon	1 (4¼ in) (2.3 oz)	262	5	15	–	29	1	241
cinnamon nut	1 (4¼ in) (2.3 oz)	280	5	16	30	30	2	236
lemon	1 (4¼ in) (2.5 oz)	264	4	13	–	34	1	251
raisin	1 (4¼ in) (2.5 oz)	264	4	13	–	34	1	251
raisin nut	1 (4¼ in) (2.3 oz)	280	5	16	30	30	2	236
raspberry	1 (4¼ in) (2.5 oz)	264	4	13	–	34	1	251
strawberry	1 (4¼ in) (2.5 oz)	264	4	13	–	34	1	251
DATES								
deglet noor dried	10	240	–	0	0	–	–	–
dried chopped	1 cup	489	4	1	0	131	–	5
dried whole	10	228	2	tr	0	61	–	2
jujube dried	1 oz	75	1	tr	–	19	2	2
jujube fresh	1 oz	30	tr	tr	0	7	–	1
jujube preserved in sugar	1 oz	91	tr	tr	–	22	–	2
medjool	2–3 (1.4 oz)	120	1	0	0	31	3	10
Calavo								
Dried Pitted	5–6 (1.4 oz)	120	1	0	0	31	3	0

FOOD	PORTION	CALS	PROT	FAT	CHOL	CARB	FIBER	SOD
California Redi-Date								
Deglet Noor Dried	5–6 (1.4 oz)	120	1	0	0	31	3	0
SunDate								
Fancy Medjool	3	120	1	0	0	31	3	0

DEER (see VENISON)

DELI MEATS/COLD CUTS (see also BEEF, CHICKEN, HAM, MEAT SUBSTITUTES, TURKEY)

FOOD	PORTION	CALS	PROT	FAT	CHOL	CARB	FIBER	SOD
barbecue loaf pork & beef	1 slice	40	4	2	9	1	0	307
beerwurst beef	1 slice (4 in x ⅛ in)	75	3	7	13	tr	—	214
beerwurst beef	1 slice (2¾ in x ¹⁄₁₆ in)	20	1	2	4	tr	—	62
beerwurst pork	1 slice (4 in x ⅛ in)	55	4	4	13	tr	—	285
beerwurst pork	1 slice (2¾in x ¹⁄₁₆ in)	14	1	1	4	tr	—	74
berliner pork & beef	1 oz	65	4	4	13	1	—	368
blood sausage	1 oz	95	4	9	30	tr	—	—
bologna beef	1 oz	88	4	8	16	tr	—	278
bologna beef & pork	1 oz	89	3	8	16	1	—	289
bologna pork	1 oz	70	4	6	17	tr	—	336
braunschweiger pork	1 slice (2½ in x ¼ in)	65	2	6	28	1	—	206
braunschweiger pork	1 oz	102	4	9	44	1	—	324
corned beef loaf	1 oz	43	7	2	13	0	—	270
dried beef	1 oz	47	—	1	—	tr	—	—
dutch brand loaf pork & beef	1 oz	68	4	5	13	2	—	354
headcheese pork	1 oz	60	5	5	23	tr	—	356
honey loaf pork & beef	1 oz	36	4	1	10	2	—	374
honey roll sausage beef	1 oz	42	4	2	12	1	—	304
lebanon bologna beef	1 oz	60	6	4	20	1	—	379

FOOD	PORTION	CALS	PROT	FAT	CHOL	CARB	FIBER	SOD
liver cheese pork	1 oz	86	4	7	49	1	–	347
liverwurst pork	1 oz	92	4	8	45	1	–	–
luncheon meat beef	1 oz	87	4	7	18	1	–	377
luncheon meat pork & beef	1 oz	100	4	9	15	1	–	367
luncheon meat pork canned	1 oz	95	4	9	18	1	–	365
luncheon sausage pork & beef	1 oz	74	4	6	18	tr	–	335
luxury loaf pork	1 oz	40	5	1	10	1	–	347
mortadella beef & pork	1 oz	88	5	7	16	1	–	353
mother's loaf pork	1 oz	80	3	6	13	2	–	320
new england sausage pork & beef	1 oz	46	5	2	14	1	–	346
olive loaf pork	1 oz	67	3	5	11	3	–	421
peppered loaf pork & beef	1 oz	42	5	2	13	1	–	432
pepperoni pork & beef	1 slice (0.2 oz)	27	1	2	–	tr	–	112
pepperoni pork & beef	1 (9 oz)	1248	53	110	–	7	–	5120
pickle & pimiento loaf pork	1 oz	74	3	6	10	2	–	394
picnic loaf pork & beef	1 oz	66	4	5	11	1	–	330
salami cooked beef & pork	1 oz	71	4	6	18	1	–	302
salami hard pork	1 pkg (4 oz)	460	26	38	–	2	–	2554
salami hard pork	1 slice (⅓ oz)	41	2	4	–	3	–	226
salami hard pork & beef	1 slice (0.3 oz)	42	2	3	8	tr	–	186
salami hard pork & beef	1 pkg (4 oz)	472	26	39	89	3	–	2101
sandwich spread pork & beef	1 tbsp	35	1	3	6	2	–	152
sandwich spread pork & beef	1 oz	67	2	5	11	3	–	287

FOOD	PORTION	CALS	PROT	FAT	CHOL	CARB	FIBER	SOD
summer sausage thuringer cervelat	1 oz	98	5	8	19	1	–	412
Boar's Head								
Bologna Beef	2 oz	150	7	13	35	0	0	520
Bologna Garlic	2 oz	150	7	13	35	1	0	530
Bologna Lowered Sodium	2 oz	150	8	13	30	0	0	410
Bologna Pork & Beef	2 oz	150	7	13	35	tr	0	530
Braunschweiger Lite	2 oz	120	9	8	50	1	0	450
Head Cheese	2 oz	90	10	5	65	tr	0	420
Liverwurst Strassburger	2 oz	170	8	15	85	1	0	560
Olive Loaf	2 oz	130	6	12	20	tr	0	630
Pastrami	2 oz	90	12	4	30	2	0	620
Prosciutto	1 oz	60	8	3	15	0	0	770
Red Pastrami	2 oz	90	12	4	30	2	0	620
Salami Beef	2 oz	120	10	9	25	0	0	470
Salami Cooked	2 oz	130	8	11	40	0	0	550
Salami Genoa	2 oz	180	12	14	55	1	0	970
Salami Hard	1 oz	110	6	9	25	tr	0	490
Spiced Ham	2 oz	120	7	10	30	1	0	570
Carl Buddig								
Beef	1 pkg (2.5 oz)	100	14	5	50	1	–	1020
Corned Beef	1 pkg (2.5 oz)	100	14	5	50	tr	–	980
Pastrami	1 pkg (2.5 oz)	100	14	5	50	1	–	750
Hormel								
Pepperoni Sliced	16 slices (1 oz)	140	6	13	25	1	–	490
TAKE-OUT								
corned beef	2 oz	70	12	2	40	0	–	390
corned beef brisket	2 oz	90	11	5	35	0	–	370
DILL								
seed	1 tsp	6	tr	tr	0	1	–	tr
sprigs fresh	5	0	tr	tr	0	tr	–	1

FOOD	PORTION	CALS	PROT	FAT	CHOL	CARB	FIBER	SOD
sprigs fresh	1 cup	4	tr	tr	0	1	–	5
weed dry	1 tsp	3	tr	tr	0	1	–	2

DINNER *(see also ASIAN FOOD, PASTA DINNERS, POT PIE, SPANISH FOOD)*

Amy's

FOOD	PORTION	CALS	PROT	FAT	CHOL	CARB	FIBER	SOD
Country Dinner Vegetable Salisbury Steak	1 pkg (11 oz)	380	11	12	15	60	9	570

Banquet

FOOD	PORTION	CALS	PROT	FAT	CHOL	CARB	FIBER	SOD
Beef Patty w/ Country Style Vegetables	1 meal (9.5 oz)	310	11	20	40	22	2	1090
Boneless Pork Rib	1 meal (10 oz)	400	17	19	45	40	4	1070
Boneless White Fried Chicken	1 meal (8.25 oz)	540	16	34	60	41	3	1180
Chicken Parmigiana	1 meal (9.5 oz)	320	10	18	50	29	3	900
Chicken Fingers Meal	1 meal (7.1 oz)	740	22	43	70	67	6	1070
Chicken Fried Beef Steak	1 pkg (10 oz)	420	15	23	35	39	4	1200
Chicken Nuggets Meal	1 meal (6.75 oz)	430	14	23	50	42	4	650
Extra Helping Boneless Pork Riblet	1 meal (15.25 oz)	720	27	40	80	62	7	1590
Extra Helping Fried Beef Steak	1 meal (16 oz)	820	29	50	70	63	6	2260
Extra Helping Fried Chicken	1 meal (14.7 oz)	910	34	55	160	70	5	2400
Extra Helping Meatloaf	1 meal (16 oz)	610	29	40	110	34	6	1940
Extra Helping Salisbury Steak	1 meal (16.5 oz)	740	27	54	130	37	7	2200
Extra Helping Turkey & Gravy w/ Dressing	1 meal (17 oz)	620	28	32	80	54	10	2250
Extra Helping White Fried Chicken	1 meal (13 oz)	690	24	48	70	40	8	1900

FOOD	PORTION	CALS	PROT	FAT	CHOL	CARB	FIBER	SOD
Extra Helping Yankee Pot Roast	1 meal (14.5 oz)	410	25	20	50	33	3	1660
Family Size Brown Gravy & Salisbury Steak	1 serv	240	9	20	40	7	1	900
Family Size Brown Gravy & Sliced Beef	1 serv	140	13	8	40	5	tr	850
Family Size Chicken & Broccoli Alfredo	1 serv	270	11	12	40	28	3	540
Family Size Country Style Chicken & Dumplings	1 serv	290	12	14	40	30	7	1270
Family Size Creamy Broccoli Chicken Cheese & Rice	1 serv	280	14	14	45	25	2	980
Family Size Hearty Beef Stew	1 cup	170	10	7	30	18	4	1120
Family Size Homestyle Gravy & Sliced Turkey	2 slices	140	7	10	40	5	1	600
Family Size Mushroom Gravy Charbroiled Beef Patties	1 patty	250	11	20	35	6	2	750
Family Size Potato Ham & Broccoli Au Gratin	⅔ cup	210	7	13	30	16	2	970
Family Size Savory Gravy & Meatloaf	1 slice	120	10	13	35	7	1	750
Fish Sticks	1 meal (6.6 oz)	290	11	13	30	33	4	820
Grilled Chicken	1 meal (9.9 oz)	330	16	13	50	37	2	1210
Honey Roast Turkey Breast	1 meal (9 oz)	270	11	12	30	29	4	1310
Meatloaf	1 meal (9.5 oz)	280	12	16	60	23	3	1020
Our Original Fried Chicken	1 meal (9 oz)	470	21	27	90	35	2	1500

FOOD	PORTION	CALS	PROT	FAT	CHOL	CARB	FIBER	SOD
Pork Cutlet Meal	1 meal (10.25 oz)	420	11	25	35	36	4	1060
Salisbury Steak	1 meal (9.5 oz)	340	13	20	50	26	4	1050
Sliced Beef	1 meal (9 oz)	270	26	10	70	19	4	740
Turkey Meal	1 meal (9.25 oz)	290	15	13	35	28	6	1050
Veal Parmagiana	1 meal (8.75 oz)	330	13	14	20	37	2	860
Western Style Beef Patty	1 meal (9.5 oz)	360	14	21	40	28	3	1400
White Meat Fried Chicken	1 meal (8.75 oz)	460	18	28	100	40	2	1100
Yankee Pot Roast	1 meal (9.4 oz)	230	14	10	60	20	4	1130
Birds Eye								
Easy Recipe Creations Sweet & Sour w/ Pineapple Tidbits	1⅔ cups	200	2	1	0	45	3	330
Voila! Beef Sirloin Steak And Garlic Potatoes	1 cup	240	13	9	25	26	3	650
Voila! Chicken Alfredo	1 cup	230	15	8	20	26	2	660
Voila! Garden Herb Chicken	1 cup	310	16	15	40	28	2	540
Voila! Grilled Salsa Chicken w/ Rice	1 cup	240	14	5	25	35	3	1180
Voila! Homestyle Turkey w/ Roasted Potatoes	1 cup	200	12	6	10	24	3	830
Voila! Teriyaki	2 cups (6.4 oz)	240	13	9	25	26	2	700
Voila! Zesty Garlic Chicken	2 cups (6.2 oz)	260	15	11	25	28	1	550
Fillo Factory								
Fillo Pie Broccoli & Cheese	¼ pie (4 oz)	350	14	12	20	50	3	370

FOOD	PORTION	CALS	PROT	FAT	CHOL	CARB	FIBER	SOD
Fillo Pie Spinach & Cheese	⅓ pie (4.8 oz)	210	12	7	15	27	2	270
Healthy Choice								
Beef Pepper Steak Oriental	1 meal (9.5 oz)	260	19	5	35	34	2	520
Beef Pot Roast	1 meal (11 oz)	300	20	6	40	41	6	600
Beef Stroganoff	1 meal (11 oz)	320	22	8	60	40	7	600
Beef Teriyaki	1 meal (9.5 oz)	310	16	7	40	44	5	600
Beef Tips Francais	1 meal (9.5 oz)	300	20	7	40	40	4	520
Beef Tips Portabello	1 meal (11.25 oz)	270	23	5	40	34	7	600
Bowls Chicken Teriyaki w/ Rice	1 meal (9.5 oz)	270	17	4	30	41	4	570
Bowls Country Chicken Bake	1 meal (9.5 oz)	230	18	8	50	22	4	600
Bowls Fiesta Chicken	1 meal (9.5 oz)	220	15	2	30	34	3	550
Bowls Garlic Lemon Chicken w/ Rice	1 meal (9.5 oz)	300	18	4	40	48	4	400
Bowls Roasted Potatoes w/ Ham	1 meal (8.5 oz)	210	17	4	30	26	6	600
Bowls Southwestern Chicken & Pasta	1 meal (9.5 oz)	320	31	4	40	39	6	350
Bowls Turkey Divan	1 meal (9.5 oz)	250	18	6	30	31	4	600
Charbroiled Beef Patty	1 meal (11 oz)	310	16	9	45	40	4	550
Chicken Cantonese	1 meal (10.75)	280	22	6	50	34	2	480
Chicken Parmigiana	1 meal (11.5 oz)	330	19	8	40	46	3	490
Chicken & Vegetables Marsala	1 meal (11.5 oz)	240	20	4	30	32	3	440
Chicken Broccoli Alfredo	1 meal (11.5 oz)	300	25	7	50	34	2	530

FOOD	PORTION	CALS	PROT	FAT	CHOL	CARB	FIBER	SOD
Chicken Dijon	1 meal (11 oz)	270	23	5	40	33	6	470
Chicken Teriyaki	1 meal (11 oz)	270	16	6	40	37	6	600
Country Glazed Chicken Breast	1 meal (8.5 oz)	250	19	5	30	31	3	600
Country Herb Chicken	1 meal (12.15 oz)	320	16	8	45	44	3	540
Country Inn Roast Turkey	1 meal (10 oz)	250	20	6	40	28	4	530
Garlic Chicken Milano	1 meal (9.5 oz)	260	18	6	35	34	3	510
Grilled Chicken Sonoma	1 meal (9 oz)	230	16	4	45	30	3	530
Grilled Chicken w/ Mashed Potatoes	1 meal (8 oz)	180	16	4	45	18	3	600
Herb Baked Fish	1 meal (10.9 oz)	340	16	7	35	54	5	480
Herb Breaded Pork Patty	1 meal (8 oz)	280	18	6	30	38	4	570
Homestyle Chicken & Pasta	1 meal (9 oz)	270	21	6	35	32	5	570
Honey Glazed Chicken	1 meal (10 oz)	270	21	7	45	32	4	600
Honey Mustard Chicken	1 meal (9.5 oz)	290	21	6	40	38	1	520
Lemon Pepper Fish	1 meal (10.7 oz)	280	11	5	35	49	5	580
Mandarin Chicken	1 meal (10 oz)	280	20	3	35	44	4	520
Mesquite Beef w/ Barbecue Sauce	1 meal (11 oz)	320	21	9	55	36	5	490
Mesquite Chicken Barbecue	1 meal (10.5 oz)	310	18	5	55	48	6	480
Oriental Style Chicken & Vegetable Stir Fry	1 meal (11.9)	360	19	6	25	57	5	600
Oven Roasted Beef	1 meal (10.15 oz)	280	18	8	50	35	4	600

FOOD	PORTION	CALS	PROT	FAT	CHOL	CARB	FIBER	SOD
Roast Turkey Breast	1 meal (8.5 oz)	220	18	5	25	28	5	600
Roasted Chicken	1 meal (11 oz)	230	20	5	50	23	4	560
Sesame Chicken	1 meal (10.8 oz)	360	19	7	20	54	4	600
Shrimp & Vegetables	1 meal (11.8 oz)	270	15	6	50	39	6	560
Sweet & Sour Chicken	1 meal (11 oz)	340	15	7	25	54	3	580
Traditional Meatloaf	1 meal (12 oz)	330	15	7	35	52	6	460
Traditional Salisbury Steak	1 meal (11.5 oz)	330	18	7	50	48	6	470
Traditional Turkey Breast	1 meal (10.5 oz)	330	21	5	35	50	4	600
Tuna Casserole	1 meal (8 oz)	240	16	5	25	33	4	560
Kid Cuisine								
Circus Show Corn Dog	1 meal (8.8 oz)	490	8	20	30	70	5	800
Cosmic Chicken Nuggets	1 meal (9.1 oz)	500	18	25	45	50	5	1070
Futuristic Fish Sticks	1 meal (8.25 oz)	410	9	16	20	57	4	550
Game Time Taco Roll Up	1 meal (7.35 oz)	420	9	18	25	55	4	740
High Flying Fried Chicken	1 meal (10.1 oz)	440	18	20	70	48	3	940
Parachuting Pork Ribettes	1 meal (7.55 oz)	390	16	19	50	39	3	760
Laura's Lifestyle								
Carb Conscious Chicken Puttanesca	1 pkg (9 oz)	270	34	10	—	7	3	830
Carb Conscious Chicken Chow Mein	1 pkg (9 oz)	260	34	8	—	9	3	870
Carb Conscious Thai Chicken	1 pkg (9 oz)	280	35	8	—	11	3	840

FOOD	PORTION	CALS	PROT	FAT	CHOL	CARB	FIBER	SOD
Carb Consciuos Chicken Santa Fe	1 pkg (9 oz)	280	40	9	–	9	2	850
Lean Cuisine								
Cafe Classics Baked Chicken	1 pkg (8.6 oz)	240	17	5	30	33	3	550
Cafe Classics Baked Fish	1 pkg (9 oz)	290	20	6	40	40	2	590
Cafe Classics Beef Peppercorn	1 pkg (8.75 oz)	260	16	7	25	32	4	590
Cafe Classics Beef Portobello	1 pkg (9 oz)	220	14	7	35	24	2	590
Cafe Classics Beef Pot Roast	1 pkg (9 oz)	210	13	6	30	25	6	570
Cafe Classics Chicken Carbonara	1 pkg (9 oz)	280	17	7	30	36	4	560
Cafe Classics Chicken Medallions w/ Creamy Cheese Sauce	1 pkg (9.37 oz)	300	19	7	35	40	2	690
Cafe Classics Chicken Mediterranean	1 pkg (10.5 oz)	260	17	4	20	38	4	690
Cafe Classics Chicken & Vegetables	1 pkg (10.5 oz)	240	19	5	30	30	4	690
Cafe Classics Chicken In Peanut Sauce	1 pkg (9 oz)	260	20	6	30	32	4	690
Cafe Classics Chicken In Wine Sauce	1 pkg (8.1 oz)	220	20	5	45	23	2	690
Cafe Classics Chicken L'Orange	1 pkg (9 oz)	230	20	2	40	33	2	300
Cafe Classics Chicken Parmesan	1 pkg (10.9 oz)	300	21	6	35	41	5	600
Cafe Classics Chicken Piccata	1 pkg (9 oz)	300	14	9	30	41	2	590

FOOD	PORTION	CALS	PROT	FAT	CHOL	CARB	FIBER	SOD
Cafe Classics Chicken w/ Basil Cream Sauce	1 pkg (8.5 oz)	260	17	7	35	33	2	650
Cafe Classics Country Vegetables & Beef	1 pkg (9 oz)	210	11	4	25	33	3	590
Cafe Classics Fiesta Chicken	1 pkg (9.25 oz)	270	17	5	30	40	3	690
Cafe Classics Glazed Chicken	1 pkg (8.5 oz)	240	22	6	55	25	0	480
Cafe Classics Glazed Turkey Tenderloins	1 pkg (9 oz)	260	14	5	25	41	4	640
Cafe Classics Grilled Chicken	1 pkg (9.4 oz)	250	22	5	40	29	3	690
Cafe Classics Herb Roasted Chicken	1 pkg (8 oz)	190	17	4	35	22	4	690
Cafe Classics Honey Mustard Chicken	1 pkg (8 oz)	270	19	4	35	40	1	690
Cafe Classics Honey Roasted Chicken	1 pkg (8.5 oz)	270	13	6	25	41	5	550
Cafe Classics Honey Roasted Pork	1 serv (9.5 oz)	250	17	6	45	32	3	590
Cafe Classics Meatloaf w/ Whipped Potatoes	1 pkg (9.4 oz)	260	20	7	45	28	4	600
Cafe Classics Oriental Beef	1 pkg (9.25 oz)	210	14	4	25	30	2	530
Cafe Classics Oven Roasted Beef	1 pkg (9.25 oz)	260	18	8	50	28	4	590
Cafe Classics Roasted Turkey Breast	1 pkg (9.75 oz)	270	13	2	25	49	3	590
Cafe Classics Salisbury Steak	1 pkg (9.5 oz)	280	24	8	60	29	4	590
Cafe Classics Southern Beef Tips	1 pkg (8.75 oz)	270	16	6	35	37	4	480
Everyday Favorites Chicken Florentine	1 pkg (8 oz)	220	13	5	25	32	3	640

FOOD	PORTION	CALS	PROT	FAT	CHOL	CARB	FIBER	SOD
Everyday Favorites Chicken Chow Mein	1 pkg (9 oz)	240	14	4	35	37	3	590
Everyday Favorites Homestyle Turkey	1 pkg (9.4 oz)	240	22	5	40	27	3	590
Everyday Favorites Hunan Beef & Broccoli	1 pkg (8.5 oz)	240	11	4	20	40	2	690
Everyday Favorites Mandarin Chicken	1 pkg (9 oz)	260	15	5	35	38	2	570
Everyday Favorites Roasted Chicken	1 pkg (8.1 oz)	260	14	7	20	34	4	640
Everyday Favorites Stuffed Cabbage	1 pkg (9.5 oz)	210	9	8	20	25	5	590
Everyday Favorites Swedish Meatballs	1 pkg (9.1 oz)	290	22	7	45	35	4	590
Everyday Favorites Vegetable Lasagna	1 pkg (10.5 oz)	260	15	7	20	36	5	590
Hearty Portions Cheese & Spinach Manicotti	1 serv	370	25	8	35	50	8	850
Hearty Portions Chicken & Barbecue Sauce	1 serv	370	20	6	40	60	6	840
Hearty Portions Homestyle Beef Stroganoff	1 serv	350	23	9	30	44	9	850
Hearty Portions Jumbo Rigatoni w/ Meatballs	1 serv	440	25	9	35	64	7	820
Hearty Portions Oriental Glazed Chicken	1 serv	370	21	2	35	66	4	850
Hearty Portions Roasted Chicken w/ Mushrooms	1 serv	330	23	4	40	49	4	740
Skillet Sensations Beef Teriyaki & Rice	1 serv	280	14	3	25	48	5	700

FOOD	PORTION	CALS	PROT	FAT	CHOL	CARB	FIBER	SOD
Skillet Sensations Chicken Primavera	1 serv	320	20	5	30	50	4	790
Skillet Sensations Chicken Oriental	1 serv	280	17	3	15	46	6	790
Skillet Sensations Fiesta Beef & Rice	1 serv	300	19	4	25	48	6	760
Skillet Sensations Garlic Chicken	1 serv	340	20	5	20	56	4	730
Skillet Sensations Herb Chicken & Roasted Potatoes	1 serv	270	18	5	40	39	5	790
Skillet Sensations Roasted Turkey	1 serv	220	14	2	25	37	6	790
Skillet Sensations Savory Beef & Vegetables	1 serv	290	18	7	35	38	9	1440
Skillet Sensations Three Cheese Chicken	1 serv	370	26	10	50	45	3	820
Luzianne								
Cajun Creole Dirty Rice	1 serv	160	4	1	0	35	0	680
Cajun Creole Etouffee	1 serv	200	5	1	0	42	1	1030
Cajun Creole Gumbo	1 serv	160	4	1	0	33	1	760
Cajun Creole Jambalaya	1 serv	200	5	1	0	43	1	690
Marie Callender's								
Beef Stroganoff w/ Noodles	1 meal (13 oz)	600	20	27	70	59	4	1140
Beef Tips In Mushroom Sauce	1 meal (13 oz)	430	25	19	50	39	6	1020
Breaded Chicken Parmigiana	1 meal (16 oz)	860	30	32	50	63	5	920
Breaded Fish w/ Mac & Cheese	1 meal (12 oz)	550	22	28	60	53	3	1400
Cheesy Rice w/ Chicken & Broccoli	1 meal (12 oz)	390	24	13	55	44	6	1220

FOOD	PORTION	CALS	PROT	FAT	CHOL	CARB	FIBER	SOD
Chicken & Dumplings	1 meal (14 oz)	390	17	20	130	34	4	1650
Chicken & Noodles	1 meal (13 oz)	520	21	30	80	42	5	1320
Chicken Cordon Bleu	1 meal (13 oz)	610	23	28	75	58	6	1920
Chicken Fried Beef Steak & Gravy	1 meal (15 oz)	650	20	37	50	50	7	2260
Chicken Teriyaki	1 meal (13 oz)	510	24	12	55	71	2	1510
Country Fried Chicken & Gravy	1 meal (16 oz)	620	24	30	75	63	6	2300
Country Fried Pork Chop	1 meal (15 oz)	540	23	28	65	50	8	2240
Escalloped Noodles & Chicken	1 meal (13 oz)	740	21	46	90	60	5	1600
Glazed Chicken	1 meal (13 oz)	490	25	25	90	40	1	2130
Grilled Southwestern Style Chicken	1 meal (14 oz)	410	24	11	80	43	6	2020
Grilled Chicken & Mashed Potatoes	1 meal (10 oz)	340	24	16	90	20	1	1090
Grilled Chicken Breast & Rice Pilaf	1 meal (11.75 oz)	360	20	14	40	36	4	1070
Grilled Chicken In Mushroom Sauce	1 meal (14 oz)	480	32	15	65	54	7	1030
Grilled Turkey Breast & Rice Pilaf	1 meal (11.75 oz)	310	22	10	40	34	4	940
Herb Roasted Chicken & Mashed Potatoes	1 meal (14 oz)	580	42	34	205	26	7	2100
Homestyle Turkey & Noodles	1 meal (12 oz)	600	18	35	90	52	5	1570
Honey Roasted Chicken	1 meal (14 oz)	440	45	17	140	27	7	1170

FOOD	PORTION	CALS	PROT	FAT	CHOL	CARB	FIBER	SOD
Honey Smoked Ham Steak w/ Macaroni & Cheese	1 meal (14 oz)	490	29	13	80	63	5	2310
Meatloaf & Gravy w/ Mashed Potatoes	1 meal (14 oz)	540	23	30	95	42	5	1570
Old Fashioned Beef Pot Roast & Gravy	1 meal (15 oz)	500	23	17	110	55	3	1460
Roast Beef	1 meal (14.5 oz)	390	24	19	70	30	11	1240
Sirloin Salisbury Steak & Gravy	1 meal (14 oz)	550	30	25	85	51	6	1660
Skillet Meal Au Gratin Potatoes	⅔ cup (5 oz)	190	7	10	30	19	2	400
Skillet Meal Beef Pot Roast	½ pkg	290	20	9	60	33	5	1200
Skillet Meal Beef Stroganoff	½ pkg	310	21	11	60	31	5	1290
Skillet Meal Chicken & Rice w/ Broccoli & Cheese	½ pkg	440	30	14	70	47	8	1450
Skillet Meal Chicken Teriyaki	½ pkg	340	21	1	30	61	5	1140
Skillet Meal Herb Chicken	½ pkg	290	22	4	35	42	5	1030
Skillet Meal Roasted Chicken & Vegetables	½ pkg	260	21	6	40	30	7	1020
Skillet Meal White & Wild Rice In Cheese Sauce	1 cup	300	11	13	35	35	2	750
Swedish Meatballs	1 meal (12.5 oz)	520	28	26	65	44	3	1020
Sweet & Sour Chicken	1 meal (14 oz)	570	23	15	40	66	7	700
Turkey w/ Gravy & Dressing	1 meal (14 oz)	500	31	19	80	52	4	2040
Morton								
Breaded Chicken Pattie	1 meal (6.75 oz)	290	10	17	35	24	4	840

FOOD	PORTION	CALS	PROT	FAT	CHOL	CARB	FIBER	SOD
Chicken Nuggets	1 meal (7 oz)	340	12	19	30	31	2	470
Chili Gravy w/ Beef Enchilada & Tamale	1 meal (10 oz)	270	7	9	10	40	7	1000
Fried Chicken	1 meal (9 oz)	470	20	30	90	30	3	1100
Gravy & Charbroiled Beef Patty	1 meal (9 oz)	310	10	18	20	26	5	1210
Gravy & Salisbury Steak	1 meal (9 oz)	310	7	20	30	24	3	1100
Gravy & Turkey w/ Stuffing	1 meal (9 oz)	240	10	10	40	27	4	1200
Tomato Sauce w/ Meat Loaf	1 meal (9 oz)	250	9	13	20	24	3	1200
Veal Parmagiana w/ Tomato Sauce	1 meal (8.75 oz)	290	8	15	25	30	4	950
Nature's Choice								
Broccoli Parmesan Alfredo	1 pkg (12 oz)	270	20	9	10	29	5	960
Nature's Entree								
Hearty Stew	1 pkg (12 oz)	290	18	9	10	34	3	960
Tuscany White Bean	1 pkg (12 oz)	330	21	8	5	42	4	920
Patio								
Ranchera	1 pkg (13 oz)	470	13	22	35	55	9	2470
Swanson								
Beef Pot Roast	1 pkg (14 oz)	320	19	8	35	44	4	1200
Chicken Parmigiana w/ Spaghetti	1 pkg (11 oz)	380	17	17	25	41	5	700
Turkey Breast & Stuffing Dinner	1 pkg (11.7 oz)	350	15	11	35	43	4	1080
Tamarind Tree								
Alu Chole	1 pkg (9.2 oz)	350	12	6	0	63	9	620
Channa Dal Masala	1 pkg (9.2 oz)	340	13	5	0	62	10	700

FOOD	PORTION	CALS	PROT	FAT	CHOL	CARB	FIBER	SOD
Dal Makhini	1 pkg (9.2 oz)	330	14	6	5	55	14	670
Dhingri Mutter	1 pkg (9.2 oz)	290	8	5	0	53	7	680
Navratan Korma	1 pkg (9.2 oz)	430	12	15	5	60	7	700
Palak Paneer	1 pkg (9.2 oz)	380	14	15	35	46	6	640
Saag Chole	1 pkg (9.2 oz)	370	14	10	0	55	13	800
Vegetable Jalfrazi	1 pkg (9.2 oz)	310	8	6	0	57	7	600
Weight Watchers								
Smart Ones Swedish Meatballs	1 pkg (9 oz)	280	19	70	30	34	3	690
Yves								
Veggie Country Stew	1 pkg (10.5 oz)	170	17	0	0	24	7	1020
DIP								
Cabot								
Bac'n Horseradish	2 tbsp	50	1	5	15	1	0	190
Clam	2 tbsp	50	1	5	15	1	0	120
French Onion	2 tbsp	50	1	5	15	1	0	190
Ranch	1 tbsp	50	1	5	15	1	0	160
Salsa Grande	2 tbsp	50	1	5	15	1	0	130
Veggie	2 tbsp	50	1	5	15	2	0	125
Fritos								
Bean	2 tbsp (1.2 oz)	40	2	1	0	6	0	140
Chili Cheese	1.2 oz	45	1	3	<5	3	0	310
French Onion	2 tbsp (1.1 oz)	60	1	5	15	4	0	230
Hot Bean	2 tbsp (1.2 oz)	40	2	1	0	5	1	170
Jalapeno & Cheddar Cheese	2 tbsp (1.2 oz)	50	1	4	5	4	0	300
Gringo Billy's								
Guacamole Mix	1 tsp	10	0	0	0	2	1	40
Guiltless Gourmet								
Black Bean Mild	2 tbsp	30	2	0	0	5	2	115
Black Bean Spicy	2 tbsp	30	2	0	0	5	2	110

FOOD	PORTION	CALS	PROT	FAT	CHOL	CARB	FIBER	SOD
Racquet								
Hot Cheddar Jalapeno	2 tbsp	30	0	3	0	1	0	270
Ruffles								
French Onion	2 tbsp	70	1	5	0	4	1	240
Ranch	2 tbsp (1.2 oz)	70	1	6	0	4	0	300
Snyder's Of Hanover								
Microwavable Hot Nacho	2 tbsp	48	1	3	3	5	0	270
Microwavable Mild Cheese	2 tbsp	45	2	3	5	2	0	250
Mustard Pretzel	2 tbsp	60	1	2	0	12	0	0
Sour Cream & Onion	2 tbsp	60	1	5	15	2	0	220
Utz								
Fat Free Sour Cream & Onion	2 tbsp (1.1 oz)	30	1	0	0	7	0	210
Jalapeno & Cheddar	2 tbsp (1 oz)	30	0	3	0	2	0	250
Low Fat Desert Garden	2 tbsp (1.1 oz)	40	1	2	0	5	0	210
Low Fat Salsa Con Queso	2 tbsp (1 oz)	40	1	2	0	5	0	240
Mild Cheddar	2 tbsp (1 oz)	45	2	3	5	2	0	250
Sour Cream & Onion	2 tbsp (1 oz)	60	1	5	15	2	0	220
Walden Farms								
Low Carb Bruschetta	2 tbsp	35	0	3	0	0	0	90
Low Carb Pesto Bruschetta	1 tsp	10	0	1	0	9	0	20
DOCK								
fresh cooked	3½ oz	20	2	1	0	3	–	3
raw chopped	½ cup	15	1	tr	0	2	–	3
DOLPHINFISH								
fresh baked	3 oz	93	20	1	80	0	–	96
fresh fillet baked	5.6 oz	174	38	1	149	0	–	179

FOOD	PORTION	CALS	PROT	FAT	CHOL	CARB	FIBER	SOD
DOUGHNUTS								
cake type unsugared	1 (1.6 oz)	198	2	11	18	23	1	257
chocolate glazed	1 (1.5 oz)	175	2	8	–	24	1	143
chocolate sugared	1 (1.5 oz)	175	2	8	–	24	1	143
chocolate coated	1 (1.5 oz)	204	2	13	–	21	1	185
creme filled	1 (3 oz)	307	6	21	20	26	–	262
french cruller glazed	1 (1.4 oz)	169	1	8	5	24	–	142
frosted	1 (1.5 oz)	204	2	13	–	21	1	185
honey bun	1 (2.1 oz)	242	4	14	4	27	1	205
jelly	1 (3 oz)	289	5	16	22	33	–	249
old fashioned	1 (1.6 oz)	198	2	11	18	23	1	257
sugared	1 (1.6 oz)	192	2	10	14	23	1	181
wheat glazed	1 (1.6 oz)	162	3	9	9	19	–	160
wheat sugared	1 (1.6 oz)	162	3	9	9	19	–	160
yeast glazed	1 (2.1 oz)	242	4	14	4	27	1	205
Entenmann's								
Frosted Mini	1 (1 oz)	150	1	11	<5	12	tr	90
Snack & Smile								
Mini Donuts Chocolate	6	370	4	19	10	45	2	350
Mini Donuts Glazed	6	340	3	16	20	46	tr	220
Mini Donuts Powdered Sugar	6	320	4	13	10	46	1	360
Super								
Donut Chocolate	1 (2.2 oz)	210	4	11	10	26	1	240
Donut Honey Wheat	1 (2.2 oz)	230	5	11	10	29	tr	260
DRINK MIXERS								
whiskey sour mix not prep	1 pkg (0.6 oz)	64	tr	0	0	16	–	46
whiskey sour mix	2 oz	55	0	0	0	14	0	66
Baja Bob's								
Bloody Mary Mix Lean & Mean	4 oz	20	0	0	0	4	0	420
Pina Colada	4 oz	30	1	1	0	4	1	80
Sugar Free Margarita Mix	4 oz	10	0	0	0	tr	–	80

FOOD	PORTION	CALS	PROT	FAT	CHOL	CARB	FIBER	SOD
Sugar Free Margarita Mix Desert Lime	4 oz	10	0	0	0	tr	0	45
Sugar Free Margarita Mix Wild Strawberry	4 oz	10	0	0	0	tr	—	80
Sweet-n-Sour Mix	4 oz	10	0	0	0	tr	—	80
Daily's								
Bloody Mary Original	1 serv (6 oz)	50	0	0	0	14	—	1040
Margarita Daiquri Strawberry	1 serv (4 oz)	180	0	0	0	47	2	65
Margarita Green Demon	1 serv (3 oz)	80	0	0	0	19	—	45
Pina Colada	1 serv (3 oz)	160	0	2	0	37	1	115
Ocean Spray								
Bloody Mary Mix	4 oz	40	0	0	0	10	—	950
Margarita Mix	4 oz	160	0	0	0	40	—	35
Sour Mix	4 oz	140	0	0	0	34	—	35
DRUM								
freshwater fillet baked	5.4 oz	236	35	10	126	0	—	148
freshwater baked	3 oz	130	19	5	70	0	—	82
DUCK								
w/ skin roasted	1 cup (4.9 oz)	472	27	40	118	0	0	83
w/ skin w/ bone leg roasted	3 oz	184	23	10	97	0	—	94
w/ skin w/o bone breast roasted	3 oz	172	21	9	116	0	—	71
w/o skin roasted	1 cup (4.9 oz)	281	33	16	125	0	0	91
w/o skin w/ bone leg braised	1 cup (6.1 oz)	310	51	10	183	0	—	188
w/o skin w/o bone breast broiled	1 cup (6.1 oz)	244	48	4	249	0	—	183
wild w/ skin w/ skin raw	½ duck (9.5 oz)	571	47	41	216	0	—	152

FOOD	PORTION	CALS	PROT	FAT	CHOL	CARB	FIBER	SOD
wild w/o skin breast raw	½ breast (2.9 oz)	102	16	4	–	0	–	47
Grimaud Farms								
Muscovy Duck Confit	1 serv (3 oz)	170	20	10	95	tr	–	140
Maple Leaf Farms								
Breast Filet	4 oz	360	17	33	60	0	0	370
Leg Quarters	4 oz	420	15	33	90	0	0	95
Orange Breast Filet	4 oz	320	15	28	75	1	–	280

DUMPLING
Health Is Wealth
Potstickers Chicken Free	2 (1.6 oz)	80	4	4	0	11	1	300
Potstickers Pork Free	2 (1.6 oz)	80	4	4	0	11	1	300
Potstickers Vegetable	2 (1.6 oz)	90	7	3	0	11	5	190
Steamed Dumpling	2 (1.6 oz)	50	7	2	0	12	1	310

DURIAN
fresh	3.5 oz	141	3	2	0	29	–	1

EEL
fresh cooked	1 fillet (5.6 oz)	375	38	24	257	0	–	104
fresh cooked	3 oz	200	20	13	137	0	–	55
raw	3 oz	156	16	10	107	0	–	43
smoked	3.5 oz	330	19	28	–	0	0	–

EGG (see also EGG DISHES, EGG SUBSTITUTES)
CHICKEN
fresh	1	75	6	5	213	1	–	63
frozen	1	75	6	5	213	1	–	63
frozen	1 cup	363	30	24	1033	3	–	307
hard cooked	1	77	6	5	213	1	–	62
hard cooked chopped	1 cup	210	17	14	578	2	–	169
poached	1	74	6	5	212	1	–	140
white only	1 cup	121	26	0	0	2	–	399
white only	1	17	4	0	0	tr	–	55

FOOD	PORTION	CALS	PROT	FAT	CHOL	CARB	FIBER	SOD
Eggology								
100% Organic Egg Whites	¼ cup	30	7	0	0	1	—	100
Gold Circle Farms								
Cage Free	1 large	70	6	5	215	tr	—	70
Horizon Organic								
Medium	1 (1.5 oz)	70	6	4	190	1	—	55
Land O Lakes								
Brown Extra Large	1 (2 oz)	80	7	5	240	1	—	70
OTHER POULTRY								
duck	1 (2.5 oz)	130	9	10	619	1	0	102
duck 100 year old	1 (1 oz)	49	4	3	173	1	—	154
duck preserved hard core	1 (1.8 oz)	80	6	6	220	1	0	350
duck preserved soft core	1 (1.8 oz)	80	7	6	220	1	0	350
duck salted	1 (1 oz)	54	4	4	184	2	—	769
goose	1 (5 oz)	267	20	19	—	2	—	—
quail	1 (9 g)	14	1	1	76	tr	—	—
turkey	1 (2.7 oz)	135	9	9	737	1	—	—
EGG DISHES								
TAKE-OUT								
cheese omelette as prep w/ 2 eggs	1 (6.8 oz)	519	31	44	—	tr	0	—
deviled	2 halves	145	6	13	280	1	—	180
omelette plain	1 serv (3.5 oz)	172	15	13	350	tr	0	245
salad	½ cup	307	13	28	562	2	—	565
scotch egg	1 (4.2 oz)	301	14	21	—	16	2	—
scrambled plain	2 (3.3 oz)	199	13	15	400	2	0	211
scrambled w/ whole milk & margarine	1 serv	365	24	27	774	5	—	616
sunny side up	1	91	6	7	211	1	—	162
EGG ROLLS								
egg roll wrapper fresh	1	83	3	tr	3	16	—	162
Chun King								
Chicken Mini	6	210	6	9	15	25	2	650

FOOD	PORTION	CALS	PROT	FAT	CHOL	CARB	FIBER	SOD
Chicken Restaurant Style	1 (3 oz)	190	6	9	20	22	2	550
Pork & Shrimp Mini	6	210	6	9	15	27	2	540
Shrimp Mini	6	190	5	6	10	28	2	730
Shrimp Restaurant Style	1 (3 oz)	180	5	7	15	25	2	490
Health Is Wealth								
Broccoli	1 (3 oz)	150	4	5	5	23	2	560
Oriental Vegetable	1 (3 oz)	160	4	4	0	23	2	390
Oriental Chicken Free	1 (3 oz)	120	8	4	0	21	2	390
Pizza	1 (3 oz)	200	7	9	0	23	3	470
Spinach	1 (3 oz)	180	7	8	0	20	3	300
Spring Rolls	1 (1.6 oz)	70	2	2	0	10	5	200
Veggie	1 (3 oz)	130	4	4	0	21	3	550
La Choy								
Chicken Mini	6	210	6	9	15	25	2	650
Chicken Restaurant Style	1 (3 oz)	210	6	9	15	25	2	550
Pork Restaurant Style	1 (3 oz)	220	5	11	10	24	2	390
Pork & Shrimp Bite Size	12	210	6	10	10	25	2	540
Pork & Shrimp Mini	6	210	6	9	15	27	2	540
Shrimp Mini	6	190	5	6	10	28	2	730
Shrimp Restaurant Style	1 (3 oz)	180	5	7	15	25	2	490
Sweet & Sour Chicken Restaurant Style	1 (3 oz)	220	6	9	15	29	2	550
Vegetable w/ Lobster Mini	6	190	5	7	5	27	2	440
Loompya								
Lumpia Chicken & Vegetables	2	170	8	1	10	31	2	150
Pagoda								
Sweet & Sour Chicken	1 (2.7 oz)	170	6	6	5	25	2	260
TAKE-OUT								
chicken	1 (3 oz)	140	7	4	15	20	4	510

FOOD	PORTION	CALS	PROT	FAT	CHOL	CARB	FIBER	SOD
lobster	1 (4.8 oz)	270	8	7	0	43	6	460
lumpia vegetable & shrimp	2 (3 oz)	120	4	0	10	26	2	300
meat & shrimp	1 (4.8 oz)	320	10	12	10	41	4	470
pork & shrimp	1 (5 oz)	300	13	10	15	41	7	890
shrimp	1 (3 oz)	170	6	5	<5	24	5	420
spicy pork	1 (3 oz)	200	6	9	5	23	3	410
vegetable	1 (3 oz)	170	5	4	0	28	4	520
EGG SUBSTITUTES								
frozen	1 cup	384	27	27	5	8	—	479
frozen	¼ cup	96	7	7	1	2	—	120
liquid	1½ oz	40	6	2	tr	tr	—	83
liquid	1 cup (8.8 oz)	211	30	8	3	2	—	444
powder	0.7 oz	88	11	3	113	4	—	158
powder	0.35 oz	44	5	1	57	2	—	79
Better'n Eggs								
Fat Free Cholesterol Free	¼ cup (2 oz)	30	6	0	0	1	0	100
Deb-El								
Just Whites	2 tsp	12	3	0	—	0	0	51
Egg Beaters								
Egg Substitute	¼ cup	30	6	0	0	1	0	115
Morningstar Farms								
Breakfast Sandwich Bagel Scramblers Pattie Cheese	1 (5.9 oz)	320	28	5	10	40	4	900
Scramblers	¼ cup (2 oz)	35	6	0	0	2	0	95
Quick Eggs								
Fat Free Cholesterol Free	¼ cup	30	6	0	0	1	0	80
EGGNOG								
eggnog	1 cup	342	10	19	149	34	—	138
eggnog	1 qt	1368	39	76	596	138	—	553
eggnog flavor mix as prep w/ milk	9 oz	260	8	8	33	39	—	163
Oberweis								
Egg Nog	½ cup	240	3	15	40	25	0	70

FOOD	PORTION	CALS	PROT	FAT	CHOL	CARB	FIBER	SOD
TAKE-OUT								
eggnog	1 cup	306	5	22	63	16	0	95
EGGNOG SUBSTITUTES								
Silk								
Nog	½ cup	90	3	2	0	15	0	75
EGGPLANT								
cubed cooked	1 cup	28	1	tr	0	7	3	3
raw cut up	½ cup (1.4 oz)	11	tr	tr	0	2	–	1
slices grilled	4 (7 oz)	38	2	0	0	0	–	–
whole peeled raw	1 (1 lb)	117	5	1	0	28	–	14
Progresso								
Caponata	2 tbsp (1 oz)	25	0	2	0	2	2	130
TastyBite								
Punjab Eggplant	½ pkg (5 oz)	130	5	8	0	9	4	780
TAKE-OUT								
baba ghannouj	¼ cup	55	2	4	0	5	–	95
caponata	2 tbsp (1 oz)	30	1	2	0	3	–	115
iman bayildi eggplant w/ onion & tomato	1 serv (15.6 oz)	345	3	28	0	25	2	552
indian eggplant runi	1 serv	180	2	14	0	13	1	228
moussaka	1 cup	237	–	13	97	–	–	432
papoutsakis little shoes	1 serv (15.5 oz)	245	12	16	40	15	1	751
ELDERBERRIES								
fresh	1 cup	105	1	1	0	27	–	–
ELDERBERRY JUICE								
elderberry	7 oz	76	4	0	0	16	–	2
ELK								
roasted	3 oz	124	26	2	62	0	–	52
EMU								
cooked	3 oz	130	–	–	111	–	–	97
ENDIVE								
fresh	3.5 oz	9	2	tr	0	tr	2	53
raw chopped	½ cup	4	tr	tr	0	1	–	6

FOOD	PORTION	CALS	PROT	FAT	CHOL	CARB	FIBER	SOD

ENERGY BARS (see also CEREAL BARS, NUTRITION SUPPLEMENTS)

AllGoode Organics

FOOD	PORTION	CALS	PROT	FAT	CHOL	CARB	FIBER	SOD
Amazin' Peanut Raisin	1 bar	210	7	11	0	25	3	80
Banana Nut Nirvana	1 bar	190	5	8	0	30	3	5
Cashew Almond Passion	1 bar	210	7	9	0	25	3	50
Chocolate Peanut Pleasure	1 bar	200	5	9	5	29	3	15
Honey Nut Harvest	1 bar	210	7	9	0	29	3	50
Nutty Chocolate Apricot	1 bar	200	6	10	5	26	5	15

Atkins

FOOD	PORTION	CALS	PROT	FAT	CHOL	CARB	FIBER	SOD
Advantage Almond Brownie	1 bar (1.6 oz)	220	21	8	5	21	7	105
Advantage Chocolate Coconut	1 bar (1.6 oz)	230	19	11	2	21	9	100
Advantage Chocolate Decadence	1 bar (1.6 oz)	220	17	11	2	25	11	65
Advantage Chocolate Mocha Crunch	1 bar (1.6 oz)	220	20	10	2	22	10	120
Advantage Chocolate Peanut Butter	1 bar (1.6 oz)	240	19	12	2	21	10	125
Advantage Cookies 'N Creme	1 bar (1.6 oz)	220	18	11	2	22	11	200
Advantage S'mores	1 bar (1.6 oz)	220	17	10	0	26	11	130
Morning Start Apple Crisp	1 bar	170	11	9	–	13	6	70
Morning Start Blueberry Muffin	1 bar	160	12	7	–	16	7	80
Morning Start Chocolate Chip Crisp	1 bar	160	12	7	–	14	5	110

Back To Nature

FOOD	PORTION	CALS	PROT	FAT	CHOL	CARB	FIBER	SOD
10th Tee Chocolate Fudge	1 bar	200	7	6	0	31	1	40

FOOD	PORTION	CALS	PROT	FAT	CHOL	CARB	FIBER	SOD
10th Tee Peanut Honey	1 bar	260	6	6	0	32	2	64
1st Tee Chocolate Peanut	1 bar	290	9	8	0	44	1	105
1st Tee Oatmeal Raisin	1 bar	280	9	7	0	44	1	150
Balance								
Big Bar Honey Peanut	1 bar	310	22	10	5	33	tr	270
Chocolate Banana + Antioxidants	1 bar	200	14	6	5	22	1	135
Chocolate Mint + Antioxidants	1 bar	200	14	6	<5	23	0	200
Gold Caramel Nut Blast	1 bar	210	15	7	0	22	tr	110
Gold Chocolate Peanut Butter	1 bar	210	15	7	0	22	tr	125
Gold Rocky Road	1 bar	210	15	7	0	23	1	70
Gold Triple Chocolate Chaos	1 bar	200	15	6	0	22	tr	85
Gold Crunch Chocolate Chocolate	1 bar	210	15	6	0	23	tr	150
Gold Crunch Chocolate Mint Cookie	1 bar	210	15	6	0	23	tr	160
Gold Crunch S'mores	1 bar	210	15	7	0	23	0	160
Honey Peanut + Ginseng	1 bar	200	15	6	<5	22	tr	190
Lemon Meringue + Calcium	1 bar	190	14	6	0	22	0	150
Original Almond Brownie	1 bar	200	14	6	<5	23	2	115
Original Chocolate	1 bar	200	14	6	<5	22	tr	180
Original Chocolate Raspberry Fudge	1 bar	200	14	6	0	22	1	90
Original Honey Peanut	1 bar	200	14	6	<5	24	tr	180
Original Mocha Chip	1 bar	200	14	6	0	23	tr	125

FOOD	PORTION	CALS	PROT	FAT	CHOL	CARB	FIBER	SOD
Original Peanut Butter	1 bar	200	14	6	<5	22	1	230
Original Yogurt Honey Peanut	1 bar	200	15	6	<5	22	tr	190
Outdoor Chocolate Crisp	1 bar	200	15	6	<5	21	3	140
Outdoor Crunchy Peanut	1 bar	200	15	6	<5	21	2	140
Outdoor Honey Almond	1 bar	200	15	6	<5	21	3	140
Outdoor Nut Berry	1 bar	200	15	6	<5	21	2	75
Satisfaction Apple Cinnamon Oatmeal	1 bar	280	12	5	0	47	6	260
Satisfaction Chocolate Crisp	1 bar	280	12	6	0	47	6	270
Satisfaction Chocolate Peanut	1 bar	280	11	6	0	48	6	320
Satisfaction Peanut Butter Crisp	1 bar	280	12	6	0	47	6	350
Yogurt Berry + Antioxidants	1 bar	200	14	6	5	22	0	120
Be Natural								
Almond & Apricot	1 bar	218	4	14	0	21	4	34
Almond & Coconut	1 bar	248	4	18	0	19	1	40
Banana & Wheat Bran	1 bar	201	2	9	0	29	4	35
Fruit & Nut Delight	1 bar	225	6	14	0	21	3	72
Macadamia & Apricot	1 bar	224	2	15	0	21	3	37
Nut Delight	1 bar	266	8	20	0	20	3	86
Sesame Nut Split	1 bar	256	7	17	0	20	2	110
Walnut & Date	1 bar	147	2	9	0	29	1	55
Yogurt Coated Almond & Apricot	1 bar	233	4	14	0	23	2	60
Yogurt Coated Fruit & Nut	1 bar	190	4	12	0	19	1	40
Benecol								
Chocolate Crisp	1 bar (1.2 oz)	130	3	3	5	23	2	60

FOOD	PORTION	CALS	PROT	FAT	CHOL	CARB	FIBER	SOD
Peanut Crisp	1 bar (1.2 oz)	140	3	4	5	23	1	105
Better Bar								
Chocolate Coated Caramel Pecan	1 bar (1.8 oz)	180	18	4	0	15	0	35
Chocolate Coated Peanut	1 bar (1.8 oz)	180	18	4	0	15	0	35
Yogurt Coated Raspberry	1 bar (1.8 oz)	180	18	3	0	15	0	35
Boost								
Chocolate Crunch	1 bar (1.5 oz)	190	4	7	<5	29	tr	90
Breakthru								
Organic Chocolate Fudge	1 bar (2.1 oz)	230	10	3	0	39	3	120
Organic Cinnamon Crunch	1 bar (2.1 oz)	220	12	3	0	37	3	160
Organic Honey Graham	1 bar (2.1 oz)	220	12	3	0	37	3	160
Organic Mocha Fudge	1 bar (2.1 oz)	230	10	3	0	39	3	120
Carb Options								
Chocolate Chip	1 bar	200	16	8	<5	17	tr	200
Chocolate Peanut	1 bar	200	16	8	<5	17	tr	240
Cinnamon Delight	1 bar	200	16	8	<5	17	0	200
Carbolite								
Chocolate Peanut Butter Sugar Free	1 bar (1 oz)	144	tr	12	4	2	0	28
CarbWise								
Chocolate S'Mores Crunch	1 bar	240	20	9	0	24	1	330
Centrum								
Energy Chocolate Nougat	1 (1.98 oz)	220	8	5	0	34	tr	185
Energy Chocolate Peanut Butter	1 (1.98 oz)	220	8	5	0	34	tr	185
Choice								
Berry Almond Crispy	1 bar	50	2	1	0	10	0	25
Fudge Brownie	1 bar	140	6	5	<5	19	3	80
Peanut Butter Crispy	1 bar	60	1	2	0	10	tr	35

FOOD	PORTION	CALS	PROT	FAT	CHOL	CARB	FIBER	SOD
Peanutty Chocolate	1 bar	140	6	5	<5	19	3	80
Clif Bar								
Apricot	1 bar (2.4 oz)	220	8	3	0	43	5	90
Carrot Cake	1 bar (2.4 oz)	240	10	4	0	43	5	150
Chocolate Brownie	1 bar (2.4 oz)	240	10	4	0	41	6	150
Chocolate Almond Fudge	1 bar (2.4 oz)	230	10	5	0	36	5	140
Chocolate Chip	1 bar (2.4 oz)	240	10	4	0	41	5	170
Chocolate Chip Peanut Crunch	1 bar (2.4 oz)	240	12	5	0	39	5	290
Cookies'N Cream	1 bar (2.4 oz)	230	10	4	0	39	5	180
Cranberry Apple Cherry	1 bar (2.4 oz)	220	8	2	0	44	5	135
Crunchy Peanut Butter	1 bar (2.4 oz)	240	12	5	0	39	5	290
GingerSnap	1 bar (2.4 oz)	230	10	4	0	42	6	140
Deliciously Slim								
Chocolate Fudge Cake	1 bar (2.1 oz)	200	20	6	0	22	tr	220
DrSoy								
Double Chocolate	1 bar (1.76 oz)	180	12	3	0	27	1	170
Ensure								
All Flavors	1 bar (2.1 oz)	230	9	6	<5	35	1	135
Extend								
Chocolate Chip Crunch	1 bar (1.4 oz)	160	3	3	0	31	tr	80
Peanut Butter Crunch	1 bar (1.4 oz)	160	4	3	0	30	0	85
Fast Fuel Up								
Natural Chocolate Espresso	1 bar (2.3 oz)	300	8	19	0	32	3	55

FOOD	PORTION	CALS	PROT	FAT	CHOL	CARB	FIBER	SOD
Natural Chocolate Crunch	1 bar (2.3 oz)	300	8	19	0	32	3	55
Organic Chocolate Espresso	1 bar (1.8 oz)	230	6	15	0	24	2	40
Organic Chocolate Crunch	1 bar (1.8 oz)	230	6	15	0	24	2	40
Gatorade								
All Flavors	1 bar (2.3 oz)	260	8	5	0	46	2	160
GeniSoy								
Soy Protein Arctic Frost Crispy Chocolate Mint	1 bar (2.2 oz)	230	14	5	0	33	2	150
Soy Protein Dutch Crunch Sour Apple Crisp	1 bar (2.2 oz)	230	14	5	0	33	1	160
Soy Protein Fair Trade Arabica Cafe Mocha Fudge	1 bar (2.2 oz)	220	14	4	0	33	1	150
Soy Protein New York Style Blueberry Cheesecake	1 bar (2.2 oz)	220	14	4	0	34	1	160
Soy Protein Obsession Fudge Cookies & Cream	1 bar (2.2 oz)	230	14	5	0	33	2	250
Soy Protein Pure Golden Honey Creamy Peanut Yogurt	1 bar (2.2 oz)	230	14	5	0	33	1	160
Soy Protein Southern Style Chunky Peanut Butter Fudge	1 bar (2.2 oz)	240	14	6	0	32	1	130
Soy Protein Ultimate Chocolate Fudge Brownie	1 bar (2.2 oz)	230	14	5	0	33	2	210
Xtreme Carrot Cake Quake	1 bar (1.6 oz)	190	9	7	0	24	1	90

FOOD	PORTION	CALS	PROT	FAT	CHOL	CARB	FIBER	SOD
Xtreme Peanut Butter Fix	1 bar (1.6 oz)	200	9	8	0	23	2	190
Xtreme Raspberry Rush	1 bar (1.6 oz)	190	9	7	0	24	2	90
Xtreme Rocky Roadtrip	1 bar (1.6 oz)	190	9	7	0	23	2	130
Glucerna								
All Flavors	1 bar (1.3 oz)	140	6	4	<5	24	4	75
Hansen's								
Chocolate Banana Crunch	1 bar	180	3	3	0	37	2	45
Chocolate Orchard Crunch	1 bar	170	2	3	0	37	2	30
Natural Bar Tropical Fruit Crunch	1 bar	170	3	3	0	35	1	60
Natural Bar Yogurt Strawberry Crunch	1 bar	190	2	3	0	38	1	60
HeartBar								
Cranberry	1 bar (1.8 oz)	190	13	3	0	27	3	95
Original	1 bar (1.76 oz)	180	14	3	0	26	3	140
Hi-Lo								
Chocolate Caramel	1 bar (1.76 oz)	200	16	8	<5	20	0	150
Chocolate Mint	1 bar (2.1 oz)	200	20	6	0	23	tr	210
Chocolate Peanut Butter	1 bar (2.1 oz)	210	20	7	0	22	0	250
Chocolate Raspberry	1 bar (2.1 oz)	200	20	6	0	22	tr	220
Ideal								
Mixed Berry Tart	1 bar (1.7 oz)	200	15	7	0	20	0	240
Jenny Craig								
Meal Bar Chocolate Peanut	1 bar (2 oz)	220	10	5	0	33	1	240
Meal Bar Lemon Meringue	1 bar (2 oz)	210	10	5	0	31	0	130
Meal Bar Milk Chocolate	1 bar (2 oz)	210	10	5	0	33	1	180
Meal Bar Oatmeal Raisin	1 bar (1.97 oz)	210	10	3	0	35	3	75

FOOD	PORTION	CALS	PROT	FAT	CHOL	CARB	FIBER	SOD
Meal Bar Yogurt Peanut	1 bar (2 oz)	220	10	5	0	33	0	270
Kashi								
GoLean Chocolate Almond Toffee	1 (2.7 oz)	290	13	6	0	45	–	250
GoLean Cookies 'N Cream	1 (2.7 oz)	290	13	6	0	50	6	200
GoLean Frosted Spice Cake	1 (2.7 oz)	290	13	5	0	49	6	200
GoLean Honey Vanilla Yogurt	1 (2.7 oz)	290	13	5	0	49	6	160
GoLean Malted Chocolate Chip	1 (2.7 oz)	290	13	6	20	49	6	200
GoLean Mocha Java	1 (2.7 oz)	290	13	6	0	50	6	190
GoLean Oatmeal Raisin Cookie	1 (2.7 oz)	280	13	5	0	49	6	140
GoLean Peanut Butter & Chocolate	1 (2.7 oz)	290	13	6	0	48	5	280
GoLean Strawberries 'N Cream	1 (2.7 oz)	290	13	5	0	50	6	200
GoLean Strawberry Vanilla Yogurt	1 (2.7 oz)	280	11	4	0	53	6	75
GoLean Crunchy Chocolate Caramel Karma	1 (1.6 oz)	140	8	3	20	26	5	180
GoLean Crunchy Chocolate Peanut Bliss	1 (1.8 oz)	270	9	4	0	30	5	220
GoLean Crunchy Sublime Lemon Lime	1 (1.8 oz)	670	9	3	0	32	5	220
Lean Body For Her								
Chocolate Honey Peanut	1 bar (1.76 oz)	190	16	7	0	10	tr	135
Luna								
Chai Tea	1 bar (1.7 oz)	180	10	4	0	27	2	125
Chocolate Pecan Pie	1 bar (1.7 oz)	180	10	5	0	24	2	125
LemonZest	1 bar (1.7 oz)	180	10	4	0	24	2	50

FOOD	PORTION	CALS	PROT	FAT	CHOL	CARB	FIBER	SOD
Nutz Over Chocolate	1 bar (1.7 oz)	180	10	5	0	24	2	100
Sesame Raisin Crunch	1 bar (1.7 oz)	170	10	3	0	26	2	125
S'Mores	1 bar (1.7 oz)	180	10	4	0	26	2	125
Toasted Nuts 'n Cranberry	1 bar (1.7 oz)	170	10	3	0	26	2	130
Tropical Crisp	1 bar (1.7 oz)	180	10	5	0	24	2	135
Met-Rx								
Big 100 Gram Bar Peanut Butter	1 bar (3.5 oz)	340	26	4	15	52	2	135
Source/One Chocolate Cheesecake	1 bar (2.1 oz)	160	15	5	5	21	tr	50
Momentum								
Chocolate Caramel Nut	1 bar	150	12	6	0	16	3	110
Chocolate Peanut Butter	1 bar	150	12	6	0	16	2	150
Double Chocolate	1 bar	150	12	6	0	17	2	160
Moto Bar								
Bodacious Banana Split	1 bar	300	8	6	0	54	6	240
Charming Cherry Almond	1 bar (2.9 oz)	300	8	6	0	54	3	200
Cozy Pumpkin Pie	1 bar	300	8	6	0	54	6	200
Jazzy Peanut Butter & Jelly	1 bar	300	10	3	0	52	4	200
Kooky Cappuccino	1 bar	300	8	6	0	54	8	200
Luscious Lemon Blueberry	1 bar	300	10	5	0	54	4	280
Saucy Apple Cinnamon	1 bar	280	8	4	0	54	6	300
Zany Cranberry Orange	1 bar	300	8	5	0	54	4	250
New You								
Chocolate Crisp	1 bar (1.65 oz)	180	10	4	0	25	3	170

FOOD	PORTION	CALS	PROT	FAT	CHOL	CARB	FIBER	SOD
NuGo								
Banana Chocolate Protein	1 bar	190	11	3	0	26	3	220
Blue Berry Boom	1 bar	180	11	3	0	26	3	250
Chocolate Blast	1 bar	180	11	3	0	26	3	250
Coffee Break	1 bar	180	11	3	0	26	3	250
Orange Smoothie Protein	1 bar	190	17	3	0	25	1	220
Peanut Butter Pleaser	1 bar	180	11	3	0	26	3	250
Nutiva								
Flaxseed & Raisin Organic	1 bar (1.4 oz)	280	14	19	0	12	6	10
Hempseed Bar Organic	1 bar (1.4 oz)	210	9	14	0	11	5	5
Nutribar								
Chocolate Covered Belgian Chocolate	1 bar (2.3 oz)	252	13	8	–	33	2	255
Chocolate Covered Caramel	1 bar (2.3 oz)	261	13	8	–	34	tr	280
Chocolate Covered Chocolate Fudge	1 bar (2.3 oz)	267	14	8	5	35	2	300
Chocolate Covered Hazelnut	1 bar (2.3 oz)	261	13	8	–	34	1	295
Chocolate Covered Mocha Almond	1 bar (2.3 oz)	261	13	8	–	34	tr	280
Chocolate Covered Peanut	1 bar (2.3 oz)	262	13	9	–	34	1	255
Yogurt Covered Peach Apricot	1 bar (2.3 oz)	261	13	8	–	34	tr	260
Yogurt Covered Raspberry	1 bar (2.3 oz)	261	13	8	–	34	tr	260
Yogurt Covered Wildberry	1 bar (2.3 oz)	261	13	8	–	34	tr	260
Odwalla Bar!								
Peanut Crunch	1 bar (2.2 oz)	260	8	7	0	40	3	180
Peacekeeper								
Nuts About Peace All Flavors	1 bar (1.4 oz)	180	4	10	0	17	2	0

FOOD	PORTION	CALS	PROT	FAT	CHOL	CARB	FIBER	SOD
PermaLean								
Protein Crunch Chocoholic Chocolate	1 bar (1.8 oz)	170	21	3	0	10	tr	65
Protein Crunch Chocolate Raspberry	1 bar (1.8 oz)	180	21	2	10	9	0	35
Protein Crunch Stark Raving Peanutz	1 bar (1.8 oz)	180	21	4	0	9	0	75
PowerBar								
Apple Cinnamon	1 bar (2.3 oz)	230	10	3	0	45	3	90
Banana	1 bar (2.3 oz)	230	9	2	0	45	3	90
Chocolate	1 bar (2.3 oz)	230	10	2	0	45	3	90
Essentials Chocolate	1 bar (1.9 oz)	180	10	4	0	28	3	105
Harvest Apple Crisp	1 bar (2.3 oz)	240	7	4	–	–	–	–
Harvest Blueberry	1 bar (2.3 oz)	240	7	4	0	45	4	80
Harvest Strawberry	1 bar (2.3 oz)	240	7	4	0	45	4	80
Malt-Nut	1 bar (2.3 oz)	230	10	3	0	45	3	90
Mocha	1 bar (2.3 oz)	230	10	3	0	45	3	90
Oatmeal Raisin	1 bar (2.3 oz)	230	10	3	0	45	3	120
Peanut Butter	1 bar (2.3 oz)	230	10	3	0	45	3	110
Power Gel Strawberry Banana	1 pkg	110	0	0	0	28	–	50
Pria Chocolate Honey Graham	1 bar (1 oz)	110	5	3	–	16	–	80
Pria Chocolate Peanut Crunch	1 bar (1 oz)	110	5	4	–	16	–	80
Pria Double Chocolate Cookie	1 bar (1 oz)	110	5	3	–	16	–	90

FOOD	PORTION	CALS	PROT	FAT	CHOL	CARB	FIBER	SOD
Pria French Vanilla Crisp	1 bar (1 oz)	110	5	3	–	16	–	80
Vanilla Crisp	1 bar (2.3 oz)	230	9	3	0	45	3	90
Wild Berry	1 bar (2.3 oz)	230	10	3	0	45	3	90
Pure Protein								
Blueberry Cheesecake	1 bar	190	20	3	5	23	0	40
Revival								
Soy Apple Cinnamon Celebration	1 bar	200	21	5	0	28	1	260
Soy Autumn Frost Low Carb	1 bar	200	21	5	0	28	1	260
Soy Chocolate Raspberry Zing Low Carb	1 bar	200	19	5	0	28	2	240
Soy Chocolate Temptation	1 bar	220	16	3	0	30	tr	270
Soy Marshmallow Krunch	1 bar	220	17	3	0	33	tr	270
Soy Peanut Butter Chocolate Pal	1 bar	240	16	5	0	32	1	260
Soy Peanut Butter Pal	1 bar	240	17	5	0	31	tr	280
Slim-Fast								
Crispy Peanut Caramel	1 bar	120	1	4	<5	21	tr	80
Dutch Chocolate	1 bar	140	5	5	5	20	2	80
Meal On-The-Go Apple Cobbler	1 bar	220	8	5	<5	33	2	150
Meal On-The-Go Chocolate Cookie Dough	1 bar	220	8	5	<5	35	2	180
Meal On-The-Go Honey Peanut	1 bar	220	8	5	<5	34	2	160
Meal On-The-Go Milk Chocolate Peanut	1 bar	220	8	5	<5	36	2	120

FOOD	PORTION	CALS	PROT	FAT	CHOL	CARB	FIBER	SOD
Meal On-The-Go Oatmeal Raisin	1 bar	220	8	5	<5	36	2	100
Meal On-The-Go Rich Chocolate Brownie	1 bar	220	8	5	<5	34	2	150
Meal On-The-Go Toasted Oat & Spice	1 bar	220	8	5	<5	35	2	140
Peanut Butter	1 bar	150	6	5	5	19	2	80
Peanut Butter Crunch	1 bar	130	1	4	0	21	tr	80
Rich Chewy Caramel	1 bar	120	tr	4	5	22	2	65
Snickers								
Marathon Chewy Chocolate Peanut	1	220	13	7	5	27	2	240
Marathon Multi Grain Crunch	1	220	9	7	5	32	2	210
SoBe								
Milk Chocolate	1 bar (1.75 oz)	240	2	14	15	28	tr	50
Strive								
Crunchy Chocolate Smores	1 bar (2.1 oz)	200	20	9	0	25	0	320
Sweet Success								
Chewy Chocolate Brownie	1 bar (1.2 oz)	120	2	4	3	23	3	35
Think!								
Apple Spice	1 bar (2 oz)	205	5	3	62	40	7	36
Chocolate Almond Coconut Raisin	1 bar (2 oz)	243	6	7	9	39	2	160
Chocolate Fruit Harvest	1 bar (2 oz)	217	5	3	38	43	7	42
Zoe								
Flax & Soy Apple Crisp	1 bar (1.83 oz)	180	8	6	–	–	–	–
ZonePerfect								
Honey Peanut	1 bar (1.8 oz)	200	14	7	0	22	1	150

FOOD	PORTION	CALS	PROT	FAT	CHOL	CARB	FIBER	SOD
ENERGY DRINKS								
AMP								
Energy Drink	1 can (8.4 oz)	120	0	0	0	32	0	75
Arizona								
Extreme Energy Shot	1 bottle (8.3 oz)	130	0	0	0	34	–	25
Atkins								
Cafe Au Lait	1 can (11 oz)	170	20	9	15	5	3	170
Chocolate	1 can (11 oz)	170	20	9	15	5	3	140
Chocolate Royale	1 can (11 oz)	170	20	9	15	6	1	170
Strawberry	1 can (11 oz)	170	20	9	15	4	2	140
Vanilla	1 can (11 oz)	170	20	9	15	4	2	140
Balance								
Chocolate as prep w/ 2% milk	1 serv	310	22	11	25	32	2	420
Vanilla as prep w/ 2% milk	1 serv	310	22	11	25	32	2	420
Bawls								
Guarana	1 bottle (10 oz)	120	0	0	0	32	–	35
Guaranexx Sugar Free	1 bottle (10 oz)	0	0	0	0	0	0	15
BooKoo								
Energy Drink	8 oz	110	–	0	0	27	–	200
Zero Carb	8 oz	0	0	0	0	0	0	200
Boost								
High Protein Vanilla	1 can (8 oz)	240	15	6	10	33	0	170
Vanilla	8 oz	240	10	4	5	41	0	130
Brain Twist								
Flu & Cold Defense All Flavors	8 oz	70	–	0	0	16	–	–
Choice								
Chocolate	1 can (8 oz)	220	9	10	0	24	3	200
Chocolate Fudge Sugar Free	1 pkg (11 oz)	125	10	3	<5	11	9	150
French Vanllia Sugar Free	1 pkg (11 oz)	100	10	3	<5	7	6	130

FOOD	PORTION	CALS	PROT	FAT	CHOL	CARB	FIBER	SOD
Strawberries'n Cream Sugar Free	1 pkg (11 oz)	100	10	3	<5	7	6	130
Vanilla	1 can (8 oz)	220	9	10	0	24	3	200
Crunk								
Energy Drink	1 can	120	0	0	0	29	–	120
Fuze								
Energize Blackberry Grape	8 oz	100	0	0	0	26	–	15
Energize Exotic Punch	8 oz	100	0	0	0	26	–	15
Energize Mojo Mango	8 oz	100	0	0	0	28	–	15
Essential Cranberry Grapefruit	8 oz	90	0	0	0	25	–	5
Focus Orange Carrot	8 oz	90	0	0	0	24	–	20
Refresh Banana Colada	8 oz	90	0	0	0	24	–	15
Refresh Mixed Berry	8 oz	90	0	0	0	25	–	15
Refresh Peach Mango	8 oz	90	0	0	0	24	–	15
Replenish Agave Cactus	8 oz	90	0	0	0	24	–	25
Slenderize Tropical Punch	8 oz	10	0	0	0	2	–	5
Stamina Grape & Aronia Punch	8 oz	80	0	0	0	23	–	10
Vitaboost Citrus Starfruit Punch	8 oz	90	0	0	0	24	–	10
Gatorade								
All Flavors	1 cup (8 oz)	50	0	0	0	14	–	110
Nutrition Shake All Flavors	1 can (11 oz)	370	18	6	0	62	1	290
X-Factor All Flavors	8 oz	50	0	0	0	14	–	110
GeniSoy								
Soy Protein Shake Chocolate	1 scoop (1.2 oz)	120	14	0	0	17	2	170
Soy Protein Shake Vanilla	1 scoop (1.2 oz)	130	14	0	0	18	0	180

FOOD	PORTION	CALS	PROT	FAT	CHOL	CARB	FIBER	SOD
Soy Protein Shake Strawberry Banana	1 scoop	130	14	0	0	17	1	170
Guaraviton								
Energy Drink	8 oz	98	0	0	0	20	–	–
Hansen's								
Energy Kiwi Strawberry	8 oz	120	0	0	0	30	–	15
Energy Peach	8 oz	130	0	0	0	33	–	15
Energy Punch	8 oz	120	0	0	0	30	–	15
Healthy Start Carrot Orange Antioxidant Blend	8 oz	130	1	0	0	30	–	25
Healthy Start Citrus Punch Focus Blend	8 oz	130	0	0	0	34	–	25
Healthy Start Cranberry Grape Defense Blend	8 oz	110	0	0	0	28	–	26
Healthy Start Tropical Orange Vitamix Blend	8 oz	110	0	0	0	30	–	30
Happy Bunny								
Spaz Juice	1 can (8.4 oz)	110	0	0	0	28	0	10
Healthy Pleasures								
Chocolate Irish Cream	1 bottle (10.5 oz)	260	12	2	6	45	0	320
High Voltage								
Sugar Free	8 oz	5	0	0	0	2	–	55
Hype								
Classic Energy	1 can (8.3 oz)	110	0	0	0	26	–	0
Impulse								
Energy Drink	1 can (8.3 oz)	110	1	0	0	28	–	200
Sugar Free	1 can (8.3 oz)	5	tr	0	0	1	–	–
Invigor8								
Energy Boost	1 can	110	0	0	0	27	1	50
Nutrition Boost	1 can	110	0	0	0	27	1	50

FOOD	PORTION	CALS	PROT	FAT	CHOL	CARB	FIBER	SOD
Jones Soda								
Lemon Lime Energy	1 can (8.4 oz)	140	1	0	0	33	0	220
Orange Energy	1 can (8.4 oz)	140	1	0	0	33	0	220
Sugar Free Energy	1 can (8.4 oz)	10	1	0	0	2	–	135
Jugular								
Energy Drink	1 can (8.3 oz)	49	3	0	0	9	–	46
KaBoom								
All Flavors	8 oz	105	0	0	0	26	0	3
Kashi								
GoLean Shake Mix Vanilla	2 scoops	220	22	0	0	32	7	105
GoLean Shake Mix Woman Chocolate	2 scoops	220	22	1	0	31	7	100
Shake Chocolate	1 can	230	15	3	0	38	7	310
Shake Vanilla	1 can	220	15	3	0	36	7	330
Kindercal								
Vanilla	1 can (8 oz)	250	7	11	5	32	0	88
Krank'd								
All Flavors	1 bottle (16 oz)	80	0	0	0	18	–	48
Lolli's Pop								
Cheery Energy Drink	1 bottle	170	0	0	0	45	–	10
Passion Stimulating Elixir	1 bottle	140	0	0	0	35	–	10
Natural Ovens								
Ultra Omega Balance	1 tbsp	75	3	5	3	5	4	10
Zesty Flax Energy Mix	1 tbsp	40	2	2	0	5	3	2
New York Minute								
Energy Drink	1 can (8.4 oz)	130	0	0	0	33	–	215
Nitro2Go								
High Energy	1 can	110	0	0	0	28	–	190
High Energy Lite	1 can	20	0	0	0	5	0	180

FOOD	PORTION	CALS	PROT	FAT	CHOL	CARB	FIBER	SOD
NOS								
High Performance	8 oz	110	1	0	0	28	–	115
NutraShake								
Citrus	1 pkg (4 oz)	200	6	0	0	44	–	30
Citrus Free	1 serv (4 oz)	200	6	0	0	44	0	110
Vanilla	1 serv (8 oz)	400	12	12	36	62	–	120
Vanilla No Added Sugar	1 serv (4 oz)	200	7	8	18	25	–	75
Odwalla								
Blueberry B Monster	8 fl oz	140	0	0	0	33	2	15
C Monster	8 fl oz	150	2	1	0	33	2	25
Femme Vitale	8 fl oz	130	1	0	0	29	1	10
Glorious Morning	8 fl oz	130	2	0	0	31	3	20
Mango Tango	8 fl oz	150	1	2	0	31	0	55
Mo Beta	8 fl oz	140	1	0	0	34	1	40
Serious Energy	8 fl oz	150	1	0	0	36	1	35
Strawberry C Monster	8 fl oz	150	2	0	0	34	tr	40
Super Protein	8 fl oz	170	9	1	0	33	2	90
Superfood	8 fl oz	140	2	1	0	32	2	50
Wellness	8 fl oz	150	2	1	0	33	1	35
Orange County Choppers								
High Octane Fuel	1 can (8.4 oz)	110	0	0	0	28	–	10
Peep One								
Erotic Drink	1 can (8.3)	109	1	tr	0	27	–	112
Pimp Juice								
Energy Drink	1 can	140	0	0	0	35	–	5
Pink								
Diet	1 can	10	0	0	0	2	–	135
Piranha								
Phunky Fruit Punch	1 can (8.4 oz)	140	0	0	0	35	0	10
Pit Bull								
Energy Drink	1 can (8.4 oz)	110	tr	0	0	28	–	200
Sugar Free	1 can (8.4 oz)	0	0	0	0	0	0	210

FOOD	PORTION	CALS	PROT	FAT	CHOL	CARB	FIBER	SOD
Pounds Off								
Dark Chocolate Ecstasy	1 can (11 oz)	200	11	3	0	39	6	220
French Vanilla	1 can (11 oz)	220	12	3	0	41	5	460
Powerade								
Fruit Punch	8 fl oz	70	0	0	0	19	–	55
Lemon Lime	8 fl oz	70	0	0	0	19	–	55
Mountain Blast	8 fl oz	70	0	0	0	19	–	55
Pure Power								
Energy Drink	1 can (8.4 oz)	110	0	0	0	28	–	210
Shotz	1 can (5.75 oz)	80	1	0	0	19	0	150
Raw Dawg								
Energy Drink	8 oz	110	0	0	0	27	–	110
Sugar Free	8 oz	0	0	0	0	0	0	110
Red Bull								
Energy Drink	1 can (8.3 oz)	110	0	0	0	28	–	200
Sugar Free	1 can	10	tr	0	0	3	–	200
Red Eye								
Classic	1 bottle (12 oz)	208	0	0	0	50	–	0
Extreme	1 bottle (12 oz)	140	0	0	0	37	–	0
Gold	1 bottle (12 oz)	208	0	0	0	49	–	0
Passion	1 bottle (12 oz)	149	0	0	0	37	–	0
Platinum	1 bottle (12 oz)	149	0	0	0	37	–	0
RESQ								
Energy Drink	1 can (8 oz)	126	1	0	0	30	–	–
Rip It								
Energy Fuel	8 oz	130	1	0	0	32	–	130
Energy Lite	8 oz	0	1	0	0	0	–	130
Rockstar								
Energy Cola	8 oz	120	0	0	0	30	–	35

FOOD	PORTION	CALS	PROT	FAT	CHOL	CARB	FIBER	SOD
Slim-Fast								
Chocolate as prep w/ fat free milk	1 serv	190	14	1	9	32	2	240
Chocolate Malt as prep w/ fat free milk	1 serv	190	14	1	8	32	2	250
JumpStart Chocolate as prep w/ fat free milk	1 serv	240	18	2	14	39	5	280
Strawberry as prep w/ fat free milk	1 serv	190	14	1	9	32	2	260
Vanilla as prep w/ fat free milk	1 serv	190	14	1	9	32	2	260
Snapple								
Meal Replacement All Flavors	1 bottle (11.5 oz)	210	7	0	0	43	5	110
SoBe								
Adrenaline Rush	1 can (8.3 oz)	140	1	0	0	36	—	60
Black & Blue Berry Brew	8 oz	120	0	0	0	31	—	24
Courage Cherry Citrus	8 oz	110	0	0	0	33	—	25
Drive	8 oz	120	0	0	0	32	—	15
Elixir Cranberry Grapefruit	8 oz	110	0	0	0	29	—	10
Elixir Orange Carrot 3C	8 oz	90	0	0	0	24	—	20
Elixir Pomegranate Cranberry	8 oz	100	0	0	0	26	—	27
Energy	8 oz	120	0	0	0	32	—	5
Fuerte	8 oz	130	0	0	0	35	—	10
Karma	8 oz	120	0	0	0	33	—	5
Long John Lizard's Grape Grog	8 oz	120	0	0	0	31	—	25
Power	8 oz	120	0	0	0	32	—	5
Synergy All Flavors	1 can (11.5 oz)	120	32	0	0	29	—	20
Tsunami	8 oz	110	0	0	0	29	—	20

FOOD	PORTION	CALS	PROT	FAT	CHOL	CARB	FIBER	SOD
Wisdom	8.5 oz	110	0	0	0	30	—	5
Zen Blend	8.5 oz	90	0	0	0	24	—	5
Source Burn								
Energy Drink	8 oz	140	0	0	0	36	—	20
Sugar Free	8 oz	10	1	0	0	0	0	15
Stevita								
All Flavors	2 tsp	0	0	0	0	0	0	0
Sweet Success								
Creamy Milk Chocolate	1 can	200	10	3	4	36	3	230
Creamy Milk Chocolate as prep w/ skim milk	1 serv	180	11	1	6	36	6	240
Tornado								
Energy Drink	8 oz	110	1	0	0	30	—	130
TwinLab								
Hydra Fuel	16 oz	132	0	0	0	33	—	50
Nitro Fuel	16 oz	460	15	0	0	100	—	—
Ultra Fuel	16 oz	400	0	0	0	100	—	55
Vipa								
Energy Drink	1 can (12 oz)	0	0	0	0	0	0	30
Wired								
Energy Drink	8 oz	110	0	0	0	29	—	225
Sugar Free	8 oz	5	2	0	0	2	—	210
X 3000 Taurine	8 oz	110	2	0	0	26	—	210
XO								
Balance	8 oz	50	0	0	0	13	—	—
Berry	1 bottle	90	tr	0	0	22	—	140
Citrus	1 bottle	90	tr	0	0	22	—	135
Defense	8 oz	40	0	0	0	9	—	0
Diet	1 bottle	15	tr	0	0	2	—	125
Endurance	8 oz	50	0	0	0	14	—	0
Energy	8 oz	40	0	0	0	9	—	0
Essential	8 oz	40	0	0	0	9	—	0
Focus	8 oz	40	0	0	0	9	—	0
Grape	1 Bottle	90	tr	0	0	21	—	130
Multi-V	8 oz	40	0	0	0	9	—	0
Original	1 bottle	110	tr	0	0	28	—	85
Peach	1 bottle	90	tr	0	0	21	—	130
Power-C	8 oz	40	0	0	0	9	—	0

FOOD	PORTION	CALS	PROT	FAT	CHOL	CARB	FIBER	SOD
Rescue	8 oz	40	0	0	0	9	–	0
Revive	8 oz	50	0	0	0	13	–	0
Stress-B	8 oz	40	0	0	0	9	–	0
Vanilla	1 bottle	90	tr	0	0	21	–	65
XS Energy								
Citrus Blast	1 can (8.4 oz)	8	2	0	0	0	0	24
Cranberry Grape	1 can (8.4 oz)	8	2	0	0	0	0	24
Electric Lemon Blast	1 can (8.4 oz)	16	2	0	0	2	–	24
Tropical Blast	1 can (8.4 oz)	8	2	0	0	0	0	24
YET								
Your Energy Drink	1 can	8	2	0	0	0	–	46

ENGLISH MUFFIN
READY-TO-EAT

FOOD	PORTION	CALS	PROT	FAT	CHOL	CARB	FIBER	SOD
apple cinnamon	1	138	4	2	0	28	–	255
crumpets	1 (1.5 oz)	80	3	0	0	16	tr	270
granola	1	155	6	1	0	31	–	275
mixed grain	1	155	6	1	0	31	–	275
plain	1	134	4	1	0	26	–	265
plain toasted	1	133	4	1	0	26	–	262
raisin cinnamon	1	138	4	2	0	28	–	255
sourdough	1	134	4	1	0	26	–	265
wheat	1	127	5	1	0	26	–	218
whole wheat	1	134	6	1	0	27	4	420
Milton's								
Multi-Grain	1 (2 oz)	150	4	1	0	33	3	180
Pepperidge Farm								
Original	1	130	5	1	0	26	2	250
Thomas'								
Blueberry	1	140	4	1	0	29	1	210
Carb Consider	1	100	7	2	<5	23	9	220
Hearty Grains Honey Wheat	1	130	5	1	0	27	2	190
Original	1	120	4	1	0	25	1	200
Raisin Bran	1	150	4	2	0	30	2	200
Raisin Cinnamon	1	140	4	1	0	30	1	180

FOOD	PORTION	CALS	PROT	FAT	CHOL	CARB	FIBER	SOD
Sourdough	1	120	4	1	0	25	1	190
Super Size	1 (3.2 oz)	200	7	2	0	41	2	310
TAKE-OUT								
w/ butter	1 (2.2 oz)	189	5	6	13	30	—	386
w/ cheese & sausage	1 (4 oz)	393	15	24	59	29	—	1036
w/ egg cheese & canadian bacon	1 (4.8 oz)	289	17	13	234	28	2	729
w/ egg cheese & sausage	1 (5.8 oz)	487	22	31	274	31	—	1135
EPAZOTE								
fresh	1 tbsp (1 g)	tr	0	0	0	tr	tr	tr
fresh sprig	1 (2 g)	1	tr	tr	0	tr	tr	1
EPPAW								
raw	½ cup	75	2	1	0	16	—	6
FALAFEL								
Near East								
Falafel as prep	2½ patties	230	10	16	0	18	5	560
TAKE-OUT								
falafel	1 (1.2 oz)	57	2	3	0	5	—	50
FAT (see also BUTTER, BUTTER SUBSTITUTES, MARGARINE, OIL)								
beef cooked	1 oz	193	3	20	27	0	—	12
beef suet	1 oz	242	tr	27	19	0	—	—
beef tallow	1 tbsp (13 g)	115	0	13	14	0	—	0
chicken	1 tbsp	115	0	13	11	0	—	—
chicken	1 cup	1846	0	205	174	0	—	—
cocoa butter	1 tbsp	120	0	14	0	0	0	—
duck	1 tbsp (13 g)	115	0	13	13	0	0	0
goose	1 oz	257	0	29	—	0	—	—
goose	1 tbsp	115	0	13	13	0	—	—
lamb new zealand	1 oz	182	2	19	25	0	—	6
lard	1 tbsp (13 g)	115	0	13	12	0	—	0
lard	1 cup (205 g)	1849	0	205	195	0	—	tr
nutmeg butter	1 tbsp	120	0	14	—	0	0	—
pork backfat	1 oz	230	1	25	16	0	0	3
pork cooked	1 oz	178	3	18	26	0	0	10
salt pork	1 oz	212	23	23	25	0	—	404

FOOD	PORTION	CALS	PROT	FAT	CHOL	CARB	FIBER	SOD
shortening	1 tbsp	113	0	13	0	0	0	—
shortening	1 cup	1812	0	205	0	0	0	—
turkey	1 tbsp	115	0	13	13	0	—	—
ucuhuba butter	1 tbsp	120	0	14	—	0	0	—

FAT SUBSTITUTES
Smucker's
Baking Healthy 100% Fat Free	1 tbsp	30	0	0	0	7	0	7

FAVA BEANS
Progresso
Fava Beans	½ cup (4.6 oz)	110	6	1	0	20	5	250

FEIJOA
fresh	1 (1.75 oz)	25	1	tr	0	5	—	2
puree	1 cup	119	3	2	0	26	—	7

FENNEL
fresh bulb	1 (8.2 oz)	72	3	tr	0	17	—	122
fresh sliced	1 cup	27	1	tr	0	6	—	45
leaves	1 oz	7	tr	tr	—	1	1	25
seed	1 tsp	7	tr	tr	0	1	—	2

FENUGREEK
seed	1 tsp	12	1	tr	0	2	—	2

FIBER
Apple Fiber
Pure	2 tbsp (7 g)	16	—	0	0	7	4	—

Benefiber
Supplement	1 pkg (4 g)	20	0	0	0	4	3	20

Choice
Fiber Burst Lemon Lime	3 pieces	45	1	1	0	12	3	0
Fiber Burst Tropical Fruit	3 pieces	45	1	1	0	11	3	0

Metamucil
Fiber Wafers Apple Crisp	2	120	2	5	0	17	6	20

ND Labs
Pure Apple Fiber	1 tbsp (7 g)	16	0	0	0	7	4	—

FOOD	PORTION	CALS	PROT	FAT	CHOL	CARB	FIBER	SOD
FIDDLEHEAD FERNS								
fresh	3.5 oz	34	5	tr	0	6	–	1
FIGS								
calimyrna	3 (5.4 oz)	120	1	0	0	28	4	0
canned in heavy syrup	3	75	tr	tr	0	19	–	1
canned in light syrup	3	58	tr	tr	0	15	–	1
canned water pack	3	42	tr	tr	0	11	–	1
dried california	½ cup (3.5 oz)	200	4	1	0	58	17	11
dried cooked	½ cup	140	2	1	0	16	–	6
dried whole	10	477	6	2	0	122	17	20
fresh	1 med	50	tr	tr	0	10	–	1
Jenny								
Sundried Kalamata	4	120	1	0	0	28	5	5
FIREWEED								
leaves chopped	1 cup (0.8 oz)	24	1	1	0	4	2	8
FISH *(see also individual names, FISH SUBSTITUTES, SUSHI)*								
FROZEN								
breaded fillet	1 (2 oz)	155	9	7	64	14	–	332
sticks	1 stick (1 oz)	76	4	3	31	7	–	163
Gorton's								
Baked Au Gratin	1 piece (4.6 oz)	130	14	5	50	7	–	400
Baked Broccoli Cheddar	1 piece (4.6 oz)	130	14	5	50	7	–	310
Baked Primavera	1 piece (4.6 oz)	120	15	5	50	4	–	340
Batter Dipped Portions	1 piece (2.5 oz)	170	6	11	20	12	–	390
Crunchy Golden Fillets Breaded	2 (3.8 oz)	250	10	14	35	21	–	480
Crunchy Golden Sticks	6 (3.8 oz)	250	12	13	30	21	–	340
Garlic & Herb	2 pieces (3.6 oz)	220	10	11	30	21	–	670

FOOD	PORTION	CALS	PROT	FAT	CHOL	CARB	FIBER	SOD
Garlic Butter Crumb	1 piece (4.6 oz)	170	17	9	55	5	—	350
Grilled Cajun Blackened	1 piece (3.8 oz)	120	16	6	60	1	—	240
Grilled Garlic Butter	1 piece (3.8 oz)	120	16	6	60	1	—	200
Grilled Italian Herb	1 piece (3.8 oz)	130	17	6	60	2	—	330
Grilled Lemon Butter	1 piece (3.8 oz)	120	16	6	60	1	—	380
Grilled Lemon Pepper	1 piece (3.8 oz)	120	16	6	60	1	—	160
Parmesan	2 pieces (3.6 oz)	260	10	15	30	20	—	650
Ranch	1 piece (3.6 oz)	240	9	13	30	22	—	650
Southern Fried Country Style	2 pieces (3.6 oz)	230	10	14	30	16	—	660
Tenders	3.5 pieces (4 oz)	250	11	14	30	20	—	530
Tenders Extra Crunchy	3.5 pieces (4 oz)	270	11	12	30	29	—	640
TAKE-OUT								
fish cake	1 (4.7 oz)	166	18	7	—	6	—	—
jamaican brown fish stew	1 serv	426	48	22	84	9	2	419
kedgeree	5.6 oz	242	21	11	—	15	1	—
mousse	1 serv (3.5 oz)	185	13	14	—	3	tr	540
stew	1 cup (7.9 oz)	157	19	4	—	10	—	—
taramasalata	2 tbsp	124	1	14	10	1	—	182

FISH OIL

FOOD	PORTION	CALS	PROT	FAT	CHOL	CARB	FIBER	SOD
cod liver	1 tbsp	123	0	14	78	0	—	—
herring	1 tbsp	123	0	14	104	0	—	—
menhaden	1 tbsp	123	0	14	71	0	—	—
salmon	1 tbsp	123	0	14	66	0	—	—
sardine	1 tbsp	123	0	14	97	0	—	—

FOOD	PORTION	CALS	PROT	FAT	CHOL	CARB	FIBER	SOD
shark	1 oz	270	0	29	–	0	0	–
whale	1 oz	270	0	29	–	0	0	–

FISH PASTE
| fish paste | 2 tsp | 15 | 1 | 1 | – | tr | 0 | – |

FISH SUBSTITUTES
Loma Linda
| Ocean Platter not prep | ½ cup (0.9 oz) | 90 | 14 | 1 | 0 | 8 | 4 | 450 |

Worthington
| Fillets | 2 (3 oz) | 180 | 16 | 10 | 0 | 8 | 4 | 750 |

FLAXSEED
Arrowhead
| Organic Flax Seeds | ¼ cup | 140 | 5 | 9 | 0 | 10 | 6 | 0 |

Bite Me
| Flax Bar | 1 bar (1.8 oz) | 242 | 7 | 11 | 0 | 30 | 12 | 79 |

Bob's Red Mill
| Flax Seed Meal | 2 tbsp | 60 | 3 | 5 | 0 | 4 | 4 | 0 |

Cracker Flax
| Organic Apple Raisin | 1 oz | 130 | 6 | 5 | 5 | 16 | 9 | 55 |

Hodgson Mill
| Milled | 2 tbsp | 60 | 3 | 1 | 0 | 4 | 4 | 0 |

FLOUNDER
FRESH
| cooked | 3 oz | 99 | 21 | 1 | 58 | 0 | – | 89 |
| cooked | 1 fillet (4.5 oz) | 148 | 31 | 2 | 86 | 0 | – | 133 |

TAKE-OUT
| battered & fried | 3.2 oz | 211 | 13 | 11 | 31 | 15 | – | 484 |
| breaded & fried | 3.2 oz | 211 | 13 | 11 | 31 | 15 | – | 484 |

FLOUR
buckwheat whole groat	1 cup (4.2 oz)	402	15	4	0	85	12	13
corn masa	1 cup (4 oz)	416	11	4	0	87	11	6
cottonseed low fat	1 oz	94	14	tr	0	10	–	10
peanut defatted	1 cup	196	31	tr	0	21	–	108
peanut defatted	1 oz	92	15	tr	0	10	–	50
peanut low fat	1 cup	257	20	13	0	19	–	0

FOOD	PORTION	CALS	PROT	FAT	CHOL	CARB	FIBER	SOD
potato	1 cup (6.3 oz)	628	14	1	0	143	–	61
rice brown	1 cup (5.5 oz)	574	11	4	0	121	7	13
rice white	1 cup (5.5 oz)	578	9	2	0	127	4	1
rye dark	1 cup (4.5 oz)	415	18	3	0	88	29	2
rye light	1 cup (3.6 oz)	374	9	1	0	82	15	2
rye medium	1 cup (3.6 oz)	361	10	2	0	79	15	3
sesame low fat	1 oz	95	14	tr	0	10	–	11
triticale whole grain	1 cup (4.6 oz)	439	17	2	0	95	19	3
white all-purpose	1 cup (4.4 oz)	455	13	1	0	95	2	3
white bread	1 cup (4.8 oz)	495	16	2	0	99	3	3
white cake unsifted	1 cup (4.8 oz)	496	11	1	0	107	2	3
white self-rising	1 cup (4.4 oz)	443	12	1	0	93	3	1588
white unbleached	1 cup (4.4 oz)	455	13	1	0	95	3	3
whole wheat	1 cup (4.2 oz)	407	16	2	0	87	15	6
All Trump								
Flour	¼ cup (1 oz)	100	4	0	0	22	tr	0
Arrowhead								
Whole Grain Oat	⅓ cup	120	5	3	0	18	3	0
Betty Crocker								
Softasilk Velvet Cake Flour	¼ cup (1 oz)	100	2	0	0	23	tr	0
Gold Medal								
All Purpose	¼ cup (1 oz)	100	3	0	0	22	tr	0
Better For Bread	¼ cup (1 oz)	100	4	0	0	22	tr	0
Organic All Purpose	¼ cup (1 oz)	100	3	0	0	22	tr	0
Self Rising	¼ cup (1 oz)	100	3	0	0	22	tr	400

FOOD	PORTION	CALS	PROT	FAT	CHOL	CARB	FIBER	SOD
Unbleached	¼ cup (1 oz)	100	3	0	0	22	tr	0
Wondra	¼ cup	100	3	0	0	23	tr	0
Heckers								
All Purpose Unbleached	¼ cup	100	3	0	0	22	tr	0
Whole Wheat	¼ cup	100	4	1	0	21	3	0
Hodgson Mill								
White Unbleached Organic	¼ cup (1 oz)	100	3	0	0	23	3	0
Whole Wheat Graham Organic	¼ cup (1 oz)	100	3	1	0	22	3	0
La Pina								
Flour	¼ cup (1 oz)	100	2	0	0	23	1	0
Red Band								
All Purpose	¼ cup (1 oz)	100	2	0	0	23	tr	0
Self-Rising	¼ cup (1 oz)	100	2	0	0	22	tr	400
Robin Hood								
All Purpose	¼ cup (1 oz)	100	3	0	0	22	tr	0
Self-Rising	¼ cup (1 oz)	100	3	0	0	22	tr	0
Unbleached	¼ cup (1 oz)	100	3	0	0	22	tr	0
Whole Wheat	¼ cup (1 oz)	90	4	1	0	21	3	0

FRENCH BEANS

| dried cooked | 1 cup | 228 | 12 | 1 | 0 | 43 | 17 | 11 |

FRENCH FRIES (see POTATO)

FRENCH TOAST
FROZEN

| french toast | 1 slice (2 oz) | 126 | 4 | 4 | 48 | 19 | 2 | 292 |

TAKE-OUT

plain	1 slice	151	7	7	75	16	–	311
sticks	5 (4.9 oz)	513	8	29	75	58	3	499
w/ butter	2 slices (4.7 oz)	356	10	19	116	36	–	513

FROG'S LEGS
TAKE-OUT

| as prep w/ seasoned flour &fried | 1 (0.8) | 70 | 4 | 5 | 12 | 15 | – | – |

FOOD	PORTION	CALS	PROT	FAT	CHOL	CARB	FIBER	SOD

FRUIT DRINKS *(see also individual names)*

FROZEN

Tree Of Life

Organic Smoothie Banana Raspberry Strawberry	⅔ cup (5 oz)	90	1	0	0	23	3	0
Organic Smoothie Mango Strawberry Raspberry	⅔ cup (5 oz)	70	1	0	0	18	4	0
Organic Smoothie Strawberry Banana	⅔ cup (5 oz)	90	7	0	0	23	3	0
Organic Smoothie Strawberry Blueberry Banana	⅔ cup (5 oz)	90	1	0	0	22	3	0

READY-TO-DRINK

| fruit punch | 6 fl oz | 87 | tr | tr | 0 | 22 | – | 41 |
| pineapple & orange drink | 8 fl oz | 125 | 3 | 0 | 0 | 29 | – | 9 |

Apple & Eve

| Apple Cranberry | 8 oz | 120 | 1 | 0 | 0 | 30 | – | 20 |

Ceres

Cranberry & Kiwi	8 oz	110	0	0	0	28	0	14
Medley	8 oz	130	0	0	0	31	2	10
Youngberry	8 oz	120	0	0	0	30	0	10

Champion Lyte

| All Flavors | 1 bottle | 0 | 0 | 0 | 0 | 0 | 0 | 55 |

Citrus Squeeze

| California Punch | 8 oz | 130 | 0 | 0 | 0 | 33 | – | 85 |
| Florida Punch | 8 oz | 120 | 0 | 0 | 0 | 30 | – | 100 |

Del Monte

Peach Raspberry	5.5 fl oz	160	1	0	0	40	3	10
Pineapple Banana Orange	5.5 fl oz	170	1	0	0	44	1	10
Strawberry Peach Banana	5.5 fl oz	150	1	0	0	39	1	10

Dole

Apple Berry Burst	8 fl oz	120	0	0	0	31	–	20
Cranberry Apple	8 fl oz	120	0	0	0	30	–	35
Fruit Fiesta	8 fl oz	140	0	0	0	34	–	20

FOOD	PORTION	CALS	PROT	FAT	CHOL	CARB	FIBER	SOD
Fruit Punch	1 carton (10 oz)	160	0	0	0	39	—	25
Mountain Cherry	8 fl oz	150	0	0	0	30	—	30
Orange Peach Mango	8 oz	120	1	0	0	28	—	35
Orange Strawberry Banana	8 oz	120	1	0	0	28	—	30
Orchard Peach	8 oz	140	1	0	0	34	—	35
Pineapple Orange	8 oz	120	2	0	0	27	—	20
Pineapple Orange Strawberry	8 oz	130	0	0	0	32	—	20
Tropical Fruit	8 oz	160	0	0	0	38	0	30
Eden								
Organic Apple Cherry Juice	8 oz	120	0	0	0	30	1	15
Fresh Samantha								
Banana Strawberry	1 cup (8 oz)	130	4	0	0	11	6	24
Carrot Orange	1 cup (8 oz)	100	4	0	0	8	4	24
Desperately Seeking C	1 cup (8 oz)	110	4	0	0	9	7	0
Protein Blast	1 cup (8 oz)	160	9	1	—	10	8	24
Super Juice	1 cup (8 oz)	140	4	1	—	11	8	0
The Big Bang	1 cup (8 oz)	100	2	0	0	8	8	0
Guzzler								
Citrus Punch	8 fl oz	140	tr	0	0	25	—	10
Island Punch	8 fl oz	140	0	0	0	29	0	30
Hansen's								
Fruit Punch 100% Juice	1 box (4.23 oz)	60	0	0	0	15	—	5
Juice Slam Wild Berry	1 box	120	0	0	0	29	—	15
Smoothie Apricot Nectar	1 can	170	1	0	0	43	—	50
Smoothie Cranberry Twist	1 can	180	0	0	0	45	—	50
Smoothie Energy Island Blast	1 can	170	1	0	0	40	—	40
Smoothie Guava Strawberry	1 can	170	0	0	0	43	—	50

FOOD	PORTION	CALS	PROT	FAT	CHOL	CARB	FIBER	SOD
Smoothie Mango Pineapple	1 can	170	0	0	0	43	—	50
Smoothie Peach Berry	1 can	170	0	0	0	43	—	50
Smoothie Pineapple Coconut	1 can	180	0	0	0	43	—	50
Smoothie Strawberry Banana	1 can	180	0	0	0	44	—	50
Smoothie Tropical Passion	1 can	170	0	0	0	44	—	50
Smoothie Whipped Orange	1 can	180	0	0	0	44	—	50
Smoothie Lite Cranberry Raspberry	1 can	50	0	0	0	13	—	45
Juicy Juice								
Apple Grape	1 box (8.45 oz)	140	0	0	0	34	0	15
Berry	1 box (8.45 oz)	130	0	0	0	37	0	15
Punch	1 box (4.23 oz)	70	0	0	0	17	0	10
Punch	1 box (8.45 oz)	140	0	0	0	34	0	15
Tropical	1 box (8.45 oz)	140	0	0	0	34	0	15
Langers								
100% Juice Pineapple Coconut	8 oz	140	0	3	0	28	1	55
Blueberry Cranberry	8 oz	135	0	0	0	34	—	10
Cranberry Berry	8 oz	135	0	0	0	34	—	10
Cranberry Fuji	8 oz	160	0	0	0	39	—	10
Cranberry Grape	8 oz	165	0	0	0	41	—	10
Cranberry Orange	8 oz	130	0	0	0	33	—	10
Diet Cranberry Berry	8 oz	30	0	0	0	8	—	10
Diet Cranberry Grape	8 oz	30	0	0	0	8	—	10
Fruit Punch Cocktail	8 oz	120	0	0	0	30	—	14

FOOD	PORTION	CALS	PROT	FAT	CHOL	CARB	FIBER	SOD
Kiwi Raspberry Cocktail	8 oz	120	0	0	0	29	—	0
Kiwi Strawberry Cocktail	8 oz	120	0	0	0	29	—	0
Mango Orange	8 oz	130	0	0	0	33	—	0
Mixed Berry 100% Juice	8 oz	120	0	0	0	30	—	15
Pineapple Orange Guava	8 oz	130	0	0	0	30	—	0
Ruby Orange	8 oz	130	0	0	0	33	—	10
Tropical Ruby	8 oz	135	0	0	0	34	—	10
White Cranberry Raspberry	8 oz	120	0	0	0	28	—	10
Mott's								
Berry	1 box (8 oz)	100	0	0	0	26	—	10
Fruit Punch	1 box (8 oz)	110	0	0	0	27	—	15
Fruit Punch	8 fl oz	130	0	0	0	32	—	0
Naked Juice								
Berry Blast	8 oz	120	1	0	0	30	1	10
Blue Machine	8 oz	150	1	1	—	40	8	30
Green Machine	8 oz	130	1	0	0	33	1	15
Power C	8 oz	120	1	1	—	29	3	15
Protein Zone	8 oz	210	17	4	20	27	tr	135
Red Machine	8 oz	160	2	3	—	32	4	15
Strawberry Banana C	8 oz	120	2	0	0	28	3	5
Very Berry	8 oz	130	2	0	0	30	1	10
Well Being	8 oz	210	17	4	—	29	1	130
Nantucket Nectars								
Orangic Blueberry Banana	8 oz	120	0	0	0	30	—	30
Organic Banana Mango Carrot	8 oz	120	0	0	0	30	—	30
Organic Cranberry Orange	8 oz	130	0	0	0	31	—	30
Peach Orange	8 oz	130	0	0	0	31	1	25
Pomegranate Pear	8 oz	110	0	0	0	28	0	30
Oberweis								
Fruit Punch	8 oz	120	0	0	0	30	0	5

FOOD	PORTION	CALS	PROT	FAT	CHOL	CARB	FIBER	SOD
Ocean Spray								
Citrus Splash Spritzer	8 oz	160	0	0	0	40	—	50
Cran*Grape	8 oz	170	0	0	0	41	0	35
Cran*Raspberry	8 oz	140	0	0	0	36	0	35
Cran*Strawberry	8 oz	140	0	0	0	36	tr	35
Cranapple	8 oz	160	0	0	0	41	tr	35
Grape Cranberry	8 oz	170	—	0	0	41	—	35
Kiwi Strawberry	8 oz	120	0	0	0	31	0	35
Mandarin Magic	8 oz	120	0	0	0	31	0	60
Orange Citrus Spritzer	8 oz	160	0	0	0	41	—	50
Ruby Tangerine Spritzer	8 oz	160	0	0	0	41	—	50
White Cranberry Apple Juice	8 oz	120	—	0	0	30	—	35
Wildberry Spritzer	8 oz	160	0	0	0	41	—	50
Odwalla								
Blackberry Fruit Shake	8 fl oz	140	1	0	0	35	1	0
Carrot Orange Apple	8 fl oz	100	2	0	0	23	1	80
Orange Pina Smoothie	8 fl oz	140	0	0	0	33	1	10
Rooty Fruity	8 fl oz	110	0	1	0	24	0	90
Strawberry Banana	8 fl oz	120	1	1	0	31	3	0
Purity Organic								
Citrus Punch	8 oz	123	tr	tr	—	33	tr	tr
Snapple								
Diet Cranberry Raspberry	8 fl oz	10	0	0	0	2	—	10
Final Fruit Fireworks	8 oz	120	0	0	0	29	—	10
Fruit Punch	8 fl oz	110	0	0	0	29	—	10
Go Bananas	8 oz	120	0	0	0	30	—	10
Kiwi Strawberry	8 fl oz	110	0	0	0	28	—	10
Pie	8 oz	120	0	0	0	31	—	35
Snapricot Orange	8 oz	120	0	0	0	30	—	10
Soy20								
All Flavors	1 bottle (12 oz)	90	0	0	0	22	—	10

FOOD	PORTION	CALS	PROT	FAT	CHOL	CARB	FIBER	SOD
V8								
Splash Berry Blend	8 oz	110	0	0	0	28	–	40
FRUIT MIXED (see also individual names)								
CANNED								
fruit cocktail in heavy syrup	½ cup	93	1	tr	0	24	–	7
fruit cocktail juice pack	½ cup	56	1	tr	0	15	–	4
fruit cocktail water pack	½ cup	40	1	tr	0	10	–	5
fruit salad in heavy syrup	½ cup	94	tr	tr	0	24	–	7
fruit salad in light syrup	½ cup	73	tr	tr	0	19	–	7
fruit salad juice pack	½ cup	62	1	tr	0	16	–	7
fruit salad water pack	½ cup	37	tr	tr	0	10	–	4
mixed fruit in heavy syrup	½ cup	92	tr	tr	0	24	–	5
tropical fruit salad in heavy syrup	½ cup	110	1	tr	0	29	–	3
Del Monte								
Cherry Mixed Light Syrup	½ cup (4.4 oz)	90	1	0	0	22	1	10
Chunky Mixed Fruit Naturals	½ cup (4.4 oz)	60	0	0	0	15	1	10
Chunky Mixed In Extra Light Syrup	½ cup (4.4 oz)	60	0	0	0	15	1	10
Chunky Mixed In Heavy Syrup	½ cup (4.5 oz)	100	0	0	0	24	1	10
Citrus Salad	½ cup (4.4 oz)	80	0	0	0	20	0	20
Fruit Cocktail Fruit Naturals	½ cup (4.4 oz)	60	0	0	0	15	1	10
Fruit Cocktail In Extra Light Syrup	½ cup (4.4 oz)	60	0	0	0	15	1	10
Fruit Cocktail In Heavy Syrup	½ cup (4.5 oz)	100	0	0	0	24	1	10

FOOD	PORTION	CALS	PROT	FAT	CHOL	CARB	FIBER	SOD
Fruit Cup Fruit Naturals Mixed	1 pkg (4 oz)	50	0	0	0	13	1	10
Fruit Cup Mixed In Extra Light Syrup	1 pkg (4 oz)	50	0	0	0	13	1	10
Fruit Salad In Extra Light Syrup	½ cup (4.5 oz)	70	1	0	0	22	2	5
Fruit To Go Fruity Combo	1 pkg (4 oz)	70	1	0	0	18	1	10
Fruit To Go Wild Berry Jumble	1 pkg (4 oz)	80	1	0	0	20	1	10
Orchard Select California Mixed	½ cup (4.5 oz)	80	1	0	0	19	1	10
Orchard Select Premium Mixed	½ cup (4.4 oz)	80	tr	0	0	20	tr	10
Snack Cups Strawberry Banana Peaches	1 pkg	70	tr	0	0	17	tr	10
Snack Cups Tropical Fruit	1 pkg	70	tr	0	0	18	tr	5
SunFresh Ambrosia Salad	½ cup	70	0	0	0	16	1	25
Tropical Fruit Salad	½ cup (4.3 oz)	60	0	0	0	16	1	15
Tropical Fruit Salad In Light Syrup	½ cup (4.4 oz)	80	0	0	0	21	1	10
Very Cherry Mixed Fruit	½ cup (4.4 oz)	90	1	0	0	22	1	10
Dole								
FruitBowls Tropical Fruit	1 pkg (4 oz)	60	tr	0	0	16	2	10
Tropical Fruit Salad	½ cup (4.3 oz)	80	tr	0	0	20	1	10
Mott's								
Fruitsations Banana	1 pkg (4 oz)	90	0	0	0	23	–	0
Fruitsations Cherry	1 pkg (4 oz)	70	0	0	0	19	–	0
Fruitsations Mango Peach	1 pkg (4 oz)	70	0	0	0	22	–	0
Fruitsations Mixed Berry	1 pkg (4 oz)	90	0	0	0	22	1	0

FOOD	PORTION	CALS	PROT	FAT	CHOL	CARB	FIBER	SOD
Fruitsations Pear	1 pkg (4 oz)	90	0	0	0	23	–	0
Fruitsations Strawberry	1 pkg (4 oz)	80	0	0	0	19	–	10
Fruitsations Tropical Fruit	1 pkg (4 oz)	70	0	0	0	19	–	0
Hearlthy Harvest Peach Medley	1 pkg (3.9 oz)	50	0	0	0	13	1	0
SunFresh								
Ambrosia Salad	½ cup (4.5 oz)	70	0	0	0	16	1	25
Mixed Fruit In Light Syrup	½ cup (4.6 oz)	90	1	0	0	20	2	25
Tropical Salad In Extra Light Syrup	½ cup (4.5 oz)	80	1	0	0	20	0	10
DRIED								
mixed	11 oz pkg	712	7	1	0	188	–	52
Paradise								
Old English Fruit & Peel Mix	1 tbsp (0.8 oz)	70	6	0	0	18	1	15
Sun-Maid								
Tropical Medley	¼ cup (1.4 oz)	130	1	0	0	32	1	10
FROZEN								
mixed fruit sweetened	1 cup	245	4	tr	0	61	–	8
Birds Eye								
Mixed Fruit	½ cup	90	1	0	0	23	–	5
Tree Of Life								
Organic Mixed Berries	¾ cup (5 oz)	60	0	0	0	16	3	0
FRUIT SNACKS								
fruit leather	1 bar (0.8 oz)	81	tr	1	0	18	–	18
fruit leather pieces	1 pkg (0.9 oz)	92	tr	2	0	21	–	109
fruit leather pieces	1 oz	97	tr	2	0	22	–	114
fruit leather rolls	1 sm (0.5 oz)	49	tr	tr	0	12	–	8
fruit leather rolls	1 lg (0.7 oz)	73	tr	1	0	18	–	13
Betty Crocker								
Fruit By The Foot All Flavors	1 roll	80	0	2	–	17	–	50
CoolFruits								
Apple Grape	1 bar (0.5 oz)	51	tr	tr	0	12	1	0

FOOD	PORTION	CALS	PROT	FAT	CHOL	CARB	FIBER	SOD
Apple Strawberry	1 bar (0.5 oz)	51	tr	tr	0	12	1	0
Wild Blueberry	1 bar (0.5 oz)	51	tr	tr	0	12	1	0
Sunbelt								
Fruit Jammers	1 pkg (1 oz)	100	0	1	0	23	0	15
Sunkist								
100% Fruit Roll All Flavors	1 (0.5 oz)	50	0	0	0	12	1	10

GARLIC

FOOD	PORTION	CALS	PROT	FAT	CHOL	CARB	FIBER	SOD
clove	1	4	tr	tr	0	1	–	1
fresh chopped	1 tsp	4	tr	tr	0	tr	1	0
powder	1 tsp	9	tr	tr	0	2	–	1
Dorot								
Frozen Crushed Cubes	1 cube (4 g)	5	0	0	0	1	0	40
McCormick								
Garlic Salt	¼ tsp	0	0	0	0	0	0	250

GEFILTE FISH

FOOD	PORTION	CALS	PROT	FAT	CHOL	CARB	FIBER	SOD
sweet	1 piece (1.5 oz)	35	4	1	12	3	–	220

GELATIN
MIX

FOOD	PORTION	CALS	PROT	FAT	CHOL	CARB	FIBER	SOD
low calorie	½ cup	8	2	0	0	0	0	9
mix as prep	½ cup (4.7 oz)	80	2	0	0	19	–	57
mix not prep	1 pkg (3 oz)	324	7	0	0	77	–	216
mix w/ fruit	½ cup (3.7 oz)	73	1	tr	0	18	–	30
powder unsweetened	1 pkg (7 g)	23	6	0	–	0	–	14

READY-TO-EAT
Hunt's

FOOD	PORTION	CALS	PROT	FAT	CHOL	CARB	FIBER	SOD
Snack Pack Gels Cherry	1 serv (3.5 oz)	100	0	0	0	25	0	42
Snack Pack Gels Raspberry Berry	1 serv (3.5 oz)	100	0	0	0	25	0	42
Snack Pack Gels Strawberry	1 serv (3.5 oz)	100	0	0	0	25	0	42
Snack Pack Gels Strawberry Orange	1 serv (3.5 oz)	100	0	0	0	25	0	42

FOOD	PORTION	CALS	PROT	FAT	CHOL	CARB	FIBER	SOD
Swiss Miss								
Gels Berry Strawberry	1 pkg (3.5 oz)	79	1	0	0	18	0	38
Gels Berry Lemon	1 pkg (3.5 oz)	79	1	0	0	18	0	38
Gels Raspberry Orange	1 pkg (3.5 oz)	79	1	0	0	18	0	38
Gels Strawberry Raspberry	1 pkg (3.5 oz)	79	1	0	0	18	0	38

GIBLETS

FOOD	PORTION	CALS	PROT	FAT	CHOL	CARB	FIBER	SOD
capon simmered	1 cup (5 oz)	238	38	8	629	0	–	80
chicken floured & fried	1 cup (5 oz)	402	47	19	647	6	–	164
chicken simmered	1 cup (5 oz)	228	37	7	570	1	–	85
turkey simmered	1 cup (5 oz)	243	39	7	606	3	–	85

GINGER

FOOD	PORTION	CALS	PROT	FAT	CHOL	CARB	FIBER	SOD
ground	1 tsp (1.8 g)	6	tr	tr	0	1	–	1
pickled	0.5 oz	5	tr	0	0	1	tr	52
root fresh	5 slices	8	tr	tr	0	2	–	1
root fresh	¼ cup	17	tr	tr	0	4	–	3
Eden								
Pickled w/ Shiso Leaves	1 tbsp	15	0	0	0	3	1	340
McCormick								
Crystallized	¼ tsp	15	0	0	0	3	–	0

GINKGO NUTS

FOOD	PORTION	CALS	PROT	FAT	CHOL	CARB	FIBER	SOD
canned	1 oz	32	1	tr	0	6	–	87
dried	1 oz	99	3	tr	0	21	–	4
raw	1 oz	52	1	tr	0	11	–	1

GINSENG

FOOD	PORTION	CALS	PROT	FAT	CHOL	CARB	FIBER	SOD
dried	1 oz	90	5	tr	–	20	2	16
fresh	1 oz	28	1	tr	–	6	tr	5

GIZZARDS

FOOD	PORTION	CALS	PROT	FAT	CHOL	CARB	FIBER	SOD
chicken simmered	1 cup (5 oz)	222	5	5	281	2	–	97
turkey simmered	1 cup (5 oz)	236	43	6	336	1	–	79

FOOD	PORTION	CALS	PROT	FAT	CHOL	CARB	FIBER	SOD
GNOCCHI								
Bellino								
w/ Potato	1 cup	240	5	1	0	55	2	550
GOAT								
roasted	3 oz	122	23	3	64	0	–	73
GOOSE								
w/ skin roasted	6.6 oz	574	47	41	172	0	–	132
w/ skin roasted	½ goose (1.7 lbs)	2362	195	170	708	0	–	543
w/o skin roasted	½ goose (1.3 lbs)	1406	171	75	569	0	–	447
w/o skin roasted	5 oz	340	41	18	138	0	–	108
GOOSEBERRIES								
canned in light syrup	½ cup	93	1	tr	0	24	–	3
fresh	1 cup	67	1	1	0	15	–	1
GRAPE JUICE								
bottled	1 cup	155	1	tr	0	38	–	7
frzn sweetened as prep	1 cup	128	tr	tr	0	32	–	5
frzn sweetened not prep	6 oz	386	1	1	0	96	–	15
grape drink	6 oz	84	0	0	0	22	–	12
Ceres								
Hanepoot White Grape	8 oz	130	0	0	0	33	0	10
Daily								
Drink	8 oz	110	0	0	0	27	–	30
Hansen's								
White Grape 100% Juice	1 box (4.23 oz)	90	0	0	0	22	–	10
Juicy Juice								
Drink	1 box (4.23 oz)	70	0	0	0	17	–	10
Drink	1 box (8.45 oz)	140	0	0	0	34	0	15
Keto								
Kooler	½ tsp	0	0	0	0	0	0	0

FOOD	PORTION	CALS	PROT	FAT	CHOL	CARB	FIBER	SOD
Langers								
Cocktail	8 oz	160	0	0	0	40	–	15
Mott's								
100% Juice	1 box (8 oz)	130	0	0	0	33	–	15
Grape Juice	8 fl oz	130	0	0	0	31	–	10
Nantucket Nectars								
Organic Concord Grape	8 oz	130	0	0	0	33	–	30
Welch's								
100% Juice	8 oz	170	0	0	0	42	–	20
100% White	8 oz	160	0	0	0	39	–	20
GRAPE LEAVES								
canned	1 (4 g)	3	tr	tr	0	tr	0	114
fresh raw	1 (3 g)	3	tr	tr	0	1	tr	tr
TAKE-OUT								
dolmas	5 (4.2 oz)	200	2	11	0	23	2	570
GRAPEFRUIT								
CANNED								
juice pack	½ cup	46	1	tr	0	11	–	9
unsweetened	1 cup	93	1	tr	0	22	–	3
water pack	½ cup	44	1	tr	0	11	–	2
SunFresh								
Red & White	½ cup (4.4 oz)	45	1	0	0	9	2	15
FRESH								
pink	½	37	1	tr	0	9	1	0
pink sections	1 cup	69	1	tr	0	18	1	1
red	½	37	1	tr	0	9	–	0
red sections	1 cup	69	1	tr	0	18	–	1
white	½	39	1	tr	0	10	1	0
white sections	1 cup	76	2	tr	0	19	1	0
GRAPEFRUIT JUICE								
fresh	1 cup	96	1	tr	0	23	–	2
frzn as prep	1 cup	102	1	tr	0	24	–	2
frzn not prep	6 oz	302	4	1	0	72	–	6
sweetened	1 cup	116	1	tr	0	28	–	4
Fresh Samantha								
Juice	1 cup (8 oz)	90	1	0	0	7	0	0

FOOD	PORTION	CALS	PROT	FAT	CHOL	CARB	FIBER	SOD
Langers								
Diet Ruby Red	8 oz	40	0	0	0	9	–	10
Ruby Red	8 oz	130	0	0	0	33	–	10
Mott's								
100% Juice	8 fl oz	110	2	0	0	27	–	10
Ocean Spray								
100% Juice Pink	8 oz	110	tr	0	0	28	0	35
100% White Juice	8 oz	100	1	0	0	24	tr	35
Ruby Drink	8 oz	120	–	0	0	30	–	35
Ruby Red Drink	8 oz	130	0	0	0	33	0	35
Odwalla								
Juice	8 fl oz	90	2	0	0	20	0	5
GRAPES								
fresh	10	36	tr	tr	0	9	tr	1
thompson seedless in heavy syrup	½ cup	94	1	tr	0	25	–	7
thompson seedless water pack	½ cup	48	1	tr	0	13	–	7
Chiquita								
Grapes	1½ cups (4.8 oz)	90	1	1	0	24	1	0
GRAVY								
CANNED								
au jus	1 cup	38	3	tr	1	6	–	–
beef	1 can (10 oz)	155	11	7	9	14	–	1630
beef	1 cup	124	9	6	7	11	–	1305
chicken	1 cup	189	5	14	5	13	–	1375
mushroom	1 cup	120	3	6	0	13	–	1259
turkey	1 cup	122	6	5	5	12	–	–
Campbell's								
Beef	¼ cup	29	1	1	1	4	tr	421
Brown	¼ cup	46	1	3	tr	4	1	350
Chicken	¼ cup	42	1	2	3	4	1	244
Turkey	¼ cup	29	1	1	2	3	tr	289
Heinz								
Home Style Chicken	¼ cup	25	0	1	0	4	0	340
MIX								
au jus as prep w/ water	1 cup	32	1	1	1	4	–	964

FOOD	PORTION	CALS	PROT	FAT	CHOL	CARB	FIBER	SOD
brown as prep w/ water	1 cup	75	2	2	2	13	–	1076
chicken as prep	1 cup	83	3	2	3	14	–	1133
mushroom as prep	1 cup	70	2	1	1	14	–	1402
onion as prep w/ water	1 cup	77	2	1	tr	16	–	1013
pork as prep	1 cup	76	2	2	3	13	–	1235
turkey as prep	1 cup	87	3	2	3	15	–	1498
Bournvita								
Extract	2 heaping tsp	34	1	1	–	7	–	–
Bovril								
Extract	1 heaping tsp	9	2	0	–	tr	0	–
Durkee								
Au Jus as prep	¼ cup	5	0	0	0	1	0	320
Brown as prep	¼ cup	10	0	1	0	3	0	250
Brown Mushroom as prep	¼ cup	15	1	0	0	3	0	300
Brown Onion as prep	¼ cup	15	1	0	0	4	0	290
Chicken as prep	¼ cup	20	1	1	0	4	0	350
Country as prep	¼ cup	35	1	2	0	5	0	370
Homestyle as prep	¼ cup	15	1	1	0	3	0	240
Onion as prep	¼ cup	10	1	0	0	3	0	310
Pork as prep	¼ cup	10	1	0	0	3	0	240
Sausage as prep	¼ cup	35	1	2	0	5	0	570
Swiss Steak as prep	¼ cup	15	0	0	0	4	0	370
Turkey as prep	¼ cup	20	1	0	0	4	0	270
French's								
Au Jus as prep	¼ cup	5	0	0	0	1	0	220
Brown as prep	¼ cup	10	0	1	0	3	0	250
Chicken as prep	¼ cup	25	1	1	0	4	0	250
Country as prep	¼ cup	35	1	2	0	5	0	370
Herb Brown as prep	¼ cup	15	1	1	0	3	0	350
Homestyle as prep	¼ cup	10	0	1	0	3	0	230
Mushroom as prep	¼ cup	10	0	1	0	3	0	250
Onion	¼ cup	15	0	1	0	4	0	260
Pork as prep	¼ cup	10	0	1	0	3	0	250
Turkey as prep	¼ cup	20	1	0	0	4	0	270

FOOD	PORTION	CALS	PROT	FAT	CHOL	CARB	FIBER	SOD
Loma Linda								
Gravy Quik Brown	1 tbsp (5 g)	20	tr	0	0	4	0	370
Gravy Quik Chicken	1 tbsp (5 g)	20	1	0	0	3	0	410
Quik Gravy Country	1 tbsp (5 g)	25	tr	1	0	4	0	250
Quik Gravy Mushroom	1 tbsp (5 g)	15	tr	0	0	3	tr	300
Quik Gravy Onion	1 tbsp (5 g)	20	tr	0	0	3	tr	230
Marmite								
Extract	1 heaping tsp	9	2	0	–	tr	–	–
McCormick								
Au Jus Natural as prep	¼ cup	5	0	0	–	1	–	310
Beef & Herb as prep	¼ cup	30	1	1	<5	3	–	290
Brown as prep	¼ cup	20	tr	1	–	3	–	340
Chicken as prep	¼ cup	20	0	0	–	4	–	330
Onion as prep	¼ cup	20	tr	1	–	3	–	340
Pork as prep	¼ cup	20	0	–	–	4	–	320
Turkey as prep	¼ cup	20	0	0	–	3	–	350
GREAT NORTHERN BEANS								
canned	1 cup	299	19	1	0	55	13	11
dried cooked	1 cup	209	15	1	0	37	12	4
Eden								
Organic	½ cup (4.6 oz)	110	5	1	0	20	8	65
GREEN BEANS								
CANNED								
green beans	½ cup	13	1	tr	0	3	1	170
italian	½ cup	13	1	tr	0	3	1	170
italian low sodium	½ cup	13	1	tr	0	3	1	1
low sodium	½ cup	13	1	tr	0	3	1	1
Del Monte								
Cut	½ cup (4.2 oz)	20	1	0	0	4	2	390
Cut Italian	½ cup (4.2 oz)	30	1	0	0	6	3	390
Cut No Salt Added	½ cup (4.2 oz)	20	1	0	0	4	2	10
French Style	½ cup (4.2 oz)	20	1	0	0	4	2	390
French Style No Salt Added	½ cup (4.2 oz)	20	1	0	0	4	2	10

FOOD	PORTION	CALS	PROT	FAT	CHOL	CARB	FIBER	SOD
French Style Seasoned	½ cup (4.2 oz)	20	1	0	0	4	2	360
Whole	½ cup (4.2 oz)	20	1	0	0	4	2	390
S&W								
Blue Lake Cut	½ cup (4.2 oz)	20	1	0	0	4	2	340
French Style	½ cup (4.2 oz)	20	1	0	0	4	2	340
Whole Small	½ cup (4.2 oz)	20	1	0	0	4	2	390
Veg-All								
French Style	½ cup	20	tr	0	0	4	2	400
FRESH								
cooked	½ cup	22	1	tr	0	5	–	2
raw	½ cup	17	1	tr	0	4	1	3
FROZEN								
cooked	½ cup	18	1	tr	0	4	–	9
italian cooked	½ cup	18	1	tr	0	4	–	9
Birds Eye								
Cut	½ cup	25	–	0	0	–	2	0
Italian	½ cup	35	–	0	0	–	3	0
Fresh Like								
Cut	3.5 oz	29	1	tr	–	7	1	6
French Cut	3.5 oz	29	1	tr	–	7	1	6
Tree Of Life								
Cut	⅔ cup (2.8 oz)	25	1	0	0	4	2	10

GREENS
Ready Pac

Microwave Leafy Greens as prep	½ cup	15	2	0	0	2	2	100

GROUNDCHERRIES

fresh	½ cup	37	1	tr	0	8	–	–

GROUPER

cooked	1 fillet (7.1 oz)	238	50	3	95	0	–	107
cooked	3 oz	100	21	1	40	0	–	45
raw	3 oz	78	16	1	31	0	–	45

GUAR GUM
Bob's Red Mill

Guar Gum	1 tbsp	20	0	0	0	6	6	2

FOOD	PORTION	CALS	PROT	FAT	CHOL	CARB	FIBER	SOD
GUAVA								
fresh	1	45	1	1	0	11	–	2
guava sauce	½ cup	43	tr	tr	0	11	–	4
GUAVA JUICE								
Ceres								
Guava	8 oz	120	0	0	0	29	0	5
Nantucket Nectars								
Guava	8 oz	130	0	0	0	33	0	5
GUINEA HEN								
w/ skin raw	½ hen (12.1 oz)	545	81	22	–	0	–	–
w/o skin raw	½ hen (9.3 oz)	292	55	7	166	0	–	–
HADDOCK								
fresh cooked	1 fillet (5.3 oz)	168	36	1	110	0	–	131
fresh cooked	3 oz	95	21	1	63	0	–	74
fresh raw	3 oz	74	16	1	49	0	–	58
roe raw	1 oz	37	7	tr	103	tr	–	–
smoked	3 oz	99	21	1	65	0	–	649
smoked	1 oz	33	7	tr	21	0	–	214
TAKE-OUT								
breaded & fried	1 piece (3.5 oz)	187	23	9	63	3	tr	350
HAKE								
raw	3.5 oz	84	17	1	–	0	–	101
HALIBUT								
atlantic & pacific cooked	½ fillet (5.6 oz)	223	42	5	65	0	–	110
atlantic & pacific cooked	3 oz	119	23	2	35	0	–	59
atlantic & pacific raw	3 oz	93	18	2	27	0	–	46
greenland baked	5.6 oz	380	29	28	94	0	–	163
greenland baked	3 oz	203	16	15	50	0	–	87

FOOD	PORTION	CALS	PROT	FAT	CHOL	CARB	FIBER	SOD
HAM								
canned extra lean roasted	3 oz	116	18	4	26	tr	0	965
center slice country style lean roasted	4 oz	220	31	9	80	tr	0	3045
chopped canned	1 oz	68	5	5	14	tr	—	387
ham & cheese loaf	1 oz	73	9	6	16	1	—	762
ham & cheese spread	1 tbsp	37	2	3	9	tr	—	179
ham salad spread	1 tbsp	32	1	2	6	2	—	137
minced	1 oz	75	5	6	20	1	—	353
patty cooked	1 patty (2 oz)	203	8	18	43	1	0	632
prosciutto	1 oz	55	8	2	20	tr	0	765
sliced extra lean 5% fat	1 oz	37	5	1	13	tr	—	405
sliced regular 11% fat	1 oz	52	5	3	16	1	—	373
steak boneless extra lean	1 (2 oz)	69	11	2	26	0	0	720
westphalian smoked	1 oz	105	5	10	—	0	—	398
Alpine Lace								
Boneless Cooked 98% Fat Free	2 slices (2 oz)	60	9	1	25	2	0	530
Honey Ham 98% Fat Free	2 slices (2 oz)	60	9	1	25	2	0	530
Smoked Virginia 98% Fat Free	2 slices (2 oz)	60	9	1	25	2	0	400
Armour								
Star Canned	1 oz	34	—	1	11	—	—	—
Boar's Head								
Black Forest Smoked	2 oz	60	10	1	30	2	0	580
Cappy	2 oz	60	10	2	15	3	0	530
Deluxe	2 oz	60	9	1	25	2	0	590
Deluxe Lowered Sodium	2 oz	50	10	1	20	tr	0	460

FOOD	PORTION	CALS	PROT	FAT	CHOL	CARB	FIBER	SOD
Maple Glazed Honey	2 oz	60	10	1	20	3	0	570
Pepper	2 oz	60	10	1	20	2	0	610
Rosemary & Sundried Tomato	2 oz	70	10	3	10	2	0	590
Sweet Slice Smoked	3 oz	100	15	3	30	1	0	780
Virgina	2 oz	60	9	1	25	3	0	590
Virginia Smoked	2 oz	60	9	1	25	2	0	590
Carl Buddig								
Ham Sliced w/ Natural Juices	1 pkg (2.5 oz)	120	12	7	40	1	—	980
Honey Ham Sliced w/ Natural Juice	1 pkg (2.5 oz)	120	12	7	40	3	—	760
Lean Slices Oven Roasted Honey Ham	1 pkg (2.5 oz)	90	13	2	35	4	—	850
Lean Slices Smoked	1 pkg (2.5 oz)	80	14	2	35	1	—	850
Hillshire								
Deli Select Honey Ham	6 slices (2 oz)	60	10	2	25	2	0	600
Oscar Mayer								
Lunchables Ham Bagels	1 pkg	410	16	10	40	64	2	890
Lunchables Ham Wraps	1 pkg	430	15	13	35	64	2	1050
Wampler								
Black Forest	2 oz	60	10	2	25	2	—	650

HAM DISHES
TAKE-OUT

FOOD	PORTION	CALS	PROT	FAT	CHOL	CARB	FIBER	SOD
croquettes	1 (3.1 oz)	217	12	14	77	11	tr	475
salad	½ cup	287	16	23	237	5	tr	671

HAM SUBSTITUTES
Yves

FOOD	PORTION	CALS	PROT	FAT	CHOL	CARB	FIBER	SOD
Veggie Ham Deli Slices	1 serv (2.2 oz)	80	14	0	0	6	1	480

FOOD	PORTION	CALS	PROT	FAT	CHOL	CARB	FIBER	SOD
HAMBURGER								
Kid Cuisine								
Buckaroo Beef Patty Sandwich w/ Cheese	1 meal (8.5 oz)	410	12	15	30	58	4	600
TAKE-OUT								
double patty w/ bun	1 reg	544	30	28	99	43	—	554
double patty w/ cheese & bun	1 reg	457	28	28	110	22	—	635
double patty w/ cheese & double bun	1 reg	461	22	22	80	44	—	892
double patty w/ cheese ketchup mayonnaise onion pickle tomato & bun	1 reg	416	21	21	60	35	—	1051
double patty w/ ketchup mayonnaise onion pickle tomato & bun	1 reg	649	30	35	94	53	—	920
double patty w/ ketchup cheese mayonnaise mustard pickle tomato & bun	1 lg	706	38	44	141	40	—	1149
double patty w/ ketchup mustard mayonnaise onion pickle tomato & bun	1 lg	540	34	27	122	40	—	791
double patty w/ ketchup mustard onion pickle & bun	1 reg	576	32	32	102	39	—	742
single patty w/ bacon ketchup cheese mustard onion pickle & bun	1 lg	609	32	37	112	37	—	1044

FOOD	PORTION	CALS	PROT	FAT	CHOL	CARB	FIBER	SOD
single patty w/ bun	1 reg	275	12	12	36	31	–	387
single patty w/ bun	1 lg	400	23	23	71	25	–	474
single patty w/ cheese & bun	1 reg	320	15	15	50	32	–	500
single patty w/ cheese & bun	1 lg	608	30	33	96	47	–	1589
single patty w/ ketchup cheese ham mayonnaise pickle tomato & bun	1 lg	745	40	48	122	38	–	1713
single patty w/ ketchup mustard mayonnaise onion pickle tomato & bun	1 reg	279	13	13	26	27	–	504
triple patty w/ cheese & bun	1 lg	769	56	51	161	27	–	1211
triple patty w/ ketchup mustard pickle & bun	1 lg	693	50	41	142	29	–	713

HAMBURGER SUBSTITUTES (see also MEAT SUBSTITUTES)

Amy's

FOOD	PORTION	CALS	PROT	FAT	CHOL	CARB	FIBER	SOD
All American Burger	1 (2.5 oz)	120	10	3	0	15	3	390
California Burger	1.(2.5 oz)	130	6	5	0	19	5	430
Chicago Burger	1 (2.5 oz)	160	10	5	5	20	3	390

Boca Burgers

FOOD	PORTION	CALS	PROT	FAT	CHOL	CARB	FIBER	SOD
Flamed Grilled	1	120	14	4	<5	6	4	370

Dr. Praeger's

FOOD	PORTION	CALS	PROT	FAT	CHOL	CARB	FIBER	SOD
California Burger	1 (2.7 oz)	100	8	3	0	10	4	190

Franklin Farms

FOOD	PORTION	CALS	PROT	FAT	CHOL	CARB	FIBER	SOD
Veggiburger Portabella	1 (3 oz)	120	15	2	0	11	4	460

Gardenburger

FOOD	PORTION	CALS	PROT	FAT	CHOL	CARB	FIBER	SOD
Classic Greek	1 (2.5 oz)	120	6	3	10	17	2	310
Fire Roasted Vegetable	1 (2.5 oz)	120	7	3	10	17	2	270

Harmony Farms

FOOD	PORTION	CALS	PROT	FAT	CHOL	CARB	FIBER	SOD
Soy Burger Onion	1 (2.5 oz)	90	10	3	0	7	3	230

FOOD	PORTION	CALS	PROT	FAT	CHOL	CARB	FIBER	SOD
Soy Burgers Garlic	1 (2.5 oz)	110	12	3	0	10	23	240
Soy Burgers Mushroom	1 (2.5 oz)	110	11	3	0	9	3	320
Soy Burgers Original	1 (2.5 oz)	110	12	3	0	7	4	250
Lightlife								
Barbecue Grilles	1 patty (2.7 oz)	120	10	4	0	11	0	180
Lemon Grilles	1 patty (2.7 oz)	140	11	6	0	11	0	280
Light Burgers	1 (3 oz)	130	16	1	0	12	2	410
Tamari Grilles	1 patty (2.7 oz)	120	11	5	0	9	0	260
Loma Linda								
Patty Mix not prep	⅓ cup (0.9 oz)	90	14	1	0	7	5	480
Redi-Burger	⅜ in slice (3 oz)	120	18	3	0	7	4	450
Vege-Burger	¼ cup (1.9 oz)	70	11	2	0	2	2	115
Morningstar Farms								
Better'n Burger	1 (2.7 oz)	80	13	0	0	8	3	360
Garden Grille	1 patty (2.5 oz)	120	6	3	<5	18	4	280
Garden Veggie Patties	1 patty	100	10	3	0	9	4	350
Hard Rock Cafe Veggie Burger	1 (3 oz)	170	6	8	0	18	3	340
Harvest Burger	1	140	18	4	0	8	5	390
Harvest Burger Italian Style	1 patty (3.2 oz)	140	17	5	0	8	5	370
Harvest Burger Southwestern	1 (3.2 oz)	140	16	4	0	9	5	370
Spicy Black Bean Burger	1 (2.7 oz)	110	11	1	0	16	5	470
Natural Touch								
Garden Veggie Pattie	1 (2.4 oz)	110	10	3	0	8	3	280
Okara Pattie	1 (2.2 oz)	110	11	5	0	4	3	360

FOOD	PORTION	CALS	PROT	FAT	CHOL	CARB	FIBER	SOD
Original Veggie Burger Kit not prep	¼ pkg (0.8 oz)	80	14	0	0	6	4	360
Southwestern Veggie Burger Kit not prep	¼ pkg (0.9 oz)	90	12	0	0	9	4	360
Spicy Black Bean Burger	1 (2.7 oz)	100	11	1	0	15	5	330
Vegan Burger	1 (2.7 oz)	70	11	0	0	6	3	370
Superburgers								
Vegan Organic Original	1 (3 oz)	98	10	2	0	14	2	350
Vegan Organic Smoked	1 (3 oz)	98	10	2	0	14	2	350
Vegan Organic TexMex	1 (3 oz)	110	10	1	0	14	3	195
V'dora								
Vegetable BurgerLites	1 (3.3 oz)	58	4	0	0	4	0	98
Worthington								
Granburger not prep	3 tbsp (0.6 oz)	60	10	1	0	3	2	410
Prosage Patties	1 (1.3 oz)	80	9	3	0	3	2	300
Yves								
Black Bean & Mushroom Burgers	1 (3 oz)	100	12	0	0	13	7	450
Garden Vegetable Patties	1 (3 oz)	90	11	0	0	11	7	470
Veggie Burger	1 (3 oz)	119	16	2	0	9	4	480
HAZELNUTS								
dried blanched	1 oz	191	4	19	0	5	–	1
dried unblanched	1 oz	179	4	18	0	4	–	1
dry roasted unblanched	1 oz	188	3	19	0	5	–	1
oil roasted unblanched	1 oz	187	4	18	0	5	2	1

FOOD	PORTION	CALS	PROT	FAT	CHOL	CARB	FIBER	SOD
Low Carb Creations								
Soft Hazelnut Brittle	2 pieces (1 oz)	160	5	12	0	16	1	160
Torras								
Hazelnut Chocolate Spread	1 tsp	27	tr	2	1	3	0	3
Twist								
Sugar Free Chocolate Hazelnut Spread	2 tbsp	180	1	14	0	2	0	0
HEART								
beef simmered	3 oz	148	24	5	164	tr	—	54
chicken simmered	1 cup (5 oz)	268	11	11	350	tr	—	69
lamb braised	3 oz	158	21	7	212	2	—	54
pork braised	1	191	30	7	285	1	0	45
pork braised	1 cup	215	34	7	320	1	0	51
turkey simmered	1 cup (5 oz)	257	39	9	327	3	—	79
veal braised	3 oz	158	25	6	150	tr	—	50
HEARTS OF PALM								
canned	1 cup (5.1 oz)	41	4	1	0	7	—	622
canned	1 (1.2 oz)	9	1	tr	0	2	—	141
HEMP								
HempNut								
Shelled Hempseed	1 oz	162	9	13	0	3	2	3
Nutiva								
Hempseed	1½ tbsp (0.5 oz)	70	4	5	0	3	2	0

HERBAL TEA (see ICED TEA, TEA/HERBAL TEA)

FOOD	PORTION	CALS	PROT	FAT	CHOL	CARB	FIBER	SOD
HERBS/SPICES (see also individual names)								
cajun seasoning	1 tbsp	19	1	1	—	3	1	5
chinese five spice	1 tsp	7	0	tr	—	2	tr	1
curry powder	1 tsp	6	tr	tr	0	1	—	1
garam masala	1 tsp	8	tr	tr	0	1	—	2
poultry seasoning	1 tsp	5	tr	tr	0	1	—	tr
pumpkin pie spice	1 tsp	6	tr	tr	0	1	—	1
Eden								
Furikake Seasoning	½ tsp	5	0	0	0	1	1	25

FOOD	PORTION	CALS	PROT	FAT	CHOL	CARB	FIBER	SOD
Gringo Billy's								
Meat Rubs Chipotle	¼ tsp	0	0	0	0	0	0	151
Meat Rubs Ultimate	¼ tsp	0	0	0	0	0	0	155
Tuna Seasoning	1 tsp	5	0	1	0	1	1	92
Instant India								
Curry Paste Cilantro Garlic	2 tbsp (1 oz)	110	2	3	0	4	0	140
Curry Paste Ginger Garlic	2 tbsp (1 oz)	90	1	3	0	8	0	570
McCormick								
Big'n Season Buffalo Wings	1 tbsp (8 g)	30	0	0	–	5	–	710
Big'n Season Chicken	1 tbsp (6 g)	20	tr	0	–	3	–	460
Big'n Season Pot Roast	1 tsp	10	tr	0	–	1	–	390
Blends Bon Appetit	¼ tsp	0	0	0	0	0	0	300
Cajun Seasoning	¼ tsp	0	0	0	0	0	0	80
Greek Seasoning	¼ tsp	0	0	0	0	0	0	20
Jamaican Jerk Seasoning	¼ tsp	0	0	0	0	0	0	125
Meat Loaf Seasoning	1 tsp (4 g)	15	0	0	–	2	–	350
Seafood Seasoning	¼ tsp	0	0	0	0	0	0	110
Mrs. Dash								
Classic Italian	¼ tsp	0	0	0	0	0	0	0
Extra Spicy	¼ tsp	0	0	0	0	0	0	0
Garlic & Herb	¼ tsp	0	0	0	0	0	0	0
Grilling Blend Mesquite	¼ tsp	0	0	0	0	0	0	0
Grilling Blend Original Chicken	¼ tsp	0	0	0	0	0	0	0
Grilling Blend Original Steak	¼ tsp	0	0	0	0	0	0	0
Lemon Pepper	¼ tsp	0	0	0	0	0	0	0
Minched Onion Medley	¼ tsp	0	0	0	0	0	0	0
Original Blend	¼ tsp	0	0	0	0	0	0	0
Table Blend	¼ tsp	0	0	0	0	0	0	0
Tomato Basil Garlic	¼ tsp	0	0	0	0	0	0	0

FOOD	PORTION	CALS	PROT	FAT	CHOL	CARB	FIBER	SOD
HERRING								
atlantic cooked	3 oz	172	20	10	65	0	–	98
atlantic cooked	1 fillet (5 oz)	290	33	17	110	0	–	165
atlantic raw	3 oz	134	15	8	51	0	–	76
pacific baked	3 oz	213	18	15	84	0	–	81
pacific fillet baked	5.1 oz	360	30	26	142	0	–	137
roe canned	1 oz	34	6	1	–	tr	–	–
roe raw	1 oz	37	7	tr	103	tr	–	–
smoked	3.5 oz	210	22	14	70	0	0	550
TAKE-OUT								
atlantic kippered	1 fillet (1.4 oz)	87	10	5	33	0	–	367
atlantic pickled	½ oz	39	2	3	2	1	–	131
fried	1 serv (3.5 oz)	233	23	15	69	2	0	100
HICKORY NUTS								
dried	1 oz	187	4	18	0	5	–	0
HOMINY								
CANNED								
white	1 cup (5.6 oz)	482	2	1	0	23	4	336
Van Camp								
Golden	½ cup (4.3 oz)	80	4	1	0	17	1	540
White	½ cup (4.3 oz)	80	1	1	0	16	1	530
HONEY								
honey	1 cup (11.9 oz)	1031	1	0	0	279	–	12
honey	1 tbsp (0.7 oz)	64	tr	0	0	17	–	1
orange blossom	1 tbsp	60	0	0	0	17	0	0
wild honey	1 tbsp	60	0	0	0	17	–	0
Steel's								
Sugar Free	1 tbsp	24	0	0	0	6	0	0
SueBee								
Clover	1 tbsp	60	0	0	0	17	–	0

FOOD	PORTION	CALS	PROT	FAT	CHOL	CARB	FIBER	SOD
HONEYDEW								
FRESH								
cubed	1 cup	60	1	tr	0	16	—	17
wedge	⅒	46	1	tr	0	12	—	13
Chiquita								
Wedge	⅒ melon (4.7 oz)	50	1	0	0	13	1	35
HORSE								
roasted	3 oz	149	24	5	58	0	—	47
HORSERADISH								
japanese wasabi	¼ tsp	1	—	—	0	tr	0	0
wasabi root raw	1 (5.9 oz)	184	8	1	0	40	12	29
wasabi root raw sliced	1 cup (4.6 oz)	142	6	1	0	31	10	22
Boar's Head								
Horseradish	1 tsp (5 g)	5	0	0	0	0	0	30
Eden								
Wasabi Powder	1 tsp	10	0	0	0	1	1	0
HOT CHOCOLATE								
mix as prep w/ water	7 oz	103	3	1	—	23	—	149
mix w/ equal as prep w/ water	7 oz	48	4	tr	—	9	—	173
Carnation								
Hot Cocoa 70 Calorie	1 pkg (0.7 oz)	70	3	0	0	15	tr	140
Hot Cocoa Double Chocolate Meltdown	1 pkg (1.2 oz)	150	2	4	0	27	1	170
Hot Cocoa Fat Free Raspberry	1 pkg (0.3 oz)	30	2	0	0	4	1	150
Hot Cocoa Fat Free w/ Marshmallows	1 pkg (0.4 oz)	45	7	0	0	10	tr	100
Hot Cocoa Lactose Free	1 pkg (1 oz)	120	1	2	0	25	1	115

FOOD	PORTION	CALS	PROT	FAT	CHOL	CARB	FIBER	SOD
Hot Cocoa Marshmallow Blizzard	1 pkg (1.5 oz)	180	2	2	<5	39	tr	140
Hot Cocoa Milk Chocolate	3 tbsp (1 oz)	110	2	1	<5	24	tr	95
Hot Cocoa Rich Chocolate as prep w/ 2% milk	1 pkg	200	tr	8	21	27	tr	288
Hot Cocoa Rich Chocolate Fat Free	1 pkg (0.3 oz)	25	2	0	0	4	1	135
Hot Cocoa Rich Chocolate No Sugar Added	3 tbsp (0.5 oz)	50	4	0	<5	8	tr	140
Hot Cocoa Rich Chocolate w/ Marshmallows	3 tbsp (1 oz)	110	1	1	<5	24	tr	95
Country Choice								
Irish Chocolate Mint	1 pkg	100	3	0	0	23	tr	160
Royal Chocolate	1 pkg	100	3	0	0	23	tr	160
Soy Cocoa Irish Chocolate Mint	1 pkg	100	2	1	0	23	1	130
Soy Cocoa Royal Chocolate	1 pkg	100	2	1	0	23	1	130
Keto								
Hot Cocoa	1 tsp	12	1	0	0	2	1	–
Low Carb Creations								
Cocoa as prep	1 cup	30	0	2	0	3	0	70
White Hot Chocolate	1 cup	25	0	2	0	3	0	50
Nestle								
Hot Cocoa Rich Chocolate	1 pkg (1 oz)	110	1	1	0	24	tr	60
Hot Cocoa Rich w/ Marshmallows	1 pkg (1 oz)	110	1	1	0	24	tr	60
Sipper Sweets								
Sugar Free Low Carb Mix	1 serv	50	1	3	0	3	0	80
Swiss Miss								
Caramel Cream	1 serv	110	1	3	0	21	tr	140
Hot Cocoa & Cream	1 serv	153	2	5	6	25	1	159

FOOD	PORTION	CALS	PROT	FAT	CHOL	CARB	FIBER	SOD
Hot Cocoa Chocolate Sensation	1 serv	148	2	4	tr	27	1	171
Hot Cocoa Diet	1 serv	22	2	tr	tr	4	1	185
Hot Cocoa Fat Free	1 serv	52	4	tr	0	9	1	185
Hot Cocoa Fat Free Marshmallow Lovers	1 serv	65	3	tr	0	13	1	155
Hot Cocoa Lite	1 serv	76	2	1	0	18	2	177
Hot Cocoa Marshmallow Lovers	1 serv	142	2	3	2	27	1	152
Hot Cocoa Milk Chocolate No Sugar Added	1 serv	55	2	1	1	10	1	164
Hot Cocoa Rich Chocolate	1 serv	110	2	2	1	23	1	140
Hot Cocoa w/ Marshmallows No Sugar Added	1 serv	56	3	1	1	10	1	146
Hot Cocoa White Chocolate	1 serv	109	3	1	1	21	tr	128
Milk Chocolate	1 pkg	120	1	3	0	22	1	160
Milk Chocolate w/ Marshmallows	1 pkg	120	1	3	tr	23	tr	150
Premiere Hot Cocoa Almond Mocha	1 serv	144	2	3	1	28	1	207
Premiere Hot Cocoa Raspberry Truffle	1 serv	144	2	3	1	28	1	220
Premiere Hot Cocoa Suisse Truffle	1 serv	142	2	2	1	28	1	225
Rich Hot Cocoa No Sugar Added	1 serv	54	2	1	1	10	1	165
Sidewalk Cafe Cappuccino	1 serv	119	3	4	1	18	1	35
Sidewalk Cafe Cinnamon	1 serv	126	3	4	1	21	1	46
Sidewalk Cafe French Vanilla	1 serv	121	3	4	1	19	tr	32

FOOD	PORTION	CALS	PROT	FAT	CHOL	CARB	FIBER	SOD
Sidewalk Cafe Mocha	1 serv	120	3	4	1	20	1	43
TAKE-OUT								
hot cocoa	1 cup	218	9	9	33	26	–	123
mexican hot chocolate	1 cup	173	10	6	18	20	1	150

HOT DOG

FOOD	PORTION	CALS	PROT	FAT	CHOL	CARB	FIBER	SOD
beef	1 (1.5)	142	5	13	27	1	–	462
beef	1 (2 oz)	180	7	16	35	1	–	585
beef & pork	1 (1.5 oz)	144	5	13	22	1	–	504
beef & pork	1 (2 oz)	183	6	17	29	1	–	639
chicken	1 (1.5 oz)	116	6	9	45	3	–	617
pork cheesefurter smokie	1 (1.5 oz)	141	6	12	29	1	–	465
turkey	1 (1.5 oz)	102	6	8	48	1	–	642
Armour								
Star Jumbo Beef	1	190	6	18	30	–	–	590
Boar's Head								
Beef	1 (2 oz)	160	7	14	30	1	0	440
Beef Lite	1 (1.6 oz)	90	7	6	25	0	0	270
Pork & Beef	1 (2 oz)	150	7	14	25	0	0	460
Health Is Wealth								
Uncured Beef	1 (1.5 oz)	80	6	6	20	1	–	340
Uncured Chicken	1 (1.5 oz)	100	8	8	30	1	–	320
Healthy Choice								
Beef Low Fat	1 (1.8 oz)	70	6	3	15	7	0	440
Low Fat Turkey Pork Beef	1 (1.4 oz)	60	5	2	10	5	–	350
Kid Cuisine								
Mystical Mini Corn Dogs	4 pieces	230	8	14	35	18	0	600
Oscar Mayer								
Fat Free Turkey & Beef	1 (1.8 oz)	40	6	0	15	3	0	490
Light Beef	1 (1.6 oz)	90	5	6	20	2	–	490
Wampler								
Chicken	1 (2 oz)	120	7	11	60	0	1	480
TAKE-OUT								
corndog	1	460	17	19	79	56	–	972

FOOD	PORTION	CALS	PROT	FAT	CHOL	CARB	FIBER	SOD
w/ bun chili	1	297	14	13	51	31	—	480
w/ bun plain	1	242	10	15	44	18	—	671

HOT DOG SUBSTITUTES
Lightlife
Smart Deli Jumbo's	1 link (2.7 oz)	80	16	0	0	4	1	590
Smart Dogs	1 (1.5 oz)	45	9	0	0	2	0	230
Tofu Pups	1 (1.4 oz)	60	8	3	0	2	0	140
Wonder Dogs	1 (1.5 oz)	60	9	2	0	2	0	320

Loma Linda
Big Franks	1 (1.8 oz)	110	10	7	0	2	2	240
Big Franks Low Fat	1 (1.8 oz)	80	11	3	0	3	2	220
Corn Dogs	1 (2.5 oz)	150	7	4	0	22	3	500

Morningstar Farms
America's Original Veggie Dog	1 (2 oz)	80	11	1	0	6	1	580
Meatfree Corn Dog	1 (2.5 oz)	150	7	4	0	22	3	500
Meatfree Mini Corn Dog	4 (2.7 oz)	170	11	5	0	21	1	580

Natural Touch
Vege Frank	1 (1.6 oz)	100	10	6	0	2	2	470

Quorn
Meat-Free Dogs	1 (1.5 oz)	70	5	4	5	3	2	250

Yves
Good Dog	1 (1.8 oz)	70	13	2	0	2	1	460
Tofu Dogs	1 (1.3 oz)	45	9	1	0	2	0	240
Veggie Dogs	1 (1.6 oz)	60	11	0	0	1	1	400
Veggie Dogs Chili	1 (1.6 oz)	50	10	0	0	3	2	360
Veggie Dogs Jumbo	1 (2.7 oz)	100	16	2	0	7	2	480
Veggie Dogs Jumbo Hot N' Spicy	1 (2.7 oz)	106	19	2	0	4	2	480

HUMMUS
hummus	1 cup	420	12	21	0	50	—	599

Athenos
Travelers Hummus & Pita	1 pkg	325	8	13	0	48	3	750

Guiltless Gourmet
Original	2 tbsp	35	1	2	0	4	1	115
Roasted Garlic	2 tbsp	35	1	2	0	4	1	115

FOOD	PORTION	CALS	PROT	FAT	CHOL	CARB	FIBER	SOD
TAKE-OUT								
hummus	⅓ cup	140	4	7	0	17	–	200
HYACINTH BEANS								
dried cooked	1 cup	228	16	1	0	40	–	13
ICE CREAM AND FROZEN DESSERTS *(see also* ICES AND ICE POPS, PUDDING POPS, SHERBET, YOGURT FROZEN)*								
chocolate	½ cup (4 fl oz)	143	3	7	22	19	–	50
dixie cup chocolate	1 (3.5 fl oz)	125	2	6	20	16	–	44
dixie cup strawberry	1 (3.5 fl oz)	112	2	5	17	16	–	35
dixie cup vanilla	1 (3.5 fl oz)	116	2	6	25	14	–	46
strawberry	½ cup (4 fl oz)	127	2	6	19	18	–	40
vanilla	½ cup (4 fl oz)	132	2	7	29	16	–	53
vanilla soft serve	½ cup	111	4	2	10	19	–	62
Atkins								
Endulge Butter Pecan	½ cup	170	2	15	40	12	4	40
Endulge Chocolate	½ cup	140	2	12	45	13	5	20
Endulge Chocolate Peanut Butter Swirl	½ cup	170	3	14	40	14	5	70
Endulge Vanilla	½ cup	140	2	12	45	13	4	30
Endulge Vanilla Fudge	½ cup	140	2	10	40	14	4	30
Endulge Bars Chocolate Fudge	1 bar	130	2	11	40	12	5	20
Endulge Bars Chocolate Fudge Swirl	1 bar	180	3	16	30	12	4	25
Endulge Bars Peanut Butter Swirl	1 bar	180	2	17	30	12	4	25
Endulge Bars Vanilla Fudge Swirl	1 bar	180	2	16	30	12	4	25
Better Than Ice Creme								
Soy Vanilla as prep	½ cup	110	1	3	0	21	0	83

FOOD	PORTION	CALS	PROT	FAT	CHOL	CARB	FIBER	SOD
Bon Bons								
Dark Chocolate	5 pieces	190	2	13	15	16	0	35
Milk Chocolate	5 pieces	200	2	14	10	17	0	35
Breyers								
Almond Joy	½ cup	140	4	5	30	20	tr	75
Banana Fudge Chunk	½ cup	170	2	9	20	21	tr	40
Butter Almond	½ cup	160	4	10	20	14	tr	85
Butter Pecan	½ cup	170	3	11	20	14	0	115
Butter Pecan Homemade	½ cup	170	3	11	50	18	0	70
Butter Pecan No Sugar Added	½ cup	120	3	7	10	15	tr	115
Caramel Praline Crunch	½ cup	180	2	9	20	22	0	75
Caramel Toffee Crunch	½ cup	180	3	9	50	22	0	100
CarbSmart Chocolate	½ cup	130	2	10	25	10	3	50
CarbSmart Strawberry	½ cup	130	2	9	25	10	3	25
CarbSmart Vanilla	½ cup	130	2	9	25	10	3	25
Cherry Chocolate Chip	½ cup	150	3	8	20	18	0	45
Cherry Vanilla	½ cup	140	2	8	20	16	0	30
Chocolate	½ cup	150	3	8	20	17	tr	35
Chocolate 98% Fat Free	½ cup	90	3	2	5	21	4	50
Chocolate Caramel No Sugar Added	½ cup	110	3	4	10	16	tr	55
Chocolate Chip	½ cup	160	3	9	20	17	0	40
Chocolate Chip Cookie Dough	½ cup	170	3	9	25	20	0	55
Chocolate Rainbow	½ cup	140	3	7	20	16	0	40
Coffee	½ cup	140	3	8	20	15	0	40
Cookies & Cream	½ cup	160	3	8	20	18	tr	50
Creamsicle	½ cup	130	2	5	15	20	0	35
Deep Chocolate Fudge	½ cup	200	3	12	30	21	1	60

FOOD	PORTION	CALS	PROT	FAT	CHOL	CARB	FIBER	SOD
Dulce De Leche	½ cup	150	3	7	20	20	0	105
French Vanilla	½ cup	150	3	8	50	15	0	45
French Vanilla Light	½ cup	120	3	4	35	18	0	50
French Vanilla No Sugar Added	½ cup	110	3	5	35	14	0	60
Fresa Banana	½ cup	140	2	5	15	20	0	35
Heath English Toffee	½ cup	190	2	9	20	22	0	120
Hershey w/ Almonds	½ cup	170	3	8	15	24	tr	65
Ice Cream Cake Oreo	1 slice	190	3	10	30	21	tr	100
Ice Cream Cake Vanilla	1 slice	190	3	11	40	19	0	40
Klondike Sandwich	½ cup	160	3	7	20	21	0	70
Mint Chocolate Chip	½ cup	160	3	9	20	17	0	40
Mint Chocolate Chip Light	½ cup	130	3	5	10	20	0	45
Mint Oreo	½ cup	170	2	7	15	23	0	75
Mocha Almond Fudge	½ cup	170	4	9	15	18	2	45
Oreo	½ cup	160	3	6	20	20	0	80
Peach	½ cup	130	2	6	15	17	0	25
Peanut Butter & Fudge	½ cup	170	4	10	20	17	tr	80
Reese's Peanut Butter Cups	½ cup	180	3	9	15	22	0	75
Rocky Road	½ cup	160	3	8	20	20	tr	60
SpongeBob Cookie Dough	½ cup	160	2	7	15	21	0	95
Strawberry	½ cup	120	2	6	15	15	0	30
Strawberry Shortcake	½ cup	160	2	6	15	23	0	40
Turtle Sundae	½ cup	190	3	11	30	20	tr	70
Vanilla	½ cup	140	3	8	20	15	0	40
Vanilla Calcium Rich	½ cup	130	3	7	20	14	0	40
Vanilla Fudge Twirl	½ cup	140	3	7	20	18	tr	45
Vanilla Homemade	½ cup	140	2	8	40	16	0	60
Vanilla Lactose Free	½ cup	130	2	7	20	14	0	35

FOOD	PORTION	CALS	PROT	FAT	CHOL	CARB	FIBER	SOD
Vanilla Light	½ cup	110	3	3	10	17	0	50
Vanilla Light 2% Milk	½ cup	130	3	5	30	18	0	60
Vanilla No Sugar Added	½ cup	100	3	5	15	15	0	45
Vanilla Caramel Brownie	½ cup	170	3	9	50	20	0	90
Vanilla Fudge Brownie	½ cup	180	3	9	25	19	tr	80
Vanilla Fudge Twirl No Sugar Added	½ cup	110	3	4	10	19	tr	50
Wild Berry Swirl	½ cup	140	2	8	20	16	0	35
Butterfinger								
Bar	1 (2.5 oz)	190	2	13	15	16	0	35
Carnation								
Cup Chocolate	1 (3 oz)	140	2	8	25	16	0	40
Cup Chocolate Malt	1 (12 oz)	270	7	6	20	48	1	130
Cup Strawberry	1 (3 oz)	100	1	5	20	12	0	25
Cup Vanilla	1 (3 oz)	100	1	6	20	11	0	30
Cup Vanilla	1 (5 oz)	170	2	10	35	19	0	50
Cup Vanilla Malt	1 (12 oz)	260	6	6	20	48	0	130
Sundae Cup Strawberry	1 (5 oz)	200	2	8	30	29	0	55
Sunday Cup Chocolate	1 (5 oz)	210	2	9	30	30	1	55
Cool Creations								
Cookies & Cream Sandwich	1 (3.5 oz)	240	2	11	15	34	1	250
Mickey Mouse Bar	1 (2.5 oz)	120	2	8	15	10	0	25
Mini Sandwich	1 (2.3 oz)	110	1	5	10	16	0	70
Dippin' Dots								
Dipping Dots Chocolate	⅝ cup (3 oz)	190	4	9	40	22	0	70
Drumstick								
Cone Chocolate	1 (4.6 oz)	320	6	17	25	36	2	90
Cone Chocolate Dipped	1 (4.6 oz)	320	5	16	25	40	1	90
Cone Vanilla	1 (4.6 oz)	340	6	19	20	35	2	90

FOOD	PORTION	CALS	PROT	FAT	CHOL	CARB	FIBER	SOD
Cone Vanilla Caramel	1 (4.6 oz)	360	6	20	25	38	2	100
Cone Vanilla Fudge	1 (4.6 oz)	360	5	20	20	39	2	100
Edy's								
3 Musketeers	½ cup	160	3	7	20	22	–	50
Dreamery Banana Split	½ cup	240	3	11	60	31	1	45
Dreamery Black Raspberry Avalanche	½ cup	270	4	16	80	27	1	50
Dreamery Caramel Toffee Bar Heaven	½ cup	290	4	16	75	32	0	90
Dreamery Cashew Praline Parfait	½ cup	280	4	16	75	30	0	75
Dreamery Chocolate Truffle Explosion	½ cup	280	5	15	8	31	1	85
Dreamery Chocolate Peanut Butter Chunk	½ cup	310	7	18	50	29	2	110
Dreamery Coney Island Waffle Cone	½ cup	310	4	18	70	32	1	55
Dreamery Cool Mint	½ cup	300	4	17	75	32	1	55
Dreamery Deep Dish Apple Pie	½ cup	280	3	15	75	34	0	95
Dreamery Dulce De Leche	½ cup	270	4	14	70	32	0	70
Dreamery Grandma's Cookie Dough	½ cup	300	4	17	75	32	0	80
Dreamery Harvest Peach	½ cup	230	3	13	70	25	0	35
Dreamery New York Strawberry Cheesecake	½ cup	260	4	15	80	27	0	70

FOOD	PORTION	CALS	PROT	FAT	CHOL	CARB	FIBER	SOD
Dreamery Nothing But Chocolate	½ cup	280	5	14	65	34	1	70
Dreamery Nuts About Malt	½ cup	290	5	17	70	29	1	65
Dreamery Raspberry Brownie A La Mode	½ cup	270	3	14	75	34	1	60
Dreamery Strawberry Fields	½ cup	220	3	12	65	26	1	35
Dreamery Tiramisu	½ cup	260	4	13	75	31	0	150
Dreamery Vanilla	½ cup	260	5	15	70	25	0	55
Grand Black Cherry Vanilla	½ cup	140	2	7	25	17	—	25
Grand Blue Ribbon Chocolate Cake	½ cup	180	3	10	25	20	—	60
Grand Butter Pecan	½ cup	170	3	10	25	16	—	70
Grand Cherry Chocolate Chip	½ cup	160	2	8	25	19	—	40
Grand Chocolate	½ cup	150	3	8	25	16	—	35
Grand Chocolate Caramel Swirl	½ cup	170	2	9	25	19	—	45
Grand Chocolate Chips	½ cup	170	3	9	25	18	—	45
Grand Chocolate Fudge Mousse	½ cup	160	2	8	25	19	—	45
Grand Chocolate Fudge Sundae	½ cup	170	3	9	20	20	—	50
Grand Coffee	½ cup	140	2	8	25	15	—	40
Grand Cookie Dough	½ cup	180	3	9	25	21	—	65
Grand Cookies'N Cream	½ cup	160	3	8	25	19	—	50
Grand Double Fudge Brownie	½ cup	170	2	9	30	19	—	45

FOOD	PORTION	CALS	PROT	FAT	CHOL	CARB	FIBER	SOD
Grand Espresso Chip	½ cup	150	2	8	25	17	—	50
Grand French Vanilla	½ cup	160	2	9	50	17	—	40
Grand French Vanilla Fudge Pie	½ cup	160	2	8	45	20	—	55
Grand Mint Chocolate Chips	½ cup	170	3	9	25	18	—	45
Grand Neapolitan	½ cup	140	2	7	25	16	—	35
Grand Nutty Cone Crunch	½ cup	180	3	10	25	19	—	45
Grand Real Strawberry	½ cup	130	2	6	20	16	—	30
Grand Rocky Road	½ cup	170	3	10	25	17	—	30
Grand Spumoni	½ cup	150	3	8	25	16	—	40
Grand Strawberry Cupcake	½ cup	140	2	6	25	19	—	40
Grand Tin Roof Sundae	½ cup	170	3	9	25	18	—	50
Grand Ultimate Caramel Cup	½ cup	170	2	8	20	22	—	55
Grand Vanilla	½ cup	140	2	8	25	15	—	30
Grand Vanillaberry Bar	½ cup	130	2	5	20	19	—	25
Grand Light Butter Pecan	½ cup	120	3	5	20	16	—	60
Grand Light Chocolate Raspberry Escape	½ cup	130	3	5	15	19	—	45
Grand Light Chocolate Fudge Mousse	½ cup	120	3	4	20	17	—	45
Grand Light Cookie Dough	½ cup	130	3	5	20	19	—	65
Grand Light Cookies'N Cream	½ cup	120	3	4	15	18	—	60
Grand Light Crazy For Caramel	½ cup	120	3	4	15	19	—	55

FOOD	PORTION	CALS	PROT	FAT	CHOL	CARB	FIBER	SOD
Grand Light French Silk	½ cup	130	3	5	15	19	—	50
Grand Light Mint Chocolate Chips	½ cup	120	3	5	20	17	—	50
Grand Light Peanut Butter Cups	½ cup	120	3	5	20	17	—	50
Grand Light Rocky Road	½ cup	120	3	4	20	17	—	40
Grand Light S'Mores & More	½ cup	130	3	4	15	22	—	60
Grand Light Strawberry Shortcake	½ cup	110	2	4	20	18	—	40
Grand Light Vanilla	½ cup	100	3	3	20	15	—	45
Homemade All Natural Vanilla	½ cup	130	3	7	30	14	—	55
Homemade Brownies A La Mode	½ cup	150	3	7	30	18	—	65
Homemade Chocolate Chip Cookie Jar	½ cup	180	3	10	25	19	—	90
Homemade Chocolate Chip Mousse	½ cup	170	3	9	30	19	—	60
Homemade Double Chocolate Chunk	½ cup	170	3	9	30	19	—	55
Homemade Mint Chocolate Chunk	½ cup	170	3	9	25	18	—	65
Homemade Old Fashioned Butter Pecan	½ cup	160	3	10	30	15	—	90
Homemade Strawberries & Cream	½ cup	120	2	6	25	15	—	45
Homemade Vanilla Custard	½ cup	150	4	8	55	15	—	55
M&M's Almond	½ cup	180	3	10	25	21	—	55
betsy ross	1 serv	206	0	0	0	5	0	3

FOOD	PORTION	CALS	PROT	FAT	CHOL	CARB	FIBER	SOD
M&M's Chocolate Brownie Sundae	½ cup	180	3	9	25	22	—	55
M&M's Mint	½ cup	200	3	11	25	21	—	60
M&M's Vanilla	½ cup	180	3	9	25	22	—	50
Milky Way	½ cup	160	3	7	25	21	—	70
Snickers	½ cup	180	3	9	25	21	—	70
Snickers Cruncher	½ cup	190	3	10	25	21	—	65
Twix	½ cup	190	3	9	25	23	—	70
Twix Peanut Butter	½ cup	190	3	11	25	20	—	80
Flintstones								
Cool Cream	1 (2.75 oz)	90	1	2	5	18	0	30
Push-Up	1	120	1	6	20	15	0	25
Pebbles Treats	(2.75 oz)							
Good Humor								
Bar Oreo	1 (4 oz)	250	3	15	15	28	tr	160
Bar Reese's Peanut Butter	1 (4 oz)	310	4	21	20	27	tr	90
Bar Toasted Almond	1 (3 oz)	180	2	10	5	22	tr	35
Bar Vanilla Dark Chocolate	1 (3 oz)	190	2	13	10	15	tr	35
Bar Vanilla Milk Chocolate	1 (3 oz)	180	2	13	15	15	0	45
Bar Candy Center Crunch	1 (4 oz)	310	3	23	15	24	tr	85
Bar Strawberry Shortcake	1 (4 oz)	230	2	12	10	30	tr	90
Chocolate Eclair Bar	1 (4 oz)	220	2	11	10	30	tr	85
Cone Premium Sundae	1 (4.3 oz)	270	4	15	15	29	tr	95
Cone Strawberry Shortcake	1 (4.3 oz)	230	2	10	5	34	tr	85
Giant Sandwich Neapolitan	1 (6 oz)	250	4	10	20	37	tr	210
Giant Sandwich Vanilla	1 (6 oz)	250	4	10	20	36	0	210
King Cone	1 (4.6 fl oz)	250	4	13	15	30	tr	100
King Cone Giant	1 (8 oz)	190	7	21	40	44	tr	160
Number 1 Bar	1 (4 oz)	200	2	11	10	21	tr	50
Sandwich Chocolate Chip Cookie	1 (4.5 oz)	290	3	13	20	41	1	210

FOOD	PORTION	CALS	PROT	FAT	CHOL	CARB	FIBER	SOD
Sandwich Vanilla	1 (3.5 oz)	160	3	6	10	25	0	160
Sundae Twist Cup	1 (6 oz)	160	2	3	10	33	0	100
Haagen-Dazs								
Bars Chocolate & Almonds	1 (3.7 oz)	380	6	27	90	27	2	65
Bars Chocolate & Dark Chocolate	1 (3.6 oz)	350	5	24	65	28	2	45
Bars Chocolate Peanut Butter Swirl	1 (3 oz)	320	6	23	60	21	2	65
Bars Coffee & Almond Crunch	1 (3.7 oz)	370	5	27	90	27	tr	80
Bars Cookies & Cream Crunch	1 (3.6 oz)	370	5	26	85	30	tr	100
Bars Dulce De Leche Caramel	1 (3.7 oz)	370	4	24	75	34	0	90
Bars Tropical Coconut	1 (3.5 oz)	340	5	24	90	25	0	70
Bars Vanilla & Almonds	1 (3.7 oz)	380	6	28	90	26	1	70
Bars Vanilla & Dark Chocolate	1 (3.6 oz)	350	5	24	85	27	1	50
Bars Vanilla & Milk Chocolate	1 (3.5 oz)	340	5	24	90	25	tr	65
Butter Pecan	½ cup	310	5	23	110	21	tr	110
Cappuccino Commotion	½ cup	310	5	21	100	25	1	90
Cherry Vanilla	½ cup	240	4	15	100	23	0	60
Chocolate	½ cup	270	5	18	115	22	1	60
Chocolate Brownie w/ Walnuts	½ cup	290	5	19	100	25	1	75
Chocolate Chocolate Fudge	½ cup	290	5	18	100	27	tr	90
Chocolate Chocolate Chip	½ cup	300	5	20	105	26	2	55
Chocolate Swiss Almond	½ cup	300	4	20	100	24	2	55
Cinnamon	½ cup	250	4	17	110	20	0	65
Coffee	½ cup	270	5	18	120	21	0	70
Coffee Mocha Chip	½ cup	290	5	19	110	25	tr	75

FOOD	PORTION	CALS	PROT	FAT	CHOL	CARB	FIBER	SOD
Cookie Dough Chip	½ cup	310	4	20	95	29	0	125
Cookies & Cream	½ cup	270	5	17	105	23	0	90
Creme Caramel Pecan	½ cup	320	5	20	95	29	0	120
Dulce De Leche Caramel	½ cup	290	5	17	100	28	0	95
Low Fat Chocolate	½ cup	170	7	3	30	29	tr	50
Low Fat Coffee Fudge	½ cup	170	5	3	25	32	0	95
Low Fat Strawberry	½ cup	150	5	2	15	28	0	40
Low Fat Vanilla	½ cup	170	7	3	20	29	0	50
Macadamia Brittle	½ cup	300	4	20	110	25	0	110
Mango	½ cup	250	4	14	85	28	tr	50
Mint Chip	½ cup	300	5	19	105	26	tr	85
Pineapple Coconut	½ cup	230	4	12	90	25	0	55
Pistachio	½ cup	290	5	20	110	22	tr	80
Rum Raisin	½ cup	270	4	17	110	22	0	60
Strawberry	½ cup	250	4	16	95	23	tr	65
Vanilla	½ cup	270	5	18	120	21	0	70
Vanilla Chocolate Chip	½ cup	310	5	20	105	26	tr	75
Vanilla Fudge	½ cup	290	5	18	100	25	0	95
Vanilla Swiss Almond	½ cup	300	5	20	105	24	tr	75
Healthy Choice								
Butter Pecan Crunch	½ cup	120	3	2	5	22	tr	60
Cappuccino Chocolate Chunk	½ cup	120	3	2	10	22	1	60
Cappuccino Mocha Crunch	½ cup	120	3	2	5	22	tr	55
Cherry Chocolate Chunk	½ cup	110	3	2	<5	19	tr	55
Chocolate Chocolate Chunk	½ cup	120	3	2	5	21	2	45
Coconut Cream Pie	½ cup	120	3	2	5	23	1	75
Cookies Creme De Mint	½ cup	130	3	2	5	24	tr	60
Cookies 'N Cream	½ cup	120	3	2	5	21	tr	90
Fudge Brownie	½ cup	120	3	2	5	22	tr	55

FOOD	PORTION	CALS	PROT	FAT	CHOL	CARB	FIBER	SOD
Mint Chocolate Chip	½ cup	120	3	2	5	21	tr	50
Old Fashioned Blueberry Hill	½ cup	120	2	2	<5	23	1	50
Old Fashioned Butterscotch Blonde	½ cup	140	3	2	10	26	tr	75
Old Fashioned Cherry Vanilla	½ cup	120	2	2	5	22	tr	50
Old Fashioned Strawberry	½ cup	110	2	2	0	20	1	35
Peanut Butter Cup	½ cup	110	3	2	5	19	tr	65
Praline & Caramel	½ cup	130	3	2	5	25	tr	70
Praline Caramel Cluster	½ cup	130	3	2	<5	25	tr	70
Rocky Road	½ cup	140	3	2	5	28	tr	60
Turtle Fudge Cake	½ cup	130	3	2	<5	25	2	60
Vanilla	½ cup	100	3	2	5	18	tr	50
Vanilla Bean	½ cup	110	3	2	5	19	tr	45
Wild Raspberry Truffle	½ cup	120	3	2	6	22	tr	55
Hershey's								
Butter Pecan	½ cup	170	3	9	35	15	0	80
French Vanilla	½ cup	170	3	10	70	17	0	90
Vanilla Chocolate Strawberry	½ cup	160	3	9	35	18	0	60
Klondike								
Bar Almond	1	300	4	21	20	24	0	70
Bar Cappuccino	1	280	3	19	20	24	0	70
Bar Caramel & Peanut	1	290	4	19	15	25	tr	150
Bar Caramel Crunch	1	270	3	17	25	26	0	80
Bar Chocolate	1	280	3	19	20	23	tr	55
Bar Dark Chocolate	1	280	3	19	20	24	tr	55
Bar Heath	1	300	3	20	20	26	0	100
Bar Krunch	1	280	3	19	20	25	0	90
Bar Oreo	1	160	2	10	10	17	tr	95
Bar Original	1	280	3	19	20	24	0	75

FOOD	PORTION	CALS	PROT	FAT	CHOL	CARB	FIBER	SOD
Bar Peppermint Patty	1	280	3	19	20	24	tr	55
Bar Reese's	1	220	3	15	15	20	tr	65
Big Bear Sandwich Neapolitan	1	300	5	12	25	42	1	230
Big Bear Sandwich Vanilla	1	300	5	12	25	42	tr	240
Big Bear Cone Vanilla	1	330	6	20	15	33	1	95
Big Bear Cone Vanilla Caramel	1	360	6	21	15	36	1	120
Big Bear Cone Vanilla Fudge	1	380	6	20	15	38	1	90
CarbSmart Fudge Bar	1	60	2	7	20	9	1	45
CarbSmart Ice Cream Bar	1	130	2	15	15	9	2	40
Choco Taco	1	290	4	16	10	35	1	115
Cone Oreo	1	250	3	12	15	32	1	95
Cone Reese's	1	290	4	15	15	33	tr	140
Cookie Sandwich Chips	1	470	7	20	30	66	2	65
Cookie Sandwich Oreo	1	230	3	9	10	34	2	310
Minis	2 pieces	170	2	11	15	15	0	45
Sandwich Double Decker	1	370	6	14	30	54	1	330
Slim-A-Bear 98% Fat Free Sandwich Vanilla	1	130	4	2	5	28	3	120
Slim-A-Bear No Sugar Added Cone Vanilla	1	270	8	15	5	31	4	110
Slim-A-Bear No Sugar Added Fudge Bar	1	90	3	2	5	22	4	90
Slim-A-Bear No Sugar Added Reduced Fat Bar Vanilla	1	160	4	9	5	21	4	75

FOOD	PORTION	CALS	PROT	FAT	CHOL	CARB	FIBER	SOD
Slim-A-Bear No Sugar Added Sandwich Vanilla	1	120	4	3	5	25	2	230
Sundae Cup	1	280	6	17	35	26	tr	75
Nestle Crunch								
Chocolate	1 bar (3 oz)	200	2	14	15	17	0	40
Crunch King	1 (4 oz)	270	3	19	20	21	0	45
Nuggets	8 pieces	310	4	21	20	25	0	60
Reduced Fat	1 (2.5 oz)	130	3	7	5	14	0	40
Vanilla	1 bar (3 oz)	200	2	14	15	16	0	40
NutraShake								
High Calorie High Protein All Flavors	1 serv (4 oz)	200	6	10	60	24	—	217
Popsicle								
Bar Col Crunch Chocolate Eclair	1 (3 oz)	160	2	8	5	20	tr	70
Bar Col Crunch Strawberry Shortcake	1 (3 oz)	170	1	9	5	21	0	60
Bar Snoopy	1 (3.5 oz)	150	2	8	15	16	0	45
Bar Sprinklers	1 (2.1 oz)	130	1	6	10	18	0	25
Cone Crispy	1 (2.5 oz)	150	2	7	5	20	0	60
Creamsicle Pop	1 (1.75 oz)	70	1	2	5	13	0	20
Cup Cookies & Cream	1 (10 oz)	310	5	13	30	45	1	160
Fruit Juicee Cups	1 (4 oz)	80	0	0	0	20	—	0
Ice Cream Bar Vanilla	1 (3 oz)	160	2	11	15	15	1	35
Ice Cream Pops Minis	2 (2.8 oz)	190	2	13	15	18	0	35
Sandwich Cookie Rugrats	1 (2.5 oz)	140	2	6	10	20	tr	80
Sandwiches Minis	1 (2 oz)	100	2	4	5	15	0	95
Scribblers Ice Cream Pops	2 (2.4 oz)	130	3	5	15	17	0	45
Swirl Bar Bubble Gum	1 (2.6 oz)	60	0	0	0	13	—	0
WWE Bar	1 (3.6 oz)	180	2	8	10	23	tr	95

FOOD	PORTION	CALS	PROT	FAT	CHOL	CARB	FIBER	SOD
X-Men Wolverine Bar	1 (4 oz)	100	0	0	0	25	—	15
Rice Dream								
Cappuccino	½ cup (3.2 oz)	150	tr	6	0	23	1	100
Carob	½ cup (3.2 oz)	150	1	6	0	24	2	100
Carob Almond	½ cup (3.2 oz)	170	1	8	0	24	2	95
Cherry Vanilla	½ cup (3.2 oz)	150	tr	6	0	24	1	90
Cocoa Marble Fudge	½ cup (3.2 oz)	150	1	6	0	25	2	100
Cookies N' Dream	½ cup (3.2 oz)	170	1	7	0	26	1	100
Mint Chocolate Chip	½ cup (3.2 oz)	170	1	8	0	26	1	95
Neapolitan	½ cup (3.2 oz)	150	1	6	0	24	2	100
Orange Vanilla Swirl	½ cup (3.2 oz)	250	tr	6	0	23	1	100
Strawberry	½ cup (3.2 oz)	140	tr	5	0	24	1	85
Vanilla Swiss Almond	½ cup (3.2 oz)	180	1	8	0	25	1	95
Rice Dream Supreme								
Cappuccino Almond Fudge	½ cup (3.2 oz)	170	1	8	0	24	2	95
Cherry Chocolate Chunk	½ cup (3.2 oz)	170	1	7	0	27	1	85
Chocolate Almond Chunk	½ cup (3.2 oz)	170	2	8	0	25	2	95
Chocolate Fudge Brownie	½ cup (3.2 oz)	170	1	7	0	28	2	95
Double Espresso Bean	½ cup (3.2 oz)	160	1	7	0	24	1	100
Mint Chocolate Cookie	½ cup (3.2 oz)	170	1	8	0	26	1	100
Peanut Butter Cup	½ cup (3.2 oz)	180	3	8	0	25	2	105

FOOD	PORTION	CALS	PROT	FAT	CHOL	CARB	FIBER	SOD
Pralines N' Dream	½ cup (3.2 oz)	180	1	9	0	25	1	95
Silhouette								
The Skinny Cow Low Fat Ice Cream Sandwich Vanilla	1	130	5	2	0	23	2	145
Slim-Fast								
Chocolate Fudge Bar	1 bar	110	3	2	10	22	tr	80
Ice Cream Sandwich Chocolate	1	130	3	2	<5	27	tr	150
Ice Cream Sandwich Vanilla	1	130	3	1	<5	27	tr	150
Starbucks								
Caramel Cappuccino Swirl	½ cup	240	4	12	65	30	0	100
Classic Coffee	½ cup	230	5	12	65	26	0	50
Coffee Almond Fudge	½ cup	250	5	13	60	29	1	65
Frappuccino Bar Java Fudge	1 bar	130	4	2	5	25	4	50
Frappuccino Bar Mocha	1 bar	120	4	2	10	22	3	50
Java Chip	½ cup	250	4	13	60	29	0	55
Low Fat Latte	½ cup	170	5	3	10	30	0	60
Mud Pie	½ cup	240	4	11	55	32	1	85
White Chocolate Latte	½ cup	280	5	15	60	31	0	60
Tofutti								
Cuties Chocolate	1 (1.4 oz)	130	2	5	0	16	0	110
Monkey Bars Peanut Butter	1 bar (2.5 oz)	220	3	13	0	22	tr	105
Turkey Hill								
Black Cherry	½ cup	140	2	7	25	18	0	30
Black Raspberry	½ cup	140	—	7	30	18	—	35
Butter Pecan	½ cup	170	2	11	30	16	0	50
Chocolate Marshmallow	½ cup	160	—	7	30	24	—	30
Chocolate Mint Chip	½ cup	180	—	11	30	18	—	40

FOOD	PORTION	CALS	PROT	FAT	CHOL	CARB	FIBER	SOD
Chocolate Peanut Butter Cup	½ cup	180	–	11	30	18	–	60
Colombian Coffee	½ cup	140	–	8	30	16	–	35
Cookies 'N Cream	½ cup	160	2	9	30	19	0	60
Death By Chocolate	½ cup	160	–	8	30	21	–	35
Dutch Chocolate	½ cup	150	–	8	30	19	–	30
Egg Nog	½ cup	150	–	8	45	17	–	35
Fat Free No Sugar Added Caramel Fudge Decadence	½ cup	100	–	0	0	23	–	75
Fat Free No Sugar Added Cherry Vanilla Fudge	½ cup	90	–	0	0	20	–	80
Fat Free No Sugar Added Dutch Chocolate	½ cup	90	–	0	0	20	–	70
Fat Free No Sugar Added Vanilla Bean	½ cup	90	–	0	0	20	–	60
Fudge Ripple	½ cup	140	–	7	30	20	–	70
Light Butter Pecan	½ cup	130	3	6	15	17	0	80
Light Choco Mint Chip	½ cup	140	3	5	15	19	0	75
Light Tin Lissie Sundae	½ cup	140	–	5	10	21	–	120
Light Vanilla & Chocolate	½ cup	110	3	3	15	18	0	60
Light Vanilla Bean	½ cup	110	3	3	15	18	0	65
Neapolitan	½ cup	150	2	8	30	18	0	30
Orange Swirl	½ cup	140	–	6	20	19	–	25
Original Vanilla	½ cup	140	–	8	30	16	–	35
Peanut Butter Ripple	½ cup	170	–	11	30	16	–	60
Philadelphia Style Butter Almond	½ cup	180	–	12	35	15	–	105
Philadelphia Style Chocolate	½ cup	170	–	10	35	18	–	40
Philadelphia Style Mint Chocolate Chip	½ cup	180	–	11	35	18	–	50

FOOD	PORTION	CALS	PROT	FAT	CHOL	CARB	FIBER	SOD
Philadelphia Style Sweet Cherry Vanilla	½ cup	160	–	8	30	18	–	50
Philadelphia Style Vanilla Bean	½ cup	170	–	10	35	16	–	50
Rocky Road	½ cup	170	3	8	30	23	0	40
Rum Raisin	½ cup	150	–	7	30	19	–	30
Sandwich Choco Mint Chip	1	200	–	8	25	27	–	180
Sandwiches Vanilla	1	190	–	8	25	26	–	180
Strawberries 'N Cream	½ cup	140	–	6	25	19	–	30
Sundae Cones Rocky Road	1	340	–	19	25	37	–	110
Sundae Cones Tin Roof Sundae	1	290	–	17	25	30	–	135
Tin Roof Sundae	½ cup	160	2	9	30	19	0	70
Vanilla & Chocolate	½ cup	150	2	8	30	17	0	35
Vanilla Bean	½ cup	140	2	8	30	16	0	35
TAKE-OUT								
cone vanilla light soft serve	1 (4.6 oz)	164	4	6	28	24	–	92
gelato chocolate hazelnut	½ cup (5.3 oz)	370	9	29	92	26	2	49
gelato vanilla	½ cup (3 oz)	211	3	15	151	18	0	78
sundae caramel	1 (5.4 oz)	303	7	9	25	49	–	195
sundae hot fudge	1 (5.4 oz)	284	6	9	21	48	–	182
sundae strawberry	1 (5.4 oz)	269	6	8	21	45	–	92

ICE CREAM CONES AND CUPS

FOOD	PORTION	CALS	PROT	FAT	CHOL	CARB	FIBER	SOD
sugar cone	1	40	1	tr	0	8	tr	32
wafer cone	1	17	tr	tr	0	3	tr	6
Frookie								
Chocolate Crunch	1 (0.4 oz)	50	1	1	0	10	tr	10
Honey Crunch	1 (0.4 oz)	45	1	1	0	9	tr	20
Keebler								
Chocolatey Cone	1 (0.4 oz)	50	tr	1	0	10	0	40
Fudge Dipped Cup	1 (0.3 oz)	35	0	2	0	6	0	20
Ice Creme Cup	1 (0.2 oz)	15	0	0	0	4	0	20
Sugar Cone	1 (0.4 oz)	50	tr	1	0	10	0	15

FOOD	PORTION	CALS	PROT	FAT	CHOL	CARB	FIBER	SOD
Waffle Bowl	1 (0.4 oz)	50	tr	1	0	10	0	25
Waffle Cone	1 (0.4 oz)	50	tr	1	0	10	0	25

ICE CREAM TOPPINGS

FOOD	PORTION	CALS	PROT	FAT	CHOL	CARB	FIBER	SOD
butterscotch	2 tbsp (1.4 oz)	103	1	tr	—	27	—	143
caramel	2 tbsp (1.4 oz)	103	1	tr	—	27	—	143
marshmallow cream	1 oz	88	1	tr	0	23	—	13
marshmallow cream	1 jar (7 oz)	615	3	tr	0	157	—	90
pineapple	2 tbsp (1.5 oz)	106	tr	0	0	28	—	26
pineapple	1 cup (11.5 oz)	861	1	—	0	226	—	214
strawberry	2 tbsp (1.5 oz)	107	tr	tr	0	28	—	9
strawberry	1 cup (11.5 oz)	863	1	1	0	225	—	73
walnuts in syrup	2 tbsp (1.4 oz)	167	2	9	0	22	—	—
Colac								
Passion Fruit	1 tbsp	31	0	0	0	13	0	0
Strawberry	1 tbsp	31	0	0	0	13	0	0
Hershey's								
Chocolate Shoppe Caramel	2 tbsp	100	tr	0	0	25	—	95
Chocolate Shoppe Double Chocolate	1 tbsp	60	tr	1	0	12	—	30
Chocolate Shoppe Hot Fudge	1 tbsp	70	tr	3	<5	10	—	80
Chocolate Shoppe Hot Fudge Fat Free	2 tbsp	100	1	0	0	23	—	135
Sprinkles Candy Coated Milk Chocolate	1 tbsp	70	tr	3	<5	10	—	10

FOOD	PORTION	CALS	PROT	FAT	CHOL	CARB	FIBER	SOD
Reese's								
Sprinkles Peanut Butter & Milk Chocolate	1 tbsp	70	1	4	0	10	–	25
Smucker's								
Plate Scrapers Caramel	2 tbsp	100	1	0	0	25	–	105
Steel's								
Sugar Free Butterscotch	2 tbsp	60	0	0	0	21	0	10
Sugar Free Chocolate Fudge	2 tbsp	45	2	3	10	5	2	15
Sugar Free Hot Fudge	2 tbsp	65	1	3	0	18	1	13
Sugar Free Peanut Butter Fudge	2 tbsp	75	2	6	7	5	2	41
ICED TEA								
MIX								
instant artificially sweetened lemon flavored as prep w/ water	8 oz	5	tr	0	0	1	–	24
instant sweetened lemon flavor as prep w/ water	9 oz	87	tr	tr	0	22	–	–
instant unsweetened lemon flavor as prep w/ water	8 oz	4	tr	0	0	0	–	14
Atkins								
Sugar Free Lemon not prep	2 tbsp	0	0	0	0	0	0	5
Carb Options								
Lemon as prep	1 serv	0	0	0	0	0	0	0
Nestea								
100% Tea	2 tsp (1 g)	0	0	0	0	tr	0	0
100% Tea Decafe	2 tsp (1 g)	0	0	0	0	tr	0	0
Ice Teasers Lemon	1 serv (0.5 oz)	5	0	0	0	1	0	0

FOOD	PORTION	CALS	PROT	FAT	CHOL	CARB	FIBER	SOD
Ice Teasers Orange	1 serv (0.5 oz)	5	0	0	0	1	0	0
Ice Teasers Wild Cherry	1 serv (0.5 oz)	5	0	0	0	1	0	0
Lemon	2 tsp (1 g)	5	0	0	0	1	0	0
Lemon & Sugar	2 tbsp (0.7 oz)	80	0	0	0	19	0	0
Lemonade Tea	2 tbsp (0.7 oz)	80	0	0	0	19	0	0
Sugar Free	2 tbsp (0.7 oz)	5	0	0	0	1	0	0
Sugar Free Decafe	1 tbsp (0.7 oz)	5	0	0	0	1	0	0
Sun Tea	1 tsp (1 g)	0	0	0	0	tr	0	0
READY-TO-DRINK								
Apple & Eve								
Lemon Fruit	8 fl oz	100	0	0	0	25	–	20
Peach Fruit	8 fl oz	100	0	0	0	25	–	20
Raspberry Fruit	8 fl oz	100	0	0	0	25	–	20
Tangerine Fruit	8 fl oz	100	0	0	0	25	–	20
Fuze								
LemonAID	8 oz	70	0	0	0	19	–	15
Slenderize Cranberry Raspberry	8 oz	7	0	0	0	2	–	10
Vitamin Tea Diet Peach	8 oz	5	0	0	0	1	0	5
Vitamin Tea Green Tea w/ Ginseng	8 oz	60	0	0	0	16	–	5
Vitamin Tea Lemon	8 oz	70	0	0	0	18	–	5
White Tea	8 oz	60	0	0	0	15	–	0
White Tea No Carb Diet Pomegranate	8 oz	0	0	0	0	0	0	0
Glaceau Vitamin Water								
Determination	8 oz	50	0	0	0	13	–	0
Leadership	8 oz	50	0	0	0	13	–	0
Perseverance	8 oz	50	0	0	0	13	–	0
Vital-T	8 oz	50	0	0	0	13	–	0
Hansen's								
Chai	8 oz	150	0	0	0	38	–	15

FOOD	PORTION	CALS	PROT	FAT	CHOL	CARB	FIBER	SOD
China Black	8 oz	90	0	0	0	25	–	15
Green	8 oz	70	0	0	0	18	–	15
Green Diet Lemon	8 oz	0	0	0	0	0	–	15
Green Diet Peach	8 oz	0	0	0	0	0	–	15
Green Lemon	8 oz	70	0	0	0	18	–	15
Green Peach	8 oz	70	0	0	0	18	–	15
Oolong	8 oz	70	0	0	0	25	–	15
Spice	8 oz	90	25	0	0	24	–	15
Hawaiian								
Iced Tea	1 can	120	0	0	0	35	0	50
Honest Tea								
Assam	8 oz	17	0	0	0	5	–	10
Black Forest Berry	8 oz	25	0	0	0	8	–	5
Gold Rush	8 oz	9	0	0	0	3	–	10
Green Dragon	8 oz	30	0	0	0	9	–	5
Kashmiri Chai	8 oz	17	0	0	0	6	–	0
Lori's Lemon	8 oz	30	0	0	0	9	–	5
Moroccan Mint	8 oz	17	0	0	0	5	–	5
Peach Oo-La-Long	8 oz	30	0	0	0	9	–	5
Inko's								
White Tea	1 bottle (16 oz)	56	0	0	0	14	–	tr
White Tea Hint O'Mint	1 bottle	0	0	0	0	0	–	tr
Mad River								
Red Tea w/ Guarana	8 oz	90	0	0	0	24	–	10
New Leaf								
All Flavors	8 oz	75	0	0	0	19	–	0
Oregon Chai								
Original Latte	1 bottle (9.5 oz)	150	2	4	15	26	0	50
Republic Of Tea								
No Carb Unsweetened All Flavors	1 bottle (12 oz)	0	0	0	0	0	0	0
Snapple								
Diet Lemon	8 fl oz	0	0	0	0	1	–	10
Diet Peach	8 fl oz	0	0	0	0	1	–	10
Diet Raspberry	8 fl oz	0	0	0	0	1	–	10

FOOD	PORTION	CALS	PROT	FAT	CHOL	CARB	FIBER	SOD
Diet Lime Green Tea	8 fl oz	0	0	0	0	1	–	10
Kiwi Teawi	8 fl oz	100	0	0	0	26	–	10
Lemon	8 fl oz	100	0	0	0	25	–	10
Lime Green Tea	8 fl oz	100	0	0	0	25	–	10
Peach	8 fl oz	100	0	0	0	26	–	10
Raspberry	8 fl oz	100	0	0	0	26	–	10
Very Cherry	8 fl oz	100	0	0	0	25	–	10
SoBe								
Lemon	8 oz	90	0	0	0	25	–	5
Soy20								
Lemon Green Tea	1 bottle (12 oz)	90	0	0	0	22	–	10
Sweet Leaf Tea								
Diet Sweet	8 oz	0	0	0	0	0	–	10
Hibiscus Herbal	8 oz	25	0	0	0	8	–	10
Lemon & Lime	8 oz	0	0	0	0	0	–	0
Mint & Honey Green	8 oz	60	0	0	0	15	–	0
Peach	8 oz	75	0	0	0	19	–	10
Raspberry & Tangerine	8 oz	75	0	0	0	19	–	0
Sweet Tea	8 oz	75	0	0	0	19	–	0
T42								
A Classic Earl Grey	8 oz	60	0	0	0	14	–	5
Herbal All Flavors	8 oz	70	0	0	0	18	–	5
Jamaican Ginger Green Tea	8 oz	70	0	0	0	16	–	6
Wake-Up Blend English Breakfast	8 oz	45	0	0	0	11	–	5
With Lemon	8 oz	60	0	0	0	14	–	0
Tradewinds								
Diet Green Tea	8 oz	0	0	0	0	0	0	0
Diet Raspberry	8 oz	0	0	0	0	0	0	0
Mango Green Tea	8 oz	80	0	0	0	20	–	0
Turkey Hill								
Blueberry Oolong w/ Vitamins C & E	1 cup	100	–	0	0	24	–	–
Decaffeinated	1 cup	80	–	0	0	20	–	–

FOOD	PORTION	CALS	PROT	FAT	CHOL	CARB	FIBER	SOD
Decaffeinated Orange	1 cup	10	–	0	0	2	–	–
Diet	1 cup	0	0	0	0	0	–	–
Diet Decaffeinated	1 cup	0	0	0	0	0	–	0
Diet Green Tea w/ Ginseng & Honey	1 cup	5	–	0	0	tr	–	–
Green Tea w/ Ginseng & Honey	1 cup	70	17	0	0	17	–	–
Lemon	1 cup	100	–	0	0	24	–	–
Mint Tea w/ Chamomile	1 cup	90	–	0	0	21	–	–
Oolong w/ Ginkgo Biloba & Ginseng	1 cup	100	–	0	0	25	–	–
Orange	1 cup	100	–	0	0	25	–	–
Peach	1 cup	110	–	0	0	28	–	–
Raspberry Tea	1 cup	110	0	0	0	28	–	0
Regular	1 cup	90	0	0	0	22	–	0
XS Energy								
Energy Tea Berry Typhoon	1 can (8.4 oz)	12	2	0	0	1	–	30

ICES AND ICE POPS

FOOD	PORTION	CALS	PROT	FAT	CHOL	CARB	FIBER	SOD
fruit & juice bar	1 (3 fl oz)	75	1	tr	0	19	–	3
gelatin pop	1 (1.5 oz)	31	1	0	0	7	–	20
ice coconut pineapple	½ cup (4 fl oz)	109	0	3	0	23	–	34
ice fruit w/ Equal	1 bar (1.7 oz)	12	tr	0	0	3	–	3
ice lime	½ cup (4 fl oz)	75	tr	0	0	31	–	–
ice pop	1 (2 fl oz)	42	0	0	0	11	–	7
Breyers								
Fruit Bars No Sugar Added	1 (1.75 oz)	25	0	0	0	5	0	0
Juice Bar Strawberry	1 (3.75 oz)	120	0	0	0	30	tr	10
Soft Frozen Cup Lemonade	1 pkg (12 oz)	290	0	0	0	74	–	25
Soft Frozen Cup Strawberry	1 pkg (12 oz)	260	0	0	0	66	–	25

FOOD	PORTION	CALS	PROT	FAT	CHOL	CARB	FIBER	SOD
Carnation								
Cup Orange Sherbet	1 (3 oz)	90	1	1	5	19	0	20
Cup Orange Sherbet	1 (5 oz)	150	1	2	5	32	0	30
Cold Fusion								
Protein Juice Bar All Flavors	1 bar (3.8 oz)	130	11	0	0	23	0	0
Cool Creations								
Ice Pop	1 pop (2 oz)	50	0	0	0	13	0	5
Mickey Mouse Bar	1 (4 oz)	170	2	11	15	17	0	40
Surprise Pops	1 (2 oz)	60	0	0	0	14	0	5
CoolFruits								
Fruit Juice Freezer Pops Grape & Cherry	3 pops (3 oz)	70	0	0	0	18	0	10
Dole								
Fruit'n Juice Coconut	1 bar (4 oz)	210	3	7	10	33	0	50
Fruit'n Juice Lemonade	1 bar (4 oz)	120	1	0	0	28	0	55
Fruit'n Juice Lime	1 bar (4 oz)	110	0	0	0	28	0	55
Fruit'n Juice Peach Passion	1 bar (2.5 oz)	70	0	0	0	17	0	5
Fruit'n Juice Pineapple Coconut	1 bar (4 oz)	150	1	4	0	27	0	5
Fruit'n Juice Pineapple Orange Banana	1 bar (4 oz)	110	0	0	0	26	0	5
Fruit'n Juice Pineapple Orange Banana	1 bar (2.5 oz)	70	0	0	0	16	0	5
Fruit'n Juice Raspberry	1 bar (2.5 oz)	70	0	0	0	16	0	5
Fruit'n Juice Strawberry	1 bar (4 oz)	110	0	0	0	26	0	5
Fruit'n Juice Strawberry	1 bar (2.5 oz)	70	0	0	0	17	0	5
Grape No Sugar Added	1 bar (1.75 oz)	25	0	0	0	6	0	5

FOOD	PORTION	CALS	PROT	FAT	CHOL	CARB	FIBER	SOD
Raspberry	1 bar (1.75 oz)	45	0	0	0	11	0	5
Raspberry No Sugar Added	1 bar (1.75 oz)	25	0	0	0	6	0	5
Strawberry	1 bar (1.75 oz)	45	0	0	0	11	0	5
Strawberry No Sugar Added	1 bar (1.75 oz)	25	0	0	0	6	0	5
Edy's								
Fruit Bars Strawberry	1 (3 oz)	80	0	0	0	21	0	0
Sherbet Berry Rainbow	½ cup	130	1	1	5	29	–	35
Sherbet Lime	½ cup	130	1	2	5	28	–	35
Sherbet Orange Cream	½ cup	120	2	2	10	23	–	40
Sherbet Raspberry	½ cup	130	1	1	5	28	–	35
Sherbet Starburst Orange & Cherry	½ cup	150	1	2	5	33	–	40
Sherbet Starburst Strawberry	½ cup	160	1	3	5	33	–	40
Sherbet Swiss Orange	½ cup	150	1	3	5	30	–	40
Sherbet Tropical Rainbow	½ cup	130	1	1	5	29	–	35
Sorbet Coconut	½ cup	140	1	3	5	28	0	20
Sorbet Lemon	½ cup	140	0	0	0	35	0	20
Sorbet Mandarin Orange	½ cup	130	0	0	0	32	0	25
Sorbet Peach	½ cup	130	0	0	0	32	1	10
Sorbet Raspberry	½ cup	130	0	0	0	33	1	15
Sorbet Strawberry	½ cup	120	0	0	0	31	0	10
Whole Fruit Bars Creamy Coconut	1 bar	120	3	3	0	21	–	40
Whole Fruit Bars Lemonade	1 bar	80	0	0	0	20	–	0
Whole Fruit Bars Lime	1 bar	80	0	0	0	20	–	0
Whole Fruit Bars Tangerine	1 bar	80	0	0	0	20	–	0

FOOD	PORTION	CALS	PROT	FAT	CHOL	CARB	FIBER	SOD
Whole Fruit Bars Wild Berry	1 bar	80	0	0	0	21	—	0
Flintstones								
Push-Up Sherbet Treats	1 (2.75 oz)	100	1	2	5	20	0	25
Good Humor								
Great White	1 (3 oz)	70	0	0	0	18	—	0
Hyper Stripe	1 (2.7 oz)	80	0	0	0	19	—	10
Haagen-Dazs								
Sorbet Chocolate	½ cup	120	2	0	0	28	2	70
Sorbet Mango	½ cup	120	0	0	0	31	tr	0
Sorbet Orange	½ cup	120	0	0	0	30	tr	0
Sorbet Orchard Peach	½ cup	130	0	0	0	33	tr	0
Sorbet Raspberry	½ cup	120	0	0	0	30	2	0
Sorbet Strawberry	½ cup	120	0	0	0	30	1	0
Sorbet Zesty Lemon	½ cup	120	0	0	0	31	tr	0
Sorbet Bar Chocolate	1 (2.7 oz)	80	1	0	0	20	1	50
Sorbet Bars Raspberry & Vanilla Yogurt	1 (2.5 oz)	90	2	0	0	21	tr	15
Sorbet Bars Strawberry & Vanilla Ice Cream	1 (2.5 oz)	110	1	5	35	15	0	20
Natural Choice								
Organic Banana	½ cup (3.6 oz)	110	0	0	0	28	tr	0
Organic Blueberry	½ cup (3.6 oz)	100	0	0	0	27	tr	0
Organic Kiwi	½ cup (3.6 oz)	110	0	0	0	28	tr	10
Organic Lemon	½ cup (3.6 oz)	110	0	0	0	28	tr	10
Organic Mango	½ cup (3.6 oz)	110	0	0	0	28	tr	10
Organic Strawberry	½ cup (3.6 oz)	110	0	0	0	28	tr	10
Organic Strawberry Kiwi	½ cup (3.6 oz)	110	0	0	0	28	tr	10

FOOD	PORTION	CALS	PROT	FAT	CHOL	CARB	FIBER	SOD
Popsicle								
All Natural Ice Pops	1 (1.75 oz)	50	0	0	0	12	—	5
Bar Bart Simpson	1 (4 oz)	110	0	1	—	26	—	20
Bar Dora The Explorer	1 (4 oz)	100	0	0	0	25	—	15
Bar Fruti Holanda Lemon Lime	1 (3 oz)	90	0	0	0	23	—	15
Bar Fruti Holanda Strawberry	1 (3 oz)	90	0	0	0	23	—	5
Bar Incredible Hulk	1 (4 oz)	100	0	0	0	25	—	15
Bar Jimmy Neutron	1 (4 oz)	100	0	0	0	25	—	15
Bar Mega Warheads	1 (4 oz)	110	0	1	0	26	0	20
Bar Power Ranger	1 (4 oz)	100	0	0	0	23	—	15
Bar Spider Man	1 (4 oz)	100	0	0	0	25	—	15
Bar SpongeBob	1 (4 oz)	100	0	0	0	25	—	15
Big Stick Pops Big Reds	1 (3.5 oz)	70	0	0	0	17	—	0
Big Stick Pops Cherry Pineapple	1 (3.5 oz)	50	0	0	0	12	0	5
Bubble Play	1 (4 oz)	100	0	0	0	28	—	15
Creamsicle Bar	1 (2.5 oz)	100	1	3	5	18	0	30
Creamsicle Sugar Free	2 (3.3 oz)	40	1	2	0	10	6	0
Creamsicle Pop No Sugar Added	1 (1.75 oz)	25	tr	0	0	6	0	20
Cup Cherry	1 (12 oz)	240	0	0	0	62	—	10
Cup Frostee Fudge	1 (10 oz)	280	7	11	35	41	2	95
Cup Lemon	1 (12 oz)	230	0	0	0	60	—	10
Cup Screwball	1 (3.75 oz)	110	0	0	0	27	—	15
Firecracker	1 (1.6 oz)	35	0	0	0	9	—	0
Fruita Holanda Coconut Bar	1 (3 oz)	120	0	3	—	25	tr	75
Fudgsicle Bar	1 (2.5 oz)	90	3	2	5	16	tr	65
Fudgsicle Bar Fat Free	1 (1.75 oz)	60	3	0	0	13	tr	50
Fudgsicle Pop	1 (1.75 oz)	60	2	1	5	11	tr	45
Fudgsicle Pops No Sugar Added	2 (1.75 oz)	90	3	1	0	19	1	85
Minis Fudge Bar	2 (2.4 oz)	80	3	2	0	16	tr	60
Pop Great White	1 (1.75 oz)	45	0	0	0	11	—	0

FOOD	PORTION	CALS	PROT	FAT	CHOL	CARB	FIBER	SOD
Pop Lick-A-Color	1 (2 oz)	50	0	0	0	13	–	0
Pop Sherbet Cyclone	1 (1.8 oz)	50	1	1	0	11	0	10
Pop Towering Tornado	1 (3.5 oz)	90	0	0	0	21	–	0
Pop Ups Orange Burst	1 (2.75 oz)	80	tr	1	<5	19	0	15
Pop Ups Reckless Rainbow	1 (2.75 oz)	90	tr	1	<5	19	0	15
Pop Ups SpongeBob	1 (2.75 oz)	90	1	2	5	17	0	20
Pops Tropical Sugar Free	1	15	0	0	0	3	–	0
Pops Wild Bunch	2 (2.2 oz)	60	0	0	0	14	–	5
Rainbow Floats	1 (1.75 oz)	60	1	2	5	11	0	15
Rainbow Pops	1 (1.75 oz)	45	0	0	0	11	–	0
Scribblers Juice Pops	2 (2.4 oz)	60	0	0	0	16	–	0
Shots	1 serv (1.7 oz)	40	0	1	–	9	–	0
Snow Cone	1 (7 oz)	30	0	0	0	7	–	5
Sugar Free Pops Orange Cherry Grape	1 (1.75 oz)	15	0	0	0	3	–	0
Super Mario Bros Bar	1 (4 oz)	100	0	0	0	25	–	15
Swirl Bar Cotton Candy	1 (2.6 oz)	60	0	0	0	13	–	0
Tingle Twister Ice Pops	1 (1.75 oz)	45	0	0	0	11	–	0
Torpedo Pop Cherry	1 (1.75 oz)	35	0	0	0	8	–	0
Silhouette								
Fat Free Fudge Bars	1	90	–	0	0	–	–	–

JACKFRUIT

fresh	3.5 oz	70	1	tr	0	4	–	2

JALAPENO (see PEPPERS)

JAM/JELLY/PRESERVES

all flavors jam	1 pkg (0.5 oz)	34	tr	0	0	9	tr	–

FOOD	PORTION	CALS	PROT	FAT	CHOL	CARB	FIBER	SOD
all flavors jam	1 tbsp (0.7 oz)	48	tr	0	0	13	tr	—
all flavors jelly	1 tbsp (0.7 oz)	52	tr	0	0	14	tr	—
all flavors jelly	1 pkg (0.5 oz)	38	tr	0	0	10	tr	—
all flavors preserves	1 pkg (0.5 oz)	34	tr	0	0	9	tr	—
all flavors preserves	1 tbsp (0.7 oz)	48	tr	0	0	13	tr	—
apple butter	1 cup (9.9 oz)	519	tr	1	0	135	—	1
apple butter	1 tbsp (0.6 oz)	33	0	0	0	9	—	0
apple jelly	1 tbsp (0.7 oz)	52	tr	0	0	14	tr	7
apple jelly	1 pkg (0.5 oz)	38	tr	0	0	10	tr	5
apricot jam	0.5 oz	36	tr	0	0	9	—	—
blackberry jam	0.5 oz	34	tr	0	0	8	—	—
cherry jam	0.5 oz	36	tr	0	0	9	—	—
linganberry jam	0.5 oz	23	tr	tr	—	6	tr	—
orange jam	0.5 oz	35	tr	0	0	9	—	2
orange marmalade	1 tbsp (0.7 oz)	49	tr	0	0	13	—	11
orange marmalade	1 pkg (0.5 oz)	34	0	0	0	9	—	8
plum jam	0.5 oz	34	tr	0	0	9	—	—
quince jam	0.5 oz	43	0	0	0	8	—	—
raspberry jam	0.5 oz	35	tr	0	0	9	—	—
raspberry jelly	0.5 oz	37	0	0	0	9	—	—
red currant jam	0.5 oz	34	1	0	0	8	—	—
red currant jelly	0.5 oz	38	0	0	0	9	—	1
rose hip jam	0.5 oz	36	tr	0	0	9	—	1
strawberry jam	1 tbsp (0.7 oz)	48	tr	0	0	13	tr	8
strawberry jam	1 pkg (0.5 oz)	34	tr	0	0	9	tr	6
strawberry preserve	1 pkg (0.5 oz)	34	tr	0	0	9	tr	6
strawberry preserve	1 tbsp (0.7 oz)	48	tr	0	0	13	tr	8

FOOD	PORTION	CALS	PROT	FAT	CHOL	CARB	FIBER	SOD
Colac								
Jelly All Flavors	1 tbsp	37	0	0	0	15	0	0
Eden								
Cherry Butter	1 tbsp	35	0	0	0	9	1	0
Organic Apple Butter	1 tbsp	20	0	0	0	5	0	0
Jok'n'Al								
Low Carb Fruit Spreads All Flavors	1 tbsp	10	0	0	0	3	0	0
Polaner								
All Fruit Peach	1 tbsp	40	0	0	0	8	–	0
All Fruit Raspberry	1 tbsp	40	0	0	0	10	–	0
Sarabeth's								
Spreadable Fruit Orange Apricot	1 tbsp	30	0	0	0	8	–	0
Spreadable Fruit Peach Apricot	1 tbsp	40	0	0	0	96	1	0
Spreadable Fruit Strawberry Raspberry	1 tbsp	40	0	0	0	10	tr	<5
Smucker's								
Concord Grape Jelly	1 tbsp	50	0	0	0	13	–	5
Peach Preserves	1 tbsp	50	0	0	0	13	–	0
Simply Fruit Red Raspberry	1 tbsp	40	0	0	0	10	–	0
Welch's								
Grape Jam	1 tbsp	50	0	0	0	13	–	10
Wild Thyme Farms								
Fruit Spreads Blackberry Currant Ginger	1 tsp	8	0	0	0	2	–	0
Fruit Spreads Mango Apricot	1 tsp	7	0	0	0	2	–	0

JAPANESE FOOD (see ASIAN FOOD, SUSHI)

JAVA PLUM

FOOD	PORTION	CALS	PROT	FAT	CHOL	CARB	FIBER	SOD
fresh	3	5	tr	tr	0	1	–	1
fresh	1 cup	82	1	tr	0	21	–	18

FOOD	PORTION	CALS	PROT	FAT	CHOL	CARB	FIBER	SOD

JELLY *(see JAM/JELLY/PRESERVES)*

JUTE
cooked	1 cup	32	3	tr	0	6	2	10

KALE
chopped cooked	½ cup	21	1	tr	0	4	–	15
frzn chopped cooked	½ cup	20	2	tr	0	4	–	10
raw chopped	½ cup	21	1	tr	0	3	–	15
scotch chopped cooked	½ cup	18	1	tr	0	4	–	29

KEFIR
kefir	7 oz	132	6	8	–	10	–	92

KETCHUP
banana	1 tsp	10	0	0	0	2	0	75
ketchup	1 pkg (0.2 oz)	6	tr	tr	0	2	tr	71
ketchup	1 tbsp	16	tr	tr	0	4	tr	178
low sodium	1 tbsp	16	tr	tr	0	4	tr	3
Atkins								
Ketch-A-Tomato	1 tbsp	10	0	0	0	2	1	160
Del Monte								
Ketchup	1 tbsp (0.5 oz)	15	0	0	0	4	0	190
Healthy Choice								
Ketchup	1 tbsp (0.5 oz)	9	tr	tr	0	2	tr	97
Heinz								
Ketchup	1 tbsp	15	0	0	0	4	0	190
No Salt	1 tbsp	20	0	0	0	5	0	0
One Carb	1 tbsp	5	0	0	0	1	0	190
Organic	1 tbsp	20	0	0	0	5	0	190
Hunt's								
Ketchup	1 tbsp	15	0	0	0	4	0	180
No Salt	1 tbsp	20	0	0	0	4	0	0
Squeeze	1 tbsp	15	0	0	0	4	0	180
Keto								
Ketchup	1 tbsp	4	0	0	0	1	0	15
Muir Glen								
Organic	1 tbsp (0.6 oz)	15	0	0	0	3	0	190
Smucker's								
Tomato	1 tbsp	25	0	0	0	7	–	110

FOOD	PORTION	CALS	PROT	FAT	CHOL	CARB	FIBER	SOD
Steel's								
Sugar Free	1 tbsp	10	0	0	0	0	0	40
Stokelys								
Tomato	1 tbsp	15	0	0	0	4	—	190
Tree Of Life								
Ketchup	1 tbsp (0.5 oz)	10	0	0	0	3	—	25
Walden Farms								
Calorie Free	1 tbsp	0	0	0	0	0	0	170
KIDNEY								
beef simmered	3 oz	122	22	3	329	0	—	114
lamb braised	3 oz	117	20	3	481	1	—	128
pork cooked	3 oz	128	22	4	408	0	0	68
pork cooked	1 cup	211	36	7	672	0	0	112
veal braised	3 oz	139	22	5	672	0	—	93
KIDNEY BEANS								
canned	1 cup	207	13	1	0	38	9	889
dried cooked	1 cup	225	15	1	0	40	11	4
Bush's								
Light Red	½ cup	110	7	0	0	20	7	260
Eden								
Organic Cannellini	½ cup (4.6 oz)	100	6	1	—	17	5	40
Hunt's								
Kidney Beans	½ cup (4.5 oz)	94	6	1	0	20	5	484
Progresso								
Dark Red	½ cup (4.5 oz)	110	8	0	0	20	6	340
Red	½ cup (4.6 oz)	110	7	1	0	20	8	280
S&W								
Dark Red Premium	½ cup (4.6 oz)	100	7	1	0	23	6	460
Van Camp								
Dark Red	½ cup (4.6 oz)	90	6	0	0	20	6	760
Light Red	½ cup (4.6 oz)	90	6	0	0	20	6	390
KIWIS								
fresh	1 med	46	1	tr	0	11	3	4
Chiquita								
Fresh	2 med (5.2 oz)	100	2	1	0	24	4	0

FOOD	PORTION	CALS	PROT	FAT	CHOL	CARB	FIBER	SOD
KNISH								
Gabila's								
Potato	1 (4.5 oz)	170	6	6	0	29	5	440
TAKE-OUT								
cheese & blueberry	1 (7 oz)	378	24	13	40	40	–	–
cheese & cherry	1 (7 oz)	378	24	13	40	40	–	–
everything	1 (7 oz)	221	7	8	0	34	–	–
kashe	1 (7 oz)	270	7	8	0	45	–	–
potato	1 lg (7 oz)	332	8	12	72	49	1	470
potato	1 med (3.5 oz)	166	4	6	36	25	tr	235
potato w/ broccoli & cheese	1 (7 oz)	312	12	15	24	33	–	–
potato w/ spinach & mushroom	1 (7 oz)	214	6	8	0	32	–	–
KOHLRABI								
raw sliced	½ cup	19	1	tr	0	4	–	14
sliced cooked	½ cup	24	1	tr	0	5	–	17
KRILL								
fresh	1 oz	22	3	1	–	tr	0	119
KUMQUATS								
fresh	1	12	tr	tr	0	3	–	1
LAMB								
cubed lean only braised	3 oz	190	29	7	92	0	–	60
cubed lean only broiled	3 oz	158	24	6	77	0	–	65
ground broiled	3 oz	240	21	17	82	0	–	69
leg lean & fat Choice roasted	3 oz	219	22	14	79	14	–	56
loin chop w/ bone lean & fat Choice broiled	1 chop (2.3 oz)	201	16	15	64	0	–	49
loin chop w/ bone lean only Choice broiled	1 chop (1.6 oz)	100	14	5	44	0	–	39
new zealand lean & fat cooked	3 oz	259	21	19	93	0	–	39

FOOD	PORTION	CALS	PROT	FAT	CHOL	CARB	FIBER	SOD
new zealand lean only cooked	3 oz	175	25	8	93	0	–	43
rib chop lean & fat Choice broiled	3 oz	307	19	25	84	0	–	64
rib chop lean only Choice broiled	3 oz	200	24	11	78	0	–	73
shank lean & fat Choice braised	3 oz	206	24	11	90	0	–	61
shank lean & fat Choice roasted	3 oz	191	22	11	77	0	–	55
shoulder chop w/ bone lean & fat Choice braised	1 chop (2.5 oz)	244	21	17	84	0	–	51
shoulder chop w/ bone lean only Choice braised	1 chop (1.9 oz)	152	19	8	66	0	–	41
sirloin lean & fat Choice roasted	3 oz	248	21	21	82	0	–	58

LAMB DISHES
TAKE-OUT

FOOD	PORTION	CALS	PROT	FAT	CHOL	CARB	FIBER	SOD
couscous lamb	1 serv	275	–	80	8	–	–	460
curry	¾ cup	345	26	17	89	22	–	258
lamb fattoush salad	1 serv	606	–	31	109	–	–	924
lamb tagine casserole	1 serv	261	–	12	57	–	–	381
moroccan pilaf w/ bulgur	1 serv	327	–	13	54	–	–	303
moussaka	5.6 oz	312	15	21	–	16	1	–
sambousa lamb & vegetable pocket	1	645	–	54	38	–	–	317
stew	¾ cup	124	10	5	29	11	2	140

LAMBSQUARTERS

FOOD	PORTION	CALS	PROT	FAT	CHOL	CARB	FIBER	SOD
chopped cooked	½ cup	29	3	1	0	5	–	–

LEEKS

FOOD	PORTION	CALS	PROT	FAT	CHOL	CARB	FIBER	SOD
chopped cooked	¼ cup	8	tr	tr	0	2	–	3
cooked	1 (4.4 oz)	38	1	tr	0	9	–	13
freeze dried	1 tbsp	1	tr	0	0	tr	–	0

FOOD	PORTION	CALS	PROT	FAT	CHOL	CARB	FIBER	SOD
raw	1 (4.4 oz)	76	2	tr	0	18	–	25
raw chopped	¼ cup	16	tr	tr	0	4	–	5

LEMON
fresh	1 med	22	1	tr	0	12	–	3
peel	1 tbsp	0	tr	tr	0	1	–	0
wedge	1	5	tr	tr	0	3	–	1

LEMON CURD
lemon curd made w/ egg	2 tsp	29	tr	1	–	4	0	–
lemon curd made w/ starch	2 tsp	28	tr	–	–	6	0	–

LEMON EXTRACT
Virginia Dare
Extract	1 tsp	22	–	0	0	–	–	–

LEMON GRASS
fresh	1 cup (2.4 oz)	66	1	tr	0	17	0	4
fresh	1 tbsp (5 g)	5	tr	tr	0	1	0	tr

LEMON JUICE
bottled	1 tbsp	3	tr	tr	0	1	–	3
fresh	1 tbsp	4	tr	0	0	1	–	0
frzn	1 tbsp	3	tr	tr	0	1	–	0
Canarino								
Italian Hot Lemon Beverage	1 cup	0	0	0	0	0	0	0
Realemon								
Juice	1 tsp (5 ml)	0	0	0	0	0	–	0

LEMONADE
FROZEN
as prep w/ water	1 cup	100	tr	tr	0	26	–	8
not prep	1 can (6 oz)	397	1	tr	0	103	–	8
MIX								
powder as prep w/ water	9 fl oz	113	0	tr	0	29	–	19
powder w/ equal	1 pitcher (67 oz)	40	tr	0	0	10	–	58
Keto								
Kooler Pink	½ tsp	0	0	0	0	0	0	0

FOOD	PORTION	CALS	PROT	FAT	CHOL	CARB	FIBER	SOD
Low Carb Creations								
Lemonade as prep	1 serv	10	0	0	0	2	0	0
Raspberry as prep	1 serv	10	0	0	0	2	0	0
Sipper Sweets								
Sugar Free Low Carb	1 serv	8	0	0	0	1	0	0
READY-TO-DRINK								
Hansen's								
Sparkling	8 fl oz	100	0	0	0	25	–	10
Sparkling Pink	8 fl oz	120	0	0	0	31	–	10
Langers								
Raspberry Lemonade	8 oz	120	0	0	0	29	–	0
White Cranberry Lemonade	8 oz	120	0	0	0	30	–	15
Minute Maid								
Chilled	8 fl oz	110	0	0	0	28	–	25
Ocean Spray								
Spritzer	8 oz	160	0	0	0	41	–	50
Odwalla								
Pure Squeezed	8 fl oz	96	0	0	0	24	0	0
Strawberry Quencher	8 fl oz	110	0	0	0	28	0	0
Purity Organic								
Lemonade	8 oz	123	tr	tr	–	33	tr	tr
Snapple								
Diet Pink	8 fl oz	20	0	0	0	4	–	10
Lemonade	8 fl oz	120	0	0	0	30	–	10
Pink	8 fl oz	120	0	0	0	29	–	10
T42								
Lemonade	8 oz	90	0	0	0	25	–	10
Pink	8 oz	90	0	0	0	25	–	10
Three Drinks								
Sparkling	12 oz	12	0	0	0	3	–	20
Turkey Hill								
Lemonade	1 cup	120	0	0	0	29	–	0
Raspberry	1 cup	120	–	0	0	29	–	–
Strawberry Kiwi	1 cup	120	–	0	0	29	–	–
Zeigler's								
Old Fashioned	8 oz	120	0	0	0	30	0	25

FOOD	PORTION	CALS	PROT	FAT	CHOL	CARB	FIBER	SOD
LENTILS								
dried cooked	1 cup	231	18	1	0	40	—	4
Natural Touch								
Lentil Rice Loaf	1 in slice (3.2 oz)	170	8	9	0	14	4	370
Near East								
Lentil Pilaf as prep	1 cup	200	11	3	9	36	8	630
Shiloh Farms								
Organic Green not prep	¼ cup (1.6 oz)	150	11	0	0	27	7	15
TastyBite								
Bengal Lentils	½ pkg (5 oz)	190	7	5	0	30	1	150
Jodhpur Lentils	½ pkg (5 oz)	190	6	9	0	22	2	600
Madras Lentils	½ pkg (5 oz)	130	6	7	22	12	5	860
TAKE-OUT								
indian sambar	1 serv	236	15	5	10	37	9	189
middle eastern lentil salad	1 serv (4.5 oz)	158	—	3	0	—	—	382
yemiser selatta ethiopian lentil salad	1 serv (3 oz)	115	4	7	0	11	2	536
LETTUCE *(see also SALAD)*								
arugula	½ cup (0.4 oz)	3	tr	tr	0	tr	tr	3
bibb	1 head (6 oz)	21	2	tr	0	4	2	8
boston	1 head (6 oz)	21	2	tr	0	4	2	8
boston	2 leaves	2	tr	tr	0	tr	tr	1
cornsalad field salad	1 cup (1.9 oz)	7	1	tr	0	1	1	2
iceberg	1 head (19 oz)	70	5	1	0	11	5	48
iceberg	1 leaf	3	tr	tr	0	tr	tr	2
looseleaf shredded	½ cup	5	tr	tr	0	1	—	3
romaine shredded	½ cup	4	tr	tr	0	1	tr	2
Dole								
Iceberg	1 cup (3 oz)	15	1	0	0	3	1	10
Romaine	1½ cups (3 oz)	15	1	0	0	2	2	5
Shredded	1½ cup (3 oz)	15	1	0	0	3	1	10

FOOD	PORTION	CALS	PROT	FAT	CHOL	CARB	FIBER	SOD
Earthbound Farm								
Romaine Salad Organic	1½ cups (2.9 oz)	15	3	0	0	3	1	5
Green Giant								
Hearts Of Romaine	6 leaves	20	1	1	0	3	1	140
Ready Pac								
Baby Arugula	4 cups	20	2	1	0	3	2	25
Bella Romaine	1½ cups	15	1	0	0	2	1	5
LILY ROOT								
dried	1 oz	89	2	1	–	21	tr	25
fresh	1 oz	32	1	tr	–	8	tr	3
LIMA BEANS								
CANNED								
large	1 cup	191	12	tr	0	36	–	809
lima beans	½ cup	88	5	tr	0	17	5	312
Del Monte								
Green	½ cup (4.4 oz)	80	4	0	0	15	4	390
Eden								
Organic Baby	½ cup (4.6 oz)	100	6	1	0	17	4	35
S&W								
Small Green	½ cup (4.4 oz)	80	4	0	0	15	4	390
Veg-All								
Baby Green	½ cup	90	4	1	0	15	3	330
DRIED								
baby cooked	1 cup	229	15	1	0	42	17	5
cooked	½ cup	104	6	tr	0	20	–	14
large cooked	1 cup	217	15	1	0	39	14	4
FROZEN								
cooked	½ cup	94	6	tr	0	18	–	26
fordhook cooked	½ cup	85	5	tr	0	16	–	45
Birds Eye								
Baby	½ cup	130	7	0	0	24	6	115
Fordhook	½ cup	100	6	0	0	19	5	10
Fresh Like								
Baby	3.5 oz	138	7	1	–	25	2	106

FOOD	PORTION	CALS	PROT	FAT	CHOL	CARB	FIBER	SOD
LIME								
fresh	1	20	tr	tr	0	7	—	1
LIME JUICE								
bottled	1 tbsp	3	tr	tr	0	1	—	2
fresh	1 tbsp	4	tr	tr	0	1	—	0
limeade	1 can (6 oz)	408	tr	tr	0	108	—	—
FROZEN								
Odwalla								
Summertime Lime	8 fl oz	90	0	0	0	23	0	10
Realime								
Juice	1 tsp (5 ml)	0	0	0	0	0	—	0
LING								
blue raw	3.5 oz	83	17	1	—	0	—	—
fresh baked	3 oz	95	21	1	—	0	—	147
fresh fillet baked	5.3 oz	168	37	1	—	0	—	261
LINGCOD								
baked	3 oz	93	19	1	57	0	—	64
fillet baked	5.3 oz	164	34	2	101	0	—	114
LIQUOR/LIQUEUR *(see also* BEER AND ALE, CHAMPAGNE, WINE*)*								
7&7	1 serv	178	0	0	0	19	0	21
alabama slammer	1 serv	103	tr	tr	0	7	tr	tr
amaretto sour	1 serv	295	2	tr	0	57	4	98
angel's kiss	1 serv	85	tr	1	5	5	0	4
anisette	1 oz	111	—	0	0	11	0	—
antifreeze	1 serv	177	1	tr	0	31	tr	2
apricot brandy	1 oz	96	—	0	0	9	0	—
apricot sour	1 serv	164	tr	tr	0	8	tr	5
aquavit	1 oz	65	0	0	—	0	0	—
b 52	1 serv	247	1	4	0	25	0	24
b&b	1 serv	75	0	0	0	0	0	tr
bahama breeze	1 serv	70	tr	tr	0	9	tr	2
bahama mama	1 serv	153	1	tr	0	23	tr	2
bailey's & amaretto	1 serv	184	1	5	0	16	0	29
banana colada	1 serv	376	2	1	0	64	3	4
bay breeze	1 serv	173	1	tr	0	18	tr	2
bend me over	1 serv	242	1	tr	0	32	tr	33
benedictine	1 oz	104	—	0	0	11	0	—
betsy ross	1 serv	206	tr	0	0	5	0	3

FOOD	PORTION	CALS	PROT	FAT	CHOL	CARB	FIBER	SOD
black devil	1 serv	220	tr	tr	0	1	tr	43
black russian	1 serv	184	0	tr	0	12	0	3
bloody mary	1 serv	150	1	tr	0	5	1	332
blue whale	1 serv	222	tr	tr	0	23	0	63
bourbon & soda	1 serv (4 oz)	105	0	0	0	0	0	16
bourbon sour	1 serv	166	tr	tr	0	8	tr	5
brandy	2 oz	255	–	–	–	–	–	–
brandy alexander	1 serv	266	1	6	20	12	0	17
brandy sour	1 serv	164	tr	tr	0	8	tr	5
bushwacker	1 serv	286	tr	5	0	27	tr	23
campari	2 oz	245	–	–	–	–	–	–
cherry hering	2 oz	245	–	–	–	–	–	–
coffee liqueur	1 serv (1.5 oz)	175	tr	tr	0	24	0	4
coffee w/ cream liqueur	1 serv (1.5 oz)	154	1	7	7	10	0	43
cognac	1 oz	67	0	0	0	tr	0	–
cosmopolitan	1 serv	126	tr	tr	0	7	tr	1
creme de almonde	1 oz	102	–	–	–	–	–	–
creme de banana	1 oz	99	–	–	–	–	–	–
creme de cassis	1 oz	82	–	–	–	–	–	–
creme de menthe	1 serv (1.5 oz)	186	0	tr	0	21	0	3
curacao liqueur	1 oz	81	–	0	0	9	0	–
daiquiri	1 serv	187	0	0	0	15	0	7
daiquiri banana	1 serv	277	1	tr	0	32	1	7
dark & stormy	1 serv	64	0	0	0	0	0	tr
doctor pepper	1 serv	95	0	0	0	12	0	1
drambuie	2 oz	225	–	–	–	–	–	–
frozen daiquiri	1 serv	393	–	2	–	–	–	–
frozen daiquiri pineapple	1 serv	186	1	tr	0	28	2	3
frozen tequila screwdriver	1 serv	159	1	tr	0	17	1	2
fuzzy navel	1 serv	247	1	tr	0	10	tr	2
gibson	1 serv (4 oz)	254	–	–	–	–	–	–
gimlet vodka	1 serv	150	tr	tr	0	6	1	3
gin	1 serv (1.5 oz)	110	0	0	0	0	0	1

FOOD	PORTION	CALS	PROT	FAT	CHOL	CARB	FIBER	SOD
gin & tonic	1 serv (7.5 oz)	171	0	0	0	16	–	10
gin ricky	1 serv	114	tr	tr	0	1	tr	38
grasshopper	1 serv	275	1	5	15	26	0	13
happy hawaiian	1 serv	434	2	8	0	60	tr	50
harvey wallbanger	1 serv	198	1	tr	0	16	tr	2
head banger	1 serv	165	0	0	0	4	0	tr
hot buttered rum	1 serv	219	tr	4	10	15	4	48
hot toddy	1 serv	188	tr	1	0	13	5	9
hurricane	1 serv	205	tr	tr	0	19	tr	2
kamikaze	1 serv	136	0	0	0	2	0	2
long island iced tea	1 serv	292	tr	tr	0	7	0	33
lynchburg lemonade	1 serv	465	tr	tr	0	85	1	38
mai tai	1 serv	165	tr	tr	0	17	tr	51
manhattan	1 serv	171	tr	tr	0	3	tr	9
margarita	1 serv	173	0	0	0	11	0	3
margarita strawberry	1 serv	106	tr	tr	0	11	1	1
martini apple	1 serv	147	tr	tr	0	4	tr	2
martini rum	1 serv	131	tr	0	0	tr	tr	1
martini vodka	1 serv	135	tr	tr	0	1	tr	45
mellow yellow	1 serv	95	0	0	0	4	0	0
mexican grasshopper	1 serv	638	1	19	66	52	0	29
mint julep	1 serv	136	tr	tr	0	17	tr	3
mississippi mud	1 serv	496	3	12	45	46	0	46
mudslide	1 serv	566	2	10	0	46	0	65
narragansett	1 serv	168	0	0	0	2	0	5
nutcracker	1 serv	730	2	10	0	64	0	65
old fashioned	1 serv	223	tr	tr	0	4	tr	5
orange crush	1 serv	461	0	tr	0	65	tr	5
pain killer	1 serv	277	1	tr	0	20	tr	5
peppermint pattie	1 serv	344	tr	tr	0	37	0	7
pina colada	1 serv (4.5 oz)	262	1	3	0	40	tr	9
planter's cocktail	1 serv	105	tr	0	0	3	tr	1
planter's punch	1 serv	233	2	tr	0	34	4	33
presbyterian	1 serv	170	tr	0	0	8	tr	26
purple passion	1 serv	215	tr	tr	0	22	0	14

FOOD	PORTION	CALS	PROT	FAT	CHOL	CARB	FIBER	SOD
rob roy	1 serv	171	tr	0	0	3	tr	13
rum	1 serv (1.5 oz)	97	0	0	0	0	0	0
rum boogie	1 serv	134	tr	tr	0	12	tr	3
rum cola	1 serv	209	tr	tr	0	21	tr	8
rum highball	1 serv	170	0	0	0	11	0	9
rum punch	1 serv	448	1	1	0	88	1	12
rusty nail	1 serv	159	0	0	0	6	0	tr
salty dog	1 serv	210	1	tr	0	19	tr	3
scotch & soda	1 serv	104	tr	0	0	tr	tr	38
screwdriver rum	1 serv	166	1	tr	0	16	tr	2
sea breeze	1 serv	207	tr	tr	0	19	tr	3
sex on the beach	1 serv	190	tr	tr	0	18	tr	2
singapore sling	1 serv (4 oz)	115	–	–	–	–	–	–
slippery nipple	1 serv	142	tr	2	0	11	0	16
sloe gin fizz	1 serv (2.5 oz)	132	0	0	0	4	0	1
snake bite	1 serv	362	0	0	0	22	0	7
sour rum	1 serv	156	tr	tr	0	8	tr	5
southern comfort	1 serv (1.5 oz)	184	–	–	–	–	–	–
swizzle rum	1 serv	187	0	0	0	15	0	44
tequila	1 serv (1.5 oz)	117	–	–	–	–	–	–
tequila gimlet	1 serv	150	tr	tr	0	6	1	3
tequila sour	1 serv	156	tr	tr	0	8	tr	5
tequila stinger	1 serv	221	0	tr	0	14	0	2
tequila sunrise	1 serv (6.8 oz)	232	1	tr	0	24	0	120
tom collins	1 serv (7.5 oz)	121	tr	0	0	3	–	39
vermouth cassis	1 serv	97	tr	tr	0	5	tr	54
vodka	1 serv (1.5 oz)	97	0	0	0	0	0	0
vodka sour	1 serv	138	tr	tr	0	3	tr	1
vodka stinger	1 serv	378	0	tr	0	28	0	4
whiskey	1 serv (1.5 oz)	105	0	0	0	tr	0	0
whiskey sour	1 serv	159	tr	0	0	6	tr	8

FOOD	PORTION	CALS	PROT	FAT	CHOL	CARB	FIBER	SOD
white russian	1 serv	290	tr	8	31	17	0	12
zombie	1 serv	235	tr	tr	0	10	tr	5

LITCHI JUICE
Ceres
| Litchi | 8 oz | 120 | 0 | 0 | 0 | 30 | 0 | 10 |

LIVER (see also PATE)
beef braised	3 oz	137	21	4	331	3	—	59
beef pan-fried	3 oz	184	23	7	410	7	—	90
chicken stewed	1 cup (5 oz)	219	34	8	883	1	—	71
duck raw	1 (1.5 oz)	60	8	2	227	2	—	—
goose raw	1 (3.3 oz)	125	15	4	—	6	—	132
lamb braised	3 oz	187	26	7	426	2	—	48
lamb fried	3 oz	202	22	11	419	3	—	105
pork braised	3 oz	140	22	4	302	3	0	42
sheep raw	3.5 oz	131	21	4	—	0	—	95
turkey simmered	1 cup (5 oz)	237	34	8	876	5	—	89
veal braised	3 oz	140	18	6	477	2	—	45
veal fried	3 oz	208	25	10	280	3	—	112

LIVER SUBSTITUTES
Sabra
| Vegetarian Liver | 1 oz | 70 | 1 | 7 | 14 | 1 | 1 | 87 |

LOBSTER
northern cooked	1 cup	142	30	1	104	2	—	551
northern cooked	3 oz	83	17	1	61	1	—	323
northern raw	3 oz	77	77	1	81	tr	—	—
northern raw	1 lobster (5.3 oz)	136	28	1	143	1	—	—
spiny steamed	3 oz	122	22	2	76	3	—	193
spiny steamed	1 (5.7 oz)	233	43	3	146	5	—	370
Progresso								
Lobster Sauce	½ cup (4.3 oz)	100	3	7	5	6	2	430

TAKE-OUT
| newburg | 1 cup | 485 | 46 | 27 | 455 | 13 | — | 127 |

LOGANBERRIES
| frzn | 1 cup | 80 | 2 | tr | 0 | 19 | — | 1 |

FOOD	PORTION	CALS	PROT	FAT	CHOL	CARB	FIBER	SOD
LONGANS								
fresh	1	2	tr	0	0	tr	–	0
LOQUATS								
fresh	1	5	tr	tr	0	1	–	0
LOTUS								
root raw sliced	10 slices	45	2	tr	0	14	–	33
root sliced cooked	10 slices	59	1	tr	0	14	–	40
seeds dried	1 oz	94	4	1	0	18	–	1
Eden								
Root	1 serv (0.3 oz)	35	1	0	0	8	2	25
LOX (see SALMON)								
LUPINES								
dried cooked	1 cup	197	26	5	0	16	–	7
LYCHEES								
fresh	1	6	tr	tr	0	2	–	0
MACADAMIA NUTS								
dry roasted w/ salt	10–12 nuts (1 oz)	200	2	22	0	4	1	80
oil roasted	1 oz	204	2	22	0	4	–	3
Hawaiian Host								
Chocolate Covered	1 piece (0.5 oz)	53	1	6	2	8	tr	15
Keto								
Chocolately Covered	1 oz	171	2	19	–	6	4	–
Maranatha								
Macadamia Butter	2 tbsp	230	3	24	–	5	3	0
Mauna Loa								
Chocolate Trio	9 pieces	200	2	15	5	19	2	10
Dry Roasted Salted	¼ cup	200	2	21	0	4	2	60
Dry Roasted Unsalted	¼ cup	200	2	21	0	4	2	0
Honey Roasted	¼ cup	210	2	21	0	6	2	35
Kona Coffee Glazed	¼ cup	190	2	15	<5	10	1	55
Maui Onion & Garlic	¼ cup	200	2	16	0	18	3	0

FOOD	PORTION	CALS	PROT	FAT	CHOL	CARB	FIBER	SOD
Milk Chocolate Coated	13 pieces	200	2	12	5	25	1	10
Milk Chocolate Toffee	7 pieces	210	2	13	5	23	1	70

MACE
| ground | 1 tsp | 8 | tr | 1 | 0 | 1 | — | 1 |

MACKEREL
CANNED
| jack | 1 can (12.7 oz) | 563 | 84 | 23 | 285 | 0 | — | 1368 |
| jack | 1 cup | 296 | 44 | 12 | 150 | 0 | — | 720 |

DRIED
Eden
| Bonito Flakes | 2 tbsp | 4 | 1 | 0 | 1 | 0 | 0 | 4 |

FRESH
atlantic cooked	3 oz	223	20	15	64	0	—	71
atlantic raw	3 oz	174	16	12	60	0	—	76
jack baked	3 oz	171	22	9	51	0	—	94
jack fillet baked	6.2 oz	354	45	18	106	0	—	194
king baked	3 oz	114	22	2	58	0	—	172
king fillet baked	5.4 oz	207	40	4	105	0	—	312
pacific baked	3 oz	171	22	9	51	0	—	94
pacific fillet baked	6.2 oz	354	45	18	106	0	—	194
spanish cooked	3 oz	134	20	5	62	0	—	56
spanish cooked	1 fillet (5.1 oz)	230	34	9	107	0	—	96
spanish raw	3 oz	118	16	5	65	0	—	50

SMOKED
| atlantic | 3.5 oz | 296 | 19 | 24 | 93 | 0 | — | 384 |

MALANGA
| fresh | ½ cup | 137 | 2 | tr | — | 32 | — | — |

MALT
| nonalcoholic | 12 fl oz | 32 | 1 | 0 | 0 | 5 | — | — |
Skyy
| Blue | 1 bottle | 235 | — | — | — | 35 | — | — |
| Sport | 1 bottle | 160 | — | — | — | 15 | — | — |

FOOD	PORTION	CALS	PROT	FAT	CHOL	CARB	FIBER	SOD
MALTED MILK								
chocolate as prep w/ milk	1 cup	229	9	9	34	30	–	172
chocolate flavor powder	3 heaping tsp (¾ oz)	79	1	1	1	18	–	53
natural flavor as prep w/ milk	1 cup	237	10	10	37	27	–	223
natural flavor powder	3 heaping tsp (¾ oz)	87	2	2	4	19	–	103
MAMMY-APPLE								
fresh	1	431	4	4	0	106	–	127
MANGO								
fresh	1	135	1	1	0	35	–	4
Del Monte								
In Extra Light Syrup	½ cup (4.4 oz)	100	0	1	0	25	0	5
Tomorrow's Tropicals								
Fresh	½ (3.6 oz)	70	0	1	0	17	1	0
MANGO JUICE								
Ceres								
Mango	8 oz	120	0	0	0	30	1	10
Fresh Samantha								
Mango Mama	1 cup (8 oz)	120	2	0	0	10	8	0
Guzzler								
Mango Passion	8 fl oz	140	0	0	0	22	–	30
Langers								
Mongo Mango	8 oz	120	0	0	0	30	–	0
Naked Juice								
Mighty Mango	8 oz	120	1	0	0	30	0	15
Snapple								
Mango Madness	8 fl oz	110	0	0	0	29	–	10
MARGARINE								
squeeze	1 tsp	34	tr	4	0	0	–	37
stick corn	1 stick (4 oz)	815	1	91	0	1	–	1070
stick corn	1 tsp	34	0	4	0	0	–	44
tub corn	1 tsp	34	0	4	0	0	–	51
tub diet	1 tsp	17	0	2	0	0	–	46

FOOD	PORTION	CALS	PROT	FAT	CHOL	CARB	FIBER	SOD
Benecol								
Single Serve Light	1 pkg (0.3 oz)	30	–	3	0	–	–	65
Tub Light	1 tbsp (0.5 oz)	45	–	5	0	–	–	110
Tub Regular	1 tbsp (0.5 oz)	80	–	9	0	–	–	110
Blue Bonnet								
Light Stick	1 tbsp	50	0	5	0	tr	–	90
Soft Spread	1 tbsp	60	0	7	0	0	0	110
Soft Spread Light	1 tbsp	40	0	5	0	tr	–	90
Stick	1 tbsp	80	0	9	0	0	0	110
Brummel & Brown								
Spread Make With Yogurt	1 tbsp (0.5 oz)	45	0	5	0	0	0	90
I Can't Believe It's Not Butter								
Spray	5 sprays	0	0	0	0	0	0	0
Take Control								
Light	1 tbsp	45	0	5	<5	0	–	85
Spread	1 tbsp (0.5 oz)	80	0	8	<5	0	0	85

MARINADE (see SAUCE)

MARJORAM

FOOD	PORTION	CALS	PROT	FAT	CHOL	CARB	FIBER	SOD
dried	1 tsp	2	tr	tr	0	tr	–	tr

MARLIN

FOOD	PORTION	CALS	PROT	FAT	CHOL	CARB	FIBER	SOD
raw	3 oz	110	20	3	–	0	0	–

MARSHMALLOW

FOOD	PORTION	CALS	PROT	FAT	CHOL	CARB	FIBER	SOD
marshmallow	1 reg (0.3 oz)	23	tr	0	0	6	–	3
marshmallow	1 cup (1.6 oz)	146	1	tr	0	37	–	22
Gol D Lite								
Sugar Free	⅓ pkg (0.9 oz)	51	0	0	0	19	0	0

MATZO

FOOD	PORTION	CALS	PROT	FAT	CHOL	CARB	FIBER	SOD
egg	1 (1 oz)	111	4	1	–	22	1	6
egg & onion	1 (1 oz)	111	3	1	–	22	1	81
plain	1 (1 oz)	112	3	tr	0	24	1	0
whole wheat	1 (1 oz)	99	4	tr	0	22	3	1

FOOD	PORTION	CALS	PROT	FAT	CHOL	CARB	FIBER	SOD
Eddyleon								
Dark Chocolate Coated Egg Matzo	1 oz	97	27	3	8	17	1	7
Milk Chocolate Coated Egg Matzo	1 oz	97	3	4	8	16	1	7
Manischewitz								
Matzo Meal	¼ cup (1 oz)	130	3	0	0	23	1	0
MAYONNAISE								
mayonnaise	1 cup	1577	2	175	130	6	–	1250
mayonnaise	1 tbsp	99	tr	11	8	tr	–	78
reduced calorie	1 tbsp	34	0	3	4	2	–	75
reduced calorie	1 cup	556	1	46	58	38	–	1193
sandwich spread	1 tbsp	60	tr	5	12	3	–	–
Blue Plate								
Squeeze	1 tbsp	100	0	11	10	0	0	80
Hellman's								
Mayonnaise	1 tbsp	100	0	11	5	0	–	80
MAYONNAISE-TYPE SALAD DRESSING								
mayonnaise-type salad dressing	1 tbsp	57	tr	5	4	4	–	–
mayonnaise-type salad dressing	1 cup	916	2	78	60	56	–	1670
reduced calorie w/o cholesterol	1 tbsp	68	7	7	0	2	–	49
reduced calorie w/o cholesterol	1 cup	1084	tr	107	0	36	–	794
Carb Options								
Whipped Dressing	1 tbsp	50	0	5	5	0	0	105
Nasoya								
Nayonaise	1 tbsp	35	0	4	0	1	0	115
Nayonaise Dijon	1 tbsp	30	0	3	0	1	0	140
MEAT STICKS								
jerky beef	1 lg piece (0.7 oz)	67	8	3	22	3	–	569
jerky beef	1 oz	96	11	4	32	4	–	815
smoked	1 oz	156	6	14	38	2	–	420
smoked	1 (0.7 oz)	109	4	10	26	1	–	293

FOOD	PORTION	CALS	PROT	FAT	CHOL	CARB	FIBER	SOD
Big Ones								
BBQ	1 (1 oz)	130	5	12	35	1	0	680
Hot n'Spicy	1 (1 oz)	130	6	12	35	1	0	580
Original	1 (1 oz)	130	5	12	35	1	0	620
Teriyaki	1 (1 oz)	130	6	12	35	2	0	440
Jack Link's								
Kippered Beefsteak Teriyaki	1 oz	80	13	1	25	5	0	440
Lowrey's								
Smokehouse Tender Hickory Smoked	1 pkg (1 oz)	80	10	2	25	5	0	710
Smokehouse Tender Original	1 pkg (1 oz)	60	11	1	25	2	1	750
Smokehouse Tender Peppered	1 pkg (1 oz)	60	11	1	25	2	1	720
Oberto								
Beef Jerky	1 pkg (1.3 oz)	100	15	1	25	8	–	780
Rustlers Roundup								
Beef Jerky	1 serv (5 g)	20	2	2	5	tr	tr	115
Flamin' Hot	1 serv (8 g)	40	2	3	10	1	tr	140
Smoky Steak	1 serv (0.8 oz)	60	8	2	20	1	0	580
Spicy	1 serv (0.5 oz)	70	3	6	20	1	tr	250

MEAT SUBSTITUTES *(see also* BACON SUBSTITUTES, CANADIAN BACON SUBSTITUTES, CHICKEN SUBSTITUTES, HAMBURGER SUBSTITUTES, SAUSAGE SUBSTITUTES, TURKEY SUBSTITUTES)

FOOD	PORTION	CALS	PROT	FAT	CHOL	CARB	FIBER	SOD
simulated meat product	1 oz	88	11	1	0	11	–	3
Frieda's								
Soyrizo	4 tbsp (1.9 oz)	120	7	9	0	5	3	440
SoyTaco	1 oz	50	4	3	0	3	2	180
Ken & Robert's								
Veggie Pockets	1 (4.5 oz)	250	8	8	0	40	5	490
Veggie Pockets Bar B Que	1 (4.5 oz)	290	10	8	0	45	5	450

FOOD	PORTION	CALS	PROT	FAT	CHOL	CARB	FIBER	SOD
Veggie Pockets Broccoli & Cheddar	1 (4.5 oz)	250	9	8	0	38	4	490
Veggie Pockets Greek	1 (4.5 oz)	250	10	8	0	37	4	450
Veggie Pockets Indian	1 (4.5 oz)	260	8	8	0	40	5	490
Veggie Pockets Pizza	1 (4.5 oz)	270	9	8	0	41	4	490
Veggie Pockets Pot Pie	1 (4.5 oz)	250	8	9	0	38	2	410
Veggie Pockets Potato & Cheddar	1 (4.5 oz)	260	6	8	0	42	2	370
Veggie Pockets Santa Fe	1 (4.5 oz)	250	8	8	0	39	5	550
Veggie Pockets Tex Mex	1 (4.5 oz)	260	9	8	0	46	6	490
Lightlife								
Foney Baloney	3 slices (1.5 oz)	60	8	3	0	2	0	240
Gimme Lean Beef	2 oz	70	9	0	0	8	1	240
Smart Deli Bologna	3 slices (1.5 oz)	50	10	0	0	2	0	300
Smart Deli Ham	3 slices (1.5 oz)	50	10	0	0	2	0	300
Smart Deli Peppercorn	3 slices (1.5 oz)	45	10	0	0	1	0	300
Smart Deli Sticks Soylami	1 oz	40	9	0	0	1	0	280
Smart Deli Sticks Pepperoni	1 oz	45	9	0	0	2	0	300
Smart Ground Original	⅓ cup (1.9 oz)	70	12	0	0	5	3	180
Smart Ground Taco	⅓ cup (2 oz)	60	10	0	0	6	3	170
Loma Linda								
Dinner Cuts	2 slices (3.2 oz)	90	17	2	0	3	2	500
Nuteena	⅜ in slice (1.9 oz)	160	6	13	0	6	2	120
Sandwich Spread	¼ cup (1.9 oz)	80	4	5	0	7	3	260

FOOD	PORTION	CALS	PROT	FAT	CHOL	CARB	FIBER	SOD
Savory Dinner Loaf Mix not prep	⅓ cup (0.9 oz)	90	14	2	0	7	5	560
Swiss Stake	1 piece (3.2 oz)	120	9	6	0	8	4	430
Tender Bits	6 pieces (3 oz)	110	11	5	0	7	3	440
Tender Rounds	6 pieces (2.8 oz)	120	14	5	0	5	3	330
Vita Burger Chunks not prep	¼ cup (0.7 oz)	70	10	1	0	6	3	350
Vita Burger Granules	3 tbsp (0.7 oz)	70	10	1	0	6	3	350
Morningstar Farms								
Burger Style Recipe Crumbles	⅔ cup (1.9 oz)	80	10	3	0	4	2	210
Ground Meatless	½ cup (1.9 oz)	60	10	0	0	4	2	260
Harvest Burger Recipe Crumbles	½ cup (2 oz)	70	12	0	0	5	3	200
Quarter Prime	1 patty (3.4 oz)	140	24	2	0	6	3	370
Natural Touch								
Dinner Entree	1 patty (3 oz)	220	19	15	0	2	2	380
Loaf Mix not prep	4 tbsp (1 oz)	100	14	1	0	10	7	700
Stroganoff Mix not prep	4 tbsp (0.8 oz)	90	5	4	10	10	3	610
Taco Mix not prep	3 tbsp (0.6 oz)	60	8	1	0	5	3	590
Vegan Burger Crumbles	½ cup (1.9 oz)	60	10	0	0	4	2	260
Quorn								
Grounds	⅔ cup (3 oz)	80	13	3	0	5	4	220
Soy7								
Burger Bits as prep	½ cup	60	9	1	0	5	2	340
Burger Mix as prep	1 serv (3.2 oz)	120	16	3	0	9	3	400
Recipe Strips as prep	¾ cup	70	11	1	0	7	3	340
Taco Mix as prep	¼ cup	70	11	1	0	6	3	100

FOOD	PORTION	CALS	PROT	FAT	CHOL	CARB	FIBER	SOD
Worthington								
Beef Style Meatless	⅜ in slice (1.9 oz)	110	9	7	0	4	3	620
Bolono	3 slices (2 oz)	80	10	4	0	2	2	720
Choplets	2 slices (3.2 oz)	90	17	2	0	3	2	500
Corned Beef Meatless	4 slices (2 oz)	140	10	9	0	5	2	520
Country Stew	1 cup (8.4 oz)	210	13	9	0	20	5	830
Dinner Roast	¾ in slice (3 oz)	180	12	12	<5	5	3	580
FriPats	1 patty (2.2 oz)	130	14	6	0	4	3	320
Multigrain Cutlets	2 slices (3.2 oz)	100	15	2	0	5	4	390
Numete	⅜ in slice (1.9 oz)	130	6	10	0	5	3	270
Prime Stakes	1 piece (3.2 oz)	120	10	7	0	4	4	440
Prosage Roll	⅝ in slice (1.9 oz)	140	10	10	0	2	2	390
Protose	⅜ in slice (1.9 oz)	130	13	7	0	5	3	280
Yves								
Veggie Bologna	4 slices (2.2 oz)	70	15	0	0	2	0	460
Veggie Ground Italian	⅓ cup (2 oz)	60	10	0	0	4	3	270
Veggie Ground Round Italian	⅓ cup (1.9 oz)	60	10	0	0	4	3	270
Veggie Ground Round Original	2 oz	60	10	0	0	4	3	270
Veggie Pizza Pepperoni Slices	1 serv (1.7 oz)	70	14	0	0	4	3	480
Veggie Salami Deli Slices	1 serv (2.2 oz)	90	17	0	0	5	1	390
MELON								
melon balls frzn	1 cup	55	1	tr	0	14	–	53

FOOD	PORTION	CALS	PROT	FAT	CHOL	CARB	FIBER	SOD
SunFresh								
Melon Salad In Extra Light Syrup	½ cup (4.5 oz)	45	0	0	0	10	2	15

MEXICAN FOOD *(see SALSA, SPANISH FOOD, TORTILLA)*

MILK
CANNED
condensed sweetened	1 cup	982	24	27	104	166	–	389
condensed sweetened	1 oz	123	3	3	13	21	–	49
evaporated	½ cup	169	9	10	37	13	–	122
evaporated skim	½ cup	99	10	tr	5	14	–	147
Carnation								
Evaporated	2 tbsp	40	2	2	10	3	–	30
Evaporated Fat Free	2 tbsp	25	2	0	0	4	–	40
Sweetened Condensed	⅓ cup	330	3	8	10	22	0	45
Pet								
Evaporated	2 tbsp	40	2	2	10	3	–	30

DRIED
buttermilk	1 tbsp	25	2	tr	5	3	–	34
nonfat instantized	1 pkg (3.2 oz)	244	32	tr	12	47	–	499
Carnation								
Nonfat	⅓ cup	80	8	0	<5	12	0	125
Sanalac								
Powder	¼ cup (0.8 oz)	85	8	tr	6	13	0	117

REFRIGERATED
1%	1 qt	409	32	10	39	47	–	493
1%	1 cup	102	8	3	10	12	–	123
1% protein fortified	1 qt	477	39	12	39	54	–	574
1% protein fortified	1 cup	119	10	3	10	14	–	143
2%	1 qt	485	33	19	73	47	–	487
2%	1 cup	121	8	5	18	12	–	122
buffalo	7 oz	224	8	16	–	10	–	80
buttermilk	1 qt	396	32	9	34	47	–	1028
buttermilk	1 cup	99	8	2	9	12	–	257
camel	7 oz	160	10	8	–	10	–	60

FOOD	PORTION	CALS	PROT	FAT	CHOL	CARB	FIBER	SOD
donkey	7 oz	86	4	2	–	12	–	–
goat	1 qt	672	35	40	111	43	–	486
goat	1 cup	168	9	10	28	11	–	122
human	1 cup	171	3	11	34	17	–	42
indian buffalo	1 cup	236	9	17	46	13	–	127
low sodium	1 cup	149	8	8	33	11	–	6
mare	7 oz	98	4	4	–	12	–	–
nonfat	1 qt	342	33	2	18	48	–	505
nonfat	1 cup	86	8	tr	4	12	–	125
nonfat protein fortified	1 qt	400	39	2	20	55	–	578
nonfat protein fortified	1 cup	100	10	1	5	14	–	144
sheep	1 cup	264	15	17	–	13	–	108
whole	1 cup	150	8	8	33	11	–	120
Borden								
Fat Free Skim	1 cup	80	8	0	5	12	0	125
Hood								
Carb Countdown	8 oz	138	12	8	35	3	0	210
Carb Countdown 2%	8 oz	100	12	5	20	3	0	210
Carb Countdown Fat Free	8 oz	78	12	0	<5	3	0	210
Horizon Organic								
Fat Free	1 cup (8 oz)	80	8	0	4	12	0	125
Land O Lakes								
1% Low fat	1 carton (10 oz)	120	10	3	15	13	–	135
Fat Free	1 carton (10 oz)	100	10	5	5	13	–	140
Whole	1 carton (10 oz)	180	10	10	45	13	–	135
Stonyfield Farm								
Organic Whole Milk	1 cup (8 oz)	180	9	10	40	12	0	125
Organic Whole Milk Vanilla	1 cup (8 oz)	230	8	8	30	30	0	130
Turkey Hill								
Cool Moos 2% Reduced Fat	1 cup	130	8	5	20	12	–	120

FOOD	PORTION	CALS	PROT	FAT	CHOL	CARB	FIBER	SOD
Cool Moos Whole Milk	1 cup	160	8	8	35	12	—	120

MILK DRINKS

FOOD	PORTION	CALS	PROT	FAT	CHOL	CARB	FIBER	SOD
chocolate milk	1 qt	833	32	34	122	103	—	596
chocolate milk	1 cup	208	8	8	30	26	—	149
chocolate milk 1%	1 qt	630	32	10	29	104	—	607
chocolate milk 1%	1 cup	158	8	3	7	26	—	152
chocolate milk 2%	1 cup	179	8	5	17	26	—	150
strawberry flavor mix as prep w/ whole milk	9 oz	234	8	8	33	33	—	128
Cocio								
Chocolate Milk	1 bottle	225	9	7	25	32	tr	130
Garelick								
Colossal Coffee	1 cup	145	8	3	15	23	0	125
Ultimate Chocolate	1 cup	150	8	3	15	29	1	210
Hershey's								
Chocolate Milk Fat Free	1 bottle	160	10	0	5	31	tr	150
Chocolate Milk Reduced Fat	1 bottle	200	8	5	20	31	1	135
Hood								
Carb Countdown Chocolate Milk	8 oz	100	12	5	25	3	1	350
Horizon Organic								
Lowfat Chocolate Milk	1 cup (8 oz)	160	9	3	10	26	1	200
Keto								
Chocolate Milk Mix	1 scoop	36	8	1	—	3	1	80
Land O Lakes								
Chocolate	1 cup (8.4 oz)	200	8	7	30	27	0	180
Nesquik								
Chocolate Milk Reduced Fat	1 cup	200	8	5	15	32	tr	150
Quik								
Banana Lowfat	1 cup (8.4 oz)	200	7	5	20	31	0	95

FOOD	PORTION	CALS	PROT	FAT	CHOL	CARB	FIBER	SOD
Banana Powder	2 tbsp (0.8 oz)	90	0	0	0	27	0	0
Chocolate	1 cup (8.4 oz)	230	7	8	30	33	1	130
Chocolate Lowfat	1 carton (8.4 oz)	200	8	5	20	30	0	130
Cookies n Cream Powder	2 tbsp (0.8 oz)	100	1	1	0	21	1	190
Strawberry	1 cup (8.4 oz)	230	7	8	30	33	0	100
Strawberry Lowfat	1 carton (8.4 oz)	210	8	5	20	35	0	100
Strawberry Powder	2 tbsp (0.8 oz)	90	0	0	0	22	0	0
Rosa's Original								
Horchata All Flavors	8 oz	160	3	2	5	32	0	60
Turkey Hill								
Cool Moos Chocolate 1% Low fat	1 cup	180	8	3	10	32	–	180
Cool Moos Orange Cream 1% Low fat	1 cup	190	8	3	10	33	–	135
Cool Moos Strawberry 1% Low fat	1 cup	160	8	3	10	27	–	125
Cool Moos Vanilla 1% Low fat	1 cup	160	8	3	10	26	–	125

MILK SUBSTITUTES

FOOD	PORTION	CALS	PROT	FAT	CHOL	CARB	FIBER	SOD
imitation milk	1 qt	600	17	33	2	60	–	764
imitation milk	1 cup	150	4	8	tr	15	–	191
8th Continent								
Soymilk Low Fat Chocolate	1 bottle (8 oz)	140	7	3	0	23	1	190
Soymilk Low Fat Original	1 bottle (8 oz)	80	7	3	0	8	tr	170
Soymilk Low Fat Vanilla	1 bottle (8 oz)	90	7	3	0	11	tr	170

FOOD	PORTION	CALS	PROT	FAT	CHOL	CARB	FIBER	SOD
Better Than Milk								
Rice Original	2 tbsp (0.66 oz)	78	0	2	0	15	1	150
Rice Original Light	2 tbsp (0.66 oz)	66	0	0	0	17	1	144
Rice Vanilla	2 tbsp (0.66 oz)	78	0	2	0	15	1	118
Rice Vanilla Light	2 tbsp (0.66 oz)	66	0	0	0	17	1	141
Soy Carob	2 tbsp (1 oz)	90	3	2	0	18	2	165
Soy Chocolate	2 tbsp (1.1 oz)	112	3	2	0	21	1	146
Soy Light	2 tbsp (0.66 oz)	73	6	2	0	8	1	139
Soy Original	2 tbsp (0.8 oz)	100	2	3	0	16	0	100
Soy Vanilla	2 tbsp (0.7 oz)	77	6	2	0	8	1	178
Blue Diamond								
Almond Breeze Chocolate	8 oz	120	1	3	0	21	1	160
Almond Breeze Original	8 oz	60	1	2	0	8	1	150
Almond Breeze Vanilla	8 oz	90	1	3	0	15	1	150
EdenBlend								
Organic	8 oz	120	7	3	0	18	0	85
Edensoy								
Organic Light	8 oz	93	5	2	0	14	0	84
Organic Light Vanilla	8 oz	120	4	2	0	21	0	87
Galaxy								
Veggie Milk Chocolate	1 cup (8 oz)	150	9	2	0	26	1	130
Veggie Milk Original	1 cup (8 oz)	110	9	3	0	13	2	130
Hansen's								
Soy Smoothie Lemon Chiffon	8 oz	150	5	0	0	33	tr	41

FOOD	PORTION	CALS	PROT	FAT	CHOL	CARB	FIBER	SOD
Soy Smoothie Orange Dream	8 oz	150	5	0	0	31	tr	41
Harmony Farms								
Original Rice Beverage	1 cup (8 oz)	90	13	0	0	21	0	100
Harmony House								
Enriched Rice Beverage	1 cup (8 oz)	90	1	0	0	21	0	100
Enriched Soy Beverage	1 cup (8 oz)	90	13	0	0	21	0	100
Original Soy Beverage	1 cup (8 oz)	90	13	0	0	21	0	100
Keto								
Low Carb Mix	1 scoop	54	8	2	30	1	–	80
Rice Dream								
Carob	1 box (8 oz)	150	1	3	0	32	0	100
Chocolate	1 box (8 oz)	170	1	3	0	36	2	115
Chocolate Enriched	1 box (8 oz)	170	1	3	0	36	0	115
Organic Original	1 box (8 oz)	120	1	2	0	25	0	90
Organic Original Enriched	1 box (8 oz)	120	1	2	0	25	0	90
Vanilla	1 box (8 oz)	130	1	2	0	28	0	90
Vanilla Enriched	1 box (8 oz)	130	1	2	0	28	0	90
Silk								
Chocolate	1 cup	140	5	4	0	23	0	75
Organic Plain	1 cup	100	7	4	0	8	0	75
Vanilla	1 bottle (11 oz)	140	8	5	0	14	0	130
Soy Dream								
Carob	8 oz	210	7	5	–	36	–	150
Chocolate Enriched	8 oz	210	7	5	–	35	–	150
Original	8 oz	140	8	5	–	14	–	140
Original Enriched	8 oz	140	8	5	–	14	–	140
Vanilla	8 oz	170	8	5	–	23	–	140
Vanilla Enriched	8 oz	140	8	5	–	23	–	160
Tree Of Life								
Original Rice Beverage	1 cup	90	13	0	0	21	0	100
Vitamite								
Non-Dairy	1 cup (8 oz)	110	3	5	0	14	0	120

FOOD	PORTION	CALS	PROT	FAT	CHOL	CARB	FIBER	SOD
Vitasoy								
1% Low Fat Vanilla Delight	8 oz	90	4	2	0	13	0	120
Carob Supreme	8 fl oz	150	8	5	0	20	tr	180
Creamy Unsweetened	8 oz	80	6	4	0	5	0	150
Creamy Original	8 fl oz	110	9	5	0	9	1	150
Enriched Light Original	8 fl oz	60	4	2	0	7	0	115
Enriched Light Vanilla	8 fl oz	90	4	2	0	13	0	105
Green Tea Soymilk	8 oz	130	7	4	0	16	1	180
Original Creamy	8 fl oz	110	7	4	0	12	1	140
Original Light	8 fl oz	60	4	2	0	7	0	115
Rich Chocolate	8 fl oz	160	7	4	0	24	1	180
Rich Cocoa	8 fl oz	150	8	5	0	21	1	180
Vanilla Light	8 fl oz	90	4	2	0	14	0	110
Vanilla Delite	8 fl oz	120	7	4	0	14	1	115
White Wave								
Mocha	1 cup	140	6	4	0	20	1	50
MILKFISH								
baked	3 oz	162	22	7	57	0	–	–
MILKSHAKE								
chocolate	10 oz	360	10	11	37	58	–	273
strawberry	10 oz	319	10	8	31	53	–	234
thick shake chocolate	10.6 oz	356	9	8	32	63	–	333
thick shake vanilla	11 oz	350	12	10	37	56	–	299
vanilla	10 oz	314	10	8	32	51	–	232
Breyers								
Quick Vanilla	1 serv (10 oz)	320	6	17	45	37	0	95
Carb Options								
Chocolate Delite	1 can (11 oz)	190	20	9	15	6	4	200
Creamy Vanilla	1 can (11 oz)	190	20	9	15	6	4	200
Hershey's								
Chocolate	1 bottle	270	10	8	20	43	tr	140
Cookies 'N' Cream	1 bottle	280	10	7	20	45	0	180
Strawberry	1 bottle	280	7	7	20	47	10	180

FOOD	PORTION	CALS	PROT	FAT	CHOL	CARB	FIBER	SOD
Vanilla Cream	1 bottle	320	9	7	20	55	0	240

MILLET
| cooked | 1 cup (6.1 oz) | 207 | 6 | 2 | 0 | 41 | 2 | 3 |

MINERAL WATER (see WATER)

MISO
dried	1 oz	86	7	3	–	10	1	2130
miso	½ cup	284	16	8	0	39	7	5036
Eden								
Organic Genmai	1 tbsp	25	2	1	0	3	tr	810
Tekka	1 tsp	5	tr	0	0	tr	0	70

MOLASSES
blackstrap	1 tbsp (0.7 oz)	47	0	0	0	12	–	11
blackstrap	1 cup (11.5 oz)	771	0	tr	0	199	–	180
molasses	1 tbsp (0.7 oz)	53	0	0	0	14	–	7
molasses	1 cup (11.5 oz)	873	0	1	0	226	–	120
Brer Rabbit								
Dark	1 tbsp	60	0	0	0	16	–	30
Mott's								
Sulphured	1 tbsp	50	0	0	0	12	–	10
Unsulphured	1 tbsp	50	0	0	0	14	–	0

MONKFISH
| baked | 3 oz | 82 | 16 | 2 | 27 | 0 | – | 20 |

MOOSE
| roasted | 3 oz | 114 | 25 | 1 | 66 | 0 | – | 58 |

MOTH BEANS
| dried cooked | 1 cup | 207 | 14 | 1 | 0 | 37 | – | 17 |

MOUSSE
FROZEN
Sara Lee
| Chocolate | ⅓ pkg (4.3 oz) | 400 | 5 | 25 | 30 | 37 | 2 | 190 |

FOOD	PORTION	CALS	PROT	FAT	CHOL	CARB	FIBER	SOD
TAKE-OUT								
chocolate	½ cup (7.1 oz)	447	9	33	299	33	–	87
orange	½ cup	87	3	5	1	19	–	24
MUFFIN								
FROZEN								
Sara Lee								
Blueberry	1 (2.2 oz)	220	3	11	15	27	tr	170
Corn	1 (2.2 oz)	260	3	14	25	30	1	220
MIX								
blueberry	1 (1¾ oz)	149	3	4	23	24	–	219
corn	1 (1.75 oz)	160	4	5	31	25	–	397
wheat bran as prep	1 (1¾ oz)	138	5	5	34	23	–	233
Betty Crocker								
Apple Cinnamon as prep	1	170	1	7	36	23	–	200
Apple Streusel as prep	1	210	2	8	18	33	–	210
Banana Nut as prep	1	170	2	6	18	27	1	240
Cranberry Orange as prep	1	150	2	5	18	25	–	150
Double Chocolate as prep	1	220	2	11	27	30	–	210
Golden Corn as prep	1	160	2	5	36	24	–	210
Lemon Poppyseed as prep	1	180	1	8	36	24	–	180
Sunkist Lemon Poppyseed as prep	1	190	2	7	18	29	–	230
Twice The Blueberries as prep	1	140	2	3	18	25	1	180
Wild Blueberry as prep	1	170	2	5	18	28	tr	270
Carbsense								
Honey Bran not prep	1 serv (1.3 oz)	120	9	4	0	16	12	120
Gold Medal								
Corn	1	160	3	6	35	25	0	270

FOOD	PORTION	CALS	PROT	FAT	CHOL	CARB	FIBER	SOD
Hodgson Mill								
Bran	¼ cup (1.3 oz)	130	4	1	0	27	3	150
Cornbread	¼ cup (1.3 oz)	130	4	1	0	28	3	240
Whole Wheat	¼ cup (1.3 oz)	130	4	1	0	27	3	560
Ketogenics								
Apple Cinnamon Bran as prep	1	190	2	10	54	10	7	210
Chocolate Chip as prep	1	215	2	14	36	10	5	210
Wild Blueberry as prep	1	190	13	14	36	10	4	210
MiniCarb								
Apple Cinnamon as prep	1	225	12	16	35	7	4	135
Sweet Corn as prep	1	225	12	16	35	80	6	245
Robin Hood								
Apple Cinnamon	1	170	3	8	35	23	0	220
Banana Nut	1	170	3	8	35	21	0	190
Blueberry	1	160	3	6	35	24	0	220
Caramel Nut	1	170	3	7	35	24	0	230
Sweet Rewards								
Low Fat Apple Cinnamon as prep	1	140	2	2	16	26	—	180
READY-TO-EAT								
blueberry	1 (2 oz)	158	3	4	17	27	2	255
corn	1 (2 oz)	174	3	5	—	29	—	297
oat bran wheat free	1 (2 oz)	154	4	4	0	28	4	224
toaster type blueberry	1	103	2	3	—	18	—	158
toaster type corn	1	114	2	4	—	19	—	142
toaster type wheat bran w/ raisins	1 (1.3 oz)	106	2	3	—	19	—	178
Atkins								
Blueberry	1 (3.5 oz)	210	14	10	0	17	6	380

FOOD	PORTION	CALS	PROT	FAT	CHOL	CARB	FIBER	SOD
Natural Ovens								
Blueberry	1 (2.5 oz)	180	4	5	0	29	2	360
Carrot Nut	1 (2.5 oz)	170	4	6	0	35	2	380
Raisin Bran	1 (2.5 oz)	170	4	3	0	36	5	300
Otis Spunkmeyer								
Apple Cinnamon	1 (4 oz)	420	6	22	70	54	tr	420
Cheese Streusel	½ muffin (2 oz)	220	3	10	25	30	tr	170
Low Fat Wild Blueberry	1 (2.25 oz)	200	3	4	35	38	tr	160
Uncle Wally's								
Chocolate Passion	1 (2 oz)	130	2	0	0	30	1	210
Cranberry Orange Supreme	1 (2 oz)	130	3	0	0	25	1	230
Fat Free Apple Cinnamon Delight	1 (2 oz)	110	3	0	0	28	1	280
Fat Free Wild Blueberry Bliss	1 (2 oz)	120	30	0	0	25	1	230
Golden Waves Of Corn	1 (2 oz)	120	3	0	0	28	1	260
Honey Raisin Bran	1 (2 oz)	130	3	0	0	29	1	210
No Nut Banana	1 (2 oz)	130	3	0	0	27	1	230
VitaMuffin								
Blue Bran	1 (2 oz)	100	3	0	0	24	4	360
Cran Bran	1 (2 oz)	100	3	0	0	24	4	360
Deep Chocolate	1 (4 oz)	200	8	3	0	50	12	460
Multi Bran	1 (2 oz)	100	3	0	0	24	4	360
VitaTops Apple Berry Bran	1 (2 oz)	100	3	0	0	25	5	140
VitaTops Blue Bran	1 (2 oz)	100	3	0	0	24	4	360
VitaTops Cran Bran	1 (2 oz)	100	3	0	0	24	4	360
VitaTops Deep Chocolate	1 (2 oz)	100	4	2	0	25	6	230
VitaTops MultiBran	1 (2 oz)	100	3	0	0	24	4	360
TAKE-OUT								
raisin bran lowfat	1 (4 oz)	270	5	1	0	61	5	560
MULBERRIES								
fresh	1 cup	61	2	1	0	14	–	14

FOOD	PORTION	CALS	PROT	FAT	CHOL	CARB	FIBER	SOD
MULLET								
striped cooked	3 oz	127	21	4	54	0	–	61
striped raw	3 oz	99	16	3	42	0	–	55
MUNG BEANS								
dried cooked	1 cup	213	14	1	0	39	–	4
MUNGO BEANS								
dried cooked	1 cup	190	14	1	1	33	–	13
MUSHROOMS								
CANNED								
chanterelle	3.5 oz	12	1	1	0	tr	6	165
pieces	½ cup	19	1	tr	0	4	–	–
straw	1 cup (6.4 oz)	58	7	1	0	8	5	699
whole	1 (0.4 oz)	3	tr	tr	0	1	–	–
DRIED								
chanterelle	1 oz	25	5	tr	0	tr	17	9
cloud ear	1 (5 g)	13	tr	tr	0	3	3	2
cloud ears	1 cup (1 oz)	80	3	tr	0	20	20	10
shitake	4 (½ oz)	44	1	tr	0	11	–	2
straw	1 piece (6 g)	2	tr	tr	0	tr	tr	21
tree ear	½ cup (0.4 oz)	36	1	tr	0	10	–	8
wood ear mok yee	½ cup (0.4 oz)	25	2	tr	–	8	4	6
Eden								
Shitake	6 (0.4 oz)	35	2	0	0	7	5	0
FRESH								
chanterelle	3.5 oz	11	2	tr	0	tr	6	3
enoki raw	1 (4 in)	2	tr	tr	0	tr	–	0
morel	3.5 oz	9	2	tr	0	0	7	2
oyster raw	1 sm (0.5 oz)	6	1	tr	0	1	tr	5
oyster raw	1 lg (5.2 oz)	55	6	1	0	9	4	46
portabella	1 serv (2 oz)	14	1	tr	0	3	–	2
raw	1 (½ oz)	5	tr	tr	0	1	tr	1
raw sliced	½ cup	9	1	tr	0	2	tr	1
shitake cooked	4 (2.5 oz)	40	1	tr	0	10	–	3
sliced cooked	½ cup	21	2	tr	0	4	1	2
whole cooked	1 (0.4 oz)	3	tr	tr	0	1	–	0

FOOD	PORTION	CALS	PROT	FAT	CHOL	CARB	FIBER	SOD
MUSKRAT								
roasted	3 oz	199	26	10	–	0	–	81
MUSSELS								
blue raw	1 cup	129	18	3	42	6	–	429
blue raw	3 oz	73	10	2	24	3	–	243
fresh blue cooked	3 oz	147	20	4	48	6	–	313
MUSTARD								
dry mustard	1 tsp	15	1	1	0	1	–	tr
organic yellow	1 tsp	5	0	0	0	0	0	70
yellow ready-to-use	1 tsp	5	tr	tr	0	tr	–	63
Boar's Head								
Delicatessen Style	1 tsp (5 g)	0	0	0	0	0	0	40
Honey	1 tsp (5 g)	10	0	0	0	2	0	25
Country Cupboard								
Smokey Garlic or Horseradish	1 tsp	10	0	0	0	2	0	5
Eden								
Organic Stone Ground	1 tsp	0	0	0	0	1	0	65
French's								
Classic Yellow	1 tsp	0	0	0	0	0	0	55
Gulden's								
Spicy Brown	1 tsp	5	0	0	0	0	–	50
Hunt's								
Mustard	1 tsp (5 g)	3	tr	tr	0	tr	tr	64
Kosciuszko								
Spicy Brown	1 tsp	5	tr	tr	0	tr	–	60
Luzianne								
Creole Mustard	1 tbsp	10	1	0	0	2	0	320
Tree Of Life								
Dijon	1 tsp (5 g)	0	0	0	0	0	–	66
Dijon Imported	1 tsp (5 g)	5	tr	0	0	tr	–	120
Stone Ground	1 tsp (5 g)	0	0	0	0	0	–	55
Yellow	1 tsp (5 g)	0	0	0	0	0	–	55
Wild Thyme Farms								
Chili Pepper Garlic	1 tsp	5	0	0	0	1	–	95
Dill Horseradish	1 tsp	5	0	0	0	1	–	50

FOOD	PORTION	CALS	PROT	FAT	CHOL	CARB	FIBER	SOD
MUSTARD GREENS								
fresh chopped cooked	½ cup	11	2	tr	0	1	–	11
fresh raw chopped	½ cup	7	1	tr	0	1	–	7
frozen chopped cooked	½ cup	14	2	tr	0	2	–	19
Birds Eye								
Chopped	1 cup	30	2	0	0	2	2	20
NATTO								
natto	½ cup	187	16	10	0	13	–	6
NAVY BEANS								
CANNED								
navy	1 cup	296	20	1	0	54	–	1173
DRIED								
cooked	1 cup	259	16	1	0	48	–	2
NECTARINE								
fresh	1	67	1	1	0	16	2	0
Chiquita								
Fresh	1 med (4.9 oz)	70	1	1	0	16	2	0
NEUFCHATEL								
neufchatel	1 pkg (3 oz)	221	8	20	65	3	–	339
neufchatel	1 oz	74	3	7	22	1	–	113
Horizon Organic								
Neufchatel	2 tbsp	70	3	6	20	tr	0	120
NOODLE DISHES *(see also* PASTA DINNERS*)*								
Hunt's								
Noodles & Chicken	1 cup (8.7 oz)	176	12	6	37	21	2	1282
Noodles & Beef	1 cup (8.7 oz)	151	10	4	17	22	5	1241
TAKE-OUT								
bami goreng indonesian noodle dish	1 cup	170	5	3	0	25	4	500
noodle pudding	½ cup	132	6	7	27	11	–	222

FOOD	PORTION	CALS	PROT	FAT	CHOL	CARB	FIBER	SOD
NOODLES								
cellophane	1 cup	492	tr	tr	0	121	—	14
chow mein	1 cup (1.6 oz)	237	4	14	0	25	2	189
egg	1 cup (38 g)	145	5	2	36	27	—	8
egg cooked	1 cup (5.6 oz)	213	8	2	53	40	2	11
japanese soba cooked	1 cup (4 oz)	113	6	tr	0	24	—	68
japanese somen cooked	1 cup (6.2 oz)	231	7	tr	0	48	—	283
korean acorn noodles not prep	2 oz	195	7	tr	—	41	tr	—
rice cooked	1 cup (6.2 oz)	192	2	tr	0	44	2	33
spinach/egg cooked	1 cup (5.6 oz)	211	8	3	53	39	4	19
Annie Chun's								
Chow Mein	2 oz	200	8	1	0	39	3	350
Rice	2 oz	210	2	0	0	50	0	75
Rice Hunan	2 oz	210	2	0	0	50	0	75
Rice Pad Thai	2 oz	210	2	0	0	50	0	75
Rice Pad Thai Basil	2 oz	210	2	0	0	50	0	75
Azumaya								
Spinach	1 cup	210	8	1	0	42	2	370
Thin Cut	1 cup	210	8	1	0	43	2	400
Wide Cut	1 cup	210	8	1	0	43	2	410
Chun King								
Chow Mein	½ cup (1 oz)	137	3	6	0	19	1	217
Eden								
Kudzu	2 oz	200	0	0	0	48	2	0
Hodgson Mill								
Four Color Veggie Egg	2 oz	200	9	2	35	37	2	25
Whole Wheat Egg not prep	2 oz	190	10	0	30	34	4	20
La Choy								
Chow Mein	½ cup (1 oz)	137	3	6	0	19	1	217

FOOD	PORTION	CALS	PROT	FAT	CHOL	CARB	FIBER	SOD
Chow Mein Crispy Wide	½ cup (1 oz)	148	3	8	0	16	1	289
Rice	½ cup (1 oz)	121	2	3	0	21	tr	378
Manischewitz								
Fine Yolk Free	1½ cups	210	8	1	0	40	2	20
Fine Egg	1½ cups	220	8	3	65	40	2	15
Wide Yolk Free	1¾ cups	210	8	1	0	40	2	20
Nasoya								
Chinese	1 cup	210	8	1	0	43	2	400
Japanese	1 cup	210	8	1	0	43	2	410
Spinach	1 cup	210	8	1	0	42	2	0
Pennsylvania Dutch								
Yolk Free Ribbons as prep	1½ cups	210	7	1	0	41	2	15
NOPALES								
cooked	1 cup (5.2 oz)	23	2	tr	0	5	—	30
raw sliced	1 cup (3 oz)	14	1	tr	0	3	—	19
NUTMEG								
ground	1 tsp	12	tr	1	0	1	—	tr

NUTRITION SUPPLEMENTS *(see also* CEREAL BARS, ENERGY BARS, ENERGY DRINKS)

FOOD	PORTION	CALS	PROT	FAT	CHOL	CARB	FIBER	SOD
Boost								
High Protein Powder Vanilla as prep w/ water	1 serv (8 oz)	200	13	1	10	36	0	190
Enlive!								
Drink All Flavors	1 box (8.1 oz)	300	10	0	<5	65	0	65
Ensure								
Supplement All Flavors	1 can (8 fl oz)	250	9	6	<5	40	0	200
GeniSoy								
Soy Natural Protein Powder	1 scoop (1 oz)	100	25	0	0	0	0	290
Glucerna								
Shakes All Flavors	1 can (8 oz)	220	10	9	<5	29	3	210

FOOD	PORTION	CALS	PROT	FAT	CHOL	CARB	FIBER	SOD
Juven								
Grape w/ Arginine, Glutamine, HMB	1 pkg (0.8 oz)	90	–	–	–	2	–	–
Orange w/ HMB	1 pkg (0.8 oz)	90	–	0	–	–	–	–
Met-Rx								
Lite	1 pkg (1.6 oz)	170	25	1	30	16	1	125
Mass Action	1 scoop (0.9 oz)	60	–	4	–	15	–	270
Original	1 pkg (2.5 oz)	250	37	2	15	22	tr	370
Protein Shake	1 can	200	25	3	10	20	2	110
Ultra	1 pkg (2.6 oz)	250	40	2	50	19	2	230
Nature Made								
CalBurst	1 piece	15	–	–	–	–	–	–
Nestle								
Additions	2⅓ tsp (0.7 oz)	100	6	5	0	9	0	90
Nutribar								
Shake Chocolate Supreme as prep w/ 2% milk	1 serv (10 oz)	262	14	8	–	34	2	290
Shake Vanilla as prep w/ 2% milk	1 (10 oz)	259	14	7	–	35	2	285
PermaLean								
Protein Powder Bodacious Berry	1 scoop (1 oz)	104	20	tr	0	1	–	tr
Protein Powder Chocoholic Chocolate	1 scoop (1 oz)	104	20	tr	0	5	–	tr
Pounds Off								
All Flavors	1 bar (2.1 oz)	210	11	5	0	32	2	25
Viactiv								
Calcium Chews	1	20	–	1	–	–	–	–
Chocolate	1	20	–	1	–	–	–	–

FOOD	PORTION	CALS	PROT	FAT	CHOL	CARB	FIBER	SOD
NUTS MIXED (see also individual names)								
dry roasted w/ peanuts	1 oz	169	5	15	0	7	–	3
dry roasted w/ peanuts salted	1 oz	169	5	15	0	7	–	223
mixed nuts chocolate covered	¼ cup (1.5 oz)	240	4	17	5	20	2	25
oil roasted w/ peanuts	1 oz	175	5	16	0	6	–	3
oil roasted w/ peanuts salted	1 oz	175	5	16	0	6	–	217
oil roasted w/o peanuts	1 oz	175	4	16	0	6	–	3
oil roasted w/o peanuts salted	1 oz	175	4	16	0	6	–	233
Here's Howe								
Royal Mixed Nuts	1 oz	180	5	17	0	7	2	160
Judy's								
Sugar Free Mixed Nut Brittle	¼ piece (1 oz)	120	2	7	<5	3	tr	30
Maranatha								
Cashew Butter	2 tbsp	210	4	20	0	8	2	5
Tamari Organic	¼ cup	160	6	14	0	7	2	140
Tamari Roasted	¼ cup	160	6	14	0	7	2	140
Mauna Loa								
Macadamia Mixed	¼ cup	190	5	15	0	8	2	60
Macadamias & Cashews	¼ cup	180	4	15	0	8	1	65
OCTOPUS								
fresh steamed	3 oz	140	25	2	82	4	–	–
OHELOBERRIES								
fresh	1 cup	39	1	tr	0	10	–	2
OIL								
almond	1 tbsp	120	0	14	0	0	0	–
almond	1 cup	1927	0	218	0	0	0	–
apricot kernel	1 tbsp	120	0	14	0	0	0	–
apricot kernel	1 cup	1927	0	218	0	0	0	–
avocado	1 tbsp	124	0	14	0	0	0	–

FOOD	PORTION	CALS	PROT	FAT	CHOL	CARB	FIBER	SOD
avocado	1 cup	1927	0	218	0	0	0	–
babassu palm	1 tbsp	120	0	14	0	0	0	–
butter oil	1 tbsp	112	tr	13	33	0	–	–
butter oil	1 cup	1795	1	204	524	0	–	–
canola	1 tbsp	124	0	14	0	0	0	–
canola	1 cup	1927	0	218	0	0	0	–
coconut	1 tbsp	117	0	14	0	0	0	–
corn	1 tbsp	120	0	14	0	0	0	–
corn	1 cup	1927	0	218	0	0	0	–
cottonseed	1 tbsp	120	0	14	0	0	0	–
cottonseed	1 cup	1927	0	218	0	0	0	–
cupu assu	1 tbsp	120	0	14	0	0	0	–
grapeseed	1 tbsp	120	0	14	0	0	0	–
hazelnut	1 tbsp	120	0	14	0	0	0	–
hazelnut	1 cup	1927	0	218	0	0	0	–
mustard	1 tbsp	124	0	14	0	0	0	–
mustard	1 cup	1927	0	218	0	0	0	–
oat	1 tbsp	120	0	14	0	0	0	–
olive	1 tbsp	119	0	14	0	0	0	0
olive	1 cup	1909	0	216	0	0	0	tr
palm	1 tbsp	120	0	14	0	0	0	–
palm	1 cup	1927	0	218	0	0	0	–
palm kernel	1 tbsp	117	0	14	0	0	0	–
palm kernel	1 cup	1879	0	218	0	0	0	–
peanut	1 tbsp	119	0	14	0	0	0	tr
peanut	1 cup	1909	0	216	0	0	0	tr
poppyseed	1 tbsp	120	0	14	0	0	0	–
pumpkin seed	1 oz	217	0	29	–	0	0	–
rice bran	1 tbsp	120	0	14	0	0	0	–
safflower	1 tbsp	120	0	14	0	0	0	–
safflower	1 cup	1927	0	218	0	0	0	–
sesame	1 tbsp	120	0	14	0	0	0	–
sheanut	1 tbsp	120	0	14	0	0	0	–
soybean	1 tbsp	120	0	14	0	0	0	0
soybean	1 cup	1927	0	218	0	0	0	tr
soybean organic	1 tbsp	120	0	14	0	0	0	0
sunflower	1 tbsp	120	0	14	0	0	0	–
sunflower	1 cup	1927	0	218	0	0	0	–
teaseed	1 tbsp	120	0	14	0	0	0	–
tomatoseed	1 tbsp	120	0	14	0	0	0	–

FOOD	PORTION	CALS	PROT	FAT	CHOL	CARB	FIBER	SOD
vegetable	1 tbsp	120	0	14	0	0	0	–
vegetable	1 cup	1927	0	218	0	0	0	–
walnut	1 tbsp	120	0	14	0	0	0	–
walnut	1 cup	1927	0	218	0	0	0	–
wheat germ	1 tbsp	120	0	14	0	0	0	–
Alpha								
Hazelnut	1 oz	257	0	29	0	0	0	–
Bertolli								
Classico	1 tbsp	120	–	14	0	–	–	–
Extra Light	1 tbsp	120	–	14	0	–	–	–
Extra Virgin	1 tbsp	120	–	14	0	–	–	–
Eden								
Olive Spanish Extra Virgin	1 tbsp	120	0	14	0	0	0	0
Enova								
Oil	1 tbsp	120	0	14	0	0	0	0
Hollywood								
Safflower	1 tbsp	120	0	14	0	0	0	0
Loriva								
5 Pepper Hot	1 tbsp	120	–	14	0	–	–	–
Avocado	1 tbsp	120	–	14	0	–	–	–
Basil Flavored	1 tbsp	120	–	14	0	–	–	–
Canola	1 tbsp	120	–	14	0	–	–	–
Canolive	1 tbsp	120	–	14	0	–	–	–
Garlic Flavored	1 tbsp	120	–	14	0	–	–	–
Grapeseed	1 tbsp	120	–	14	0	–	–	–
Olive	1 tbsp	120	–	14	0	–	–	–
Olive Organic Extra Virgin	1 tbsp	120	–	14	0	–	–	–
Peanut	1 tbsp	120	–	14	0	–	–	–
Rice Bran	1 tbsp	120	–	14	0	–	–	–
Safflower	1 tbsp	120	–	14	0	–	–	–
Sesame	1 tbsp	120	–	14	0	–	–	–
Sunflower	1 tbsp	120	–	14	0	–	–	–
Toasted Sesame	1 tbsp	120	–	14	0	–	–	–
Walnut	1 tbsp	120	–	14	0	–	–	–
Mazola								
Oil	1 tbsp	120	0	14	0	0	0	0
Monini								
Olive Extra Virgin	1 tbsp	118	0	13	0	0	0	–

FOOD	PORTION	CALS	PROT	FAT	CHOL	CARB	FIBER	SOD
Orville Redenbacher's								
Popping	1 tbsp (0.5 oz)	120	0	14	0	0	0	0
Pompeian								
Olive	1 tbsp	130	–	14	0	–	–	–
Progresso								
Olive Extra Mild	1 tbsp (0.5 oz)	120	0	14	0	0	0	0
Olive Extra Virgin	1 tbsp (0.5 oz)	120	0	14	0	0	0	0
Olive Riviera Blend	1 tbsp (0.5 oz)	120	0	14	0	0	0	0
Tree Of Life								
Olive Extra Virgin Organic	1 tbsp (0.5 g)	130	0	14	0	0	–	0
Wesson								
Canola	1 tbsp	120	0	14	1	0	0	0
OKRA								
FRESH								
raw	8 pods	36	2	tr	0	7	–	8
raw sliced	½ cup	19	1	tr	0	4	–	4
sliced cooked	8 pods	27	2	tr	0	6	–	5
sliced cooked	½ cup	25	1	tr	0	6	–	4
FROZEN								
sliced cooked	1 pkg (10 oz)	94	5	1	0	21	–	8
sliced cooked	½ cup	34	2	tr	0	8	–	3
Birds Eye								
Cut	¾ cup	25	1	0	0	5	3	35
Whole	9 pods	25	1	0	0	5	3	35
McKenzie's								
Breaded Okra	1 serv (2.8 oz)	90	3	1	0	–	3	350
OLIVES								
green	4 med	15	tr	2	0	tr	tr	312
green	3 extra lg	15	tr	2	0	tr	tr	312
green olive tapenade	1 tbsp	25	0	3	0	1	0	210
ripe	1 sm	4	tr	tr	0	tr	tr	28
ripe	1 lg	5	tr	tr	0	tr	tr	38

FOOD	PORTION	CALS	PROT	FAT	CHOL	CARB	FIBER	SOD
ripe	1 jumbo	7	tr	1	0	tr	–	75
ripe	1 colossal	12	tr	1	0	1	–	136
spanish stuffed	5 (0.5 oz)	15	0	1	0	1	0	320
Progresso								
Olive Salad (drained)	2 tbsp (0.8 oz)	25	0	3	0	1	tr	360
Vlasic								
Ripe Colossal Pitted	2 (0.6 oz)	20	0	2	0	1	0	110
Ripe Jumbo Pitted	3 (0.6 oz)	25	0	2	0	1	0	135
Ripe Large Pitted	4 (0.5 oz)	25	0	3	0	1	0	115
Ripe Medium Pitted	5 (0.5 oz)	25	0	3	0	1	0	115
Ripe Sliced	¼ cup (0.5 oz)	25	0	3	0	1	0	115
Ripe Small Pitted	6 (0.5 oz)	25	0	3	0	1	0	115

ONION
CANNED

FOOD	PORTION	CALS	PROT	FAT	CHOL	CARB	FIBER	SOD
chopped	½ cup	21	1	tr	0	5	–	416
whole	1 (2.2 oz)	12	1	tr	0	3	–	234
Boar's Head								
Sweet Vidalia In Sauce	1 tbsp	10	0	0	0	2	0	15
DRIED								
flakes	1 tbsp	16	tr	tr	0	4	–	1
powder	1 tsp	7	tr	tr	0	2	–	1
shallots	1 tbsp	3	tr	0	0	1	–	1
FRESH								
chopped cooked	½ cup	47	1	tr	0	11	–	3
raw chopped	½ cup	30	1	tr	0	7	–	2
raw chopped	1 tbsp	4	tr	tr	0	1	tr	0
scallions raw chopped	1 tbsp	2	tr	tr	0	tr	tr	1
scallions raw sliced	½ cup	16	1	tr	0	4	1	8
shallots raw chopped	1 tbsp	7	tr	tr	0	2	–	1
welsh raw	3½ oz	34	2	tr	0	7	–	–
Antioch Farms								
Vidalia	1 med	60	1	0	0	14	3	10

FOOD	PORTION	CALS	PROT	FAT	CHOL	CARB	FIBER	SOD
Nature's Harvest								
Onion	1 med (5.2 oz)	60	2	0	0	14	3	5
FROZEN								
chopped cooked	½ cup	30	tr	tr	0	7	—	12
chopped cooked	1 tbsp	4	tr	tr	0	1	—	2
rings	7 (2.5 oz)	285	4	19	0	27	—	263
rings cooked	2 (0.7 oz)	81	1	5	0	8	—	75
whole cooked	3½ oz	28	tr	tr	0	7	—	8
Birds Eye								
Diced	⅔ cup	30	tr	0	0	6	1	30
Pearl Onions In Real Cream Sauce	½ cup	60	2	2	10	8	1	280
Small Whole	17	30	—	0	0	—	1	10
McKenzie's								
Onion Rounds	1 serv (3.2 oz)	220	3	10	0	28	6	210
TAKE-OUT								
fried	½ cup (7.5 oz)	176	3	11	—	17	—	—
rings breaded & fried	8 to 9	275	4	16	14	31	—	430
OPOSSUM								
roasted	3 oz	188	26	9	—	0	—	—
ORANGE								
CANNED								
Del Monte								
Mandarin In Light Syrup	½ cup (4.5 oz)	80	0	0	0	19	1	10
Dole								
Fruit Bowls Mandarin Oranges	1 pkg	70	0	0	0	18	0	10
FRESH								
california navel	1	65	1	tr	0	16	3	1
california valencia	1	59	1	tr	0	14	3	0
florida	1	69	1	tr	0	17	4	1
peel	1 tbsp	6	tr	tr	0	2	—	0
sections	1 cup	85	2	tr	0	21	4	0

FOOD	PORTION	CALS	PROT	FAT	CHOL	CARB	FIBER	SOD
ORANGE EXTRACT								
Virginia Dare								
Extract	1 tsp	22	–	0	0	–	–	–
ORANGE JUICE								
canned	1 cup	104	1	tr	0	25	–	6
chilled	1 cup	110	2	1	0	25	–	2
fresh	1 cup	111	2	tr	0	26	–	2
frzn as prep	1 cup	112	2	tr	0	27	1	2
frzn not prep	6 oz	339	5	tr	0	81	2	7
mandarin orange	7 oz	94	2	tr	–	20	–	–
orange drink	6 oz	94	0	0	0	24	–	31
Big Juicy								
Drink	8 oz	110	0	0	0	28	–	55
Fresh Samantha								
Juice	1 cup (8 oz)	100	1	0	0	8	0	0
Horizon Organic								
Juice Pulp Free	8 fl oz	110	2	0	0	26	–	0
Juicy Juice								
Punch	1 box (8.45 oz)	130	0	0	0	33	0	15
Punch	1 box (4.23 oz)	60	0	0	0	15	0	5
Minute Maid								
Heart Wise	8 fl oz	110	2	0	0	27	–	20
Light	8 fl oz	50	0	0	0	13	–	15
Original	8 fl oz	110	2	0	0	27	–	25
Original Calcium + Vitamin D	8 fl oz	110	2	0	0	27	–	15
Plus Calcium	8 fl oz	110	2	0	0	27	–	20
Simply Orange 100%	8 fl oz	110	2	0	0	26	–	0
Simply Orange Calcium Fortified	8 fl oz	110	2	0	0	26	–	0
Simply Orange Grove Made	8 fl oz	110	2	0	0	26	–	0
Mott's								
100% Juice	8 fl oz	130	2	0	0	31	–	10
100% Juice	1 box (8 oz)	130	2	0	0	31	–	10

FOOD	PORTION	CALS	PROT	FAT	CHOL	CARB	FIBER	SOD
Naked Juice								
Just OJ	8 oz	110	2	0	0	25	0	0
NutraShake								
Fortified	1 pkg (4 oz)	50	0	0	0	12	4	0
Ocean Spray								
100% Juice	8 oz	120	0	0	0	31	0	35
Odwalla								
Organic	8 fl oz	110	2	0	0	25	–	0
Simply Orange								
Pulp Free w/ Calcium	8 oz	110	2	0	0	26	–	0
Snapple								
Orangeade	8 fl oz	120	0	0	0	29	–	10
Tropicana								
HomeStyle	8 oz	110	2	0	0	26	–	0
Light'N Healthy	8 oz	70	1	0	0	17	–	10
Original No Pulp	8 oz	110	2	0	0	26	–	0
With Calcium + Vitamin D	8 oz	110	2	0	0	26	–	0
Turkey Hill								
Orangeade	1 cup	120	–	0	0	30	–	–
TAKE-OUT								
orange julius	1 serv (24 oz)	443	2	tr	0	118	1	10

OREGANO

ground	1 tsp	5	tr	tr	0	1	–	tr

ORGAN MEATS (see BRAINS, GIBLETS, GIZZARDS, HEART, KIDNEY, LIVER, SWEETBREADS)

OSTRICH

cooked	3 oz	120	22	3	74	–	–	57

OYSTERS

canned eastern	3 oz	58	6	2	46	3	–	95
canned eastern	1 cup	170	18	6	136	10	–	277
eastern cooked	3 oz	117	12	4	93	7	–	190
eastern cooked	6 med	58	6	2	46	3	–	94
eastern raw	1 cup	170	18	6	136	10	–	277
eastern raw	6 med	58	6	2	46	3	–	94
pacific raw	1 med	41	5	1	–	2	–	53

FOOD	PORTION	CALS	PROT	FAT	CHOL	CARB	FIBER	SOD
pacific raw	3 oz	69	8	2	–	4	–	90
steamed	3 oz	138	16	4	–	8	–	180
steamed	1 med	41	5	1	–	2	–	53
Bumble Bee								
Fancy Whole	2 oz	70	7	3	45	3	0	140
Smoked	½ can (1.9 oz)	120	10	7	35	6	0	210
TAKE-OUT								
breaded & fried	6 (4.9 oz)	368	13	18	109	40	–	677
oysters rockefeller	3 oysters	66	7	2	38	5	–	80
stew	1 cup	278	15	18	100	15	tr	928

PANCAKE/WAFFLE SYRUP

FOOD	PORTION	CALS	PROT	FAT	CHOL	CARB	FIBER	SOD
low calorie	1 tbsp	12	0	0	0	3	0	–
maple	1 tbsp (0.8 oz)	52	0	0	0	13	–	2
maple	1 cup (11.1 oz)	824	tr	1	0	212	–	27
pancake syrup	1 tbsp (0.7 oz)	57	0	0	0	15	–	17
pancake syrup	1 cup (11 oz)	903	0	0	0	238	–	290
pancake syrup light	1 oz	46	0	0	0	13	–	57
pancake syrup w/ butter	1 tbsp (0.7 oz)	59	0	tr	1	15	–	20
pancake syrup w/ butter	1 cup (11 oz)	933	tr	5	14	234	–	307
Atkins								
Sugar Free	¼ cup	0	0	0	0	0	0	40
Aunt Jemima								
Original	¼ cup	210	0	0	0	52	–	120
Country Cupboard								
Boysenberry	¼ cup	0	1	0	0	0	0	0
Maple Butter	¼ cup	0	1	0	0	2	0	0
Strawberry	¼ cup	0	1	0	0	1	0	0
Keto								
Maple Butter	¼ cup	0	0	0	0	1	0	20
Ketogenics								
Zero Carb	¼ cup	0	0	0	0	0	0	40

FOOD	PORTION	CALS	PROT	FAT	CHOL	CARB	FIBER	SOD
Log Cabin								
Lite	¼ cup	100	0	0	0	25	–	130
Original	¼ cup	210	0	0	0	53	0	100
Mrs. Butterworth's								
Lite	¼ cup	100	0	0	0	25	–	130
Original	¼ cup (2 oz)	230	0	0	0	56	–	95
Smucker's								
Breakfast Syrup Sugar Free	¼ cup (2 oz)	30	0	0	0	8	–	60
Stonewall Kitchen								
Maine Maple	¼ cup	210	0	0	0	54	0	5
PANCAKES								
FROZEN								
buttermilk	1 (4-in diam)	83	2	1	3	16	–	183
plain	1 (4-in diam)	83	2	1	3	16	–	183
Golden								
Potato	1 (1.3 oz)	70	2	3	5	10	1	190
MIX								
buckwheat	1 (4 in diam)	62	2	2	20	9	–	160
buttermilk	1 (4-in diam)	74	2	1	–	14	tr	239
plain	1 (4-in diam)	74	2	1	–	14	tr	239
sugar free low sodium	1 (3 in diam)	44	1	tr	0	9	–	58
whole wheat	1 (4 in diam)	92	4	3	27	13	–	252
Atkins								
Quick Quisine Buttermilk not prep	⅓ cup	100	14	0	0	13	5	320
Quick Quisine Original not prep	¼ cup	80	13	2	5	6	3	120
Aunt Jemima								
Buttermilk Pancake & Waffle Mix not prep	⅓ cup	160	4	3	10	31	1	460
Aunt Paula's								
Pancake & Waffle Mix as prep	2	132	21	8	0	6	4	0
Betty Crocker								
Buttermilk as prep	3	200	5	3	10	20	1	540

FOOD	PORTION	CALS	PROT	FAT	CHOL	CARB	FIBER	SOD
Original as prep	3	200	6	3	10	39	2	540
Big Train								
Low Carb Pancake & Waffle Mix as prep	3	190	11	10	108	12	5	300
Bisquick								
Shake 'N Pour Blueberry as prep	3	210	6	4	0	40	1	640
Bruce								
Sweet Potato Pancakes	2	210	6	3	0	39	2	670
Carbolite								
Low Carb Mix not prep	⅓ cup	100	21	tr	–	10	tr	310
Carbsense								
Buckwheat not prep	½ cup	140	21	3	0	10	7	430
Buttermilk not prep	½ cup	140	21	3	0	10	7	320
Hodgson Mill								
Buckwheat	⅓ cup (1.8 oz)	160	5	1	0	36	5	590
Keto								
Banana not prep	⅓ cup	114	19	2	–	6	2	224
Original not prep	⅓ cup	114	19	2	–	5	2	224
Ketogenics								
Low Carb not prep	⅔ cup	185	23	4	94	15	6	400
MiniCarb								
Apple Cinnamon as prep	2	150	12	6	10	17	13	170
Robin Hood								
Buttermilk as prep	3	230	8	6	60	35	1	560
TAKE-OUT								
blueberry	1 (4 in diam)	84	2	4	21	11	–	157
plain	1 (4 in diam)	86	2	4	23	11	–	157
potato	1 (4 in diam)	78	2	6	60	4	tr	238
w/ butter & syrup	2 (8.1 oz)	520	8	14	58	91	–	1104

FOOD	PORTION	CALS	PROT	FAT	CHOL	CARB	FIBER	SOD
PAPAYA								
fresh	1	117	2	tr	0	30	—	8
fresh cubed	1 cup	54	1	tr	0	14	—	4
SunFresh								
In Extra Light Syrup	½ cup (4.5 oz)	70	1	0	0	17	1	5
PAPAYA JUICE								
nectar	1 cup	142	tr	tr	0	36	—	14
Ceres								
Papaya	8 oz	120	0	0	0	30	0	5
PAPRIKA								
paprika	1 tsp	6	tr	tr	0	1	—	1
PARSLEY								
dry	1 tbsp	1	tr	tr	0	tr	—	2
dry	1 tsp	1	tr	tr	0	tr	—	1
fresh chopped	½ cup	11	1	tr	0	2	—	17
PARSNIPS								
fresh cooked	1 (5.6 oz)	130	2	tr	0	31	—	17
fresh sliced cooked	½ cup	63	1	tr	0	15	—	8
raw sliced	½ cup	50	1	tr	0	12	—	7
PASSION FRUIT								
purple fresh	1	18	tr	tr	0	4	—	5
PASSION FRUIT JUICE								
purple	1 cup	126	1	tr	0	34	—	—
yellow	1 cup	149	2	tr	0	36	—	15
Ceres								
Passion Fruit	8 oz	120	0	0	0	31	0	10
PASTA (see also NOODLES, PASTA DINNERS, PASTA SALAD)								
DRY								
corn cooked	1 cup (4.9 oz)	176	4	1	0	39	7	0
corn spaghetti	2 oz	180	4	2	0	35	3	5
elbows	1 cup	389	13	2	0	78	—	8
elbows cooked	1 cup (4.9 oz)	197	7	1	0	40	2	1
shells small cooked	1 cup (4 oz)	162	5	1	0	33	2	1
shells small protein fortified cooked	1 cup (4 oz)	189	9	tr	0	36	—	6
spaghetti cooked	1 cup (4.9 oz)	197	7	1	0	40	2	1

FOOD	PORTION	CALS	PROT	FAT	CHOL	CARB	FIBER	SOD
spaghetti protein fortified cooked	1 cup (4.9 oz)	230	11	tr	0	44	2	7
spinach spaghetti cooked	1 cup (4.9 oz)	182	6	1	0	37	–	20
spirals cooked	1 cup (4.7 oz)	189	6	tr	0	38	2	1
vegetable cooked	1 cup (4.7 oz)	172	6	tr	0	36	6	8
whole wheat cooked	1 cup (4.9 oz)	174	7	tr	0	37	4	4
whole wheat spaghetti cooked	1 cup (4.9 oz)	174	7	1	0	37	6	4
Annie Chun's								
Soba Noodles	2 oz	200	8	1	0	39	3	390
Atkins								
All Shapes not prep	2 oz	230	36	3	0	15	9	270
Quick Quisine All Shapes as prep	¾ cup	210	4	3	0	13	8	280
Barilla								
Pastina	2 oz	210	8	2	65	40	2	20
Tortelloni Porcini Mushroom	¾ cup	240	8	8	50	32	5	335
Tortelloni Ricotta & Asparagus	¾ cup	240	7	8	60	32	5	450
Tortelloni Ricotta & Spinach	¾ cup	240	8	8	50	31	4	450
Bella Vita								
Low Carb Penne Rigate	2 oz	190	28	1	0	18	8	40
Darielle								
All Shapes not prep	2 oz	160	28	1	0	18	8	40
DaVinci								
Rotini	1 cup	210	6	1	0	43	2	0
Spaghetti	2 oz	210	6	1	0	43	2	0
Dreamfields								
All Shapes not prep	2 oz	190	7	1	0	42	4	0
Duc Amici								
Pasta Lite Low Carb Fusilli	2 oz	160	28	1	0	10	7	50
Eden								
Organic Extra Fine	2 oz	210	9	2	0	40	3	0
Organic Gemelli	2 oz	210	8	2	0	40	5	0

FOOD	PORTION	CALS	PROT	FAT	CHOL	CARB	FIBER	SOD
Organic Pesto Gemelli	2 oz	210	8	1	0	41	4	0
Organic Ribbons Saffron	2 oz	210	9	2	0	40	3	0
Organic Spaghetti Semolina	2 oz	200	8	1	0	40	2	0
Organic Spaghetti 50% Whole Grain	2 oz	210	8	1	0	41	4	0
Organic Spirals Kamut Vegetable	2 oz	210	8	2	0	40	6	45
Organic Spirals Sesame Rice	2 oz	200	8	2	0	37	4	0
Organic Spirals Mixed Grain	2 oz	210	8	2	0	41	7	15
Organic Spirals Spinach	2 oz	210	8	1	0	41	4	30
Organic Vegetable Alphabets	2 oz	200	8	1	0	40	2	15
Spirals Rye	2 oz	200	6	0	0	44	8	10
Goya								
Coditos not prep	½ cup	230	8	1	0	47	3	0
Hodgson Mill								
Four Color Veggie Bows	2 oz	200	8	1	0	41	1	15
Four Color Veggie Rotini Spirals	2 oz	200	8	1	0	41	1	15
Pastamania! Durum Wheat Fettuccine	2 oz	200	8	2	30	38	1	20
Pastamania! Fettuccine Garlic & Parsley	2 oz	200	8	2	30	38	1	20
Pastamania! Fettuccine w/ Jerusalem Artichoke	2 oz	210	8	2	0	41	2	10
Pastamania! Fettucinne w/ Mushroom	2 oz	210	8	2	35	41	2	15

FOOD	PORTION	CALS	PROT	FAT	CHOL	CARB	FIBER	SOD
Pastamania! Fusilli Tre Colore w/ Tomato & Spinach	2 oz	200	7	1	0	40	2	20
Pastamania! Sea Shell Mix	2 oz	200	8	1	0	40	1	10
Pastamania! Spinach Fettuccine	2 oz	200	8	2	40	37	2	35
Pastamania! Thin Linguine	2 oz	200	8	2	30	38	1	20
Pastamania! Tomato Spinach & Durum Wheat	2 oz	210	8	2	35	40	2	29
Spaghetti Whole Wheat not prep	2 oz	190	9	0	0	34	6	10
Whole Wheat Lasagne not prep	2 oz	190	9	0	0	34	6	10
Whole Wheat Spinach Spaghetti not prep	2 oz	190	9	1	0	35	5	25
Keto								
Elbows not prep	1.6 oz	108	22	0	0	5	1	120
Spaghetti not prep	1.3 oz	130	22	1	0	7	2	120
Lundberg								
Spaghetti Organic Brown Rice	2 oz	210	4	2	0	44	3	5
Pastalia								
Heart Health Low Carb not prep	2 oz	176	30	2	–	10	3	180
Real Torino								
Tirali not prep	1 cup (2 oz)	210	6	1	0	43	2	0
Revival								
Soy Penne	⅙ box	200	14	2	0	34	1	85
Soy Thin Spaghetti	⅙ box	200	14	2	0	34	1	85
Ronzoni								
Elbows not prep	½ cup (2 oz)	210	7	1	0	42	2	0
Healthy Harvest Whole Wheat Blend	2 oz	210	7	2	0	42	3	0
Lasagne	2½ pieces (2 oz)	210	7	1	0	42	2	0

FOOD	PORTION	CALS	PROT	FAT	CHOL	CARB	FIBER	SOD
Tradizione D'Italia All Shapes	2 oz	210	7	1	0	42	2	0
Soy7								
Pasta All Shapes	2 oz	200	13	1	0	33	2	120
Whey Cool								
High Protein Xtreme Rotini	1 serv (2 oz)	210	42	2	5	8	1	270
FRESH								
cooked	2 oz	75	3	1	33	14	–	3
spinach cooked	2 oz	74	3	1	19	14	–	3
REFRIGERATED								
Buitoni								
Angel Hair	1¼ cup	230	10	3	50	43	2	20
Fettuccine	1¼ cup	240	10	3	55	45	2	20
Fettuccine Spinach	1¼ cup	260	12	3	75	45	2	110
Linguine	1¼ cup	240	10	3	55	45	2	20
Ravioletti Beef	1 cup	300	12	7	35	46	2	370
Ravioletti Three Cheese	1 cup	270	12	6	35	43	2	330
Ravioli Four Cheese	1 serv (9 oz)	330	12	14	65	40	3	630
Ravioli Beef	1¼ cup	340	15	10	60	48	2	530
Ravioli Chicken Parmesan	1¼ cup	310	14	8	55	45	2	620
Ravioli Garden Vegetable	1 cup	250	11	5	40	39	2	500
Ravioli Light Four Cheese	1¼ cup	230	12	4	35	37	2	390
Ravioli Roasted Chicken & Garlic	1¼ cup	340	14	11	50	47	2	550
Tortellini Herb Chicken	1 cup	340	13	9	40	52	2	410
Tortellini Spinach Cheese	1 cup	330	15	8	55	49	3	510
Tortellini Three Cheese	1 cup	320	15	7	40	50	3	480
Tortelloni Cheese & Roasted Garlic	1 cup	270	12	8	35	37	2	360
Tortelloni Chicken & Prosciutto	1 cup	330	14	9	45	47	2	630

FOOD	PORTION	CALS	PROT	FAT	CHOL	CARB	FIBER	SOD
Tortelloni Mozzarella & Herb	1 cup	330	14	10	45	46	2	450
Tortelloni Mozzarella & Pepperoni	1 cup	330	15	10	45	45	2	440
Tortelloni Sun Dried Tomato	1 cup	310	12	9	25	46	3	340
Tortelloni Sweet Italian Sausage	1 cup	330	13	9	35	48	3	280

PASTA DINNERS (see also PASTA SALAD)
CANNED
Chef Boyardee

FOOD	PORTION	CALS	PROT	FAT	CHOL	CARB	FIBER	SOD
99% Fat Free Beef Ravioli	1 cup (8.6 oz)	210	9	1	15	41	3	1150
99% Fat Free Cheese Ravioli	1 cup (8.8 oz)	210	7	1	<5	44	4	860
Beef Ravioli	1 cup (8.6 oz)	230	9	5	20	37	4	1150
Beefaroni	1 cup (8.7 oz)	260	10	7	25	37	5	870
Macaroni & Cheese	½ can (7.5 oz)	180	8	2	20	35	2	1090
Mini Ravioli	1 cup (8.8 oz)	252	8	6	20	37	3	1180
Spaghetti & Meat Balls	1 cup (8.4 oz)	240	9	10	25	32	3	950
Tortellini Cheese	½ can (7 oz)	230	9	1	15	48	5	770
Tortellini Meat	½ can (7 oz)	260	10	4	30	48	4	810

Franco-American

FOOD	PORTION	CALS	PROT	FAT	CHOL	CARB	FIBER	SOD
Beef Raviolios	1 can (7.7 oz)	250	9	5	12	39	4	911
Beefy Mac	1 can (7.5 oz)	228	9	8	10	30	3	1144
Elbow Macaroni & Cheese	1 can (7.5 oz)	187	6	6	7	25	2	875
Spaghetti 'N Beef	1 can (7.5 oz)	226	10	8	14	30	3	1063
Spaghetti w/ Meatballs	1 can (7.2 oz)	249	10	9	14	33	4	917

FOOD	PORTION	CALS	PROT	FAT	CHOL	CARB	FIBER	SOD
Progresso								
Beef Ravioli	1 cup (9.1 oz)	260	9	5	5	45	4	940
Cheese Ravioli	1 cup (9.1 oz)	220	7	2	<5	43	4	930
FROZEN								
Amy's								
Bowl Stuffed Pasta Shells	1 pkg (10 oz)	300	19	12	30	30	5	740
Cannelloni w/ Vegetables	1 pkg (9 oz)	330	16	12	15	34	6	390
Lasagna Cheese	1 pkg (10.25 oz)	330	19	12	35	38	5	680
Lasagna Garden Vegetable	1 pkg (10.25 oz)	290	13	9	20	41	5	720
Macaroni & Cheese	1 pkg (9 oz)	410	16	16	50	47	3	590
Macaroni & Soy Cheese	1 pkg (9 oz)	370	16	15	0	42	4	500
Pasta & Vegetable Alfredo	1 cup	220	11	8	20	27	4	460
Pasta Primavera	1 pkg (9 oz)	300	15	11	45	37	3	670
Ravioli w/ Sauce	1 pkg (8 oz)	340	15	12	25	43	3	580
Rice Mac & Cheese	1 pkg (9 oz)	140	16	16	50	47	3	590
Skillet Meals	1 cup	250	9	11	5	27	3	480
Tofu Vegetable Lasagna	1 pkg (9.5 oz)	300	13	10	0	41	6	630
Vegetable Lasagna	1 pkg (9.5 oz)	280	14	12	20	29	3	680
Banquet								
Chicken Pasta Primavera	1 meal (9.5 oz)	320	11	12	25	40	6	840
Family Size Egg Noodles w/ Beef & Brown Gravy	1 serv	150	11	5	35	16	2	1120
Family Size Lasagna w/ Meat Sauce	1 cup	270	14	10	45	33	2	900
Family Size Macaroni & Cheese	1 cup	230	8	7	10	32	3	1290
Fettuccine Alfredo	1 meal (9.5 oz)	350	11	16	25	40	4	850

FOOD	PORTION	CALS	PROT	FAT	CHOL	CARB	FIBER	SOD
Homestyle Noodles & Chicken	1 meal (12 oz)	390	12	19	50	44	7	1080
Lasagna w/ Meat Sauce	1 meal (9.5 oz)	260	10	8	15	38	3	820
Macaroni & Cheese	1 meal (12 oz)	420	15	14	20	57	5	1330
Birds Eye								
Easy Recipe Creations Basil Herb Primavera	2¼ cup	260	9	11	25	31	3	750
Easy Recipe Creations Tortellini Parmigiana	2¼ cups	240	9	12	25	25	4	870
Pasta Secrets Italian Pesto	2⅓ cups	240	9	9	5	32	2	700
Pasta Secrets Primavera	2⅓ cups	230	9	10	10	26	3	430
Pasta Secrets Ranch	2⅓ cups	300	7	15	25	29	2	460
Pasta Secrets Three Cheese	2 cups	230	9	8	5	31	2	590
Pasta Secrets White Cheddar	2 cups	240	7	10	10	30	2	560
Pasta Secrets Zesty Garlic	2 cups	240	7	10	5	31	2	310
Healthy Choice								
Beef Macaroni	1 meal (8.5 oz)	220	12	4	20	34	5	450
Bowls Cheese & Chicken Tortellini	1 meal (8.7 oz)	250	11	5	20	40	6	600
Breaded Chicken Breast Stips w/ Macaroni & Cheese	1 meal (8 oz)	270	22	5	40	34	1	600
Cheese Ravioli Parmigiana	1 meal (9 oz)	260	11	5	20	44	6	290
Chicken Fettuccine Alfredo	1 meal (8.5 oz)	280	21	7	35	30	4	600
Fettuccine Alfredo	1 meal (8 oz)	240	11	5	20	37	2	560
Lasagna Bake	1 pkg (9 oz)	270	13	7	20	38	4	600

FOOD	PORTION	CALS	PROT	FAT	CHOL	CARB	FIBER	SOD
Macaroni & Cheese	1 meal (9 oz)	240	12	5	20	36	3	600
Manicotti w/ Three Cheeses	1 meal (11 oz)	300	15	9	35	40	5	550
Spaghetti & Sauce w/ Seasoned Beef	1 meal (10 oz)	260	14	8	30	43	5	470
Stuffed Pasta Shells	1 meal (10.35 oz)	370	18	6	20	60	5	570
Joseph's Pasta								
Grilled Chicken Ravioli w/ Roasted Red Pepper Sauce	1 pkg (14 oz)	540	36	15	150	66	6	1440
Kid Cuisine								
Magical Macaroni & Cheese	1 meal (10.6 oz)	440	10	13	15	72	4	670
Lean Cuisine								
Cafe Classics Bow Tie Pasta & Chicken	1 pkg (9.5 oz)	220	15	4	40	32	5	690
Cafe Classics Cheese Lasagna w/ Chicken Scaloppini	1 pkg (10 oz)	270	22	8	35	27	4	690
Cafe Classics Shrimp & Angel Hair Pasta	1 pkg (10 oz)	240	15	5	45	35	2	670
Everyday Favorites Alfredo Pasta Primavera	1 pkg (10 oz)	290	11	7	10	46	3	570
Everyday Favorites Angel Hair Pasta	1 pkg (10 oz)	240	9	4	5	43	4	500
Everyday Favorites Cheese Cannelloni	1 pkg (9.1 oz)	230	21	4	15	28	4	590
Everyday Favorites Cheese Lasagna Casserole	1 pkg (10 oz)	270	13	6	10	40	5	590
Everyday Favorites Cheese Ravioli	1 pkg (8.5 oz)	260	12	7	35	38	4	590
Everyday Favorites Chicken Lasagna	1 pkg (10 oz)	280	20	7	40	34	2	590

FOOD	PORTION	CALS	PROT	FAT	CHOL	CARB	FIBER	SOD
Everyday Favorites Classic Cheese Lasagna	1 pkg (11.5 oz)	290	20	6	25	38	4	590
Everyday Favorites Fettucini Alfredo	1 pkg (9.25 oz)	280	13	7	15	42	3	540
Everyday Favorites Fettucini Primavera	1 pkg (10 oz)	270	13	7	15	38	4	580
Everyday Favorites Lasagna w/ Meat Sauce	1 pkg (10.5 oz)	300	23	8	30	35	4	570
Everyday Favorites Macaroni & Cheese	1 pkg (10 oz)	290	15	7	20	42	2	630
Everyday Favorites Macaroni & Beef	1 pkg (10 oz)	270	15	4	25	43	4	590
Everyday Favorites Penne Pasta	1 pkg (10 oz)	260	9	4	0	47	5	390
Everyday Favorites Spaghetti w/ Meat Sauce	1 pkg (11.5 oz)	290	11	5	20	50	7	570
Everyday Favorites Spaghetti w/ Meatballs	1 pkg (9.5 oz)	270	16	6	20	37	4	590
Family Style Favorites Five Cheese Lasagna	1 serv (8 oz)	210	14	5	20	27	3	690
Skillet Sensations Chicken Alfredo	1 serv	280	20	6	30	36	3	590
Marie Callender's								
Cheese Ravioli In Marinara Sauce w/ Spirals & Garlic Bread	1 meal (16 oz)	750	25	29	30	96	11	1070
Extra Cheese Lasagna	1 meal (15 oz)	590	27	27	50	61	7	1230
Fettuccine Alfredo & Garlic Bread	1 meal (14 oz)	920	23	55	90	62	3	1270
Fettuccine Alfredo Supreme	1 meal (13 oz)	450	15	27	80	35	4	680

FOOD	PORTION	CALS	PROT	FAT	CHOL	CARB	FIBER	SOD
Fettuccine Primavera w/ Tortellini	1 meal (14 oz)	750	19	49	65	57	6	1130
Fettuccine w/ Broccoli & Chicken	1 meal (13 oz)	710	26	43	85	53	6	910
Lasagna w/ Meat Sauce	1 meal (15 oz)	630	29	31	75	59	3	1230
Macaroni & Cheese	1 meal (12 oz)	540	25	24	50	55	5	1930
Skillet Meal Chicken Alfredo	½ pkg	490	28	29	75	32	7	1220
Skillet Meal Penne Pasta & Meatballs	½ pkg	600	26	31	45	53	4	1360
Skillet Meal Rigatoni Vegetables In Cheese Sauce	1 cup	290	12	12	30	32	4	640
Spaghetti w/ Meat Sauce & Garlic Bread	1 meal (17 oz)	670	27	25	35	65	9	1100
Stuffed Pasta Trio	1 meal (10.5 oz)	380	15	16	50	40	5	950
Morton								
Macaroni & Cheese	1 serv (8 oz)	240	9	8	20	34	3	1190
Spaghetti w/ Meat Sauce	1 meal (8.5 oz)	200	5	6	5	30	4	750
Quorn								
Fettuccine Alfredo	1 pkg (10.5 oz)	360	17	16	45	40	4	920
Lasagna	1 pkg (10.5 oz)	360	23	12	15	43	4	910
Seeds Of Change								
Organic Lasagna Creamy Spinach	1 pkg (11 oz)	370	19	16	35	36	7	750
Slim-Fast								
Fettuccine Alfredo	1 pkg	240	10	6	20	41	5	890
Rotini w/ Tomato & Italian Herb	1 pkg	240	10	2	<5	45	4	890
Shells & Creamy Cheese Sauce	1 pkg	240	10	6	20	40	5	890

FOOD	PORTION	CALS	PROT	FAT	CHOL	CARB	FIBER	SOD
Stouffer's								
Lasagna w/ Meat Sauce	1 cup	250	17	8	30	27	2	720
Yves								
Veggie Lasagna	1 pkg (10.5 oz)	300	17	3	0	51	4	650
Veggie Macaroni	1 pkg (10.5 oz)	230	14	2	0	38	3	580
Veggie Penne	1 pkg (10.5 oz)	220	12	2	0	36	4	730
MIX								
Annie's Homegrown								
Mac & Cheese Meals	1 pkg	230	9	5	10	40	tr	560
Aramana								
Cheddar Cheeseburger as prep	1 cup	260	16	17	55	11	4	840
Creamy Chicken Alfredo as prep	1 cup	260	17	16	55	12	5	720
Mild Mexican as prep	1 cup	260	17	16	55	12	5	840
Atkins								
Quick Quisine Elbows & Cheese as prep	1 cup	250	32	7	10	17	9	500
Quick Quisine Fettuccine Alfredo as prep	1 cup	210	32	7	10	16	9	620
Quick Quisine Pesto Cream as prep	1 cup	240	32	6	5	17	10	580
Hodgson Mill								
Macaroni & Cheese Whole Wheat	1 serv	250	11	1	<5	45	6	570
Keto								
Macaroni & Cheese not prep	1 serv	112	24	10	–	5	1	20
Near East								
Angel Hair w/ Spicy Tomato as prep	1 cup	240	8	6	0	39	3	630

FOOD	PORTION	CALS	PROT	FAT	CHOL	CARB	FIBER	SOD
Radiatore Basil & Herb as prep	1 cup	240	8	6	3	39	3	380
Vermicelli Garlic & Oil as prep	1 cup	310	10	9	3	48	3	510
Whey Cool								
High Protein Macaroni & Cheese as prep	1 serv	260	46	5	15	12	1	780
SHELF-STABLE								
It's Pasta Anytime								
Penne With Tomato Italian Sausage Sauce	1 pkg (15.25 oz)	540	17	8	<5	100	12	1100
Lunch Bucket								
Lasagna 'n Meatsauce	1 pkg (7.5 oz)	160	5	3	5	29	2	850
Macaroni 'n Beef in Meatsauce	1 pkg (7.5 oz)	180	0	5	10	10	8	820
Macaroni'n Cheese	1 pkg (7.5 oz)	190	7	7	20	24	2	930
Pasta'n Chicken	1 pkg (7.5 oz)	150	5	5	20	22	2	810
Spaghetti'n Meatsauce	1 pkg (7.5 oz)	160	5	3	5	29	2	850
TAKE-OUT								
fettuccini alfredo	1 cup	715	–	170	60	–	–	735
lasagna	1 piece (2.5 in x 2.5 in)	374	22	21	107	25	2	668
lasagna vegetarian	2 cups	720	–	130	43	–	–	1740
macaroni & cheese	1 cup	230	9	10	24	26	–	730
manicotti	¾ cup (6.4 oz)	273	14	12	77	28	2	414
ravioli cheese w/ tomato sauce	2 cups	530	–	0	75	–	–	1100
rigatoni w/ sausage sauce	¾ cup	260	10	12	59	28	3	106
spaghetti w/ clam sauce	1 serv	395	–	65	16	–	–	310

FOOD	PORTION	CALS	PROT	FAT	CHOL	CARB	FIBER	SOD
spaghetti w/ marinara sauce	1 cup	260	–	0	9	–	–	955
spaghetti w/ meatballs & cheese	1 cup	407	21	19	104	38	–	696
tortellini cheese w/ tomato sauce	1 cup	470	–	15	75	–	–	945

PASTA SALAD
MIX
Kraft
Pasta Salad Italian 97% Fat Free as prep	¾ cup (4.9 oz)	190	8	2	<5	35	2	740

Suddenly Salad
Classic Pasta	¾ cup	250	7	8	0	38	2	910
Classic Pasta Reduced Fat Recipe	¾ cup	210	7	4	0	38	2	910
Garden Italian 98% Fat Free	¾ cup	140	5	1	0	28	2	520

TAKE-OUT
elbow macaroni salad	3.5 oz	160	3	5	0	26	–	590
italian style pasta salad	3.5 oz	140	3	7	0	15	–	480
mustard macaroni salad	3.5 oz	190	4	10	0	23	–	560
pasta salad w/ vegetables	3.5 oz	140	4	4	0	21	–	210

PATE
chicken liver canned	1 tbsp (13 g)	109	2	2	–	1	–	–
duck pate	1 oz	96	4	8	–	1	–	–
fish pate	1 oz	76	3	7	–	1	–	286
goose liver smoked canned	1 tbsp (13 g)	60	1	6	20	1	–	–
liver canned	1 tbsp (13 g)	41	5	4	–	tr	–	91
mushroom anchovy pate	1 can (2.25 oz)	130	2	11	5	7	1	400

FOOD	PORTION	CALS	PROT	FAT	CHOL	CARB	FIBER	SOD
pate foie gras	1 oz	127	3	13	109	1	—	211
pork pate	1 oz	107	3	10	51	1	0	189
pork pate en croute	1 oz	91	3	7	32	3	tr	214
rabbit pate	1 oz	66	5	5	21	1	—	97
shrimp	1 can (2.25 oz)	140	6	10	25	7	0	450

PEACH
CANNED

FOOD	PORTION	CALS	PROT	FAT	CHOL	CARB	FIBER	SOD
halves in heavy syrup	1 half	60	tr	tr	0	16	—	5
halves in light syrup	1 half	44	tr	tr	0	12	—	4
halves juice pack	1 half	34	tr	tr	0	9	—	3
halves water pack	1 half	18	tr	tr	0	5	—	3
peachsauce	½ cup	120	tr	0	0	32	1	0
spiced in heavy syrup	1 cup	180	1	tr	0	49	—	9
spiced in heavy syrup	1 fruit	66	tr	tr	0	18	—	3

Del Monte

FOOD	PORTION	CALS	PROT	FAT	CHOL	CARB	FIBER	SOD
Fruit Cup Diced Extra Light Syrup	1 pkg (4 oz)	50	0	0	0	13	1	10
Fruit Cup Diced In Heavy Syrup	1 serv (4 oz)	80	0	0	0	20	1	10
Fruit Cup Fruit Naturals Diced	1 pkg (4 oz)	50	0	0	0	13	1	10
Fruit Pleasures Raspberry Flavor	½ cup (4.5 oz)	80	1	0	0	20	1	10
Fruit To Go Banana Berry Peaches	1 pkg (4 oz)	70	1	0	0	17	1	10
Fruitrageous Peachy Pie	1 pkg (4 oz)	80	1	0	0	21	1	10
Fruitrageous Wild Raspberry Flavor	1 pkg (4 oz)	80	1	0	0	20	1	10
Halves Ginger Flavor	½ cup (4.5 oz)	90	0	0	0	22	1	10
Halves In Extra Light Syrup	½ cup (4.4 oz)	60	0	0	0	15	1	10

FOOD	PORTION	CALS	PROT	FAT	CHOL	CARB	FIBER	SOD
Halves	½ cup (4.5 oz)	100	0	0	0	24	1	10
Halves Melba In Heavy Syrup	½ cup (4.5 oz)	100	0	0	0	24	1	10
Orchard Select Sliced Cling	½ cup	80	tr	0	0	22	tr	10
Slice Fruit Natural	½ cup (4.4 oz)	60	0	0	0	15	1	10
Sliced In Extra Light Syrup	½ cup (4.4 oz)	60	0	0	0	14	1	10
Sliced Natural Raspberry Flavor	½ cup (4.4 oz)	80	0	0	0	20	1	10
Sliced Natural Harvest Spice Flavor	½ cup (4.5 oz)	80	1	0	0	21	1	10
Whole Spiced In Heavy Syrup	½ cup (4.2 oz)	100	0	0	0	24	1	10
Dole								
All Natural Yellow Cling Sliced	½ cup	80	1	0	0	17	tr	10
DRIED								
halves	10	311	5	1	0	80	11	9
halves	1 cup	383	6	1	0	98	13	12
halves cooked w/ sugar	½ cup	139	1	tr	0	36	—	3
halves cooked w/o sugar	½ cup	99	1	tr	0	25	—	3
FRESH								
peach	1	37	1	tr	0	10	1	0
sliced	1 cup	73	1	tr	0	19	—	1
Chiquita								
Peach	1 med (3.4 oz)	40	14	0	0	10	2	0
FROZEN								
slices sweetened	1 cup	235	2	tr	0	60	—	16
PEACH JUICE								
nectar	1 cup	134	1	tr	0	35	—	17
Ceres								
Peach	8 oz	120	0	0	0	30	0	5

FOOD	PORTION	CALS	PROT	FAT	CHOL	CARB	FIBER	SOD
PEANUT BUTTER								
chunky	2 tbsp	188	8	16	0	7	2	156
chunky	1 cup	1520	62	129	0	56	17	1255
chunky w/o salt	2 tbsp	188	8	16	0	7	2	5
chunky w/o salt	1 cup	1520	62	129	0	56	17	44
smooth	2 tbsp	188	8	16	0	7	2	153
smooth	1 cup	1517	63	128	0	53	15	1234
smooth w/o salt	2 tbsp	188	8	16	0	7	2	5
smooth w/o salt	1 cup	1517	63	129	0	53	15	44
Carb Options								
Creamy	2 tbsp	190	7	17	0	5	2	150
Jif								
Apple Cinnamon	2 tbsp (1.3 oz)	200	6	16	0	11	2	115
Berry Blend	2 tbsp (1.2 oz)	200	6	17	0	10	1	115
Chocolate Silk	2 tbsp (1.3 oz)	190	5	15	0	14	1	115
Creamy	2 tbsp	190	8	16	0	7	2	150
Extra Crunchy	2 tbsp (1.1 oz)	190	8	16	0	7	2	130
Reduced Fat Creamy	2 tbsp (1.3 oz)	190	8	12	0	15	2	250
Reduced Fat Crunchy	2 tbsp (1.3 oz)	190	8	12	0	15	2	220
Simply	2 tbsp (1.1 oz)	190	8	16	0	6	2	1
Maranatha								
Crunchy	2 tbsp	190	8	16	–	7	2	80
Salted	2 tbsp	190	8	16	0	7	2	80
P.B.								
Slices	1 slice (1 oz)	170	6	14	0	5	1	110
Peanut Butter & Co.								
Cinnamon Raisin Swirl	2 tbsp	143	10	7	0	10	2	67
Crunch Time	2 tbsp	200	7	16	0	7	2	120
Dark Chocolate Dreams	2 tbsp	175	8	12	0	8	2	82
Smooth Operator	2 tbsp	200	7	16	0	7	2	120
The Heat Is On	2 tbsp	164	9	10	0	9	2	86

FOOD	PORTION	CALS	PROT	FAT	CHOL	CARB	FIBER	SOD
White Chocolate Wonderful	1 tbsp	165	7	12	0	8	2	56
Peanut Wonder								
Low Sodium	2 tbsp	100	4	3	0	13	0	95
Regular	2 tbsp	100	4	3	0	13	0	220
Reese's								
Peanut Butter Chips	1 tbsp	80	3	4	0	7	–	35
Skippy								
Creamy	2 tbsp	190	7	17	0	7	2	150
Creamy w/ 2 slices white bread	1 sandwich	340	14	19	0	33	–	430
Reduced Fat Creamy	2 tbsp	190	7	12	0	15	2	190
Roasted Honey Nut	2 tbsp	190	7	17	0	7	2	125
Roasted Honey Nut Super Chunk	2 tbsp	190	7	17	0	7	2	125
Squeeze Stix	1 pkg	140	6	12	0	5	2	120
Squeeze Stix Chocolate	1 pkg	140	4	10	0	9	2	85
Squeez'It	2 tbsp	190	7	17	0	7	2	160
Super Chunk	2 tbsp	190	7	17	0	7	2	140
Tropical Source								
Chips Dairy Free	13 pieces (1.5 oz)	80	2	5	0	9	0	7
PEANUTS								
chocolate coated	10 (1.4 oz)	208	5	13	4	20	–	16
chocolate coated	1 cup (5.2 oz)	773	19	50	13	74	–	61
cooked	½ cup	102	4	7	0	7	–	240
dry roasted	1 cup	855	35	73	0	31	12	1187
dry roasted w/ salt	30 nuts (1 oz)	170	7	14	0	6	2	230
At Last!								
Chocolate Covered	1 pkg (0.9 oz)	150	4	11	0	18	5	15
Frito Lay								
Honey Roasted	1 serv (1.5 oz)	270	10	21	0	10	3	80

FOOD	PORTION	CALS	PROT	FAT	CHOL	CARB	FIBER	SOD
Hot	1 serv (1.1 oz)	190	7	16	0	6	2	250
Salted	1 oz	200	7	16	0	5	2	180
Judy's								
Sugar Free Coconut Peanut Brittle	¼ piece (1 oz)	90	1	5	0	2	1	0
Low Carb Creations								
Soft Peanut Brittle	2 pieces (1 oz)	140	6	10	0	8	2	150
Sweet Delight								
Peanut Roasters	⅓ pkg (1 oz)	160	7	12	0	7	3	200
PEAR								
CANNED								
halves in heavy sirup	1 cup	188	1	tr	0	49	—	13
halves in heavy syrup	1 half	68	tr	tr	0	15	—	4
halves in light syrup	1 half	45	tr	tr	0	12	—	4
halves juice pack	1 cup	123	1	tr	0	32	—	10
halves water pack	1 half	22	tr	tr	0	6	—	41
Del Monte								
Fruit Cup Diced In Heavy Syrup	1 pkg (4 oz)	80	0	0	0	20	1	10
Fruit Cup Diced Extra Light Syrup	1 pkg (4 oz)	50	0	0	0	13	1	10
Fruit To Go Peachy Peaches	1 pkg (4 oz)	70	1	0	0	17	1	10
Halves Fruit Naturals	½ cup (4.4 oz)	60	0	0	0	15	1	10
Halves In Extra Light Syrup	½ cup (4.4 oz)	60	0	0	0	15	1	10
Halves In Heavy Syrup	½ cup (4.5 oz)	100	0	0	0	24	1	10
Orchard Select Sliced Bartlett	½ cup	80	tr	0	0	20	2	10
Sliced In Extra Light Syrup	½ cup (4.5 oz)	60	0	0	0	15	1	10

FOOD	PORTION	CALS	PROT	FAT	CHOL	CARB	FIBER	SOD
DRIED								
halves	1 cup	472	3	1	0	125	–	10
halves	10	459	3	1	0	122	–	10
halves cooked w/ sugar	½ cup	196	1	tr	0	52	–	4
halves cooked w/o sugar	½ cup	163	tr	tr	0	43	–	4
FRESH								
asian	1 (4.3 oz)	51	1	tr	0	13	–	0
pear	1	98	1	1	0	25	4	1
sliced w/ skin	1 cup	97	1	1	0	25	4	1
Chiquita								
Pear	1 med (5.8 oz)	100	1	1	0	25	4	0
PEAR JUICE								
nectar	1 cup	149	tr	tr	0	39	–	9
Ceres								
Pear	8 oz	120	0	0	0	30	0	10
PEAS								
CANNED								
green	½ cup	59	4	tr	0	11	–	186
green low sodium	½ cup	59	4	tr	0	11	–	2
Del Monte								
Sweet	½ cup (4.4 oz)	60	3	0	0	13	4	390
Sweet No Salt Added	½ cup (4.4 oz)	60	3	0	0	11	4	10
Sweet Very Young Small	½ cup (4.4 oz)	60	3	0	0	10	4	360
S&W								
Petite	½ cup (4.4 oz)	70	4	0	0	12	4	330
Small	½ cup (4.4 oz)	70	4	0	0	12	4	330
Veg-All								
Tender Sweet	½ cup	60	4	1	0	10	3	370
DRIED								
split cooked	1 cup	231	16	1	0	41	–	4

FOOD	PORTION	CALS	PROT	FAT	CHOL	CARB	FIBER	SOD
FRESH								
green cooked	½ cup	67	4	tr	0	13	–	2
green raw	½ cup	58	4	tr	0	11	–	3
snap peas cooked	½ cup	34	3	tr	0	6	2	3
snap peas raw	½ cup	30	2	tr	0	5	2	3
FROZEN								
green cooked	½ cup	63	4	tr	0	11	–	70
snap peas cooked	½ cup	42	3	tr	0	7	–	4
snap peas cooked	1 pkg (10 oz)	132	9	1	0	23	–	12
Birds Eye								
Butter Peas	½ cup	110	7	1	0	20	4	10
Crowder	½ cup	120	8	1	0	22	4	10
Field Peas w/ Snaps	⅔ cup	130	9	1	0	24	4	15
Green	½ cup	70	–	0	0	–	5	125
Purple Hull Peas	½ cup	110	7	1	0	21	4	10
Sugar Snap	½ cup	40	–	0	0	–	2	10
Tiny Tender	¾ cup	40	–	0	0	–	2	40
Fresh Like								
Garden	3.5 oz	85	5	1	–	14	2	79
La Choy								
Snow Pea Pods	½ pkg (3 oz)	35	2	2	0	4	2	0
Tree Of Life								
Peas	⅔ cup (3.1 oz)	70	5	0	0	12	4	100
SHELF-STABLE								
TastyBite								
Agra Peas & Greens	½ pkg (5 oz)	260	8	14	0	26	1	380
TAKE-OUT								
pea & potato curry	1 serv (7 oz)	284	5	22	–	19	6	–
pea curry	1 serv (4.4 oz)	438	5	42	–	11	4	–
PECANS								
dry roasted	1 oz	187	2	18	0	6	–	0
dry roasted salted	1 oz	187	2	18	0	6	–	260
halves dry roasted w/ salt	20 (1 oz)	200	3	21	0	4	3	110
halves dried	1 cup	721	8	73	0	20	7	1
oil roasted	1 oz	195	2	20	0	5	–	0
oil roasted salted	1 oz	195	2	20	0	5	–	252

FOOD	PORTION	CALS	PROT	FAT	CHOL	CARB	FIBER	SOD
Keto								
Chocolately Covered	1 oz	207	3	19	–	6	5	–
Sweet Delights								
Pecan Roasters	⅓ pkg (1 oz)	210	3	21	0	4	2	100
PECTIN								
powder	¼ pkg (0.4 oz)	39	0	0	0	11	–	24
powder	1 pkg (1.75 oz)	163	tr	tr	0	45	–	100
Slim Set								
Packet	1 pkg	208	0	0	0	44	14	42
Powder	1 tbsp	3	0	0	0	1	tr	1
Sure Jell								
For Lower Sugar Recipes	1 tsp (2.8 g)	20	0	0	0	4	0	40
Fruit Pectin	1 tsp (3.6 g)	20	0	0	0	4	0	0
PEPEAO								
dried	½ cup	36	1	tr	0	10	–	8
raw sliced	1 cup	25	tr	tr	0	7	–	9
PEPPER								
black	1 tsp	5	tr	tr	0	1	–	1
cayenne	1 tsp	6	tr	tr	0	1	–	1
red	1 tsp	6	tr	tr	0	1	–	1
white	1 tsp	7	tr	tr	0	2	–	tr
McCormick								
Lemon & Pepper Seasoning Salt	¼ tsp	0	0	0	0	0	0	130
PEPPERS								
CANNED								
chili green	1 cup (5.5 oz)	29	1	tr	0	6	2	552
chili green hot chopped	½ cup	17	1	tr	0	4	–	–
chili red hot	1 (2.6 oz)	18	1	tr	0	4	–	–
chili red hot chopped	½ cup	17	1	tr	0	4	–	–
green halves	½ cup	13	1	tr	0	3	–	958
jalapeno chopped	½ cup	17	1	tr	0	3	–	995
red halves	½ cup	13	1	tr	0	3	–	958

FOOD	PORTION	CALS	PROT	FAT	CHOL	CARB	FIBER	SOD
Old El Paso								
Green Chiles Chopped	2 tbsp (1 oz)	5	0	0	0	1	1	110
Progresso								
Cherry Sliced & So Hot	2 tbsp (1 oz)	25	0	2	0	2	1	30
Hot Cherry	1 (1 oz)	10	0	0	0	2	tr	150
Pepper Salad (drained)	2 tbsp (1 oz)	15	0	1	0	1	tr	160
Roasted	1 piece (1 oz)	10	0	0	0	3	0	55
Sweet Fried w/ Onions	2 tbsp (0.9 oz)	20	0	2	0	2	1	130
Tuscan	3 (1 oz)	10	0	0	0	2	1	450
Rosarita								
Chilies Diced Green	2 tbsp (1 oz)	6	tr	tr	0	1	1	85
Chilies Green Strips	¼ cup (1.2 oz)	5	tr	tr	0	1	1	74
Chilies Whole Green	2 tbsp (1.2 oz)	5	tr	tr	0	1	1	74
Jalapeno Whole w/ Escabeche	¼ cup (1.2 oz)	8	1	tr	0	1	1	430
Jalapenos Diced	2 tbsp (1 oz)	5	tr	tr	0	1	1	121
Jalapenos Nacho Sliced	2 tbsp (1 oz)	2	tr	tr	0	1	tr	224
Vlasic								
Hot Sliced Cherry	1 oz	5	0	0	0	1	—	480
Jalapeno Sliced	1 oz	10	0	0	0	2	—	480
Mild Cherry	1 oz	5	0	0	0	1	—	480
Pepper Rings Hot	1 oz	5	0	0	0	1	—	480
Pepper Rings Mild	1 oz	5	0	0	0	1	—	480
DRIED								
ancho	1 (0.6 oz)	48	2	1	0	9	4	7
green	1 tbsp	1	tr	tr	0	tr	—	1
pasilla	1 (7 g)	24	1	1	0	4	2	6
red	1 tbsp	1	tr	tr	0	tr	—	1
FRESH								
banana	1 (4 in) (1.2 oz)	9	1	tr	0	2	1	4
banana	1 cup (4.4 oz)	33	2	1	0	7	4	16
chili green hot	1	18	1	tr	0	4	—	3

FOOD	PORTION	CALS	PROT	FAT	CHOL	CARB	FIBER	SOD
chili green hot chopped	½ cup	30	2	tr	0	7	—	5
chili red chopped	½ cup	30	2	tr	0	7	—	5
chili red hot	1 (1.6 oz)	18	1	tr	0	4	—	3
green	1 (2.6 oz)	20	1	tr	0	5	1	1
green chopped	½ cup	13	tr	tr	0	3	1	1
green chopped cooked	½ cup	19	1	tr	0	5	—	1
green cooked	1 (2.6 oz)	20	1	tr	0	5	—	1
habanero chile	1 tsp	9	1	tr	0	2	1	2
hungarian	1 (0.9 oz)	8	tr	tr	0	2	0	tr
jalapeno	1 (0.5 oz)	4	tr	tr	0	1	tr	tr
jalapeno sliced	1 cup (3.2 oz)	27	1	1	0	5	3	1
red	1 (2.6 oz)	20	1	tr	0	5	1	1
red chopped	½ cup	13	tr	tr	0	3	1	1
red chopped cooked	½ cup	19	1	tr	0	5	—	1
red cooked	1 (2.6 oz)	20	1	tr	0	5	—	1
serrano	1 (6 g)	2	tr	tr	0	tr	tr	1
serrano chopped	1 cup (3.7 oz)	34	2	tr	0	7	4	11
yellow	1 (6.5 oz)	50	2	tr	0	12	—	3
yellow	10 strips	14	1	tr	0	3	—	1
Chiquita								
Pepper	1 med (5.2 oz)	30	1	0	0	7	2	0
FROZEN								
green chopped	1 oz	6	tr	tr	0	1	—	1
red chopped	1 oz	6	tr	tr	0	1	—	1
Birds Eye								
Diced Green	¾ cup	20	1	0	0	4	2	10
PERCH								
FRESH								
cooked	3 oz	99	21	1	90	0	—	67
cooked	1 fillet (1.6 oz)	54	11	1	53	0	—	36
ocean perch atlantic cooked	3 oz	103	20	2	46	0	—	82

FOOD	PORTION	CALS	PROT	FAT	CHOL	CARB	FIBER	SOD
ocean perch atlantic cooked	1 fillet (1.8 oz)	60	12	1	27	0	–	48
ocean perch atlantic raw	3 oz	80	16	1	36	0	–	64
raw	3 oz	77	16	1	76	0	–	52
red raw	3.5 oz	114	18	4	–	0	–	80

PERSIMMONS

FOOD	PORTION	CALS	PROT	FAT	CHOL	CARB	FIBER	SOD
dried japanese	1	93	tr	tr	0	25	–	1
fresh	1	32	tr	tr	0	8	–	0
fresh japanese	1	118	1	tr	0	31	–	3

PHEASANT

FOOD	PORTION	CALS	PROT	FAT	CHOL	CARB	FIBER	SOD
breast w/o skin raw	½ breast (6.4 oz)	243	44	6	–	0	–	60
leg w/o skin raw	1 (3.6 oz)	143	24	5	–	0	–	48
roasted	3.5 oz	215	33	9	120	0	0	100
w/ skin raw	½ pheasant (14 oz)	723	91	37	–	0	–	161
w/o skin raw	½ pheasant (12.4 oz)	470	83	13	–	0	–	131

PHYLLO

FOOD	PORTION	CALS	PROT	FAT	CHOL	CARB	FIBER	SOD
phyllo dough	1 oz	85	2	2	0	15	–	137
sheet	1	57	1	1	0	10	–	92
Ekizian								
Sheets	¼ lb	433	12	9	62	76	–	287
Fillo Factory								
Fillo Dough Spelt Vegan	3 sheets (2 oz)	180	0	1	0	31	4	120
Fillo Dough Vegan	3 sheets (2 oz)	170	5	1	0	36	1	220
Fillo Dough Whole Wheat Vegan	3 sheets (2 oz)	190	6	1	0	40	3	135
Pastry Shells Vegan	3 (0.4 oz)	45	1	2	0	7	0	50

PICANTE (see SALSA)

PICKLES

FOOD	PORTION	CALS	PROT	FAT	CHOL	CARB	FIBER	SOD
dill	1 (2.3 oz)	12	tr	tr	0	3	–	833
dill low sodium	1 (2.3 oz)	12	tr	tr	0	3	1	12

FOOD	PORTION	CALS	PROT	FAT	CHOL	CARB	FIBER	SOD
dill low sodium sliced	1 slice	1	tr	tr	0	tr	tr	1
dill sliced	1 slice	1	tr	tr	0	tr	tr	77
gerkins	1 oz	6	tr	tr	0	1	—	274
kosher dill	1 (2.3 oz)	12	tr	tr	0	3	1	833
polish dill	1 (2.3 oz)	12	tr	tr	0	3	1	833
quick sour	1 (1.2 oz)	4	tr	tr	0	1	—	423
quick sour low sodium	1 (1.2 oz)	4	tr	tr	0	1	—	6
quick sour sliced	1 slice	1	tr	tr	0	tr	—	85
sweet	1 (1.2 oz)	41	tr	tr	0	11	tr	328
sweet gherkin	1 sm (½ oz)	20	tr	tr	0	5	—	107
sweet low sodium	1 (1.2 oz)	41	tr	tr	0	11	tr	6
sweet sliced	1 slice	7	tr	tr	0	2	tr	56
Claussen								
Bread 'N Butter Chips	4 slices (1 oz)	20	0	0	0	4	0	170
Deli Style Hearty Garlic Whole	½ (1 oz)	5	0	0	0	1	0	260
Kosher Dills Spears	1 spear (1.2 oz)	5	0	0	0	1	0	320
Kosher Dills Halves	1 half (1 oz)	5	0	0	0	1	0	330
Kosher Dills Mini	1 (0.8 oz)	5	0	0	0	1	0	300
Kosher Dills Whole	½ (1 oz)	5	0	0	0	1	0	330
New York Deli Style Half Sours Whole	½ (1 oz)	5	0	0	0	1	0	260
Sandwich Slices Bread 'N Butter	2 (1.2 oz)	25	0	0	0	5	0	210
Sandwich Slices Deli Style Hearty Garlic	2 (1.2 oz)	5	0	0	0	1	0	320
Sandwich Slices Kosher Dills	2 (1.2 oz)	5	0	0	0	1	0	440
Super Slices For Burgers	1 (0.8 oz)	5	0	0	0	1	0	320
Mt Olive								
Bread & Butter No Sugar Added	1 oz	0	0	0	0	tr	0	105

FOOD	PORTION	CALS	PROT	FAT	CHOL	CARB	FIBER	SOD
Vlasic								
Hamburger Dill Chips	1 oz	5	0	0	0	1	–	400
Kosher Cross Cuts	1 oz	5	0	0	0	1	–	220
Kosher Spears	1 oz	5	0	0	0	1	–	220
Kosher Whole	1 oz	5	0	0	0	1	–	220
Sweet Butter Chips	1 oz	30	0	0	0	7	–	190
Sweet Gerkins	1 oz	35	0	0	0	9	–	260
Whole Dills	1 oz	5	0	0	0	1	–	390
PIE								
FROZEN								
apple	⅛ of 9 in pie (4.4 oz)	297	2	14	0	43	2	333
blueberry	⅛ of 9 in pie (4.4 oz)	289	2	13	0	44	–	406
cherry	⅛ of 9 in pie (4.4 oz)	325	3	14	0	50	1	308
chocolate creme	⅙ of 8 in pie (4 oz)	344	3	22	6	38	–	153
coconut creme	⅙ of 7 in pie (2.2 oz)	191	1	11	0	24	1	163
lemon meringue	⅙ of 8 in pie (4.5 oz)	303	2	10	51	53	1	165
peach	⅙ of 8 in pie (4.1 oz)	261	2	12	0	39	–	316
Amy's								
Apple	1 serv (4 oz)	240	2	8	25	37	2	135
Mrs. Smith's								
Apple	1 slice (4.3 oz)	350	3	19	0	41	3	430
Blueberry	1 slice (4.6 oz)	330	3	17	0	43	3	500
Cappuccino	1 slice (4.2 oz)	300	4	13	0	45	2	260
Cherry	1 slice (4.3 oz)	320	3	17	0	41	2	490
Cherry Crumb	1 slice (4.2 oz)	320	3	12	0	52	1	250

FOOD	PORTION	CALS	PROT	FAT	CHOL	CARB	FIBER	SOD
Chocolate Cream	1 slice (4.6 oz)	340	3	18	15	43	2	380
Chocolate Mint Cream	1 slice (4.3 oz)	360	3	15	0	53	2	240
Coconut Custard	1 slice (4.4 oz)	260	6	14	70	28	tr	310
Cookies 'N Cream	1 slice (4.3 oz)	360	4	16	0	52	2	290
Dutch Apple	1 slice (4.4 oz)	330	3	13	0	50	2	300
French Silk	1 slice (4.4 oz)	560	4	40	55	48	1	280
Key West Lime	1 slice (4.3 oz)	430	5	18	15	62	1	290
Lemon Cream	1 slice (5 oz)	440	3	26	0	49	tr	180
Lemonade	1 slice (4.3 oz)	340	3	15	0	51	1	280
Mince	1 slice (4.6 oz)	380	3	17	0	53	2	520
Mixed Berry	1 slice (4.2 oz)	300	2	13	0	44	2	360
Peach	1 slice (4.6 oz)	320	3	17	0	40	2	450
Peach Lattice	1 slice (4.2 oz)	290	2	13	0	42	2	280
Peanut Butter Silk	1 slice (4.6 oz)	600	8	41	55	51	2	330
Pecan	1 slice (4.8 oz)	560	6	27	65	75	2	450
Pumpkin Custard	1 slice (4.6 oz)	270	5	13	40	35	2	330
Raspberry	1 slice (4.6 oz)	330	3	17	0	44	1	510
S'Mores Cream	1 slice (4.3 oz)	360	3	16	0	53	2	300
Strawberry Banana	1 slice (4.3 oz)	330	3	15	0	48	1	270
Sweet Potato Custard	1 slice (4.6 oz)	340	4	17	40	44	2	240

FOOD	PORTION	CALS	PROT	FAT	CHOL	CARB	FIBER	SOD
Sara Lee								
Apple 45% Reduced Fat	⅙ pie (4.5 oz)	290	4	8	<5	51	2	400
Chocolate Silk	⅕ pie (4.8 oz)	500	4	32	<5	49	<2	440
Coconut Cream	⅕ pie (4.8 oz)	480	4	31	0	47	2	430
Homestyle Apple	⅛ pie (4.6 oz)	340	3	16	0	46	1	310
Homestyle Blueberry	⅛ pie (4.6 oz)	360	3	15	0	54	2	340
Homestyle Cherry	⅛ pie (4.6 oz)	320	3	16	0	42	2	290
Homestyle Dutch Apple	⅛ pie (4.6 oz)	350	3	15	0	53	2	320
Homestyle Mince	⅛ pie (4.6 oz)	390	3	17	0	56	3	450
Homestyle Peach	⅛ pie (4.6 oz)	320	3	14	0	46	2	250
Homestyle Pecan	⅛ pie (4.2 oz)	520	5	24	45	70	3	480
Homestyle Pumpkin	⅛ pie (4.6 oz)	260	4	11	30	37	2	460
Homestyle Raspberry	⅛ pie (4.6 oz)	380	3	19	<5	48	2	330
Lemon Meringue	⅙ pie (5 oz)	350	2	11	0	59	5	460
SNACK								
apple	1 (3 oz)	266	2	14	13	33	–	325
cherry	1 (3 oz)	266	2	14	13	33	–	325
lemon	1 (3 oz)	266	2	14	13	33	–	325
TAKE-OUT								
apple	⅛ of 9 in pie (5.4 oz)	411	4	19	0	58	3	327
banana cream	⅛ of 9 in pie (5.2 oz)	398	7	20	75	49	–	355
blueberry	⅛ of 9 in pie (5.2 oz)	360	4	18	0	49	–	272
butterscotch	⅛ of 9 in pie (4.5 oz)	355	6	18	78	42	–	335

FOOD	PORTION	CALS	PROT	FAT	CHOL	CARB	FIBER	SOD
cherry	⅛ of 9 in pie (6.3 oz)	486	5	22	0	69	–	343
coconut creme	⅛ of 9 in pie (4.7 oz)	396	6	21	77	46	–	356
coconut custard	⅙ of 8 in pie (3.6 oz)	271	6	14	36	32	–	348
custard	⅛ of 9 in pie (4.5 oz)	262	7	11	87	34	2	256
lemon meringue	⅛ of 9 in pie (4.5 oz)	362	5	16	68	50	2	307
mince	⅛ of 9 in pie (5.8 oz)	477	18	18	0	79	–	419
pecan	⅙ of 8 in pie (4 oz)	452	5	21	36	65	4	480
pumpkin	⅙ of 8 in pie (3.8 oz)	229	4	10	22	30	3	308
vanilla cream	⅛ of 9 in pie (4.4 oz)	350	6	18	78	41	–	327

PIE CRUST
FROZEN

FOOD	PORTION	CALS	PROT	FAT	CHOL	CARB	FIBER	SOD
baked	9 in shell (4.4 oz)	647	6	41	–	63	–	815
baked	⅛ of 9 in pie (0.6 oz)	82	1	5	–	8	–	104
puff pastry baked	1 shell (1.4 oz)	223	3	15	0	18	–	101
Pet-Ritz								
Deep Dish	⅛ pie (0.7 oz)	90	1	5	<5	10	0	85
Regular	⅛ pie (0.6 oz)	80	tr	5	<5	9	0	60
Tart Shells	1 (1 oz)	130	1	8	0	13	0	170
MIX								
as prep	⅛ of 9 in pie (0.7 oz)	100	1	6	0	10	–	146
as prep	9 in crust (5.6 oz)	801	11	49	0	81	–	1167
Betty Crocker								
Pie Crust as prep	⅛ crust	110	1	8	0	9	–	135

FOOD	PORTION	CALS	PROT	FAT	CHOL	CARB	FIBER	SOD
MiniCarb								
Pie Crust Mix	1 slice	105	9	7	40	1	0	320
READY-TO-EAT								
chocolate cookie crumb	⅛ of 9 in pie (1 oz)	139	1	9	0	15	–	185
chocolate cookie crumb	9 in crust (7.7 oz)	1130	12	69	3	122	–	1502
graham cracker	9 in crust (8.4 oz)	1181	10	60	0	156	–	1365
graham cracker	⅛ of 9 in pie (1 oz)	148	1	8	0	20	–	171
vanilla wafer cracker crumbs	9 in crust (6.1 oz)	937	7	64	69	89	–	909
vanilla wafer cracker crumbs	⅛ of 9 in pie (0.8 oz)	119	1	8	9	11	–	116
Keebler								
Graham Single Serve	1 (0.8 oz)	120	1	6	0	15	tr	150
Reduced Fat Graham	⅛ pie (0.7 oz)	90	1	4	0	14	0	85
REFRIGERATED								
All Ready								
Crust	⅛ pie (0.9 oz)	120	tr	7	5	13	0	100
PIE FILLING								
apple	1 can (21 oz)	599	1	1	0	156	6	259
apple	⅛ can (2.6 oz)	74	tr	tr	0	19	1	32
cherry	⅛ can (2.6 oz)	85	tr	tr	0	22	–	7
cherry	1 can (21 oz)	683	3	1	0	175	–	54
pumpkin pie mix	1 cup	282	3	tr	0	71	–	561
Colac								
All Flavors	1 tbsp	19	0	0	0	7	0	0
Comstock								
Light Cherry	⅓ cup	60	0	0	0	15	1	15
Red Ruby Cherry	⅓ cup (3.1 oz)	90	0	0	0	23	1	25

FOOD	PORTION	CALS	PROT	FAT	CHOL	CARB	FIBER	SOD
Libby's								
Pumpkin Pie Mix	⅓ cup	90	tr	1	0	20	2	115
Smucker's								
Pie Glaze Strawberry	2 oz	80	0	0	0	21	—	0

PIEROGI

FOOD	PORTION	CALS	PROT	FAT	CHOL	CARB	FIBER	SOD
pierogi	¾ cup (4.4 oz)	307	11	19	49	24	—	369
Health Is Wealth								
Potato & Cheddar	2 (2.8 oz)	140	5	2	0	27	3	360
Potato & Onion	2 (2.8 oz)	140	4	2	0	27	3	300
Mrs. T's								
Broccoli & Cheddar	3 (4.2 oz)	200	6	5	10	34	2	570
Jalapeno & Cheddar	3 (4.2 oz)	190	6	3	10	34	2	550
Potato & American Cheese	3 (4.2 oz)	220	8	4	15	39	2	420
Potato & Roasted Garlic	3 (4.2 oz)	190	5	4	5	36	2	430
Potato & Cheddar	3 (4.2 oz)	180	7	3	10	34	2	430
Potato & Onion	3 (4.2 oz)	180	5	2	0	34	2	410
Rogies Cheddar & Bacon	7 (3 oz)	140	5	3	5	24	1	430
Rogies Jalapeno & Cheddar	7 (3 oz)	120	4	2	5	23	1	350
Rogies Potato & Cheddar	7 (3 oz)	130	4	2	5	24	1	350

PIGEON

FOOD	PORTION	CALS	PROT	FAT	CHOL	CARB	FIBER	SOD
w/ skin & bone	3.5 oz	169	21	10	110	0	—	90

PIGEON PEAS

FOOD	PORTION	CALS	PROT	FAT	CHOL	CARB	FIBER	SOD
dried cooked	½ cup	102	6	tr	0	20	—	5
dried cooked	1 cup	204	11	1	0	39	—	9

PIGNOLIA (see PINE NUTS)

PIG'S EARS AND FEET

FOOD	PORTION	CALS	PROT	FAT	CHOL	CARB	FIBER	SOD
ear simmered	1	184	18	12	100	tr	0	185
feet pickled	1 oz	58	4	5	26	tr	0	262
feet pickled	1 lb	921	61	73	417	tr	0	4187
feet simmered	3 oz	165	16	11	85	0	0	26

FOOD	PORTION	CALS	PROT	FAT	CHOL	CARB	FIBER	SOD
PIKE								
northern cooked	½ fillet (5.4 oz)	176	38	1	78	0	–	76
northern cooked	3 oz	96	21	1	43	0	–	42
northern raw	3 oz	75	16	1	33	0	–	33
roe raw	1 oz	37	7	tr	103	tr	–	–
walleye baked	3 oz	101	21	1	94	0	–	56
walleye fillet baked	4.4 oz	147	30	2	137	0	–	81
PILLNUTS								
canarytree dried	1 oz	204	3	23	0	1	–	1
PIMIENTOS								
canned	1 tbsp	3	tr	tr	0	1	–	2
canned	1 slice	0	tr	0	0	tr	–	0
PINE NUTS								
pignolia dried	1 tbsp	51	2	5	0	1	–	0
pignolia dried	1 oz	146	7	14	0	4	–	1
pinyon dried	1 oz	161	3	17	0	5	–	20
Progresso								
Pignoli	1 jar (1 oz)	170	10	13	0	2	0	0
PINEAPPLE								
CANNED								
chunks in heavy syrup	1 cup	199	1	tr	0	52	–	3
chunks juice pack	1 cup	150	1	tr	0	39	–	4
crushed in heavy syrup	1 cup	199	1	tr	0	52	–	3
slices in heavy syrup	1 slice	45	tr	tr	0	12	–	1
slices in light syrup	1 slice	30	tr	tr	0	8	–	1
slices juice pack	1 slice	35	tr	tr	0	9	–	1
slices water pack	1 slice	19	tr	tr	0	5	–	1
tidbits in heavy syrup	1 cup	199	1	tr	0	52	–	3
tidbits in juice	1 cup	150	1	tr	0	19	–	4
tidbits in water	1 cup	79	1	tr	0	20	–	3
Del Monte								
Chunks In Heavy Syrup	½ cup (4.3 oz)	90	0	0	0	24	1	10

FOOD	PORTION	CALS	PROT	FAT	CHOL	CARB	FIBER	SOD
Chunks In Its Own Juice	½ cup (4.3 oz)	70	0	0	0	17	1	10
Crushed In Heavy Syrup	½ cup (4.3 oz)	90	0	0	0	24	1	10
Crushed In Its Own Juice	½ cup (4.3 oz)	70	0	0	0	17	1	10
Fruit Cup Tidbits	1 pkg (4 oz)	50	1	0	0	15	1	10
Sliced In Heavy Syrup	2 slices (4.1 oz)	90	0	0	0	23	1	10
Sliced In Its Own Juice	½ cup (4 oz)	60	0	0	0	16	1	10
Spears In Its Own Juice	½ cup (4.3 oz)	70	0	0	0	17	1	10
Tidbits In Its Own Juice	½ cup (4.3 oz)	70	0	0	0	17	1	10
Wedges In Its Own Juice	½ cup (4.3 oz)	70	0	0	0	17	1	10
Dole								
All Natural Chunks	½ cup	60	0	0	0	16	tr	10
Chunks Juice Pack	½ cup	60	0	0	0	15	1	10
SunFresh								
In Lightly Sweetened Juice	½ cup	70	0	0	0	18	tr	10
FRESH								
diced	1 cup	77	1	tr	0	19	2	1
slice	1 slice	42	tr	tr	0	10	1	1
Bonita Hill								
Golden Extra Sweet	2 slices (3.9 oz)	60	1	0	0	16	1	10
Cala Fruit								
Golden Sliced	1 serv (3.5 oz)	50	0	0	0	12	1	0
Frosty Fresh								
Peeled & Cored	½ cup	60	0	0	0	14	1	0
FROZEN								
chunks sweetened	½ cup	104	tr	tr	0	27	—	2
PINEAPPLE JUICE								
canned	1 cup	139	1	tr	0	34	—	2
frzn as prep	1 cup	129	1	tr	0	32	—	3

FOOD	PORTION	CALS	PROT	FAT	CHOL	CARB	FIBER	SOD
frzn not prep	6 oz	387	3	tr	0	96	–	6
Ceres								
Pineapple	8 oz	120	0	0	0	29	2	5
Del Monte								
Juice	6 fl oz	80	1	0	0	20	0	5
Dole								
Chilled	8 oz	130	0	0	0	30	–	10

PINK BEANS
dried cooked	1 cup	252	15	1	0	47	–	3

PINTO BEANS
CANNED

pinto	1 cup	186	11	1	0	35	–	998
Eden								
Organic Spicy	½ cup (4.6 oz)	125	6	0	0	24	2	195
Progresso								
Pinto Beans	½ cup (4.6 oz)	110	7	1	0	18	7	250
DRIED								
cooked	1 cup	235	14	1	0	44	–	3
FROZEN								
cooked	3 oz	152	9	tr	0	29	–	–

PISTACHIOS
dried	1 cup	739	26	62	0	32	14	7
dry roasted	1 oz	172	4	15	0	8	–	2
dry roasted salted	1 cup	776	19	68	0	35	–	1040
dry roasted salted	1 oz	172	4	15	0	8	–	260
dry roasted w/ salt	47 nuts (1 oz)	160	6	13	0	8	3	120
with shells dry roasted unsalted	½ cup	180	6	14	0	9	3	10
American Almond								
Pistachio Paste	2 tbsp	160	4	11	0	14	2	0
Sweet Delights								
Pistachio Roasters	⅓ pkg (1 oz)	190	6	14	0	9	3	220

PITANGA
fresh	1	2	tr	tr	0	1	–	0
fresh	1 cup	57	1	1	0	13	–	5

FOOD	PORTION	CALS	PROT	FAT	CHOL	CARB	FIBER	SOD

PIZZA (see also PIZZA DOUGH, PIZZA SAUCE)

Amy's

FOOD	PORTION	CALS	PROT	FAT	CHOL	CARB	FIBER	SOD
Cheese	⅓ pie	300	12	13	15	38	2	530
Mushroom & Olive	⅓ pie	250	10	9	10	33	2	560
Pesto	⅓ pie	310	12	12	10	39	2	480
Pocket Sandwich Cheese Pizza	1 (4.5 oz)	300	14	9	15	42	4	450
Pocket Sandwich Vegetarian Pizza	1 (4.5 oz)	250	11	6	10	39	4	360
Roasted Vegetable	⅓ pie	260	6	8	0	42	2	490
Snacks Cheese	5–6 pieces	180	9	6	10	22	2	290
Soy Cheese	⅓ pie	290	12	11	0	37	2	590
Spinach	⅓ pie	300	12	12	15	38	2	590
Veggie Combo	⅓ pie	280	10	9	10	36	2	580

Appian Way

FOOD	PORTION	CALS	PROT	FAT	CHOL	CARB	FIBER	SOD
Pizza Mix Thick Crust	⅓ pie (4.2 oz)	290	10	5	10	51	2	830
Pizza Mix Thin Crust	⅓ pie (4.1 oz)	250	7	3	0	48	2	740

Banquet

FOOD	PORTION	CALS	PROT	FAT	CHOL	CARB	FIBER	SOD
Pepperoni	1 pie (6.75 oz)	490	11	23	35	56	5	790
Pizza Snack Cheese	6 pieces (7.5 oz)	200	9	8	20	24	2	360
Pizza Snack Pepperoni	6 pieces (7.5 oz)	230	8	11	20	23	2	430
Pizza Snack Pepperoni & Sausage	6 pieces (7.5 oz)	210	8	9	20	24	2	440

Health Is Wealth

FOOD	PORTION	CALS	PROT	FAT	CHOL	CARB	FIBER	SOD
Pizza Munchees	6 (3 oz)	190	2	5	0	9		560

Healthy Choice

FOOD	PORTION	CALS	PROT	FAT	CHOL	CARB	FIBER	SOD
French Bread Cheese	1 piece (6 oz)	340	22	5	15	51	5	480
French Bread Pepperoni	1 piece (6 oz)	340	24	5	20	49	6	580
French Bread Sausage	1 piece (6 oz)	320	21	5	25	48	5	580
French Bread Supreme	1 piece (6.35 oz)	330	21	5	20	51	6	580

FOOD	PORTION	CALS	PROT	FAT	CHOL	CARB	FIBER	SOD
French Bread Vegetable	1 piece (6 oz)	280	17	4	10	44	5	480
Jeno's								
Crisp 'N Tasty Cheese	1 pie (6.8 oz)	460	19	19	20	52	2	860
Kid Cuisine								
Backpacking Pizza Snack	6 pieces	230	8	11	20	23	1	480
Big League Hamburger	1 meal (8.3 oz)	400	14	11	35	61	5	550
Fire Chief Cheese	1 pie (5.2 oz)	340	19	10	20	44	2	760
Pirate Pizza w/ Cheese	1 meal (8 oz)	430	12	11	30	71	5	480
Poolside Pepperoni	1 (5.2 oz)	380	18	14	35	44	2	990
Lean Cuisine								
Everyday Favorites French Bread Cheese	1 pkg (6 oz)	320	15	7	15	48	4	580
Everyday Favorites French Bread Deluxe	1 pkg (6.1 oz)	290	16	6	25	43	3	550
Everyday Favorites French Bread Pepperoni	1 pkg (5.25 oz)	300	15	8	25	43	3	590
Everyday Favorites French Bread Sun Dried Tomatoes	1 serv (6 oz)	340	19	8	20	48	3	580
Marie Callender's								
French Bread Cheese	1 (7.2 oz)	530	28	24	60	50	4	980
French Bread Pepperoni	1 (7.5 oz)	570	29	28	65	50	4	1160
French Bread Supreme	1 (7.5 oz)	510	26	23	50	50	4	1200
Red Baron								
Deep Dish Single Pepperoni	1 pizza	460	17	25	35	41	2	910

FOOD	PORTION	CALS	PROT	FAT	CHOL	CARB	FIBER	SOD
Totino's								
Crisp Crust Cheese	½ pie	320	15	14	20	34	2	620
TAKE-OUT								
cheese	⅛ of 12 in pie	140	8	3	9	21	—	336
cheese	12 in pie	1121	61	26	74	164	—	2680
cheese deep dish individual	1 (5.5 oz)	460	15	24	20	47	2	750
cheese meat & vegetables	12 in pie	1472	104	43	165	170	—	3054
cheese meat & vegetables	⅛ of 12 in pie	184	13	5	21	21	—	382
pepperoni	12 in pie	1445	81	56	115	157	—	2133
pepperoni	⅛ of 12 in pie	181	10	7	14	20	—	267

PIZZA DOUGH

FOOD	PORTION	CALS	PROT	FAT	CHOL	CARB	FIBER	SOD
crust	1 slice (1.7 oz)	130	4	2	0	25	1	230
Betty Crocker								
Italian Herb Crust Mix	¼ crust (1.6 oz)	180	4	2	0	32	1	350
Boboli								
Thin Crust	⅕ crust (2 oz)	160	6	4	0	24	1	300
Carbsense								
Garlic & Herb as prep	1 slice	100	9	1	0	7	4	85
Keto								
Dough Mix as prep	1 slice	79	13	1	—	5	3	95
MiniCarb								
Parmesan Herb Mix as prep	1 slice	130	18	5	0	6	3	220
Robin Hood								
Crust	¼ crust	160	4	2	0	33	1	340

PIZZA SAUCE

FOOD	PORTION	CALS	PROT	FAT	CHOL	CARB	FIBER	SOD
Hunt's								
Family Favorites	¼ cup	25	1	0	0	5	1	270
Muir Glen								
Organic	¼ cup (2.2 oz)	40	1	0	0	6	2	230

FOOD	PORTION	CALS	PROT	FAT	CHOL	CARB	FIBER	SOD
Progresso								
Pizza Sauce	¼ cup (2.1 oz)	20	tr	0	0	4	1	170
PLANTAINS								
fresh uncooked	1 (6.3 oz)	218	2	1	0	57	—	7
sliced cooked	½ cup	89	1	tr	0	24	—	4
TAKE-OUT								
ripe fried	2.8 oz	214	1	7	—	38	4	—
PLUMS								
CANNED								
purple in heavy syrup	1 cup	320	1	tr	0	60	—	50
purple in heavy syrup	3	119	tr	tr	0	31	—	26
purple in light syrup	1 cup	158	1	tr	0	41	—	50
purple in light syrup	3	83	tr	tr	0	22	—	26
purple juice pack	1 cup	146	1	tr	0	38	—	3
purple juice pack	3	55	tr	tr	0	14	—	1
purple water pack	3	39	tr	tr	0	10	—	1
purple water pack	1 cup	102	1	tr	0	27	—	2
Eden								
Umeboshi Paste	1 tsp	5	0	0	0	1	0	600
Umeboshi Plums	1	5	0	0	0	1	0	710
FRESH								
plum	1	36	1	tr	0	9	—	0
sliced	1 cup	91	1	1	0	21	—	1
Chiquita								
Purple	2 med (4.6 oz)	80	1	1	0	19	2	0
POI								
poi	½ cup	134	tr	tr	0	33	—	14
POKEBERRY SHOOTS								
cooked	½ cup	16	2	tr	0	3	—	—
fresh	½ cup	18	2	tr	0	3	—	—
POLENTA								
Frieda's								
Dried Tomato	4 oz	80	2	0	0	17	2	250
Italian Herb	4 oz	80	2	0	0	17	2	45

FOOD	PORTION	CALS	PROT	FAT	CHOL	CARB	FIBER	SOD
Mexicana	4 oz	80	2	0	0	17	2	200
Original	4 oz	80	2	0	0	16	2	198
Wild Mushroom	4 oz	80	2	0	0	17	2	200
Melissa's								
Original	4 oz	80	2	0	0	16	2	198
POLLACK								
atlantic fillet baked	5.3 oz	178	38	2	137	0	—	166
atlantic baked	3 oz	100	21	1	77	0	—	94
POMEGRANATE JUICE								
fresh	1	104	1	tr	0	26	—	5
Cortas								
Concentrated Juice	1 tbsp (0.6 oz)	40	0	0	0	9	0	0
Naked Juice								
Pomegranaberry Blue	8 oz	130	1	1	—	33	2	10
Pomigranalicious	8 oz	150	1	0	—	38	0	10
POM Wonderful								
Pomegranate Blueberry	8 oz	140	1	0	0	34	0	45
Pomegranate Cherry	8 oz	140	1	0	0	33	0	35
Pomegranate Tangerine	8 oz	150	0	0	0	37	0	75
Pomegrante Juice	8 oz	140	1	0	0	35	0	30
POMPANO								
florida cooked	3 oz	179	20	10	54	0	—	65
florida raw	3 oz	140	16	8	43	0	—	55
POPCORN (see also POPCORN CAKES)								
air-popped	1 cup (0.3 oz)	31	1	tr	0	6	2	0
caramel coated	1 cup (1.2 oz)	152	1	5	—	28	2	72
caramel coated w/ peanuts	⅔ cup (1 oz)	114	2	2	0	23	1	84
cheese	1 cup (0.4 oz)	58	1	4	1	6	1	98
oil popped	1 cup (0.4 oz)	55	1	3	0	6	1	97
Chester's								
Butter	3 cups	160	2	12	0	15	2	330
Caramel Craze	¾ cup	130	1	2	0	27	1	220

FOOD	PORTION	CALS	PROT	FAT	CHOL	CARB	FIBER	SOD
Cheddar Cheese	3 cups	190	3	13	<5	17	3	300
Microwave Butter	5 cups	200	3	12	0	22	4	300
Cracker Jack								
Fat Free Butter Toffee	¾ cup	110	1	0	0	26	1	85
Fat Free Caramel	¾ cup	110	tr	0	0	26	1	70
Original	½ cup (1 oz)	120	2	2	0	23	1	70
Husman's								
Cheese Corn	2¼ cups (1 oz)	160	2	10	<5	15	1	220
Jolly Time								
America's Best 94% Fat Free	1 cup	20	tr	0	0	5	1	10
Blast O Butter	1 cup	45	1	3	0	5	1	85
Blast O Butter Light	1 cup	30	tr	2	0	4	1	75
Butter Licious	1 cup	35	tr	2	0	4	1	40
Butter Licious Light	1 cup	30	tr	2	0	4	tr	25
Crispy & White	1 cup	40	tr	3	0	4	1	40
Crispy & White Light	1 cup	25	tr	1	0	4	1	25
Healthy Pop 94% Fat Free	1 cup	20	tr	0	0	5	1	10
White Air Popped	5 cups	100	4	1	0	24	6	0
Yellow Air Popped	5 cups	100	4	1	0	24	6	0
Judy's								
Sugar Free Popcorn Nut Brittle	¼ piece (1 oz)	100	1	5	0	3	tr	45
Mauna Loa								
Macadamia Nut Butter Corn Crunch	1 oz	150	1	8	1	18	1	140
Orville Redenbacher's								
Gourmet Original	3 cups	92	3	1	0	22	5	2
Hot Air	3 cups	92	3	1	0	22	5	2
Microwave Butter	3 cups	168	2	13	0	15	4	388
Microwave Butter No Salt Added	3 cups	176	3	12	0	19	4	2
Microwave Butter Light	3 cups	122	3	6	0	20	5	357
Microwave Caramel	1 serv	179	1	10	0	23	3	47
Microwave Golden Cheddar	1 serv	169	2	13	0	15	3	373

FOOD	PORTION	CALS	PROT	FAT	CHOL	CARB	FIBER	SOD
Microwave Natural	3 cups	164	2	11	0	18	4	512
Microwave Natural No Salt Added	3 cups	174	3	12	0	19	5	2
Microwave Natural Light	3 cups	118	3	5	0	19	5	382
Microwave Smartpop	1 serv	96	3	3	0	20	5	445
Microwave Smartpop Butter Snack Size	1 bag	155	5	4	0	34	0	477
Microwave Snack Size Butter	1 bag	287	3	22	0	25	6	647
Microwave Snack Size Butter Light	1 bag	183	4	8	0	30	7	539
Microwave White Cheddar	1 serv	169	2	13	0	15	3	373
Redenbudders Microwave Herb & Garlic	1 serv	176	2	13	0	16	4	499
Redenbudders Microwave Zesty Butter	1 serv	177	2	13	0	16	4	429
Redenbudders Movie Theater Butter Light	1 serv	113	3	5	0	20	5	321
Redenbudders Movie Theater Microwave Butter	1 serv	176	2	13	0	16	4	499
Smart Pop Movie Theater Butter	1 serv	92	3	2	0	20	5	307
White	3 cups	92	3	1	0	22	5	2
Pop Secret								
94% Fat Free Butter	1 cup (5 g)	20	tr	0	0	4	tr	40
94% Fat Free Natural	1 cup (5 g)	20	tr	0	0	4	tr	40
Butter	1 cup (7 g)	35	tr	3	0	4	tr	50
Cheddar Cheese	1 cup (6 g)	30	tr	2	0	3	tr	45
Jumbo Pop Butter	1 cup (7 g)	40	tr	3	0	4	tr	55
Jumbo Pop Movie Theater Butter	1 cup (7 g)	40	tr	3	0	4	tr	55

FOOD	PORTION	CALS	PROT	FAT	CHOL	CARB	FIBER	SOD
Light Butter	1 cup (5 g)	20	tr	1	0	4	tr	45
Light Movie Theater Butter	1 cup (5 g)	25	tr	1	0	4	tr	45
Light Natural	1 cup (5 g)	25	tr	1	0	4	tr	45
Movie Theater Butter	1 cup (7 g)	40	tr	3	0	3	tr	55
Nacho Cheese	1 cup (6 g)	30	tr	2	0	3	tr	50
Natural	1 cup (7 g)	35	tr	3	0	4	tr	65
Real Butter	1 cup (7 g)	35	tr	3	0	4	tr	60
Poppycock								
The Original	½ cup	160	2	8	10	20	1	90
Smart Balance								
No Trans Fat Low Sodium Low Fat	1 cup	20	0	0	0	6	1	0
Smartfood								
Butter	3 cups	150	2	9	5	15	1	240
Low Fat Toffee Crunch	¾ cup	110	1	1	0	25	1	220
Reduced Fat Golden Butter	3⅓ cups	130	3	4	0	21	4	410
Reduced Fat White Cheddar	3 cups	140	4	6	<5	19	3	280
White Cheddar	2 cups	190	3	12	5	17	2	310
Snyder's Of Hanover								
Butter	⅝ oz	110	1	10	0	6	0	150
Utz								
Au Natural	3 cups (1 oz)	120	3	1	0	25	5	0
Butter	2 cups (1 oz)	170	2	12	0	13	3	210
Cheese	2 cups (1 oz)	150	2	10	5	14	3	250
Hulless Puff'N Corn	2 cups (1 oz)	180	1	15	0	11	0	150
Hulless Puff'N Corn Hot Cheese	1 pkg (1.75 oz)	290	3	22	0	21	0	680
Hulless Puff'N Corn Cheese	2 cups (1 oz)	170	2	12	<5	13	0	210
White Cheddar	2 cups (1 oz)	150	3	9	<5	15	3	270

POPCORN CAKES
Orville Redenbacher's

FOOD	PORTION	CALS	PROT	FAT	CHOL	CARB	FIBER	SOD
BBQ Mini	8 (0.5 oz)	55	0	1	0	12	1	124

FOOD	PORTION	CALS	PROT	FAT	CHOL	CARB	FIBER	SOD
Butter	2 (0.6 oz)	134	2	1	tr	13	2	79
Butter Mini	8 (0.5 oz)	56	2	1	1	11	1	71
Caramel	1 (0.4 oz)	34	1	tr	0	8	1	16
Caramel Mini	7 (0.5 oz)	50	1	tr	tr	12	1	24
Nacho Cheese Mini	8 (0.5 oz)	56	2	1	1	11	1	85
Peanut Crunch Mini	7 (0.5 oz)	55	2	1	tr	11	1	39
White Cheddar	2 (0.6 oz)	63	0	1	tr	13	2	83
White Cheddar MIni	8 (0.5 oz)	56	2	1	tr	12	1	67

POPOVER

FOOD	PORTION	CALS	PROT	FAT	CHOL	CARB	FIBER	SOD
home recipe as prep w/ 2% milk	1 (1.4 oz)	87	4	3	46	11	–	82
home recipe as prep w/ whole milk	1 (1.4 oz)	90	4	3	47	11	–	82
mix as prep	1 (1.2 oz)	67	3	2	–	10	–	143

POPPY SEEDS

FOOD	PORTION	CALS	PROT	FAT	CHOL	CARB	FIBER	SOD
poppy seeds	1 tsp	15	1	1	0	1	–	1
American Almond								
Baker's Style Poppy Seed Filling	2 tbsp	120	2	5	0	18	tr	15

PORGY

FOOD	PORTION	CALS	PROT	FAT	CHOL	CARB	FIBER	SOD
fresh	3 oz	77	18	tr	–	0	0	52

PORK (see also HAM, PORK DISHES)
FRESH

FOOD	PORTION	CALS	PROT	FAT	CHOL	CARB	FIBER	SOD
boston blade roast lean & fat cooked	3 oz	229	20	16	73	0	0	57
boston blade steak lean & fat cooked	3 oz	220	22	14	81	0	0	59
center loin roast lean bone in cooked	3 oz	169	23	8	67	0	0	56
center loin chop lean bone in cooked	3 oz	172	25	7	72	0	0	53
center rib chop lean & fat bone in cooked	3 oz	213	23	13	62	0	0	34

FOOD	PORTION	CALS	PROT	FAT	CHOL	CARB	FIBER	SOD
center rib roast lean & fat bone in cooked	3 oz	217	23	13	62	0	0	39
fresh ham rump lean roasted	3 oz	175	26	7	82	0	0	55
fresh ham rump lean & fat roasted	3 oz	214	25	12	82	0	0	53
fresh ham shank lean roasted	3 oz	183	24	9	78	0	0	54
fresh ham shank lean & fat roasted	3 oz	246	22	17	78	0	0	50
fresh ham whole lean roasted	3 oz	179	25	8	80	0	0	54
fresh ham whole lean roasted diced	1 cup	285	40	13	127	0	0	86
fresh ham whole lean & fat roasted	3 oz	232	23	15	80	0	0	51
fresh ham whole lean & fat roasted diced	1 cup	369	36	24	127	0	0	81
ground 97% fat free	4 oz	130	23	3	65	0	0	60
ground cooked	3 oz	252	22	18	80	0	0	62
leg loin & shoulder lean only roasted	3 oz	198	—	11	79	—	—	—
loin chop lean bone in braised	3 oz	191	21	11	71	0	0	53
loin chop lean bone in broiled	3 oz	199	22	12	71	0	0	68
loin roast lean bone in roasted	3 oz	210	23	13	79	0	0	25
loin whole lean & fat braised	3 oz	203	23	12	68	0	0	41
loin whole lean & fat broiled	3 oz	206	23	12	68	0	0	53
loin whole lean & fat roasted	3 oz	211	23	12	70	0	0	50
lungs braised	3 oz	84	14	3	329	0	0	69
pancreas cooked	3 oz	186	24	9	268	0	0	36
ribs country style lean & fat braised	3 oz	252	20	18	74	0	0	50

FOOD	PORTION	CALS	PROT	FAT	CHOL	CARB	FIBER	SOD
shoulder arm picnic lean & fat roasted	3 oz	269	20	20	80	0	0	60
shoulder whole lean & fat roasted	3 oz	248	20	18	77	0	0	58
shoulder whole lean & fat roasted diced	1 cup	394	31	29	122	0	0	92
shoulder whole lean roasted	3 oz	196	22	12	77	0	0	64
shoulder whole lean roasted diced	1 cup	311	34	18	122	0	0	101
sirloin chop lean & fat bone in braised	3 oz	208	22	13	70	0	0	43
sirloin roast lean & fat bone in cooked	3 oz	222	23	14	74	0	0	51
spareribs braised	3 oz	338	25	26	103	0	0	79
spleen braised	3 oz	127	24	3	420	0	0	91
tail simmered	3 oz	336	15	30	110	0	0	21
tenderloin lean roasted	3 oz	139	24	4	67	0	0	48
top loin chop boneless lean & fat cooked	3 oz	198	24	11	64	0	0	36
top loin roast boneless lean & fat cooked	3 oz	192	24	10	66	0	0	37
Freirich								
Porkette	4 oz	220	16	18	70	1	0	660
TAKE-OUT								
chicharrones pork cracklings fried	1 cup	844	27	72	—	22	tr	128

PORK DISHES
Hormel

FOOD	PORTION	CALS	PROT	FAT	CHOL	CARB	FIBER	SOD
Center Cut Loin Lemon Garlic	1 serv (4 oz)	130	19	5	45	1	0	690
Extra Lean Teriyaki	4 oz	140	20	4	50	5	0	400
Pork Roast Au Jus	1 serv (5 oz)	180	29	7	85	0	0	570

FOOD	PORTION	CALS	PROT	FAT	CHOL	CARB	FIBER	SOD
Smithfield								
Pulled Pork w/ Barbecue Sauce	2 oz	90	9	4	20	7	–	220
Tenderloin Garlic & Herb	3 oz	100	17	3	60	2	tr	900
Tenderloin Hickory Sweet	4 oz	110	16	3	60	6	0	480
Tyson								
Lemon Pepper Pork Roast	1 serv (3 oz)	110	19	3	30	2	0	680
TAKE-OUT								
chinese spareribs	1 serv	776	–	166	54	–	–	716
pork roast	2 oz	70	10	3	40	0	–	390
tourtiere	1 piece (4.9 oz)	451	15	34	–	21	–	–

PORK RINDS *(see SNACKS)*

POT PIE

FOOD	PORTION	CALS	PROT	FAT	CHOL	CARB	FIBER	SOD
Amy's								
Broccoli	1 (7.5 oz)	430	11	22	45	46	4	630
Country Vegetable	1 (7.5 oz)	370	12	16	40	47	4	580
Shepard's	1 (8 oz)	160	5	4	0	27	5	490
Vegetable	1 (7.5 oz)	420	9	19	50	54	4	590
Vegetable Non-Dairy	1 (7.5 oz)	320	7	9	0	50	4	590
Banquet								
Beef	1 (7 oz)	400	9	23	30	38	1	1000
Cheesy Potato & Broccoli w/ Ham	1 (7 oz)	410	9	23	25	40	2	1220
Chicken	1 (7 oz)	380	10	22	40	36	1	950
Chicken & Broccoli	1 (7 oz)	350	10	20	35	32	2	830
Family Size Hearty Chicken	1 cup	460	11	29	35	39	2	1010
Macaroni & Cheese	1 pkg (6.5 oz)	210	7	5	10	34	1	750
Turkey	1 (7 oz)	370	10	20	45	38	3	850
Vegetable Cheese	1 (7 oz)	340	6	17	10	39	1	920
Healthy Choice								
Colonial Chicken	1 (9.5 oz)	310	22	7	45	40	5	570

FOOD	PORTION	CALS	PROT	FAT	CHOL	CARB	FIBER	SOD
Lean Cuisine								
Everyday Favorites Chicken Pie	1 pkg (9.5 oz)	300	19	8	30	38	—	580
Everyday Favorites Vegetable Eggroll	1 pkg (9 oz)	300	7	5	0	57	4	610
Marie Callender's								
Beef	1 (9.5 oz)	680	16	42	20	53	1	1430
Chicken	1 (9.5 oz)	680	14	48	20	53	3	1100
Chicken & Broccoli	1 (9.5 oz)	670	16	43	25	54	4	1000
Chicken Au Gratin	1 (9.5 oz)	690	19	46	30	50	4	1300
Turkey	1 (9.5 oz)	680	13	46	15	56	5	1100
Morton								
Macaroni & Cheese	1 (6.5 oz)	210	7	5	10	34	1	750
Vegetable w/ Beef	1 (7 oz)	340	5	21	20	33	2	1380
Vegetable w/ Chicken	1 (7 oz)	320	8	18	25	32	2	1040
Vegetable w/ Turkey	1 (7 oz)	310	8	18	25	29	2	1060
Swanson								
Beef	1 (7 oz)	376	12	19	22	39	5	739
Chicken	1 (7 oz)	416	9	22	19	45	2	814
Turkey	1 (7 oz)	440	12	24	18	44	2	748
TAKE-OUT								
beef	⅓ of 9 in pie (7.4 oz)	515	21	30	42	39	—	596
chicken	⅓ of 9 in pie (8.1 oz)	545	23	31	56	42	—	594

POTATO (see also CHIPS, KNISH, PANCAKES)

FOOD	PORTION	CALS	PROT	FAT	CHOL	CARB	FIBER	SOD
CANNED								
potatoes	½ cup	54	1	tr	0	12	—	—
Del Monte								
New Sliced	⅔ cup (5.4 oz)	60	1	0	0	13	2	360
New Whole	2 med (5.5 oz)	60	1	0	0	13	2	360
S&W								
Whole Small	2 (5.5 oz)	60	1	0	0	13	2	360
FRESH								
baked skin only	1 skin (2 oz)	115	2	tr	0	27	2	12
baked w/ skin	1 (6.5 oz)	220	5	tr	0	51	—	16

FOOD	PORTION	CALS	PROT	FAT	CHOL	CARB	FIBER	SOD
baked w/o skin	1 (5 oz)	145	3	tr	0	34	2	8
baked w/o skin	½ cup	57	1	tr	0	13	1	3
boiled	½ cup	68	1	tr	0	16	1	3
microwaved	1 (7 oz)	212	5	tr	0	49	—	16
microwaved w/o skin	½ cup	78	2	tr	0	18	—	5
raw w/o skin	1 (3.9 oz)	88	2	tr	0	20	—	7
Arrowfarms								
Yukon Gold	1 med (5 oz)	100	4	0	0	26	3	0
Dole								
Idaho	1 (5.3 oz)	100	4	0	0	26	3	0
Yukon Gold								
Fresh	1 (5.3 oz)	110	—	0	0	—	—	—
FROZEN								
french fries	10 strips	111	2	4	0	17	2	15
french fries thick cut	10 strips	109	2	4	0	17	—	23
hashed brown	½ cup	170	2	9	—	22	—	27
potato puffs	½ cup	138	2	7	0	19	—	462
potato puffs as prep	1	16	tr	1	0	2	—	52
Birds Eye								
Baby Gourmet	7 (4 oz)	100	2	0	0	21	1	15
Whole	3	50	1	0	0	13	1	25
Fillo Factory								
Petite Fillo Puffs Potato & Herb	7 (4.6 oz)	280	8	8	15	44	1	250
Healthy Choice								
Cheddar Broccoli Potatoes	1 meal (10.5 oz)	330	13	7	25	53	6	550
Lean Cuisine								
Everyday Favorites Deluxe Cheddar Potato	1 pkg (10.4 oz)	250	13	6	20	37	5	590
Everyday Favorites Roasted Potatoes w/ Broccoli	1 pkg (10.25 oz)	260	12	6	15	39	7	590
Oh Boy!								
Stuffed With Cheddar Cheese	1 (5 oz)	130	3	4	<5	22	2	270

FOOD	PORTION	CALS	PROT	FAT	CHOL	CARB	FIBER	SOD
Tree Of Life								
Organic French Fries	20 pieces (3 oz)	110	2	3	0	19	1	75
MIX								
au gratin as prep	½ cup	160	6	9	29	14	–	528
instant mashed flakes as prep w/ whole milk & butter	½ cup	118	2	6	15	16	–	349
instant mashed flakes not prep	½ cup	78	2	tr	0	18	–	24
instant mashed granules as prep w/ whole milk & butter	½ cup	114	2	5	15	15	–	270
instant mashed granules not prep	½ cup	372	8	1	0	86	–	67
scalloped	½ cup	105	4	5	14	13	–	409
Betty Crocker								
Au Gratin as prep	½ cup	150	3	6	5	22	1	600
Au Gratin Low Fat Recipe	½ cup	110	3	1	<5	22	1	560
Cheddar & Bacon	½ cup	150	3	6	<5	21	1	650
Cheddar & Bacon Low Fat Recipe	½ cup	120	3	3	0	21	1	620
Cheddar & Sour Cream	½ cup	130	3	3	5	25	1	580
Chicken & Vegetable	⅔ cup	140	4	4	<5	23	2	520
Chicken & Vegetable Low Fat Recipe	⅔ cup	120	4	3	<5	23	2	510
Hash Browns	½ cup	190	3	8	0	30	3	620
Homestyle Broccoli Au Gratin	½ cup	140	3	6	<5	21	2	530
Homestyle Broccoli Au Gratin Low Fat Recipe	½ cup	110	3	3	0	21	2	530
Homestyle Cheddar Cheese	½ cup	120	3	3	<5	21	1	600

FOOD	PORTION	CALS	PROT	FAT	CHOL	CARB	FIBER	SOD
Homestyle Cheddar Cheese Stove Top Recipe	½ cup	140	3	5	5	21	1	680
Homestyle Cheesy Scalloped	½ cup	140	3	6	<5	21	2	540
Homestyle Cheesy Scalloped Low Fat Recipe	½ cup	110	3	3	<5	21	3	540
Julienne	½ cup	150	3	6	<5	21	1	630
Mashed Butter & Herb	½ cup	160	2	7	3	21	1	400
Mashed Butter & Herb Reduced Fat Recipe	½ cup	130	3	5	<5	20	1	450
Mashed Chicken & Herb	½ cup	150	3	7	<5	21	1	520
Mashed Chicken & Herb Reduced Fat Recipe	½ cup	120	3	4	0	21	1	490
Mashed Four Cheese	½ cup	150	3	7	<5	20	2	570
Mashed Four Cheese Reduced Fat Recipe	½ cup	120	3	4	0	20	2	540
Mashed Potato Buds	⅔ cup	160	3	8	<5	19	1	460
Mashed Potato Buds Reduced Fat Recipe	⅔ cup	120	3	4	0	19	1	420
Mashed Roasted Garlic	½ cup	150	3	8	<5	19	2	400
Mashed Roasted Garlic Reduced Fat Recipe	½ cup	130	3	5	0	19	2	380
Mashed Sour Cream & Chives	½ cup	150	3	7	5	21	1	440
Mashed Sour Cream & Chives Reduced Fat Recipe	½ cup	120	3	4	<5	21	1	420

FOOD	PORTION	CALS	PROT	FAT	CHOL	CARB	FIBER	SOD
Potato Shakers Original	⅔ cup	140	3	4	<5	23	2	580
Potato Shakers Original Low Fat Recipe	⅔ cup	120	3	2	<5	23	2	560
Ranch	½ cup	160	3	6	<5	25	2	610
Scalloped	½ cup	150	3	6	<5	23	1	620
Scalloped Low Fat Recipe	⅔ cup	110	3	1	0	23	1	580
Sour Cream'n Chive	½ cup	160	3	7	5	22	2	600
Three Cheese	½ cup	150	3	6	<5	23	1	600
Twice Baked Cheddar & Bacon as prep	⅔ cup	210	6	11	85	22	1	580
Twice Baked Cheddar & Bacon Low Fat Recipe	⅔ cup	130	6	3	<5	22	1	530
Hungry Jack								
Mashed Potato Flakes as prep	½ cup	160	2	7	3	21	1	240
Idahoan								
AuGratin as prep	½ cup	150	3	6	3	20	2	744
Hash Browns as prep	½ cup	160	2	8	0	18	1	110
Hash Browns Cheesy not prep	½ cup	120	2	2	0	23	2	450
Mashed Baked as prep	½ cup	110	3	3	0	19	2	450
Mashed Butter & Herb as prep	½ cup	110	2	3	0	20	1	560
Mashed Buttery Homestyle as prep	½ cup	110	2	3	0	20	1	450
Mashed Four Cheese as prep	½ cup	100	2	3	0	19	1	550
Mashed Southwest as prep	½ cup	110	2	3	0	20	2	520

FOOD	PORTION	CALS	PROT	FAT	CHOL	CARB	FIBER	SOD
Roasted Garlic as prep	½ cup	600	2	3	0	20	1	260
Scalloped as prep	½ cup	150	2	7	3	21	1	610
REFRIGERATED								
PurelyIdaho								
Cheddar Crusted	¾ cup	120	2	1	3	26	2	420
Oven Roasts	1 serv (3 oz)	70	2	0	0	17	2	0
SHELF-STABLE								
Lunch Bucket								
Scalloped w/ Ham Chunks	1 pkg (7.5 oz)	170	2	7	10	24	3	660
TastyBite								
Bombay Potatoes	½ pkg (5 oz)	190	9	8	0	22	6	720
Mumbai Pav Bhaji	½ pkg (5 oz)	229	2	6	0	23	7	121
Simla Potatoes	½ pkg (5 oz)	180	5	8	0	23	1	650
TAKE-OUT								
au gratin w/ cheese	½ cup	178	7	10	18	17	–	548
baked topped w/ cheese sauce	1	475	15	29	19	47	–	381
baked topped w/ cheese sauce & bacon	1	451	18	26	30	44	–	973
baked topped w/ cheese sauce & broccoli	1	402	14	14	20	47	–	484
baked topped w/ cheese sauce & chili	1	481	23	22	31	56	–	701
baked topped w/ sour cream & chives	1	394	7	22	23	50	–	182
cheese fries w/ ranch dressing	1 serv	3010	–	–	–	–	–	–
curry	1 serv (6 oz)	292	4	16	–	36	4	–
french fries	1 reg	235	3	12	0	29	–	124
french fries	1 lg	355	5	19	0	44	–	187
hash brown	½ cup (2.5 oz)	151	2	9	9	16	–	290
indian yogurt potatoes	1 serv	315	7	9	18	52	0	216

FOOD	PORTION	CALS	PROT	FAT	CHOL	CARB	FIBER	SOD
mashed	½ cup	111	2	4	2	18	—	309
mustard potato salad	3.5 oz	120	1	6	0	16	—	393
o'brien	1 cup	157	5	3	7	30	—	421
potato dumpling	3.5 oz	334	7	1	—	74	3	1
potato pancakes	1 (1.3 oz)	101	2	7	35	11	—	188
potato salad	½ cup	179	3	10	86	14	—	661
potato salad w/ vegetables	3.5 oz	120	2	3	0	20	—	390
red new boiled	5 sm (5 oz)	120	3	0	0	27	2	5
scalloped	½ cup	127	4	5	7	18	—	435
twice baked w/ cheese	1 half (10 oz)	392	8	18	54	48	4	810

POTATO STARCH

FOOD	PORTION	CALS	PROT	FAT	CHOL	CARB	FIBER	SOD
potato starch	1 oz	96	tr	tr	0	24	—	1

POUT

FOOD	PORTION	CALS	PROT	FAT	CHOL	CARB	FIBER	SOD
ocean baked	3 oz	86	18	1	57	0	—	66
ocean fillet baked	4.8 oz	139	29	2	91	0	—	107

PRETZELS

FOOD	PORTION	CALS	PROT	FAT	CHOL	CARB	FIBER	SOD
chocolate covered	1 oz	130	2	5	—	20	—	—
dutch twist	4 (2.1 oz)	229	6	2	0	48	2	1029
milk chocolate covered twists	4 (1 oz)	140	2	7	0	19	tr	125
pretzels	1 oz	108	3	1	0	23	1	486
rods	4 (2 oz)	229	6	2	0	48	2	1029
sticks	10	10	tr	tr	tr	2	—	48
sticks	120 (2 oz)	229	6	2	0	48	2	1029
twists	10 (2.1 oz)	229	6	2	0	48	2	1029
whole wheat	2 sm (1 oz)	103	3	1	0	23	—	58
whole wheat	2 med (2 oz)	205	6	2	0	46	—	115
Aramana								
Soy Pretzels	15 (1 oz)	100	10	3	5	12	4	330
Bachman								
Thin'n Right	12 (1 oz)	120	3	1	0	23	1	650
Gardetto's								
Mustard	1 pkg (0.5 oz)	50	1	1	0	10	tr	110

FOOD	PORTION	CALS	PROT	FAT	CHOL	CARB	FIBER	SOD
Landies Candies								
Sugar Free Chocolate	4 (1.5 oz)	220	5	12	<5	23	tr	390
Rold Gold								
Crispy's Thins	4 (1 oz)	110	3	2	0	22	1	670
Fat Free Honey Mustard	17 (1 oz)	110	3	0	0	23	1	380
Fat Free Sticks	48 (1 oz)	110	3	0	0	23	1	530
Fat Free Thins	12 pieces (1 oz)	110	2	0	0	24	1	520
Fat Free Tiny Twists	18 pieces (1 oz)	110	3	0	0	23	1	420
Honey Mustard	16 (1 oz)	110	3	1	0	22	1	370
Rods	3 (1 oz)	110	3	1	0	22	1	610
Sharp Cheddar	22 (1 oz)	110	3	1	0	22	1	370
Sour Dough Nuggets	11 (1 oz)	110	2	0	0	24	1	330
Snyder's Of Hanover								
Dips White Fudge	1 oz	130	2	6	0	19	0	80
Hard Sourdough	1 oz	100	3	0	0	22	1	240
Hard Sourdough Unsalted	1 oz	100	3	0	0	22	1	90
Logs	1 oz	110	3	1	0	21	tr	360
Mini	1 oz	120	3	0	0	25	tr	250
Mini Unsalted	1 oz	110	3	0	0	25	tr	75
Nibblers	1 oz	120	3	0	0	25	tr	200
Nibblers Honey Mustard & Onions	1 oz	130	3	3	0	23	tr	95
Nibblers Oat Bran	1 oz	130	3	3	0	23	3	170
Nibblers Unsalted	1 oz	120	3	0	0	25	tr	50
Oat Bran	1 oz	100	3	3	0	22	2	260
Old Fashioned Dipping Stix	1 oz	100	3	0	0	22	1	330
Old Tyme Unsalted	1 oz	120	3	1	0	24	1	75
Olde Tyme	1 oz	120	3	1	0	24	1	120
Olde Tyme Stix	1 oz	120	3	1	0	23	1	150
Pieces Buttermilk Ranch	1 oz	130	3	5	0	19	tr	250
Pieces Cheddar Cheese	1 oz	190	2	6	0	18	tr	260

FOOD	PORTION	CALS	PROT	FAT	CHOL	CARB	FIBER	SOD
Pieces Honey Mustard & Onions	1 oz	140	2	7	0	18	tr	240
Pieces Peppered Pizza	1 oz	150	2	8	0	16	tr	340
Rods	1 oz	120	4	2	0	24	tr	400
Snaps	24 (1 oz)	110	3	1	0	24	tr	340
Thin	1 oz	130	3	0	0	23	tr	430
Whole Wheat Honey	1 oz	120	3	1	0	24	2	20
Spinzels								
Braided	1 pkg (0.5 oz)	55	2	1	0	11	tr	200
Utz								
Country Store Stix	5 (1 oz)	110	3	1	0	22	1	470
Fat Free Hard	1 (0.8 oz)	90	2	0	0	18	tr	470
Fat Free Hard No Salt Added	1 (0.8 oz)	90	2	0	0	19	tr	50
Fat Free Sour Dough Nuggets	10 (1 oz)	100	2	0	0	22	1	470
Fat Free Stix	14 (1 oz)	100	3	0	0	23	1	280
Honey Mustard & Onion	⅓ cup (1 oz)	130	2	6	0	18	tr	270
Rods	3 (1 oz)	120	3	1	0	24	1	400
Specials	5 (1 oz)	110	3	1	0	21	1	470
Wege								
Honey Wheat	1 (0.8 oz)	120	2	2	0	24	1	20

PRUNE JUICE

canned	1 cup	181	2	tr	0	45	3	11
Ocean Spray								
100% Juice	8 oz	180	2	0	0	44	0	8

PRUNES

canned in heavy syrup	1 cup	245	2	tr	0	65	—	6
canned in heavy syrup	5	90	1	tr	0	24	—	2
dried	1 cup	385	4	1	0	101	12	6
dried	10	201	2	tr	0	53	6	3
dried cooked w/ sugar	½ cup	147	1	tr	0	39	7	2

FOOD	PORTION	CALS	PROT	FAT	CHOL	CARB	FIBER	SOD
dried cooked w/o sugar	½ cup	113	1	tr	0	30	6	2
American Almond								
Baker's Style Ledvar	2 tbsp	90	0	0	0	21	1	120
St Dalfour								
French Prunes	3	100	1	0	0	22	3	5
Sunsweet								
Dried Plums	5	100	1	0	0	24	3	5

PUDDING
MIX

FOOD	PORTION	CALS	PROT	FAT	CHOL	CARB	FIBER	SOD
banana as prep w/ 2% milk	½ cup (4.9 oz)	142	4	2	9	26	–	232
banana as prep w/ whole milk	½ cup (4.9 oz)	157	4	4	17	25	–	231
chocolate	½ cup (5 oz)	150	5	3	9	28	–	148
chocolate as prep w/ whole milk	½ cup (5 oz)	158	5	5	17	26	–	147
coconut cream	½ cup (4.9 oz)	148	4	4	9	25	–	226
instant banana as prep w/ 2% milk	½ cup (5.2 oz)	152	4	3	9	29	–	435
instant banana as prep w/ whole milk	½ cup (5.2 oz)	167	4	4	17	27	–	434
instant chocolate	½ cup (5.2 oz)	149	3	3	9	28	–	418
instant chocolate as prep w/ whole milk	½ cup (5.2 oz)	164	5	5	17	28	–	417
instant lemon	½ cup (5.2 oz)	155	4	4	9	30	–	394
instant vanilla	½ cup (5 oz)	147	2	2	9	28	–	407
lemon	½ cup (5.1 oz)	163	1	2	77	36		94
rice as prep w/ whole milk	½ cup (5.1 oz)	175	5	4	17	30	–	158
tapioca	½ cup (5 oz)	147	4	2	9	28	–	172

FOOD	PORTION	CALS	PROT	FAT	CHOL	CARB	FIBER	SOD
tapioca as prep w/ whole milk	½ cup (5 oz)	161	4	4	17	28	–	171
vanilla as prep w/ 2% milk	½ cup (4.9 oz)	141	4	2	9	26	–	224
vanilla as prep w/ whole milk	½ cup (4.9 oz)	155	2	4	17	26	–	223
Betty Crocker								
Rice as prep	1 serv	200	1	3	9	33	–	70
Jell-O								
Vanilla as prep w/ 2% milk	½ cup (5.1 oz)	150	0	3	9	30	0	408
Keto								
Banana not prep	½ scoop	62	7	3	10	3	2	105
Chocolate not prep	½ scoop	66	7	3	10	4	3	115
French Vanilla not prep	½ scoop	62	7	3	10	3	2	105
Louisiana Purchase								
Bread	1 serv (1.3 oz)	150	3	3	0	28	2	220
Lundberg								
Elegant Rice Cinnamon Raisin	½ cup (3.9 oz)	70	0	0	0	16	1	0
Elegant Rice Coconut	½ cup (3.9 oz)	70	0	2	0	13	1	0
Elegant Rice Honey Almond	½ cup (3.9 oz)	70	2	1	0	15	1	0
Uncle Ben's								
Rice Pudding Cinnamon & Raisins as prep	½ cup (1.5 oz)	160	2	1	0	37	1	150
READY-TO-EAT								
banana	1 pkg (5 oz)	180	3	5	–	30	–	278
chocolate	1 pkg (5 oz)	189	4	6	5	32	–	183
lemon	1 pkg (5 oz)	177	tr	4	0	36	–	199
rice	1 pkg (5 oz)	231	3	11	–	31	–	121
tapioca	1 pkg (5 oz)	169	3	5	–	28	–	168
vanilla	1 pkg (4 oz)	146	3	4	8	25	–	153
Boost								
Vanilla	1 pkg (5 oz)	240	7	9	<5	33	0	125

FOOD	PORTION	CALS	PROT	FAT	CHOL	CARB	FIBER	SOD
Healthy Choice								
Low Fat Chocolate Raspberry	½ cup (3.5 oz)	102	3	2	0	19	0	111
Low Fat Chocolate Almond	½ cup (3.5 oz)	109	3	2	0	21	0	109
Low Fat Double Chocolate Fudge	½ cup (3.5 oz)	101	3	1	0	20	0	116
Low Fat French Vanilla	½ cup (3.5 oz)	98	2	1	0	20	0	122
Low Fat Tapioca	½ cup (3.5 oz)	101	2	1	1	21	0	115
Hunt's								
Snack Pack Banana	1 serv (3.5 oz)	119	2	4	2	18	0	155
Snack Pack Butterscotch	1 serv (3.5 oz)	130	2	4	2	21	0	164
Snack Pack Chocolate	1 serv (3.5 oz)	143	2	5	1	22	0	139
Snack Pack Chocolate Fudge	1 serv (3.5 oz)	147	2	5	1	23	0	153
Snack Pack Chocolate Marshmallow	1 serv (3.5 oz)	134	2	5	1	21	0	212
Snack Pack Fat Free Chocolate	1 serv (3.5 oz)	86	2	tr	1	19	0	134
Snack Pack Fat Free Tapioca	1 serv (3.5 oz)	82	2	tr	0	18	0	141
Snack Pack Fat Free Vanilla	1 serv (3.5 oz)	81	2	tr	0	18	0	146
Snack Pack Lemon	1 serv (3.5 oz)	124	tr	3	0	24	0	47
Snack Pack Milk Chocolate Variety	1 serv (3.5 oz)	143	2	5	2	22	0	136
Snack Pack Swirl Chocolate Caramel	1 serv (3.5 oz)	143	2	5	1	23	0	143

FOOD	PORTION	CALS	PROT	FAT	CHOL	CARB	FIBER	SOD
Snack Pack Swirl Chocolate Peanut Butter	1 serv (3.5 oz)	146	3	6	2	21	0	156
Snack Pack Swirl Smores	1 serv (3.5 oz)	136	2	5	1	21	0	94
Snack Pack Tapioca	1 serv (3.5 oz)	125	1	4	1	21	0	144
Snack Pack Toppers Chocolate Fudge w/ Rainbow Sprinkles	1 serv (4 oz)	164	2	6	tr	25	tr	145
Snack Pack Toppers Chocolate w/ Dinosaurs	1 serv (4 oz)	161	2	6	tr	25	tr	164
Snack Pack Toppers Chocolate w/ Fun Chips	1 serv (4 oz)	176	2	6	1	28	tr	153
Snack Pack Toppers Vanilla w/ Chocolate Sprinkles	1 serv (4 oz)	164	1	6	tr	26	tr	129
Snack Pack Vanilla	1 serv (3.5 oz)	135	2	5	1	21	0	147
Imagine								
Banana	1 pkg (4 oz)	150	1	3	0	30	0	40
Butterscotch	1 pkg (4 oz)	150	1	3	0	31	0	45
Chocolate	1 pkg (4 oz)	170	1	3	0	38	1	65
Lemon	1 pkg (4 oz)	150	1	3	0	33	1	50
Jell-O								
Fat Free Chocolate Vanilla Swirl	1 serv (4 oz)	100	2	0	0	23	tr	200
Fat Free Chocolate Fudge & Caramel	1 serv (4 oz)	100	2	0	0	24	0	230
Fat Free Tapioca	1 serv (4 oz)	100	1	0	0	23	0	230
Fat Free Vanilla Caramel	1 serv (4 oz)	100	1	0	0	23	0	230
Swiss Miss								
Butterscotch	1 pkg (4 oz)	156	2	6	1	24	0	182
Chocolate	1 pkg (4 oz)	166	3	6	1	26	0	177
Chocolate Fudge	1 pkg (4 oz)	175	3	6	1	28	0	207

FOOD	PORTION	CALS	PROT	FAT	CHOL	CARB	FIBER	SOD
Fat Free Chocolate	1 pkg (4 oz)	98	2	tr	0	22	0	141
Fat Free Chocolate Fudge	1 pkg (4 oz)	101	2	tr	0	23	0	147
Fat Free Vanilla	1 pkg (4 oz)	93	2	tr	0	21	0	168
Fat Free Parfait Vanilla Chocolate	1 pkg (4 oz)	96	2	tr	0	21	0	143
Lemon Meringue Pie	1 pkg (4 oz)	150	0	3	0	30	—	60
Low Fat Tapioca	1 pkg (4 oz)	130	3	3	0	25	—	200
Low Fat Vanilla	1 serv (4 oz)	120	2	2	0	24	—	190
Milk Chocolate	1 pkg (4 oz)	166	2	6	1	26	0	165
Parfait Vanilla Chocolate	1 pkg (4 oz)	164	3	6	1	25	0	196
Swirl Chocolate Caramel	1 pkg (4 oz)	169	2	6	1	26	1	178
Swirl Chocolate Vanilla	1 pkg (4 oz)	169	2	6	1	26	0	159
Swirl Chocolate Vanilla Chocolate	1 pkg (4 oz)	169	3	6	1	26	0	159
Tapioca	1 pkg (4 oz)	138	2	4	1	24	0	180
Vanilla	1 pkg (4 oz)	156	2	6	1	24	0	181
TAKE-OUT								
blancmange	1 serv (4.7 oz)	154	4	5	—	25	tr	—
bread pudding	½ cup (4.4 oz)	212	7	7	83	31	—	291
bread w/ raisins	½ cup	180	5	5	77	31	—	185
chocolate	½ cup (5.5 oz)	221	5	6	17	40	—	137
corn	⅔ cup	181	7	9	122	21	—	92
queen of puddings	1 serv (4.4 oz)	266	6	10	—	41	tr	—
rice pudding	1 serv (6 oz)	220	6	8	—	34	tr	—
rice w/ raisins	½ cup	246	7	6	136	42	4	270
tapioca	½ cup (5.3 oz)	189	7	7	124	26	—	288
vanilla	½ cup (4.3 oz)	130	4	4	17	20	—	113
yorkshire	1 serv (3 oz)	177	6	8	57	22	tr	168

FOOD	PORTION	CALS	PROT	FAT	CHOL	CARB	FIBER	SOD
PUDDING POPS								
chocolate	1 (1.6 oz)	72	2	2	1	12	–	77
vanilla	1 (1.6 oz)	75	2	2	1	13	–	50
PUFFERFISH								
raw	3 oz	72	17	0	–	0	0	120
PUMMELO								
fresh	1	228	5	tr	0	59	–	7
sections	1 cup	71	1	tr	0	18	–	2
PUMPKIN								
butter	1 tbsp	32	0	0	0	8	–	0
canned	½ cup	41	1	tr	0	10	–	6
cooked mashed	½ cup	24	1	tr	0	6	–	2
flowers cooked	½ cup	10	1	tr	0	2	–	4
flowers raw	1	0	tr	0	0	tr	–	0
leaves cooked	½ cup	7	1	tr	0	1	–	3
leaves raw	½ cup	4	1	tr	0	tr	–	2
raw cubed	½ cup	15	1	tr	0	4	–	1
Libby's								
Puree	½ cup	40	2	1	0	9	5	5
PUMPKIN SEEDS								
dried	1 oz	154	7	13	0	5	–	5
roasted	¼ cup	296	19	24	0	8	–	10
salted & roasted	¼ cup	296	19	24	0	8	–	324
whole roasted	¼ cup	71	3	3	0	9	–	3
whole roasted	1 oz	127	5	6	0	15	–	5
whole salted roasted	¼ cup	71	3	3	0	9	–	67
PURSLANE								
cooked	1 cup	21	2	tr	0	4	–	51
fresh	1 cup	7	1	tr	0	1	–	20
QUAIL								
breast w/o skin raw	1 (2 oz)	69	13	2	–	0	–	31
w/ skin raw	1 quail (3.8 oz)	210	21	13	–	0	–	58
w/o skin raw	1 quail (3.2 oz)	123	20	4	–	0	–	67

FOOD	PORTION	CALS	PROT	FAT	CHOL	CARB	FIBER	SOD
QUICHE								
Atkins								
Crustless Bacon & Onion	1 serv	320	18	27	175	2	0	540
Crustless Four Cheese	1 serv	290	22	24	45	2	0	270
Crustless Smoked Ham & Cheese	1 serv	290	18	24	170	2	0	470
TAKE-OUT								
cheese	1 slice (3 oz)	283	11	20	–	16	1	–
lorraine	⅛ of 8 in pie	600	13	48	285	29	–	653
mushroom	1 slice (3 oz)	256	9	18	–	17	1	–
QUINCE								
fresh	1	53	tr	tr	0	14	–	4
QUINOA								
quinoa not prep	1 cup (6 oz)	636	22	10	0	117	10	36
RABBIT								
domestic w/o bone roasted	3 oz	167	25	7	70	0	–	40
wild w/o bone stewed	3 oz	147	28	3	104	0	–	38
RACCOON								
roasted	3 oz	217	25	12	–	0	–	–
RADICCHIO								
raw shredded	½ cup	5	tr	tr	0	1	–	4
RADISHES								
chinese dried	½ cup	157	5	tr	0	37	–	161
chinese raw	1 (12 oz)	62	2	tr	0	14	–	71
chinese raw sliced	½ cup	8	tr	tr	0	2	–	9
chinese sliced cooked	½ cup	13	tr	tr	0	3	–	10
daikon dried	½ cup	157	5	tr	0	37	–	161
daikon raw	1 (12 oz)	62	2	tr	0	14	–	71

FOOD	PORTION	CALS	PROT	FAT	CHOL	CARB	FIBER	SOD
daikon raw sliced	½ cup	8	tr	tr	0	2	—	9
daikon sliced cooked	½ cup	13	tr	tr	0	3	—	10
red raw	10	7	tr	tr	0	2	—	11
red sliced	½ cup	10	tr	tr	0	2	—	14
white icicle raw	1 (⅓ oz)	2	tr	tr	0	tr	—	3
white icicle raw sliced	½ cup	7	1	tr	0	1	—	8
Eden								
Daikon Dried Shredded	2 tbsp	45	1	0	0	9	3	20
Daikon Pickled	2 slices	5	0	0	0	1	0	250
TAKE-OUT								
korean kimchee	½ cup	31	2	1	—	6	—	—
moo namul saengche korean salad	1 serv (3.7 oz)	34	1	tr	0	8	2	547

RAISINS

FOOD	PORTION	CALS	PROT	FAT	CHOL	CARB	FIBER	SOD
chocolate coated	10 (0.4 oz)	39	tr	2	0	7	—	4
chocolate coated	1 cup (6.7 oz)	741	8	28	5	130	—	68
golden seedless	1 cup	437	5	1	0	115	8	17
jumbo golden	¼ cup	130	1	0	0	31	2	10
seedless	1 tbsp	27	tr	tr	0	7	—	—
seedless	1 cup	434	5	1	0	115	8	17
sultanas	1 oz	88	1	0	—	23	2	—
Dole								
CinnaRaisins	1 pkg (1 oz)	95	1	0	0	22	2	5
Mariana								
Fruit'n Yogurt Milk Chocolate Covered Raisins	32 pieces (1 oz)	130	1	5	0	20	2	40
Nestle								
Chocolate Covered	1½ tbsp	70	tr	3	0	11	tr	0
Sun-Maid								
California Golden	¼ cup	130	1	0	0	31	2	10

FOOD	PORTION	CALS	PROT	FAT	CHOL	CARB	FIBER	SOD
California Seedless	1 box (1.5 oz)	130	1	0	0	33	2	10
Tree Of Life								
Organic	¼ cup (1.4 oz)	130	1	0	0	31	2	10

RASPBERRIES

canned in heavy syrup	½ cup	117	1	tr	0	30	–	4
fresh	1 pint	154	3	2	0	36	–	0
fresh	1 cup	61	1	1	0	14	–	0
frozen sweetened	1 pkg (10 oz)	291	2	tr	0	74	–	1
frozen sweetened	1 cup	256	2	tr	0	65	–	1
frzn unsweetened	¾ cup	130	2	0	0	29	2	0
Birds Eye								
Red	5 oz	90	1	0	0	22	5	5
Tree Of Life								
Organic	⅔ cup (5 oz)	50	1	0	0	12	2	0

RASPBERRY JUICE
Dole

Country Raspberry	8 fl oz	140	0	0	0	35	–	35
Fresh Samantha								
Raspberry Dream	1 cup (8 oz)	120	2	1	–	10	8	0
Nantucket Nectars								
Organic Very Raspberry	8 oz	120	0	0	0	30	–	30

RED BEANS
CANNED
Hunt's

Small	½ cup (4.5 oz)	89	6	1	0	19	6	713
Van Camp								
Red Beans	½ cup (4.6 oz)	90	6	0	0	20	5	560

FOOD	PORTION	CALS	PROT	FAT	CHOL	CARB	FIBER	SOD
MIX								
Bean Cuisine								
Pasta & Beans Barcelona Red With Radiatore	1 serv	210	7	1	0	29	4	15
RELISH								
cranberry orange	½ cup	246	tr	tr	0	64	–	44
hamburger	1 tbsp	19	tr	tr	0	5	–	164
hamburger	½ cup	158	1	1	0	42	–	1338
hot dog	1 tbsp	14	tr	tr	0	4	–	164
hot dog	½ cup	111	2	1	0	28	–	1332
piccalilli	1.4 oz	13	tr	tr	–	2	1	–
sweet	1 tbsp	19	tr	tr	0	5	–	122
sweet	½ cup	159	tr	1	0	43	–	990
Claussen								
Sweet Pickle	1 tbsp (0.5 oz)	15	0	0	0	3	0	85
Matouk's								
Hot Chow	2 tbsp	20	0	0	0	5	0	200
Kuchela	1 tsp	9	0	1	0	tr	0	80
Vlasic								
Fancy Sweet	1 tbsp	15	0	0	0	4	–	140
RENNIN								
tablet	1 (0.9 g)	1	0	0	–	tr	–	234
RHUBARB								
fresh	½ cup	13	1	tr	0	3	–	2
frozen	½ cup	60	tr	tr	0	3	–	1
frzn as prep w/ sugar	½ cup	139	tr	tr	0	37	–	2
RICE *(see also RICE CAKES, WILD RICE)*								
arborio	½ cup	100	2	0	0	22	–	5
brown long grain cooked	1 cup (6.8 oz)	216	5	2	0	45	4	10
brown medium grain cooked	1 cup (6.8 oz)	218	5	2	0	46	4	2
glutinous cooked	1 cup (6.1 oz)	169	4	tr	0	37	2	9

FOOD	PORTION	CALS	PROT	FAT	CHOL	CARB	FIBER	SOD
starch	1 oz	98	tr	0	0	24	–	17
white long grain cooked	1 cup (5.5 oz)	205	4	tr	0	45	1	2
white long grain instant cooked	1 cup (5.8 oz)	162	3	tr	0	35	1	5
white medium grain cooked	1 cup (6.5 oz)	242	4	tr	0	53	1	0
white short grain cooked	1 cup (6.5 oz)	242	4	tr	0	53	–	0
Amy's								
Bowls Brown Rice & Vegetables	1 pkg (10 oz)	240	9	8	0	36	5	510
Birds Eye								
Rice & Broccoli In Cheese Sauce	1 pkg	290	8	9	15	15	2	1110
White & Wild w/ Green Beans	1 cup (6.6 oz)	180	4	4	10	31	2	480
Buitoni								
Risotto Garden Vegetable	1 serv	210	4	1	0	47	0	930
Risotto Portobello Mushrooms	1 serv	210	5	0	0	48	0	930
Risotto Rosemary & Potatoes	1 serv	210	4	1	10	47	2	810
Risotto Tomato Basil	1 serv	210	4	1	0	46	0	870
Carolina								
Black Beans & Rice Mix as prep	1 serv	200	7	2	0	39	5	930
Gold as prep	1 cup	160	3	0	0	37	tr	0
Spanish Rice Mix as prep	1 serv	180	4	1	0	42	2	760
Chun King								
Fried Rice Mix	½ cup (1.4 oz)	126	4	tr	0	29	1	691
Gourmet House								
Brown & White not prep	¼ cup	160	7	10	0	34	1	0

FOOD	PORTION	CALS	PROT	FAT	CHOL	CARB	FIBER	SOD
La Choy								
Fried Rice	1 cup (4.9 oz)	236	5	1	0	53	2	1024
Lundberg								
One-Step Curry	1 cup (7.4 oz)	160	5	1	0	38	5	400
Quick Brown Rice Savory Vegetarian Chicken	1 cup (2.5 oz)	260	6	3	–	53	5	910
Risotto Tomato Basil	1 serv	140	4	1	0	30	1	630
Mahatma								
Jambalaya as prep	1 cup	190	5	1	0	42	1	1120
Nacho Cheese Mix as prep	1 serv	250	6	3	5	49	tr	1260
Thai Jasmine as prep	¾ cup	160	3	0	0	36	2	0
Minute								
Instant Brown as prep	⅔ cup	170	4	2	0	34	2	10
Near East								
Creative Grains Chicken & Herb as prep	1 cup	270	8	6	0	51	6	780
Creative Grains Creamy Parmesan as prep	1 cup	280	8	8	18	48	3	790
Creative Grains Roasted Garlic as prep	1 cup	220	6	5	0	41	5	570
Creative Grains Roasted Pecan as prep	1 cup	240	6	8	0	37	4	540
Long Grain & Wild Rice Roasted Vegetable & Chicken as prep	1 cup	220	5	5	9	43	2	730
Long Grain & Wild Rice Garlic & Herb as prep	1 cup	220	5	5	9	43	2	680

FOOD	PORTION	CALS	PROT	FAT	CHOL	CARB	FIBER	SOD
Pilaf Brown Rice as prep	1 cup	210	5	5	9	41	3	670
Pilaf Chicken as prep	1 cup	220	5	5	9	43	2	800
Pilaf Mix Curry as pre	1 cup	220	4	5	9	44	2	600
Pilaf Mix Garlic & Herb as prep	1 cup	220	5	3	0	44	1	680
Pilaf Mix Long Grain & Wild as prep	1 cup	220	5	5	9	43	2	800
Pilaf Mix Rice as prep	1 cup	220	5	5	9	44	1	780
Pilaf Mix Roasted Chicken & Garlic as prep	1 cup	220	5	4	6	44	2	570
Pilaf Mix Spanish Rice as prep	1 cup	310	5	8	21	54	2	1010
Pilaf Mix Toasted Almond as prep	1 cup	230	6	6	9	40	2	640
Pilaf Mix Wild Mushroom & Herb as prep	1 cup	220	5	5	9	44	2	530
Rice Expressions								
Indian Basmati	1 cup	180	4	tr	0	40	tr	0
Organic Brown	1 cup	160	4	1	0	34	3	0
Organic Long Grain	1 cup	180	4	tr	0	40	tr	0
Organic Rice Pilaf	1 cup	170	4	3	0	32	2	470
Organic Tex Mex	1 cup	190	4	2	0	40	tr	540
River Rice								
Brown Long Grain not prep	¼ cup	150	3	1	0	32	tr	0
S&W								
Arborio as prep	¾ cup	150	3	0	0	35	tr	0
Basmati Mix as prep	¾ cup	160	3	0	0	36	0	0

FOOD	PORTION	CALS	PROT	FAT	CHOL	CARB	FIBER	SOD
Brown Long Grain not prep	¼ cup	150	3	1	0	32	1	0
Long Grain Organic not prep	¼ cup	150	3	0	0	35	0	0
Success								
Beef Mix as prep	1 cup	240	5	7	0	42	2	984
Broccoli & Cheese	½ cup	130	2	4	0	21	tr	432
Brown	1 cup	150	4	1	0	33	2	5
Brown & Wild Mix	½ cup	120	3	3	0	21	2	432
Classic Chicken	½ cup	90	2	1	0	15	1	384
Grilled Chicken & Broccoli Mix as prep	1 cup	240	5	6	0	42	1	936
Long Grain & Wild	½ cup	120	3	3	0	21	tr	480
Pilaf	½ cup	120	3	3	0	21	1	336
Red Beans & Rice Mix as prep	1 cup	300	7	7	0	51	8	960
Spanish	½ cup	120	2	3	0	21	1	408
White as prep	1 cup	190	4	0	0	44	1	5
Yellow Mix as prep	1 cup	170	3	3	0	33	1	696
TastyBite								
Pilaf Curried Vegetable	½ pkg (4.5 oz)	180	5	6	0	26	9	440
Pilaf Green Peas	½ pkg (4.5 oz)	208	6	4	0	36	4	487
Pilaf Vegetable Kofta	½ pkg (4.5 oz)	229	7	5	0	39	7	531
Uncle Ben's								
White Converted as prep	1 cup	170	4	0	0	38	—	0
Van Camp								
Spanish	½ cup (4.5 oz)	90	2	2	0	19	2	645
Water Maid								
White Medium Grain not prep	¼ cup	160	2	0	0	37	tr	0
Zatarain's								
Dirty Rice Mix as prep w/o meat and oil	½ cup	130	3	0	0	29	0	680

FOOD	PORTION	CALS	PROT	FAT	CHOL	CARB	FIBER	SOD
Red Beans & Rice as prep w/o oil	½ cup	100	4	0	0	21	4	490
TAKE-OUT								
coconut rice	1 serv	500	6	42	–	30	2	27
congee	½ cup (4.1 oz)	44	1	–	–	10	–	–
nasi goreng (fried rice)	1 serv	206	10	4	–	35	5	356
nasi goreng indonesian rice & vegetables	1 cup (4.9 oz)	130	4	0	0	28	1	530
paella	1 serv (7 oz)	308	23	16	92	17	3	580
pilaf	½ cup	84	4	3	22	11	3	362
risotto	6.6 oz	426	6	18	–	65	3	–
spanish	¾ cup	363	11	27	35	19	–	1339

RICE CAKES (see also POPCORN CAKES)
Lundberg

FOOD	PORTION	CALS	PROT	FAT	CHOL	CARB	FIBER	SOD
Nutra Farmed Brown Rice	1 (0.7 oz)	70	1	0	0	15	–	55
Nutra Farmed Sesame Tamari	1 (0.7 oz)	70	2	1	0	16	2	120
Organic Koku Semsame	1 (0.7 oz)	80	2	0	0	17	2	35

Tastemorr

FOOD	PORTION	CALS	PROT	FAT	CHOL	CARB	FIBER	SOD
Rice Crisps Caramel	7	55	tr	0	0	12	0	46

ROCKFISH

FOOD	PORTION	CALS	PROT	FAT	CHOL	CARB	FIBER	SOD
pacific cooked	3 oz	103	20	2	38	0	–	65
pacific cooked	1 fillet (5.2 oz)	180	36	3	66	0	–	114
pacific raw	3 oz	80	16	1	29	0	–	51

ROE (see also individual fish names)

FOOD	PORTION	CALS	PROT	FAT	CHOL	CARB	FIBER	SOD
fish	1 oz	11	2	tr	30	tr	–	–
fresh baked	3 oz	173	24	7	408	2	–	–
fresh baked	1 oz	58	8	2	136	1	–	–

FOOD	PORTION	CALS	PROT	FAT	CHOL	CARB	FIBER	SOD
ROLL								
FROZEN								
Pillsbury								
Dinner Rolls Crusty French	1	110	4	2	0	19	0	220
Sara Lee								
Deluxe Cinnamon Rolls w/o Icing	1 (2.7 oz)	370	5	15	40	41	1	300
READY-TO-EAT								
bialy	1 (2.2 oz)	138	14	0	0	32	1	167
brioche sweet roll	1 (3.5 oz)	410	10	23	190	41	3	495
brown & serve	1 (1 oz)	85	2	2	0	14	—	148
cheese	1 (2.3 oz)	238	5	12	—	29	—	236
cinnamon raisin	1 (2¾ in)	223	4	10	40	31	1	229
dinner	1 (1 oz)	85	2	2	0	14	—	148
egg	1 (2½ in)	107	3	2	—	18	1	191
french	1 (1.3 oz)	105	3	2	0	19	—	232
hamburger	1 (1½ oz)	123	4	2	—	22	—	241
hamburger multi-grain	1 (1½ oz)	113	4	2	0	19	2	197
hamburger reduced calorie	1 (1½ oz)	84	4	1	0	18	3	190
hard	1 (3½ in)	167	6	2	0	30	—	310
hot cross bun	1	202	5	4	—	38	1	—
hotdog	1 (1½ oz)	123	4	2	—	22	—	241
hotdog reduced calorie	1 (1½ oz)	84	4	1	0	18	3	190
hotdog whole wheat	1 (1.5 oz)	110	5	2	0	19	2	220
kaiser	1 (3½ in)	167	6	2	0	30	—	310
oat bran	1 (1.2 oz)	78	3	2	0	13	1	136
rye	1 (1 oz)	81	3	1	0	15	—	253
submarine	1 (4.7 oz)	155	5	2	tr	30	—	313
wheat	1 (1 oz)	77	2	2	0	13	—	96
whole wheat	1 (1 oz)	75	3	1	0	15	—	135

FOOD	PORTION	CALS	PROT	FAT	CHOL	CARB	FIBER	SOD
Bread Du Jour								
Cracked Wheat	1 (1.2 oz)	100	3	1	0	17	1	200
Italian	1 (1.2 oz)	90	3	1	0	16	0	190
Sourdough	1 (1.2 oz)	90	3	1	0	17	0	190
Country Kitchen								
Wheat Light	1	80	4	2	0	17	4	160
Natural Ovens								
Best Burger Bun	1	178	4	4	0	29	3	150
Better Wheat Buns	1	140	4	2	0	30	5	120
Gourmet Dinner	1	70	3	1	0	15	4	70
Pepperidge Farm								
Dinner Rolls Finger Poppy	1 (0.9 oz)	80	3	2	<5	12	tr	125
REFRIGERATED								
cinnamon w/ frosting	1	109	2	4	–	17	–	250
crescent	1 (1 oz)	98	2	4	0	14	–	341
Pillsbury								
Crescents Reduced Fat	1 (1 oz)	100	2	5	0	12	0	230
ROSE APPLE								
fresh	3.5 oz	32	1	tr	0	7	–	–
ROSE HIP								
fresh	1 oz	26	1	0	0	5	–	42
ROSELLE								
fresh	1 cup	28	1	tr	0	6	–	3
ROSEMARY								
dried	1 tsp	4	tr	tr	0	1	–	1
ROUGHY								
orange baked	3 oz	75	16	1	22	0	–	69
RUTABAGA								
cooked mashed	½ cup	41	1	tr	0	9	–	22
raw cubed	½ cup	25	1	tr	0	6	–	14
SABLEFISH								
baked	3 oz	213	15	17	53	0	-	61
fillet baked	5.3 oz	378	26	30	95	0	–	108

FOOD	PORTION	CALS	PROT	FAT	CHOL	CARB	FIBER	SOD
smoked	3 oz	218	15	17	55	0	–	626
smoked	1 oz	72	5	6	18	0	–	206

SAFFLOWER

seeds dried	1 oz	147	5	11	0	10	–	–

SAFFRON

saffron	1 tsp	2	tr	tr	0	tr	–	1

SAGE

ground	1 tsp	2	tr	tr	0	tr	–	tr

SALAD
MIX
Dole

FOOD	PORTION	CALS	PROT	FAT	CHOL	CARB	FIBER	SOD
All American Toss	2 cups (3.5 oz)	50	4	1	<5	7	2	160
American Blend	1½ cups (3 oz)	15	1	0	0	3	1	10
Classic	1½ cups (3 oz)	15	1	0	0	4	1	15
Classic Romaine Blend	1½ cups (3 oz)	15	1	0	0	3	1	10
Coleslaw	1½ cups (3 oz)	25	1	0	0	5	2	25
European Special Blend	2 cups (3 oz)	15	1	0	0	3	1	15
Garlic Caesar Complete w/ Dressing	1½ cups (3.5 oz)	180	3	15	5	8	1	420
Greek Marinade	1½ cups (3.5 oz)	100	2	8	<5	5	1	340
Greener Selection	1½ cups (3 oz)	15	1	0	0	3	1	10
Light Caesar Complete w/ Dressing	1½ cups (3.5 oz)	60	3	1	0	10	2	390
Light Herb Ranch Complete w/ Dressing	1½ cups (3.5 oz)	50	2	1	5	10	2	280

FOOD	PORTION	CALS	PROT	FAT	CHOL	CARB	FIBER	SOD
Light Roasted Garlic Caesar Complete w/ Dressing	1½ cups (3.5 oz)	60	3	1	0	11	1	400
Light Zesty Italian Complete w/ Dressing	1½ cups (3.5 oz)	50	2	1	0	11	1	290
Mediterranean Marinade	2 cups (3.5 oz)	90	1	8	0	5	1	180
Oriental Complete w/ Dressing	1½ cups (3.5 oz)	120	2	6	0	13	2	240
Romano Complete w/ Dressing	1½ cups (3.5 oz)	150	3	12	0	9	2	570
Sunflower Ranch Complete w/ Dressing	1½ cups (3.5 oz)	160	2	16	5	5	2	220
Tomato & Mozzarella Medley	2 cups (3.5 oz)	60	4	2	5	7	2	80
Triple Cheese Toss	2 cups (3.5 oz)	80	5	5	15	4	1	120
Earthbound Farm								
Baby Caesar Mix	1 pkg (5 oz)	25	2	0	0	3	2	10
Baby Greens w/ Low Fat Honey Dijon Vinaigrette & Tomato Croutons	1 serv (3.5 oz)	90	3	3	0	15	2	380
Caesar w/ Garlic Croutons	1 serv (3.5 oz)	170	3	15	10	7	1	230
Italian Salad Organic	1⅔ cups (2.9 oz)	15	1	0	0	3	1	10
Mixed Baby Greens Organic	1 pkg (4 oz)	30	3	0	0	4	2	100
Organic Baby Greens w/ Vinaigrette & Garlic Croutons	1 serv (3.5 oz)	230	3	20	0	11	1	290

FOOD	PORTION	CALS	PROT	FAT	CHOL	CARB	FIBER	SOD
Organic Baby Spinach w/ Sesame Soy Vinaigrette & Peanuts	1 serv (3.5 oz)	150	5	11	0	8	2	340
Organic Italian Salad w/ Blue Cheese Dressing & Walnuts	1 serv (3.5 oz)	190	4	17	15	4	1	210
Romaine Blend Organic	1⅔ cups (2.9 oz)	15	1	0	0	3	1	10
Fresh Express								
Baby Spinach Trio	4 cups (3 oz)	20	2	0	0	4	1	55
Fancy Field Greens	1½ cups (3 oz)	15	1	0	0	3	2	15
Original Iceberg Garden w/ Zip	1½ cups (3 oz)	15	1	0	0	3	1	10
Veggie Lover's	1½ cups (3 oz)	20	1	0	0	4	1	15
Krakus								
Bordeaux	1 pkg (5 oz)	35	2	0	0	5	2	20
Ready Pac								
All American	2.5 cups	15	1	0	0	3	1	10
Bowl Salad Chef	1 pkg	350	21	25	70	9	2	1060
Bowl Salad Chicken Caesar	1 pkg	380	26	27	75	8	2	1050
Bowl Salad Greek	1 pkg	400	6	35	20	5	3	910
Bowl Salad Spinach Bacon	1 pkg	300	17	17	155	22	1	980
Bowl Salad Spring Mix Veggie	1 pkg	330	12	23	15	18	3	1120
Caesar Romaine	1½ cups	15	1	0	0	2	1	5
Classic Crisp Salad	2¼ cups	10	tr	0	0	2	tr	5
Continental	3 cups	20	1	0	0	4	2	15
Costa Brava	3 cups	15	1	0	0	3	2	20
Healthy Green Salad	2½ cups	10	tr	0	0	2	tr	5
Lafayette	3 cups	10	0	0	0	3	1	5
Milano	3 cups	15	1	0	0	3	2	15

FOOD	PORTION	CALS	PROT	FAT	CHOL	CARB	FIBER	SOD
Organic Caesar Romaine	2¼ cups	15	tr	0	0	2	tr	20
Organic Mesclun Blend	1 pkg (4.5 oz)	35	3	0	0	7	3	40
Organic Monterey	3 cups	15	1	0	0	3	2	10
Parisian	2 cups	20	1	0	0	4	1	20
Portofino	1 pkg (5 oz)	25	3	0	0	4	2	125
Santa Barbara	3½ cups	15	1	0	0	3	tr	20
Spring Mix	1 pkg (5 oz)	35	3	0	0	7	3	40
Suddenly Salad								
Caesar	¾ cup	220	5	9	0	30	1	580
Caesar Low Fat Recipe	¾ cup	170	5	3	0	30	1	580
Italian Pepperoni	1 cup	190	6	4	0	35	2	680
Italian Pepperoni Low Fat Recipe	1 cup	180	6	2	0	35	2	680
Ranch & Bacon	¾ cup	330	7	20	15	30	1	480
Ranch & Bacon Low Fat Recipe	¾ cup	180	7	2	<5	30	1	530
TAKE-OUT								
caesar	2 cups (5 oz)	235	5	20	10	11	1	440
chef w/o dressing	1½ cups	386	24	28	244	9	–	279
tossed w/o dressing	¾ cup	16	1	0	0	3	–	27
tossed w/o dressing	1½ cups	32	3	tr	0	7	–	53
tossed w/o dressing w/ cheese & egg	1½ cups	102	9	6	98	5	–	119
tossed w/o dressing w/ chicken	1½ cups	105	17	2	72	4	–	209
tossed w/o dressing w/ pasta & seafood	1½ cups (14.6 oz)	380	16	21	50	32	–	1572
tossed w/o dressing w/ shrimp	1½ cups	107	15	2	180	7	–	487
waldorf	½ cup	79	1	6	8	6	1	49

FOOD	PORTION	CALS	PROT	FAT	CHOL	CARB	FIBER	SOD
SALAD DRESSING								
MIX								
Et Tu								
Caesar Salad Kit	1 serv	140	2	12	5	6	0	115
Good Seasons								
Italian as prep	2 tbsp	130	0	14	0	3	–	340
Italian not prep	⅛ pkg (3 g)	5	0	0	0	1	–	320
McCormick								
Mediterranean Potato Salad	1 tbsp	25	tr	0	–	4	1	460
Pasta Salad Vinagarette	1 tsp (5 g)	15	0	0	–	2	–	590
READY-TO-EAT								
blue cheese	1 tbsp	77	1	8	–	1	–	–
french	1 tbsp	67	tr	6	–	3	–	214
french reduced calorie	1 tbsp	22	0	1	1	4	–	128
italian	1 tbsp	69	tr	7	–	2	–	116
italian reduced calorie	1 tbsp	16	tr	2	1	1	–	118
russian	1 tbsp	76	tr	8	–	2	–	·133
russian reduced calorie	1 tbsp	23	tr	1	1	5	–	141
sesame seed	1 tbsp	68	1	7	0	1	–	153
thousand island	1 tbsp	59	tr	6	–	2	–	109
thousand island reduced calorie	1 tbsp	24	tr	2	2	3	–	153
Annie Chun's								
Lemongrass	2 tbsp	60	0	3	0	6	0	75
Sesame Cilantro	1 tbsp	4	0	0	0	4	0	400
Carb Options								
Italian	2 tbsp	70	0	8	0	0	0	350
Ranch	2 tbsp	150	0	17	10	0	0	210
Drew's								
Low Carb Garlic Italian	1 tbsp	80	0	9	0	0	0	90
Low Carb Lemon Tahini Goddess	1 tbsp	80	0	9	0	1	0	90
Low Carb Sesame Orange	1 tbsp	80	0	9	0	2	0	90

FOOD	PORTION	CALS	PROT	FAT	CHOL	CARB	FIBER	SOD
Hellmann's								
Citrus Splash Ruby Red Ginger	2 tbsp (1 oz)	90	0	7	–	8	–	400
LaMartinique								
Blue Cheese Vinaigrette	2 tbsp	160	2	17	5	0	0	450
Poppy Seed	2 tbsp	170	0	15	0	8	0	330
Nasoya								
Creamy Dill	2 tbsp	70	0	7	0	2	0	135
Creamy Italian	2 tbsp	60	0	6	0	2	0	180
Garden Herb	2 tbsp	70	0	7	0	2	0	140
Sesame Garlic	2 tbsp	60	0	6	0	2	0	130
Thousand Island	2 tbsp	70	0	6	0	3	0	115
Old Dutch								
Sweet & Sour	2 tbsp	50	0	0	0	13	0	480
Paul's								
No-Fat Raspberry & Balsamic	2 tbsp	20	0	0	0	5	–	45
No-Oil Orange & Basil	2 tbsp	15	0	0	0	4	0	64
Steel's								
Honey Mustard	1 tbsp	90	0	7	0	0	0	125
Sweet Ginger Lime	1 tbsp	68	0	7	0	1	1	0
Wishbone								
Italian	2 tbsp	80	0	8	0	3	0	490
TAKE-OUT								
vinegar & oil	1 tbsp	72	0	8	0	tr	–	tr

SALMON
CANNED

FOOD	PORTION	CALS	PROT	FAT	CHOL	CARB	FIBER	SOD
chum w/ bone	3 oz	120	18	5	33	0	–	414
chum w/ bone	1 can (13.9 oz)	521	79	20	144	0	–	1797
pink w/ bone	3 oz	118	17	5	–	0	–	471
pink w/ bone	1 can (15.9 oz)	631	90	27	–	0	–	2514
sockeye w/ bone	3 oz	130	17	6	37	0	–	458
sockeye w/ bone	1 can (12.9 oz)	566	76	27	161	0	–	1987

FOOD	PORTION	CALS	PROT	FAT	CHOL	CARB	FIBER	SOD
Bumble Bee								
Keta	½ cup (3.5 oz)	160	20	8	–	0	–	490
Red	½ cup (3.5 oz)	180	20	10	–	0	–	490
Chicken Of The Sea								
Pink Chunk In Water	¼ cup	60	10	2	20	0	0	280
Pink Skinless Boneless	¼ cup	60	10	2	20	0	0	280
Libby's								
Alaskan Sockeye Red	¼ cup	110	13	7	40	0	0	270
Pink Skinless Boneless	¼ cup	50	11	1	20	0	0	150
FRESH								
atlantic baked	3 oz	155	22	7	60	0	–	48
chinook baked	3 oz	196	22	11	72	0	–	51
chum baked	3 oz	131	22	4	81	0	–	54
coho cooked	3 oz	157	23	6	42	0	–	50
coho cooked	½ fillet (5.4 oz)	286	42	12	76	0	–	91
coho raw	3 oz	124	18	5	33	0	–	39
pink baked	3 oz	127	22	4	57	0	–	73
roe raw	1 oz	59	7	3	–	tr	–	–
sockeye cooked	½ fillet (5.4 oz)	334	42	17	135	0	–	102
sockeye cooked	3 oz	183	23	9	74	0	–	102
sockeye raw	3 oz	143	18	7	53	0	–	40
SMOKED								
chinook	3 oz	99	16	4	20	0	–	666
chinook	1 oz	33	5	1	7	0	–	220
Lascco								
Nova Sliced	2 oz	60	10	1	20	3	0	960
TAKE-OUT								
roulette w/ spinach stuffing	1 serv (4 oz)	160	13	6	45	10	tr	400
salmon cake	1 (3 oz)	241	18	15	104	6	–	602

FOOD	PORTION	CALS	PROT	FAT	CHOL	CARB	FIBER	SOD
SALSA								
black bean & corn	2 tbsp (1 oz)	15	1	0	0	3	tr	45
citrus	2 tbsp (1 oz)	10	0	0	0	2	0	7
peach	2 tbsp	15	0	0	0	4	0	90
Del Salsa								
Fire Roasted All Flavors	2 tbsp	8	0	0	0	2	0	70
Gringo Billy's								
Salsa Mix	1 tsp	5	0	1	0	1	1	233
Guiltless Gourmet								
Roasted Red Pepper	2 tbsp	10	0	0	0	2	0	130
Southwestern Grill	2 tbsp	15	0	0	0	2	0	115
Hunt's								
Alfresco All Varieties	2 tbsp (1.1 oz)	10	tr	tr	0	2	tr	161
Hot	2 tbsp (1.1 oz)	27	1	tr	0	6	1	236
Medium	2 tbsp (1.1 oz)	27	1	tr	0	6	1	236
Mild	2 tbsp (1.1 oz)	27	1	tr	0	6	1	236
Picante All Varieties	2 tbsp (1.1 oz)	11	1	tr	0	2	tr	256
Squeeze Mild & Medium	2 tbsp (1.1 oz)	27	1	tr	0	6	1	236
Muir Glen								
Black Bean & Corn Medium	2 tbsp (1.1 oz)	15	1	0	0	3	tr	125
Chipotle Medium	2 tbsp (1.1 oz)	10	0	0	0	2	0	125
Fire Roasted Tomato Medium	2 tbsp (1.1 oz)	10	0	0	0	2	0	125
Garlic Cilantro Medium	2 tbsp (1.1 oz)	10	0	0	0	2	0	125
Habanero Hot	2 tbsp (1.1 oz)	10	0	0	0	2	0	125
Organic Medium	2 tbsp (1.1 oz)	10	0	0	0	2	0	125

FOOD	PORTION	CALS	PROT	FAT	CHOL	CARB	FIBER	SOD
Organic Mild	2 tbsp (1.1 oz)	10	0	0	0	2	0	125
Roasted Garlic Medium	2 tbsp (1.1 oz)	10	0	0	0	2	0	125
Pace								
Picante Mild or Medium	2 tbsp	10	0	0	0	2	0	220
Thick & Chunky Mild or Medium	2 tbsp	10	0	0	0	2	0	220
Rosarita								
Extra Chunky Medium	2 tbsp (1 oz)	7	tr	tr	0	1	tr	229
Green Tomatillo Medium	2 tbsp (1 oz)	8	tr	tr	0	2	1	188
Picante Zesty Jalapeno Hot	2 tbsp (1 oz)	8	tr	tr	0	2	1	246
Picante Zesty Jalapeno Medium	2 tbsp (1 oz)	9	tr	tr	0	2	1	254
Picante Zesty Jalapeno Mild	2 tbsp (1 oz)	8	tr	tr	0	2	tr	239
Roasted Mild	2 tbsp (1 oz)	10	tr	tr	0	2	1	233
Traditional Medium	2 tbsp (1 oz)	7	tr	tr	0	2	1	234
Traditional Mild	2 tbsp (1 oz)	7	1	tr	0	1	1	247
Snyder's Of Hanover								
Mild	2 tbsp	10	0	0	0	2	0	220
Tostitos								
Con Queso	2.3 oz	80	2	5	<10	10	<2	560
Hot	2.3 oz	30	2	0	0	6	2	520
Low Fat Con Queso	2.5 oz	80	2	3	<10	8	tr	560
Medium	2.3 oz	30	2	0	0	6	2	520
Mild	2.3 oz	30	2	0	0	6	2	520
Restaurant Style	2.2 oz	30	<2	0	0	6	<2	420
Ultimate Garden	2.4 oz	30	2	0	0	6	2	460

FOOD	PORTION	CALS	PROT	FAT	CHOL	CARB	FIBER	SOD
Tree Of Life								
Medium	2 tbsp (1 oz)	10	0	0	0	2	–	30
Mild	2 tbsp (1 oz)	10	0	0	0	2	–	30
Utz								
Chunky	2 tbsp (1 fl oz)	60	2	0	0	14	4	190

SALSIFY

FOOD	PORTION	CALS	PROT	FAT	CHOL	CARB	FIBER	SOD
fresh sliced cooked	½ cup	46	2	tr	0	10	–	11
raw sliced	½ cup	55	2	tr	0	12	–	13

SALT SUBSTITUTES

FOOD	PORTION	CALS	PROT	FAT	CHOL	CARB	FIBER	SOD
Eden								
Shiso Leaf Powder	1 tsp	0	0	0	0	0	2	200
Halsosalt								
All Flavors	¼ tsp (7 g)	1	0	0	0	0	–	0
Molly McButter								
Lite Sodium	1 tsp	5	0	0	0	2	–	90
Morton								
Salt Substitute	¼ tsp (1.2 g)	tr	0	0	0	tr	–	tr
Mrs. Dash								
Onion & Herb	¼ tsp	0	0	0	0	0	0	0

SALT/SEASONED SALT

FOOD	PORTION	CALS	PROT	FAT	CHOL	CARB	FIBER	SOD
salt	1 tsp (6 g)	0	0	0	0	0	–	2325
salt	1 tbsp (18 g)	0	0	0	0	0	–	6976
Eden								
Atlantic Sea Salt	¼ tsp	0	0	0	0	0	0	467
Brittany Sea Salt	¼ tsp	0	0	0	0	0	0	552
McCormick								
Celery Salt	¼ tsp	0	0	0	0	0	0	250
Morton								
Garlic	1 tsp	3	–	tr	0	–	–	–
Iodized	1 tsp	tr	–	0	0	–	–	–
Kosher	1 tsp	0	–	0	0	–	–	–
Lite	¼ tsp (1.4 g)	tr	0	0	0	tr	–	280
Nature's Season Seasoning Blend	1 tsp	3	–	tr	0	–	–	–
Non-Iodized	1 tsp	0	–	0	0	–	–	–
Seasoned	1 tsp	4	–	tr	0	–	–	–

FOOD	PORTION	CALS	PROT	FAT	CHOL	CARB	FIBER	SOD

SANDWICHES

Amy's

FOOD	PORTION	CALS	PROT	FAT	CHOL	CARB	FIBER	SOD
Pocket Sandwich Broccoli & Cheese	1 (4.5 oz)	270	8	10	15	37	3	560
Pocket Sandwich Roasted Vegetables	1 (4.5 oz)	220	6	8	0	35	4	480
Pocket Sandwich Spinach Feta	1 (4.5 oz)	250	11	9	20	34	3	590
Pocket Sandwich Tofu Scramble	1 (4 oz)	160	11	6	0	23	tr	520
Pocket Sandwich Vegetable Pie	1 (5 oz)	300	5	9	0	45	3	490
Toaster Pops Grilled Cheese	1	180	8	8	20	19	0	220

Croissant Pockets

FOOD	PORTION	CALS	PROT	FAT	CHOL	CARB	FIBER	SOD
Chicken Parmesan	1 piece	370	11	20	15	36	4	760

Healthy Choice

FOOD	PORTION	CALS	PROT	FAT	CHOL	CARB	FIBER	SOD
Bread Stuffs Chicken & Broccoli	1 (6.1 oz)	310	17	4	25	50	2	600
Bread Stuffs Ham & Cheese w/Broccoli	1 (6.1 oz)	320	21	5	20	46	1	590
Bread Stuffs Italian Style Meatball	1 (6.1 oz)	330	16	5	20	52	4	600
Bread Stuffs Philly Beef Steak	1 (6.1 oz)	310	17	5	20	50	3	600

Hot Pockets

FOOD	PORTION	CALS	PROT	FAT	CHOL	CARB	FIBER	SOD
Four Cheese Pizza	1 (4.5 oz)	380	11	17	45	45	3	680

Lean Pockets

FOOD	PORTION	CALS	PROT	FAT	CHOL	CARB	FIBER	SOD
Chicken Fajita	1 (4.5 oz)	260	11	7	25	38	3	730

Smucker's

FOOD	PORTION	CALS	PROT	FAT	CHOL	CARB	FIBER	SOD
Uncrustables Grape	1 (2 oz)	200	7	8	0	27	2	260

TAKE-OUT

FOOD	PORTION	CALS	PROT	FAT	CHOL	CARB	FIBER	SOD
chicken fillet plain	1	515	24	29	60	39	–	957

FOOD	PORTION	CALS	PROT	FAT	CHOL	CARB	FIBER	SOD
chicken fillet w/ cheese lettuce mayonnaise & tomato	1	632	29	39	76	42	–	1238
croque monsieur	1 (12.4 oz)	765	41	46	152	43	2	1018
fish fillet w/ tartar sauce	1	431	17	55	–	41	–	615
fish fillet w/ tartar sauce & cheese	1	524	21	29	68	48	–	939
fried egg w/ cheese	1	340	16	19	291	26	–	804
fried egg w/ cheese & ham	1	348	19	16	245	31	–	1005
ham w/ cheese	1	353	21	15	58	33	–	772
roast beef submarine sandwich w/ tomato lettuce & mayonnaise	1	411	29	13	73	44	–	845
roast beef w/ cheese	1	402	32	18	77	27	–	1634
roast beef plain	1	346	22	14	52	33	–	792
steak w/ tomato lettuce salt & mayonnaise	1	459	30	14	73	52	–	798
submarine w/ salami ham cheese lettuce tomato onion & oil	1	456	22	19	35	51	–	1650
tuna salad submarine sandwich w/ lettuce & oil	1	584	30	28	47	55	–	1294

SAPODILLA

FOOD	PORTION	CALS	PROT	FAT	CHOL	CARB	FIBER	SOD
fresh	1	140	1	2	0	34	–	20
fresh cut up	1 cup	199	1	3	0	48	–	29

SAPOTES

FOOD	PORTION	CALS	PROT	FAT	CHOL	CARB	FIBER	SOD
fresh	1	301	5	1	0	76	–	21

FOOD	PORTION	CALS	PROT	FAT	CHOL	CARB	FIBER	SOD
SARDINES								
CANNED								
atlantic in oil w/ bone	2	50	6	3	34	0	–	121
atlantic in oil w/ bone	1 can (3.2 oz)	192	23	11	131	0	–	465
pacific in tomato sauce w/ bone	1	68	6	5	23	0	–	157
pacific in tomato sauce w/ bone	1 can (13 oz)	658	61	44	225	0	–	1532
Bumble Bee								
In Hot Sauce	½ can (2 oz)	109	9	8	30	tr	0	230
In Mustard	½ can (2 oz)	88	10	5	35	1	0	260
In Oil	½ can (2 oz)	125	15	7	39	0	0	240
In Water	½ can (2 oz)	83	15	3	60	0	0	190
Goya								
In Tomato Sauce	2 pieces (2.2 oz)	50	8	1	45	20	2	15
King Oscar								
In Olive Oil	1 can (3.75 oz)	150	14	11	120	0	0	340
Skinless Boneless In Soya Oil	3 pieces (1.9 oz)	120	13	7	20	0	0	350
Season								
Brisling In Water	1 can (3.75 oz)	145	14	10	120	0	0	340
FRESH								
raw	3.5 oz	135	19	5	–	0	–	100
SAUCE (see also BARBECUE SAUCE, GRAVY, PIZZA SAUCE, SPAGHETTI SAUCE)								
JARRED								
fish sauce chinese	1 tbsp	9	2	0	–	tr	0	1224
fish sauce vietnamese nuoc mam	1 tbsp	6	1	0	0	1	0	1390
hoisin	1 tbsp	35	1	1	0	7	tr	258
morroccan tagine	½ cup (4 oz)	70	2	3	0	10	1	1140
oyster	1 tbsp	8	tr	0	0	2	0	437
teriyaki	1 oz	30	2	0	0	6	–	1380

FOOD	PORTION	CALS	PROT	FAT	CHOL	CARB	FIBER	SOD
teriyaki	1 tbsp	15	1	0	0	3	–	690
A1								
Bold Steak Sauce	1 tbsp	20	0	0	0	5	–	190
Annie Chun's								
Shiitake Mushroom	1 tbsp	15	1	0	0	3	0	190
Thai Peanut	2 tbsp	120	4	7	0	10	1	230
Atkins								
Steak Sauce	1 tbsp	5	0	0	0	1	0	180
Teriyaki	1 tbsp	10	0	1	0	1	0	300
Boar's Head								
Ham Glaze Brown Sugar & Spice	2 tbsp (1.4 oz)	120	0	0	0	30	0	95
Carb Options								
Alfredo	¼ cup	110	1	10	30	2	0	390
Asian Teriyaki Marinade	1 tbsp	5	0	1	–	1	0	500
Cheese	¼ cup	90	2	8	25	2	0	480
Garden Style	½ cup	80	2	5	0	7	2	540
Steak Sauce	1 tbsp	5	0	0	0	1	0	200
Chun King								
Sweet And Sour	2 tbsp (1.2 oz)	58	tr	tr	0	14	0	104
Teriyaki	1 tbsp (0.6 oz)	17	1	tr	0	3	0	917
Teriyaki Hot	1 tbsp (0.6 oz)	17	2	tr	0	3	0	995
Consorzio								
Marinade Baja Lime	1 tbsp	60	0	6	0	3	–	140
Del Monte								
Seafood Cocktail	¼ cup (2.7 oz)	100	1	0	0	24	0	910
Sloppy Joe Hickory Flavor	¼ cup (2.4 oz)	70	1	0	0	18	0	700
Sloppy Joe Original	¼ cup (2.4 oz)	70	1	0	0	16	0	680
Fritos								
Texas-Style Chili Hearty Topping	2.3 oz	50	2	2	10	8	1	330

FOOD	PORTION	CALS	PROT	FAT	CHOL	CARB	FIBER	SOD
Utimate Taco Hearty Topping	2.3 oz	50	2	2	10	8	1	330
Gebhardt								
Enchilada Sauce	¼ cup (2.2 oz)	35	1	2	0	4	1	218
Hot Dog Chili Sauce	¼ cup (2.2 oz)	60	3	3	1	6	2	274
Hot Sauce	1 tsp (5 g)	1	tr	tr	0	tr	0	89
Gringo Billy's								
Chipotle Dipping & Grilling Sauce	1 tsp	5	0	0	0	1	0	35
Jok'n'Al								
Cocktail	¼ cup	29	0	0	0	6	–	400
Plum	1 tbsp	10	0	0	0	2	–	40
Just Rite								
Hot Dog	¼ cup (2.2 oz)	50	2	3	2	5	2	265
Kikkoman								
Teriyaki	1 tbsp	15	1	0	0	3	0	610
La Choy								
Duck Sauce Sweet & Sour	2 tbsp (1.3 oz)	61	tr	tr	0	15	0	128
Sweet & Sour	2 tbsp (1.2 oz)	58	tr	tr	0	14	0	104
Teriyaki	1 tbsp (0.6 oz)	17	1	tr	0	3	0	917
Lea & Perrins								
Worcestershire	1 tsp	5	0	0	0	1	–	65
Manwich								
Bold	¼ cup (2.2 oz)	62	1	1	0	13	1	802
Mexican	¼ cup (2.2 oz)	27	1	tr	0	5	1	552
Original	¼ cup (2.2 oz)	32	1	tr	0	6	1	365
Taco Season	¼ cup (2.2 oz)	27	1	tr	0	6	1	552
Thick & Chunky	¼ cup (2.3 oz)	44	1	tr	0	9	1	737

FOOD	PORTION	CALS	PROT	FAT	CHOL	CARB	FIBER	SOD
Matouk's								
Flambeau Sauce	1 tsp	0	0	0	0	0	0	140
McCormick								
Flavor Medleys Garlic & Herb	2 tbsp	50	0	5	–	5	–	390
Flavor Medleys Italian Herb	2 tbsp	50	0	4	–	4	–	370
Flavor Medleys Lemon Pepper	2 tbsp	50	0	4	–	4	–	450
Flavor Medleys Tomato & Basil	2 tbsp	50	0	3	–	4	–	400
Old El Paso								
Enchilada Mild	¼ cup	20	0	1	0	3	0	220
Open Range								
Hot Dog Chili	¼ cup (2.2 oz)	61	3	3	3	6	2	255
Pace								
Enchilada Sauce	¼ cup	36	0	0	0	6	0	290
Taco Sauce	¼ cup	32	0	2	0	4	0	150
Progresso								
Alfredo	½ cup (4.4 oz)	200	8	15	50	7	1	850
Sauce Arturo								
Original	¼ cup (2.2 fl oz)	50	1	1	0	8	0	680
Steel's								
Sugar Free Cocktail w/ Dill & Lemon	¼ cup	36	1	0	0	1	1	160
Sugar Free Hoisin	2 tbsp	15	1	0	0	2	1	440
Sugar Free Peanut Sauce	1 tbsp	34	2	2	–	7	5	150
Sugar Free Sweet & Sour	2 tbsp	10	0	0	0	2	0	155
Tostitos								
Beef Fiesta Nacho	2.4 oz	120	4	8	10	6	tr	500
Chicken Quesadilla Topping	2.5 oz	90	4	6	10	6	tr	600

FOOD	PORTION	CALS	PROT	FAT	CHOL	CARB	FIBER	SOD
Walden Farms								
Calorie Free Seafood Sauce	1 tbsp	0	0	0	0	0	0	290
Scampi Sauce Calorie Free	2 tbsp	0	0	0	0	0	0	130
Wild Thyme Farms								
Chili Ginger Honey	1 tbsp	30	0	0	0	8	–	0
MIX								
cheese as prep w/ milk	1 cup	307	16	17	53	23	–	1566
curry as prep w/ milk	1 cup	270	11	15	35	26	–	1276
mushroom as prep w/ milk	1 cup	228	11	10	34	24	–	1533
sour cream as prep w/ milk	1 cup	509	19	30	91	45	–	1007
stroganoff as prep	1 cup	271	12	11	38	34	–	1829
sweet & sour as prep	1 cup	294	1	tr	0	73	–	779
teriyaki as prep	1 cup	131	4	1	0	28	–	4791
white as prep w/ milk	1 cup	241	10	13	34	21	–	796
Durkee								
A La King as prep	1 cup	60	1	4	0	8	0	800
Cheese as prep	¼ cup	25	1	2	2	4	0	260
Hollandaise as prep	2 tbsp	10	0	0	0	2	0	70
White as prep	¼ cup	20	0	1	0	5	0	330
French's								
Cheese as prep	¼ cup	25	1	1	0	4	0	250
Hollandaise as prep	2 tbsp	10	0	0	0	2	0	75
Manwich								
Mix	¼ oz	22	tr	tr	0	5	tr	355
McCormick								
Bernaise Blend	1 tsp (3 g)	10	0	0	–	1	–	130
Chicken Dijon Blend	1⅓ tbsp (10 g)	40	tr	2	<5	5	–	420
Green Peppercorn Blend as prep	¼ cup	20	tr	0	–	3	–	360

FOOD	PORTION	CALS	PROT	FAT	CHOL	CARB	FIBER	SOD
Grill Mates Mesquite Marinade as prep	1 tbsp	15	0	0	–	2	–	610
Grill Mates Southwest Marinade	2 tsp (5 g)	15	0	0	–	2	tr	440
Hollandaise Blend	2 tsp (4 g)	15	0	0	15	1	–	110
Hunter Blend as prep	¼ cup	25	tr	0	–	4	–	270
Meat Marinade	1 tsp (4 g)	15	0	0	–	2	–	240
Pepper Medley Blend as prep	¼ cup	30	1	2	–	3	–	310
White Blend	2 tsp (6 g)	20	tr	1	–	3	–	300
TAKE-OUT								
bearnaise	1 oz	177	1	19	21	1	tr	257
cucumber yogurt sauce	1.5 tbsp	20	2	0	2	3	0	20

SAUERKRAUT

FOOD	PORTION	CALS	PROT	FAT	CHOL	CARB	FIBER	SOD
canned	½ cup	22	1	tr	0	5	–	780
B&G								
Sauerkraut	2 tbsp (1 oz)	6	0	0	0	1	1	180
Boar's Head								
Sauerkraut	2 tbsp (1 oz)	5	0	0	0	1	tr	180
Claussen								
Sauerkraut	¼ cup (1.1 oz)	5	0	0	0	1	1	210
Del Monte								
Bavarian Style	2 tbsp (1 oz)	15	0	0	0	4	0	180
Sauerkraut	2 tbsp (1 oz)	0	0	0	0	1	1	180
Eden								
Organic	½ cup	25	2	0	0	4	3	580
S&W								
Canned	2 tbsp (1 oz)	5	0	0	0	1	0	220
Red Cabbage	2 tbsp (1 oz)	15	0	0	0	3	0	160
Silver Floss								
Sauerkraut	½ cup	20	0	0	0	5	4	740

SAUSAGE

FOOD	PORTION	CALS	PROT	FAT	CHOL	CARB	FIBER	SOD
bierschinken	3.5 oz	174	18	11	–	tr	–	753
bierwurst	3.5 oz	258	16	21	–	0	–	–

FOOD	PORTION	CALS	PROT	FAT	CHOL	CARB	FIBER	SOD
blutwurst uncooked	3.5 oz	424	13	39	—	0	—	680
bockwurst	3.5 oz	276	12	25	—	0	—	700
bratwurst pork cooked	1 link (3 oz)	256	12	22	51	2	—	473
brotwurst pork & beef	1 link (2.5 oz)	226	10	19	44	2	—	778
chipolata	3.5 oz	342	14	32	66	1	0	747
chorizo	3.5 oz	499	20	45	70	4	tr	2300
fleischwurst	3.5 oz	305	12	29	—	0	—	829
free range chicken breakfast	2 links (2.7 oz)	110	14	6	45	1	0	570
gelbwurst uncooked	3.5 oz	363	12	33	—	0	—	640
italian pork cooked	1 (3 oz)	268	17	21	65	1	—	765
jagdwurst	3.5 oz	211	16	16	—	0	—	818
kielbasa pork	1 oz	88	8	8	19	1	—	305
knockwurst pork & beef	1 (2.4 oz)	209	8	19	39	1	—	687
mettwurst uncooked	3.5 oz	483	13	45	—	0	—	1090
plockwurst uncooked	3.5 oz	312	19	45	—	0	—	—
polish pork	1 (8 oz)	739	32	65	158	4	—	1989
pork cooked	1 link (½ oz)	48	3	4	11	tr	—	168
regensburger uncooked	3.5 oz	354	13	31	—	0	—	—
vienna canned	7 (4 oz)	315	12	28	59	2	—	1077
vienna canned	1 (½ oz)	45	2	4	8	tr	—	152
weisswurst uncooked	3.5 oz	305	11	27	—	0	—	620
zungenwurst	3.5 oz (tongue)	285	17	24	—	0	—	—
Banner								
Sausage Stomachs	2 oz	90	0	5	95	0	0	430
Sausage Tripe	2 oz	90	9	5	85	2	0	430
Bilinski's								
Chicken Bratworst With Wild Rice	1 (2 oz)	70	11	2	25	2	0	280

FOOD	PORTION	CALS	PROT	FAT	CHOL	CARB	FIBER	SOD
Chicken Cajun-Style Andouille	2 oz	80	9	4	60	1	0	300
Chicken Italian With Peppers	1 (2 oz)	70	9	4	60	1	0	270
Chicken With Apples & Chardonnay	2 oz	70	10	6	60	3	0	350
Chicken With Cilantro	2 oz	70	9	4	40	1	1	270
Chicken With Jalapenos	2 oz	70	9	4	55	0	0	270
Chicken With Pesto	2 oz	90	10	5	40	0	0	320
Chicken With Spinach	2 oz	70	9	4	40	1	1	270
Chicken With Sun-Dried Tomato	2 oz	70	10	4	40	2	0	280
Boar's Head								
Bratwurst	1 (4 oz)	300	19	25	75	0	0	650
Hot Smoked	1 (3.2 oz)	280	12	25	55	1	0	740
Kielbasa	2 oz	120	9	10	50	0	0	440
Knockwurst	1 (4 oz)	310	15	27	50	1	0	950
Brown'N Serve								
Turkey	3 (2.1 oz)	120	10	8	35	2	0	370
Jennie-O								
Italian Hot	1 (3.9 oz)	160	17	10	60	2	–	850
Jones								
Light 50% Less Fat	2 (1.6 oz)	100	7	8	25	1	–	230
Little Pork	3	190	8	17	45	1	–	420
Murray's								
Chicken Hot Italian	3 oz	130	16	7	85	1	–	670
Chicken Spinach & Garlic	3 oz	100	12	5	50	1	–	640
Chicken Sun Dried Tomato	3 oz	110	18	5	55	2	–	420
Chicken Sweet Italian	3 oz	130	16	7	85	1	–	670
Perdue								
Hot Italian Turkey Cooked	1 link (2.4 oz)	150	16	9	60	1	–	470

FOOD	PORTION	CALS	PROT	FAT	CHOL	CARB	FIBER	SOD
Sweet Italian Turkey Cooked	1 link (2.4 oz)	150	16	9	60	1	–	490
Shady Brook								
Turkey Sweet Italian	1 (2.5 oz)	110	13	7	50	1	–	570
Turkey Store								
Breakfast	2 links (2 oz)	140	8	11	45	1	–	360
Breakfast Sausage Patties Mild	2 patties (2.3 oz)	160	10	13	50	1	–	420
Wampler								
Breakfast Turkey	2 (2.4 oz)	110	13	6	45	1	–	440
Italian Turkey	1 (2.7 oz)	120	14	6	50	1	–	480
TAKE-OUT								
pork	1 patty (1 oz)	100	5	8	22	tr	–	349
pork	1 link (0.5 oz)	48	3	4	11	tr	–	168

SAUSAGE DISHES
TAKE-OUT

FOOD	PORTION	CALS	PROT	FAT	CHOL	CARB	FIBER	SOD
italian sausage w/ peppers & onions	1 cup	210	17	11	70	14	–	1120
sausage roll	1 (2.3 oz)	311	5	24	–	22	1	–

SAUSAGE SUBSTITUTES

FOOD	PORTION	CALS	PROT	FAT	CHOL	CARB	FIBER	SOD
nonmeat sausage	1 patty (38 g)	97	7	7	0	4	–	137
nonmeat sausage	1 link (25 g)	64	5	5	0	2	–	222
Boca Burgers								
Breakfast Patties	1 (1.3 oz)	70	9	3	0	4	2	300
Lightlife								
Gimme Lean	2 oz	70	9	0	0	8	1	290
Lean Links Breakfast	1 (1.2 oz)	60	4	3	0	4	0	130
Lean Links Italian	1 (1.4 oz)	60	5	2	0	5	0	160
Light	2 patties (2.3 oz)	80	11	0	0	10	1	340
Loma Linda								
Linketts	1 (1.2 oz)	70	7	5	0	1	1	160
Little Links	2 (1.6 oz)	90	8	6	0	2	2	230

FOOD	PORTION	CALS	PROT	FAT	CHOL	CARB	FIBER	SOD
Morningstar Farms								
Breakfast Links	2	60	8	2	0	2	2	340
Breakfast Patties	1 (1.3 oz)	80	10	3	0	3	2	270
Grillers	1 patty (2.2 oz)	140	14	7	0	5	3	260
Sausage Style Recipe Crumbles	⅔ cup (1.9 oz)	90	11	3	0	5	2	370
Natural Touch								
Vegan Sausage Crumbles	½ cup (1.9 oz)	60	10	0	0	4	2	300
Quorn								
Meat-Free Links	2 (1.6 oz)	70	8	3	0	2	1	210
Worthington								
Leanies	1 link (1.4 oz)	100	7	7	0	2	1	430
Prosage Links	2 (1.6 oz)	60	8	3	0	2	2	340
Yves								
Veggie Breakfast Links	1 (1.6 oz)	60	11	0	0	3	2	390
Veggie Breakfast Patties	1 (2 oz)	70	11	2	0	4	2	350

SAVORY

FOOD	PORTION	CALS	PROT	FAT	CHOL	CARB	FIBER	SOD
ground	1 tsp	4	tr	tr	0	1	–	tr

SCALLOP

FOOD	PORTION	CALS	PROT	FAT	CHOL	CARB	FIBER	SOD
raw	3 oz	75	14	1	28	2	–	137
TAKE-OUT								
breaded & fried	2 lg	67	6	3	19	3	–	144

SCONE

FOOD	PORTION	CALS	PROT	FAT	CHOL	CARB	FIBER	SOD
Finnegan's								
Irish Raisin	1 (2 oz)	170	4	4	0	31	1	290
King Arthur								
Cranberry Orange as prep	1	248	5	8	47	39	0	174
TAKE-OUT								
apricot	1	232	5	7	34	39	–	201
blueberry	1 (3 oz)	270	7	9	10	41	2	600
cheese	1 (3.5 oz)	364	10	18	–	44	2	–
orange poppy	1 (3 oz)	260	6	6	30	47	2	400

FOOD	PORTION	CALS	PROT	FAT	CHOL	CARB	FIBER	SOD
plain	1 (3.5 oz)	362	8	14	–	54	2	–
raisin	1 (3 oz)	270	6	8	10	43	2	490

SCUP

| fresh baked | 3 oz | 115 | 21 | 3 | – | 0 | – | 46 |

SEA BASS (see BASS)

SEA CUCUMBER

| dried | 1 oz | 74 | 14 | 1 | 17 | 1 | 0 | 1411 |
| fresh | 1 oz | 20 | 5 | tr | 14 | tr | 0 | 143 |

SEA TROUT (see TROUT)

SEA URCHIN

canned	1 oz	39	4	1	–	3	0	–
fresh	1 oz	36	4	1	–	3	tr	32
roe paste	1 tbsp	19	2	tr	–	3	0	658

SEAWEED

agar dried	1 oz	87	2	tr	0	23	–	29
agar fresh	1 oz	tr	tr	tr	0	2	–	3
hijiki dried	1 tbsp	9	1	0	0	2	1	–
irishmoss fresh	1 oz	14	tr	tr	0	4	–	19
kelp fresh	1 oz	12	tr	tr	0	3	–	66
kombu fresh	1 oz	12	tr	tr	0	3	–	66
laver fresh	1 oz	10	2	tr	0	1	–	14
nori fresh	1 oz	10	2	tr	0	1	–	14
nori sheet dried	1 (8 x 8 in)	5	1	0	0	1	1	18
seahair dried	1 tbsp	13	1	0	0	3	tr	–
spirulina dried	1 oz	83	16	2	0	7	–	309
spirulina fresh	1 oz	7	2	tr	0	1	–	28
tangle fresh	1 oz	12	tr	tr	0	3	–	66
wakame fresh	1 oz	13	1	tr	0	3	–	249

SEITAN (see WHEAT)

SEMOLINA

| dry | 1 cup (5.9 oz) | 601 | 21 | 2 | 0 | 122 | 7 | 2 |

SESAME

| seeds | 1 tsp | 16 | 1 | 2 | 0 | tr | – | 1 |
| sesame butter | 1 tbsp | 95 | 3 | 8 | 0 | 4 | 1 | 2 |

FOOD	PORTION	CALS	PROT	FAT	CHOL	CARB	FIBER	SOD
sesame crunch candy	20 pieces (1.2 oz)	181	4	12	0	18	–	–
sesame crunch candy	1 oz	146	3	9	0	14	–	–
tahini from roasted & toasted kernels	1 tbsp	89	3	8	0	3	–	17
tahini from stone ground kernels	1 tbsp	86	3	7	0	4	–	11
tahini from unroasted kernels	1 tbsp	85	3	8	0	3	–	0
Eden								
Organic Seaweed Gomasio	1 serv (1.5 oz)	10	0	1	0	0	0	35
Organic Gomasio	½ tsp	10	0	1	0	0	tr	40
Organic Gomasio Garlic	½ tsp	10	0	1	0	0	tr	35
Maranatha								
Raw Tahini	2 tbsp	190	6	16	0	9	3	80
Roasted Tahini	2 tbsp	210	6	16	0	10	2	80
SESBANIA								
flower	1	1	tr	0	0	tr	–	0
flowers	1 cup	5	tr	tr	0	1	–	3
flowers cooked	1 cup	23	1	tr	0	5	–	11
SHAD								
american baked	3 oz	214	18	15	–	0	–	56
roe baked w/ butter & lemon	1 oz	36	6	1	–	tr	–	21
roe raw	1 oz	37	7	tr	103	tr	–	–
SHARK								
fin dried	1 oz	32	7	tr	–	–	–	5
raw	3 oz	111	18	4	43	0	–	67
TAKE-OUT								
batter-dipped & fried	3 oz	194	16	12	50	5	–	103
SHEEPSHEAD FISH								
cooked	1 fillet (6.5 oz)	234	48	3	–	0	–	136

FOOD	PORTION	CALS	PROT	FAT	CHOL	CARB	FIBER	SOD
cooked	3 oz	107	22	1	–	0	–	62
raw	3 oz	92	17	2	–	0	–	61

SHELLFISH (see individual names, SHELLFISH SUBSTITUTES)

SHELLFISH SUBSTITUTES

crab imitation	3 oz	87	10	1	17	1	–	715
scallop imitation	3 oz	84	11	tr	18	9	–	676
shrimp imitation	3 oz	86	11	1	31	8	–	599
surimi	3 oz	84	13	1	25	6	–	122
surimi	1 oz	28	4	tr	8	2	–	40
Louis Kemp								
Crab Delights	½ cup (3 oz)	90	10	0	10	12	2	410
Lobster Delights	½ cup (3 oz)	80	8	0	10	12	0	420
Scallop Delights	13 pieces (3 oz)	80	9	0	10	12	0	550

SHELLIE BEANS

canned	½ cup	37	2	tr	0	8	–	408

SHERBET

orange	½ gal	2158	17	31	113	469	–	706
orange	½ cup (4 fl oz)	132	1	2	5	29	–	44
orange	1 bar (2.75 fl oz)	91	1	1	3	20	–	30
orange home recipe	½ cup	120	2	2	9	24	–	30
Breyers								
Orange	½ cup	120	1	2	5	26	0	35
Rainbow	½ cup	120	1	2	5	26	0	35
Turkey Hill								
Fruit Rainbow	½ cup	120	–	1	5	26	–	20
Orange Grove	½ cup	120	–	1	5	26	–	20

SHRIMP

canned	3 oz	102	20	2	147	1	–	143
canned	1 cup	154	30	3	222	1	–	216
chinese shrimp paste	1 tbsp	15	3	tr	45	1	–	2000
cooked	3 oz	84	18	1	166	0	–	190

FOOD	PORTION	CALS	PROT	FAT	CHOL	CARB	FIBER	SOD
cooked	4 large	22	5	tr	43	0	–	49
raw	4 large	30	6	tr	43	tr	–	42
raw	3 oz	90	17	1	130	1	–	126
Bumble Bee								
Medium	⅓ can (2 oz)	45	10	tr	115	0	0	650
Orleans Tiny Cocktail	½ can (3 oz)	44	–	0	114	0	0	650
Gorton's								
Popcorn Garlic & Herb	22 pieces (3.6 oz)	270	11	14	90	24	–	600
Popcorn Original	20 pieces (3.2 oz)	240	9	13	65	22	–	780
TAKE-OUT								
breaded & fried	3 oz	206	18	10	150	10	–	292
gingered	4	80	–	tr	140	–	–	920
jambalaya	¾ cup	188	11	5	50	26	8	83
scampi	2 cups	438	–	480	20	–	–	584

SMELT

FOOD	PORTION	CALS	PROT	FAT	CHOL	CARB	FIBER	SOD
rainbow cooked	3 oz	106	19	3	76	0	–	65
rainbow raw	3 oz	83	15	2	60	0	–	51

SMOOTHIE (see FRUIT DRINKS)

SNACKS

FOOD	PORTION	CALS	PROT	FAT	CHOL	CARB	FIBER	SOD
cheese puffs	1 oz	157	2	10	1	15	tr	298
corn puffs cheese	1 bag (8 oz)	1256	17	78	9	122	2	2383
corn twists cheese	1 oz	157	2	10	1	15	tr	298
corn twists cheese	1 bag (8 oz)	1256	17	78	9	122	2	2383
oriental mix	1 oz	155	6	12	0	9	–	235
pork skins	1 oz	154	17	9	27	0	–	521
pork skins barbecue	1 oz	152	16	9	33	1	–	756
trail mix	1 oz	131	4	8	0	13	–	65
trail mix	1 cup (5.3 oz)	693	21	44	0	67	–	343
trail mix tropical	1 oz	115	2	5	0	19	–	3
trail mix w/ chocolate chips	1 cup (5.1 oz)	707	21	47	–	66	–	177
trail mix w/ chocolate chips	1 oz	137	4	9	–	13	–	34

FOOD	PORTION	CALS	PROT	FAT	CHOL	CARB	FIBER	SOD
Baken-ets								
BBQ	9 (0.5 oz)	70	7	5	10	tr	tr	400
Hot N'Spicy	7 (0.5 oz)	70	8	5	20	tr	tr	440
Hot N'Spicy Cracklins	8 (0.5 oz)	80	7	5	20	tr	tr	320
Regular	9 (0.5 oz)	80	8	5	20	tr	tr	330
Regular Cracklins	8 (0.5 oz)	40	7	6	15	tr	tr	550
Barbara's Bakery								
Cheese Puffs Bakes	1½ cups (1 oz)	160	2	11	0	13	0	190
Cheese Puffs Jalapeno	¾ cup (1 oz)	150	2	10	0	16	0	130
Cheese Puffs Original	¾ cup (1 oz)	150	2	10	0	16	0	130
Bowlby's								
Bits Almond	½ cup	100	4	19	0	5	1	95
Bits Pecan	½ cup	200	4	19	0	5	1	95
Bits Ranch	½ cup	170	4	16	0	7	0	170
Bits Salsa	½ cup	170	2	16	0	7	0	230
Bits Sour Cream Onion & Dill	½ cup	170	4	16	0	7	0	190
Bits'N'Pops	¾ cup	130	1	7	13	16	1	90
Mix-Ups Country Mix	½ cup	170	5	14	0	8	1	150
Mix-Ups Nuttyest-Of-All	½ cup	160	5	13	0	8	1	130
Mix-Ups Trail Mix	½ cup	165	4	12	0	11	1	135
Bugles								
Baked Original	1⅓ cup	130	2	4	0	23	—	380
Chile Con Queso	1⅓ cups	160	2	9	0	18	—	310
Nacho	1½ cups	160	1	9	0	18	—	300
Original	1½ cups	160	1	9	0	18	tr	310
Smokin'BBQ	1⅓ cups	150	1	8	0	19	—	330
Cheetos								
Crunchy	21 pieces (1 oz)	160	2	10	0	15	tr	290
Curls	15 pieces (1 oz)	150	2	10	0	15	1	290

FOOD	PORTION	CALS	PROT	FAT	CHOL	CARB	FIBER	SOD
Flamin' Hot	21 pieces (1 oz)	160	2	10	0	15	tr	280
Nacho Cheese	23 pieces (1 oz)	160	2	10	0	15	tr	260
Puffed Balls	38 pieces (1 oz)	150	2	10	0	15	tr	300
Puffs	29 pieces (1 oz)	160	2	10	0	15	tr	370
Zig Zags	17 pieces (1 oz)	170	2	11	<5	17	tr	370
Chex Mix								
Cheddar	⅔ cup	140	3	5	0	21	2	330
Hot'N Spicy	⅔ cup	130	3	5	0	21	2	390
Nacho Fiesta	⅔ cup	120	2	4	0	22	1	350
Party Blend Bold	⅔ cup	140	3	6	0	20	2	290
Peanut Lovers	⅔ cup	140	3	6	0	19	1	370
Traditional	⅔ cup	130	2	4	0	22	1	50
Dakota Gourmet								
Amazing Corn Classic	1 pkg (1 oz)	360	10	7	0	78	5	813
Amazing Corn Cool Ranch	1 pkg (1 oz)	367	10	9	2	74	5	1073
Amazing Corn Mesquite BBQ	1 pkg (1 oz)	369	11	8	0	76	5	725
Heart Smart Toasted Corn	⅓ cup (1 oz)	110	3	2	0	22	3	280
Heart Smart Toasted Corn	1 pkg (1.75 oz)	177	5	3	0	39	2	470
Trail Mix Heart Smart	1 pkg (1.75 oz)	172	4	0	0	39	3	156
Eden								
Rice Puffs Five Flavor Arare	1 oz	110	3	0	0	24	2	160
Frito Lay								
Funyuns	13 (1 oz)	140	2	7	0	18	tr	270
Munchos	16 (1 oz)	160	1	10	0	16	1	230
Munchos BBQ	14 (1 oz)	160	1	10	0	15	1	250
Glenny's								
Soy Crisps All Flavors	5	60	2	4	0	8	1	30

FOOD	PORTION	CALS	PROT	FAT	CHOL	CARB	FIBER	SOD
Gram's Gourmet								
Crunchies Pork Rinds	⅛ pkg (0.5 oz)	70	8	5	–	0	0	190
J&J								
Microwave Pork Rinds All Flavors	1 oz	130	23	4	0	tr	0	160
Maranatha								
High Energy Mix	¼ cup	120	3	7	0	15	2	0
Organic Harvest Mix	¼ cup	150	4	9	0	15	2	0
Organic Nature Mix	¼ cup	150	4	9	0	15	2	0
Snack Attack Mix	¼ cup	140	2	8	0	16	2	0
Trail Mix Organic Raw	¼ cup	140	5	9	0	13	2	4
Trail Mix Deluxe	¼ cup	150	5	11	0	11	2	0
Trail Mix Navajo	¼ cup	140	4	9	0	13	4	3
Trail Mix Olympic w/ Chocolate	¼ cup	140	4	8	0	16	2	13
Trail Mix Organic Delight	¼ cup	150	4	10	0	12	2	3
Mauna Loa								
Tropical Nut & Fruit	¼ cup	180	3	8	0	23	2	50
Old Dutch Foods								
Baked Cheese Curls	2 cups (1.1 oz)	180	2	12	0	15	tr	340
Cheese Puffcorn Curls	2 cups (1.1 oz)	170	2	12	0	15	0	310
Planters								
Cheez Mania Original	42 pieces (1 oz)	150	2	10	<5	15	1	300
Pumpkorn								
Caramel	⅓ cup	150	9	11	0	4	2	85
Chili	⅓ cup	150	9	11	0	4	2	100
Curry	⅓ cup	150	9	11	0	4	2	100
Maple Vanilla	⅓ cup	150	9	11	0	4	2	100
Mesquite	⅓ cup	150	9	11	0	4	2	110
Original	⅓ cup	150	10	11	0	4	2	110

FOOD	PORTION	CALS	PROT	FAT	CHOL	CARB	FIBER	SOD
Robert's American Gourmet								
Pirate's Booty Puffed Rice & Corn w/ Cheddar	1 oz	120	3	3	0	22	4	137
Rold Gold								
Snack Mix Colossal Cheddar	1 pkg (1 oz)	140	3	7	0	17	1	230
Snyder's Of Hanover								
Cheese Twists	1 oz	230	1	14	0	10	0	280
Fried Pork Skins	1 oz	80	8	4	30	1	0	115
Fried Pork Skins Barbecue	1 oz	80	8	4	20	1	0	106
Kruncheez	1.25 oz	200	2	10	0	19	tr	210
Onion Toasters	1 oz	188	2	10	0	21	tr	350
Utz								
Caramel Corn Clusters	1⅛ cups (1 oz)	120	tr	2	0	24	tr	140
Cheese Balls	50 (1 oz)	150	2	9	0	16	tr	260
Cheese Curls	18 (1 oz)	150	2	9	0	16	tr	260
Cheese Curls Crunchy	30 (1 oz)	160	2	10	0	16	0	200
Cheese Curls Reduced Fat	32 (1 oz)	140	3	6	<5	18	2	300
Onion Rings	41 (1 oz)	140	1	7	0	18	0	340
Party Mix	¾ cup (1 oz)	140	2	6	0	19	1	250
Pork Cracklins	0.5 oz	90	6	7	15	0	—	300
Pork Cracklins Hot & Spicy	0.5 oz	80	8	5	15	0	—	340
Pork Rinds	0.5 oz	80	8	5	15	0	—	230
Pork Rinds BBQ	0.5 oz	80	8	5	15	0	—	280
SNAIL								
cooked	3 oz	233	41	1	110	13	—	350
raw	3 oz	117	20	tr	55	7	—	175
TAKE-OUT								
escargot cooked	5	25	4	0	15	1	0	25
SNAKE								
fresh	3 oz	78	17	tr	—	3	0	57

FOOD	PORTION	CALS	PROT	FAT	CHOL	CARB	FIBER	SOD
SNAPPER								
cooked	1 fillet (6 oz)	217	45	3	80	0	–	96
cooked	3 oz	109	22	1	40	0	–	48
raw	3 oz	85	17	1	31	0	–	54
SODA								
club	12 oz	0	0	0	0	0	–	75
cola	12 oz	151	tr	tr	0	39	–	14
cream	12 oz	191	0	0	0	49	–	43
diet cola	12 oz	2	tr	0	0	tr	–	21
diet cola w/ equal	12 oz	2	tr	0	0	tr	–	21
diet cola w/ saccharin	12 oz	2	tr	0	0	tr	–	57
ginger ale	12 oz can	124	tr	0	0	32	–	25
grape	12 oz	161	0	0	0	42	–	57
lemon lime	12 oz	149	0	0	0	38	–	41
orange	12 oz	177	0	0	0	46	–	49
pepper type	12 oz	151	0	tr	0	38	–	38
quinine	12 oz	125	0	0	0	32	–	15
root beer	12 oz	152	tr	0	0	39	–	49
shirley temple	1 serv	159	0	0	0	41	0	34
tonic water	12 oz	125	0	0	0	32	–	15
7 Up								
Diet	8 oz	0	0	0	0	0	–	30
Original	1 can	140	0	0	0	39	–	75
Plus Mixed Berry	8 oz	10	0	0	0	2	–	130
A & W								
Root Beer	1 can (12 oz)	170	0	0	0	46	–	45
Barq's								
Root Beer	1 can (12 oz)	160	0	0	0	45	–	70
Barritts								
Ginger Beer	1 bottle (12 oz)	200	0	0	0	49	–	40
Best Health								
Root Beer	1 bottle (12 oz)	165	0	0	0	42	–	35
Vanilla Cream	1 bottle (12 oz)	170	0	0	0	43	–	30

FOOD	PORTION	CALS	PROT	FAT	CHOL	CARB	FIBER	SOD
Bong Water								
Chronic Tonic	12 oz	144	0	0	0	36	—	32
Cottonmouth Quencher	12 oz	165	0	0	0	42	—	29
Green Dreams	12 oz	165	0	0	0	42	—	30
Purple Haze	12 oz	165	0	0	0	42	—	30
Briar's								
Black Cherry	1 bottle (12 oz)	180	0	0	0	45	—	35
Cream	1 bottle (12 oz)	180	0	0	0	45	—	50
Diet Root Beer	8 oz	4	0	0	0	1	—	10
Orange Cream	8 oz	120	0	0	0	31	—	30
Red Birch	8 oz	104	0	0	0	26	—	7
Root Beer	1 bottle (12 oz)	168	0	0	0	42	—	15
Canada Dry								
Ginger Ale	1 can (12 oz)	140	0	0	0	35	0	50
Tonic Water	8 fl oz	90	0	0	0	24	0	15
Capt'n Eli's								
Root Beer	8 oz	165	0	0	0	49	—	35
Chronic 187								
Orange	1 bottle (12 oz)	300	0	0	0	77	—	53
Coca-Cola								
C2	8 oz	48	0	0	0	12	—	30
Classic	1 can (12 oz)	140	0	0	0	39	—	50
Diet	1 can (12 oz)	0	0	0	0	0	—	40
Dr Pepper								
Diet	1 oz	tr	—	0	0	—	—	—
Original	1 can (12 oz)	150	0	0	0	40	—	55
Fanta								
Orange	1 can (12 oz)	160	0	0	0	44	—	50
Firefighter								
Backdraft Root Beer	8 oz	90	0	0	0	22	—	10
Courageous Cola	8 oz	90	0	0	0	20	—	10
Flashover Orange	8 oz	20	0	0	0	24	—	10
Incendiary Citrus	8 oz	90	0	0	0	23	—	10

FOOD	PORTION	CALS	PROT	FAT	CHOL	CARB	FIBER	SOD
Rolling Code Black Cherry	8 oz	90	0	0	0	23	—	10
Hansen's								
Black Cherry	8 fl oz	110	0	0	0	30	—	0
Diet All Flavors	1 can	0	0	0	0	0	—	0
Ginger Beer	8 fl oz	100	0	0	0	28	—	0
Natural Black Cherry	1 can	160	0	0	0	44	—	0
Natural Cherry Vanilla	1 can	140	0	0	0	39	—	0
Natural Creamy Rootbeer	1 can	160	0	0	0	44	—	0
Natural Ginger Ale	1 can	140	0	0	0	37	—	0
Natural Grapefruit	1 can	130	0	0	0	38	—	0
Natural Key Lime	1 can	130	0	0	0	37	—	0
Natural Kiwi Strawberry	1 can	130	0	0	0	38	—	0
Natural Mandarin Lime	1 can	130	0	0	0	37	—	0
Natural Orange Mango	1 can	170	0	0	0	46	—	0
Natural Raspberry	1 can	130	0	0	0	36	—	0
Natural Tangerine	1 can	160	0	0	0	43	—	0
Natural Tropical Passion	1 can	160	0	0	0	43	—	0
Natural Vanilla Cola	1 can	140	0	0	0	39	—	0
Orange Creme	8 fl oz	110	0	0	0	31	—	0
Sangria	8 fl oz	110	0	0	0	30	—	0
Sarsaparilla	8 fl oz	110	0	0	0	30	—	0
Sparkling Orangeade	8 fl oz	100	0	0	0	25	—	10
Vanilla Creme	8 fl oz	110	0	0	0	30	—	0
Hiball								
Club	1 bottle	5	1	0	0	0	0	20
Tonic Water	1 bottle	120	1	0	0	31	—	15
IBC								
Cream	1 bottle (12 oz)	180	0	0	0	48	—	75
Root Beer	1 can	160	0	0	0	43	—	55

FOOD	PORTION	CALS	PROT	FAT	CHOL	CARB	FIBER	SOD
Jolt								
Blue	8 oz	120	0	0	0	32	–	50
Cherry Bomb	8 oz	90	0	0	0	25	–	25
Cola	8 oz	100	0	0	0	27	–	10
Red	8 oz	120	0	0	0	33	–	40
Ultra	8 oz	0	0	0	0	0	0	30
Jones Soda								
Sugar Free All Flavors	1 bottle (12 oz)	0	0	0	0	0	–	10
Kutztown								
Birch Beer	1 bottle (12 oz)	160	0	0	0	39	–	20
Red Cream	1 bottle (12 oz)	150	0	0	0	39	–	25
Sarsaparilla	1 bottle (12 oz)	150	0	0	0	38	–	25
Like								
Cola	1 oz	13	–	0	0	–	–	–
Lucozade								
Soda	7 oz	136	0	0	0	36	0	–
Minute Maid								
Valencia Orange	1 can (12 oz)	180	0	0	0	47	–	30
Mountain Dew								
Pitch Black	8 oz	110	0	0	0	31	–	35
Olde Brooklyn								
Flatbush Orange	8 oz	130	0	0	0	33	–	25
Williamsburg Root Beer	8 oz	120	0	0	0	32	–	25
Olde Philadelphia								
Black Cherry	1 bottle (12 oz)	180	0	0	0	45	–	40
Cream	1 bottle (12 oz)	190	0	0	0	47	–	40
Cream Diet	1 bottle (12 oz)	0	0	0	0	0	–	0
Grape	1 bottle (12 oz)	180	0	0	0	45	–	40
Orange Cream	1 bottle (12 oz)	190	0	0	0	49	–	40

FOOD	PORTION	CALS	PROT	FAT	CHOL	CARB	FIBER	SOD
Pineapple	1 bottle	190	0	0	0	48	–	40
Root Beer	1 bottle (12 oz)	180	0	0	0	44	–	35
Orangina								
Sparkling Citrus	8 oz	90	0	0	0	23	–	0
Pennsylvania Dutch								
Birch Beer	8 fl oz	110	0	0	0	28	–	30
Pepsi-Cola								
Blue Berry Cola Fusion	8 fl oz	100	0	0	0	28	–	25
Diet	1 can (12 oz)	0	0	0	0	0	–	35
Edge	1 can (12 oz)	70	0	0	0	20	–	40
Regular	1 can (12 oz)	150	0	0	0	41	–	35
Vanilla	1 can	160	0	0	0	43	–	40
Vanilla Diet	1 can	0	0	0	0	0	0	25
Prism								
Green Tea Soda Cola	8 oz	105	0	0	0	26	–	7
Lemon Lime	8 oz	117	0	0	0	29	–	2
Qibla								
Cola	1 bottle (18 oz)	185	tr	tr	–	11	–	–
Diet Cola	1 bottle (18 oz)	1	0	0	0	0	0	–
Rockstar								
Energy Drink	8 oz	110	0	0	0	29	–	35
Saranac								
Diet Root Beer	1 bottle (12 oz)	35	0	0	0	9	–	55
Ginger Beer	1 bottle (12 oz)	160	0	0	0	42	–	55
Root Beer	1 bottle (12 oz)	180	0	0	0	46	–	55
Schweppes								
Ginger Ale	8 oz	120	0	0	0	34	0	60
Seagram's								
Ginger Ale	1 can (12 oz)	130	0	0	0	35	–	45

FOOD	PORTION	CALS	PROT	FAT	CHOL	CARB	FIBER	SOD
Sex Cola								
All Flavors	1 bottle (12 oz)	0	0	0	0	0	0	0
Ski								
Citrus	1 bottle (10 oz)	150	0	0	0	40	—	40
Steap								
Green Tea Soda Root Beer	8 oz	90	0	0	0	23	—	35
Organic Green Tea Soda Raspberry	8 oz	90	0	0	0	23	—	35
Stewart's								
Cream	1 bottle (12 oz)	180	0	0	0	45	—	50
Diet Cream	1 bottle (12 oz)	0	0	0	0	0	0	25
Root Beer	1 bottle (12 oz)	160	0	0	0	41	—	51
Strawberries N' Cream	1 bottle	200	0	—	—	50	—	65
Wishniak Black Cherry	1 bottle	180	0	—	—	47	—	65
Sunkist								
Orange	1 can	190	0	0	0	52	0	45
Thomas Kemper								
Black Cherry	1 bottle	177	0	0	0	40	—	40
Old Fashion Birch	1 bottle	170	0	0	0	43	—	70
Orange Cream	1 bottle	180	0	0	0	37	—	64
Pure Draft Honey Cola	1 bottle	140	0	0	0	35	—	15
Pure Draft Root Beer	1 bottle	160	0	0	0	41	—	80
Vanilla Cream	1 bottle	170	0	0	0	43	—	70
Three Drinks								
Citrus	12 oz	12	0	0	0	3	—	20
Tommyknocker								
Almond Creme	1 bottle (12 oz)	150	0	0	0	40	—	19

FOOD	PORTION	CALS	PROT	FAT	CHOL	CARB	FIBER	SOD
Key Lime Creme	1 bottle (12 oz)	180	0	0	0	45	–	29
Orange Creme	1 bottle (12 oz)	180	0	0	0	45	–	29
Root Beer	1 bottle (12 oz)	150	0	0	0	40	–	19
Root Beer Float	1 bottle (12 oz)	110	0	0	0	29	–	20
Strawberry Creme	1 bottle (12 oz)	150	0	0	0	40	–	19
Vermont Sweetwater								
Country Apple Jack	1 bottle	180	0	0	0	42	0	8
Kickin' Cow Cola	1 bottle	129	0	0	0	33	0	8
Mango Moonshine	1 bottle	180	0	0	0	42	0	8
Maple	1 bottle	101	0	0	0	27	0	2
Raspberry Rhubarb Ramble	1 bottle	180	0	0	0	42	0	8
Tangerine Cream Twister	1 bottle	180	0	0	0	42	0	8
Vermont Maple Seltzer	1 bottle	53	0	0	0	12	0	0
Virgil's								
Micro Brewed Root Beer	1 bottle (12 oz)	160	0	0	0	42	–	0
White T								
All Flavors	1 bottle (12 oz)	128	0	0	0	33	0	15
Diet All Flavors	1 bottle (12 oz)	0	0	0	0	0	0	15
Yoo-Hoo								
Original	9 fl oz	150	3	tr	0	31	tr	200
Z Cola								
No Artifical Sweeteners	8 oz	0	0	0	0	1	0	35
SOLE								
cooked	3 oz	99	21	1	58	0	–	89
cooked	1 fillet (4.5 oz)	148	31	2	86	0		133

FOOD	PORTION	CALS	PROT	FAT	CHOL	CARB	FIBER	SOD
lemon raw	3.5 oz	85	17	1	–	0	–	80
raw	3.5 oz	90	18	1	50	0	–	100
TAKE-OUT								
battered & fried	3.2 oz	211	13	11	31	15	–	484
breaded & fried	3.2 oz	211	13	11	31	15	–	484

SORGHUM

FOOD	PORTION	CALS	PROT	FAT	CHOL	CARB	FIBER	SOD
sorghum	1 cup (6.7 oz)	651	22	6	0	143	–	12

SOUFFLE

FOOD	PORTION	CALS	PROT	FAT	CHOL	CARB	FIBER	SOD
lemon chilled	1 cup	176	9	tr	2	34	–	108
raspberry chilled	1 cup	173	10	tr	3	34	–	108
spinach	1 cup	218	11	18	184	3	–	763
Atkins								
Broccoli Cheddar & Bacon	1 serv	200	12	15	205	3	1	520

SOUP
CANNED

FOOD	PORTION	CALS	PROT	FAT	CHOL	CARB	FIBER	SOD
asparagus cream of as prep w/ milk	1 cup	161	6	8	22	16	–	1041
asparagus cream of as prep w/ water	1 cup	87	1	4	5	11	–	981
beef broth ready-to-serve	1 can (14 oz)	27	5	1	1	tr	–	1294
beef broth ready-to-serve	1 cup	16	3	1	tr	tr	–	782
beef noodle as prep w/water	1 cup	84	5	3	5	9	–	952
black bean turtle soup	1 cup	218	14	1	0	40	17	922
black bean as prep w/water	1 cup	116	6	2	0	20	–	1198
celery cream of as prep w/ milk	1 cup	165	6	10	32	15	–	1010
celery cream of as prep w/ water	1 cup	90	2	6	15	9	–	949
celery cream of not prep	1 can (10¾ oz)	219	4	14	34	21	–	2308

FOOD	PORTION	CALS	PROT	FAT	CHOL	CARB	FIBER	SOD
cheese as prep w/ milk	1 cup	230	9	15	48	16	—	1020
cheese as prep w/ water	1 cup	155	5	10	30	11	—	959
cheese not prep	1 can (11 oz)	377	13	25	72	26	—	2331
chicken broth as prep w/ water	1 cup	39	5	1	1	1	—	776
chicken cream of as prep w/ milk	1 cup	191	7	11	27	15	—	1046
chicken cream of as prep w/ water	1 cup	116	3	7	10	9	—	986
chicken gumbo as prep w/ water	1 cup	56	3	1	5	8	—	955
chicken noodle as prep w/ water	1 cup	75	4	2	7	9	—	1107
chicken rice as prep w/ water	1 cup	251	4	2	7	7	—	814
clam chowder manhattan as prep w/ water	1 cup	77	2	2	3	12	—	1029
clam chowder new england as prep w/ water	1 cup	95	5	3	5	12	—	914
clam chowder new england as prep w/ milk	1 cup	163	9	7	22	17	—	992
consomme w/ gelatin not prep	1 can (10½ oz)	71	13	0	0	4	—	1550
consomme w/ gelatin as prep w/ water	1 cup	29	5	0	0	2	—	637
escarole ready-to-serve	1 cup	27	2	2	2	2	—	3865
french onion as prep w/ water	1 cup	57	4	2	0	8	—	1053
gazpacho ready-to-serve	1 cup	57	9	2	0	1	—	1183
minestrone as prep w/water	1 cup	83	4	3	2	11	—	911

FOOD	PORTION	CALS	PROT	FAT	CHOL	CARB	FIBER	SOD
mushroom cream of as prep w/ milk	1 cup	203	6	14	20	15	–	1076
mushroom cream of as prep w/ water	1 cup	129	2	9	2	9	–	1031
oyster stew as prep w/ milk	1 cup	134	6	8	32	10	–	1040
oyster stew as prep w/ water	1 cup	59	2	4	14	4	–	980
pepperpot as prep w/ water	1 cup	103	6	5	10	9	–	970
potato cream of as prep w/ milk	1 cup	148	6	6	22	17	–	1060
potato cream of as prep w/ water	1 cup	73	2	2	5	11	–	1000
scotch broth as prep w/ water	1 cup	80	5	3	5	9	–	1012
split pea w/ ham as prep w/water	1 cup	189	10	4	8	28	–	1008
tomato as prep w/ milk	1 cup	160	6	6	17	22	–	932
tomato as prep w/ water	1 cup	86	2	2	0	17	–	872
vegetarian vegetable as prep w/ water	1 cup	72	2	2	0	12	–	823
vichyssoise	1 cup	148	6	6	22	17	–	1060
Amy's								
Organic Barley	1 cup	50	1	1	0	10	2	580
Organic Black Bean Vegetable	1 cup	110	6	1	0	22	5	580
Organic Cream Of Mushroom	1 cup	120	2	9	5	10	2	590
Organic Cream Of Tomato	1 cup	100	2	2	10	17	4	590
Organic Lentil	1 cup	130	8	4	0	19	9	590
Organic Minestrone	1 cup	90	3	2	0	17	3	540

FOOD	PORTION	CALS	PROT	FAT	CHOL	CARB	FIBER	SOD
Organic No Chicken Noodle Soup	1 cup	90	5	3	0	12	2	480
Organic Vegetable	1 cup	35	1	0	0	8	1	680
Boston Market								
Chicken Broth Reduced Sodium	1 cup	15	1	1	0	1	0	760
Butterball								
Chicken Broth Reduced Sodium 99% Fat Free	1 cup	10	1	0	0	2	0	620
Campbell's								
98% Fat Free Cream Of Chicken as prep	1 cup	70	3	2	10	10	tr	890
Cheddar Cheese	1 cup	110	3	5	10	12	1	950
Cheddar Cheese as prep	1 cup	134	4	8	19	11	1	1083
Chicken Vegetable as prep	1 cup	74	3	3	9	9	1	985
Chicken Broth	½ cup	20	1	1	<5	1	0	770
Chicken Gumbo as prep	1 cup	55	2	1	5	9	1	985
Chunky Beef Barley	1 cup	160	10	3	25	22	2	920
Chunky Chicken Corn Chowder	1 cup	230	8	13	20	21	3	800
Chunky New England Clam Chowder	1 cup	240	7	13	15	23	2	890
Chunky Old Fashioned Vegetable Beef	1 cup	130	9	3	15	18	6	910
Chunky Sirloin Burger w/ Country Vegetables	1 cup	180	10	8	20	17	3	890
Chunky Classic Chicken Noodle	1 cup	100	9	3	20	16	2	860
Chunky Vegetable	1 cup	130	3	4	0	22	4	870

FOOD	PORTION	CALS	PROT	FAT	CHOL	CARB	FIBER	SOD
Clam Chowder New England as prep	1 cup	89	4	3	3	13	1	979
Classic Chicken Rice	1 cup (8.4 oz)	80	2	2	5	14	1	850
Classics Beef Noodle	1 cup	70	5	3	15	8	1	920
Classics Minestrone	1 cup	90	4	1	<5	17	3	960
Classics Old Fashioned Vegetable	1 cup	90	3	2	<5	16	2	940
Classics Vegetarian Vegetable as prep	1 cup	90	3	1	0	18	2	790
Consomme as prep	1 cup	24	5	tr	tr	1	tr	817
Cream Of Asparagus as prep	1 cup	72	2	4	2	9	1	749
Cream Of Mushroom as prep	1 cup	108	2	7	2	9	2	872
Cream Of Celery as prep	1 cup	107	2	7	2	9	1	903
Cream Of Chicken as prep	1 cup	120	3	8	10	10	1	880
Cream of Chicken w/ Herbs	1 cup	90	3	4	10	10	1	890
Fiesta Tomato as prep	1 cup	72	1	tr	1	16	1	856
Garden Vegetable as prep	1 cup	69	3	2	3	11	1	857
Green Pea as prep	1 cup	173	9	3	1	29	4	888
Healthy Request Chicken Noodle as prep	1 cup	70	3	2	15	9	0	480
Healthy Request Chicken Rice as prep	1 cup	60	2	2	10	8	tr	420
Healthy Request Cream Of Mushroom as prep	1 cup	66	2	2	4	10	1	475
Healthy Request Cream Of Chicken & Broccoli as prep	1 cup	78	3	3	6	10	1	460

FOOD	PORTION	CALS	PROT	FAT	CHOL	CARB	FIBER	SOD
Healthy Request Cream Of Chicken as prep	1 cup	70	2	3	10	12	tr	430
Healthy Request Hearty Pasta w/ Vegetables	1 cup	87	3	1	1	17	2	474
Healthy Request Tomato as prep	1 cup	91	2	2	1	18	2	456
Healthy Request Vegetable as prep	1 cup	84	3	1	1	17	2	473
Home Cookin' Chicken Vegetable	1 cup (8.4 oz)	130	6	4	10	20	3	820
Italian Tomato as prep	1 cup	105	2	tr	1	23	4	820
Kitchen Classics Bean With Bacon	1 cup	180	9	4	5	28	8	820
Kitchen Classics Chicken Noodle	1 cup	980	6	1	10	13	1	870
Kitchen Classics Chicken w/ White & Wild Rice	1 cup	100	5	1	10	18	2	800
Kitchen Classics Lentil	1 cup	120	7	1	5	23	5	750
Low Sodium Chicken w/ Noodles	1 can (10.75 oz)	162	14	5	40	16	2	85
Low Sodium Chunky Vegetable Beef	1 can (10.75 oz)	159	13	4	39	17	3	64
Low Sodium Cream of Mushroom	1 can (10.75 oz)	200	3	13	12	18	2	48
Low Sodium Green Pea	1 can (10.75 oz)	235	12	4	4	38	6	27
Low Sodium Tomato w/ Pieces	1 can (10.75 oz)	170	4	5	6	28	3	36
Ready To Serve Bean w/ Bacon 'N Ham	1 can (10.5 oz)	274	14	7	13	41	11	1299

FOOD	PORTION	CALS	PROT	FAT	CHOL	CARB	FIBER	SOD
Ready To Serve Chicken Noodle	1 cup	80	3	2	15	11	1	890
Ready To Serve Chicken w/ Rice	1 can (10.5 oz)	122	5	2	11	20	2	1132
Ready-To-Serve Vegetable Beef	1 can (10.5 oz)	143	9	1	10	26	5	1243
Savory Tomato & Dill as prep	1 cup	99	2	2	tr	20	2	811
Select Chicken & Pasta With Roasted Garlic	1 cup (8.4 oz)	100	7	1	10	16	2	840
Select Chicken Rice	1 cup	100	6	1	5	17	2	990
Select Chicken With Egg Noodles	1 cup	110	9	2	15	14	1	990
Select Creamy Potato w/ Roasted Garlic	1 cup	180	3	10	10	20	2	770
Select Fiesta Vegetable	1 cup (8.4 oz)	120	4	1	0	24	3	810
Select Herbed Chicken w/ Roasted Vegetables	1 cup	90	7	1	15	14	1	890
Select Italian Style Wedding	1 cup	110	8	3	10	16	2	840
Select Mexican Chicken Tortilla	1 cup	150	8	3	10	22	4	890
Select Roasted Chicken w/ Long Grain & Wild Rice	1 cup	130	6	1	10	17	1	890
Select Roasted Chicken w/ Rotini & Penne Pasta	1 cup	90	6	1	10	16	2	840
Select Rosemary w/ Roasted Potatoes	1 cup	110	8	1	10	18	2	820
Select Split Pea w/ Ham	1 cup (8.4 oz)	170	10	2	10	30	6	860

FOOD	PORTION	CALS	PROT	FAT	CHOL	CARB	FIBER	SOD
Select Tuscany-Style Minestrone	1 cup (8.4 oz)	190	5	9	5	21	5	870
Soup At Hand Blended Vegetable Medley	1 pkg (10.75 oz)	110	3	2	10	21	4	950
Vegetable Beef as prep	1 cup	68	5	2	8	9	2	897
College Inn								
Beef Broth 99% Fat Free	1 cup	20	4	1	0	0	0	910
Beef Broth Fat Free Lower Sodium	1 cup	15	4	0	0	0	0	450
Chicken Broth Light & Fat Free	1 cup	5	1	0	0	0	0	450
Gold's								
Borscht Unsalted	1 cup	70	1	0	0	17	1	45
Healthy Choice								
Bean & Ham	1 cup (8.7 oz)	166	9	1	4	31	7	570
Beef & Potato	1 cup (8.5 oz)	116	11	1	5	16	tr	452
Broccoli Cheddar	1 cup (8.4 oz)	116	4	2	4	22	2	304
Chicken Corn Chowder	1 cup (8.8 oz)	176	8	3	8	30	2	466
Chicken Pasta	1 cup (8.6 oz)	119	7	3	6	18	1	493
Chicken Rice	1 cup (8.4 oz)	119	9	2	6	19	3	324
Chili Beef	1 cup (9.1 oz)	189	15	2	12	32	5	441
Clam Chowder	1 cup (8.8 oz)	123	6	1	12	23	2	481
Classic Italian Bean and Pasta	1 cup (8 oz)	100	6	2	0	17	3	480
Country Vegetable	1 cup	100	4	1	0	21	5	480
Cream Of Mushroom	1 cup (8.8 oz)	77	4	1	tr	14	1	450

FOOD	PORTION	CALS	PROT	FAT	CHOL	CARB	FIBER	SOD
Cream Of Celery as prep	1 cup	73	1	2	3	14	3	366
Cream Of Chicken Vegetable	1 cup (8.9 oz)	127	7	2	10	21	1	384
Cream Of Roasted Chicken as prep	1 cup	80	2	3	4	13	3	349
Cream Of Roasted Garlic as prep	1 cup	57	1	1	2	13	3	489
Garden Vegetable	1 cup (8.6 oz)	108	5	1	tr	22	6	454
Lentil	1 cup (8.7 oz)	135	10	1	tr	28	5	472
Minestrone	1 cup (8.6 oz)	107	5	1	1	24	5	370
Old Fashioned Chicken Noodle	1 cup	110	8	2	10	17	3	480
Roasted Italian Style Chicken	1 cup	120	9	2	15	18	4	480
Split Pea & Ham	1 cup (8.8 oz)	164	11	2	7	26	5	468
Tomato Garden	1 cup (8.6 oz)	101	4	1	1	19	5	468
Turkey Wild Rice	1 cup (8.4 oz)	72	10	1	3	9	3	407
Vegetable Beef	1 cup (8.8 oz)	96	11	1	2	14	2	433
Zesty Gumbo	1 cup	100	6	2	20	16	3	480
Imagine								
Creamy Broccoli	1 serv (8 oz)	70	3	2	0	10	2	370
Creamy Butternut Squash	1 serv (8 oz)	120	2	2	0	23	2	370
Creamy Mushroom	1 serv (8 oz)	80	4	3	0	10	2	310
Creamy Potato Leek	1 serv (8 oz)	90	2	3	0	14	2	380
Creamy Sweet Corn	1 serv (8 oz)	100	4	3	0	15	1	540
Creamy Tomato	1 serv (8 oz)	90	8	2	0	17	2	520
Vegetable Broth	1 serv (8 oz)	45	0	1	0	7	1	500
Zesty Gazpacho	1 serv (8 oz)	80	tr	0	0	8	tr	720

FOOD	PORTION	CALS	PROT	FAT	CHOL	CARB	FIBER	SOD
Manischewitz								
Clear Chicken Condensed	½ cup	15	tr	1	0	2	2	740
Natural Choice								
Organic Vegan Classic Tomato	1 cup	100	2	1	0	22	2	317
Organic Vegan Classic Mushroom	1 cup	50	2	2	0	9	2	435
Organic Vegan Country Corn	1 cup	100	3	1	0	24	3	377
Organic Vegan Kabocha Squash	1 cup	60	2	1	0	14	1	370
Organic Vegan Southern Greens	1 cup	80	2	3	0	13	2	399
Organic Vegan Split Pea	1 cup	120	7	1	0	21	7	420
Organic Vegan Vegetable Curry	1 cup	110	4	4	0	17	2	392
Pacific								
Free Range Organic Chicken Broth	1 cup	5	1	0	0	1	—	570
Progresso								
99% Fat Free Beef Barley	1 cup (8.5 oz)	140	11	2	20	20	3	470
99% Fat Free Beef Vegetable	1 cup (8.5 oz)	160	11	2	10	24	3	870
99% Fat Free Chicken Rice w/ Vegetables	1 cup (8.4 oz)	110	7	2	10	16	1	780
99% Fat Free Lentil	1 cup (8.5 oz)	130	8	2	0	20	6	440
99% Fat Free Minestrone	1 cup (8.5 oz)	130	7	2	0	23	4	710
99% Fat Free Split Pea	1 cup (0.9 oz)	170	10	2	0	29	5	620
99% Fat Free Tomato Garden Vegetable	1 cup (8.6 oz)	100	3	2	0	19	2	660
99% Fat Free Vegetable	1 cup (8.4 oz)	70	2	1	0	13	2	870

FOOD	PORTION	CALS	PROT	FAT	CHOL	CARB	FIBER	SOD
99% Fat Free White Cheddar Potato	1 cup (8.6 oz)	140	4	3	5	26	2	930
Bean & Ham	1 cup (8.4 oz)	160	10	2	10	25	8	870
Beef & Vegetable	1 cup	130	10	3	20	16	2	850
Beef Barley	1 cup (8.5 oz)	130	10	4	25	13	3	780
Beef Minestrone	1 cup (8.5 oz)	140	10	3	10	18	3	970
Beef Noodle	1 cup (8.5 oz)	140	13	4	30	15	1	950
Cheese & Herb Tortellini Tomato	1 cup (8.6 oz)	140	4	3	<5	23	2	700
Chickarina	1 cup (8.3 oz)	130	8	5	20	12	tr	1010
Chicken Minestrone	1 cup (8.4 oz)	110	9	2	15	15	2	890
Chicken Vegetable	1 cup (8.4 oz)	90	7	2	15	13	2	820
Chicken & Wild Rice	1 cup (8.4 oz)	100	7	2	15	15	1	850
Chicken Barley	1 cup (8.5 oz)	110	8	2	15	16	3	850
Chicken Broth	1 cup (8.2 oz)	20	1	2	0	1	0	920
Chicken Rice w/ Vegetable	1 cup	100	6	2	10	15	1	820
Clam & Rotini Chowder	1 cup (8.8 oz)	190	7	9	10	21	0	800
Escarole In Chicken Broth	1 cup (8.1 oz)	25	1	1	<5	3	1	930
Hearty Black Bean	1 cup (8.5 oz)	170	8	2	<5	30	10	730
Hearty Penne In Chicken Broth	1 cup (8.4 oz)	80	4	1	0	14	tr	1020
Hearty Tomato	1 cup (8.7 oz)	100	2	2	0	19	1	800
Herb Rotini Vegetable	1 cup (9.1 oz)	120	5	2	0	21	4	990

FOOD	PORTION	CALS	PROT	FAT	CHOL	CARB	FIBER	SOD
Homestyle Chicken w/ Vegetable	1 cup (8.4 oz)	90	7	2	15	11	tr	900
Italian Herb Shells Minestrone	1 cup (9.1 oz)	120	5	2	0	22	4	1050
Macaroni & Bean	1 cup (8.6 oz)	160	7	4	<5	23	6	800
Manhattan Clam Chowder	1 cup (8.4 oz)	110	12	2	10	11	3	710
Meatballs & Pasta Pearls	1 cup (8.3 oz)	140	7	7	15	13	0	700
Minestrone Parmesan	1 cup (8.3 oz)	100	3	3	0	16	3	700
New England Clam Chowder	1 cup (8.4 oz)	190	6	10	15	20	1	920
Oregano Penne Italian Style Vegetable	1 cup (8.7 oz)	90	3	2	0	15	1	960
Peppercorn Penne Vegetable	1 cup (9.1 oz)	100	3	1	0	20	2	920
Potato Broccoli & Cheese	1 cup (8.8 oz)	160	5	6	<5	21	1	960
Potato Ham & Cheese	1 cup (8.6 oz)	170	6	7	10	21	1	860
Rich & Hearty Beef Pot Roast	1 cup	130	10	2	20	17	2	990
Rich & Hearty Chicken & Homestyle Noodles	1 cup	110	8	3	30	14	1	990
Roasted Garlic Pasta Lentil	1 cup (9.3 oz)	120	7	2	0	20	5	960
Rotisserie Seasoned Chicken	1 cup (8.5 oz)	100	7	2	15	15	2	920
Spicy Chicken & Penne	1 cup (8.5 oz)	110	9	2	15	14	1	950
Split Pea w/ Ham	1 cup (8.4 oz)	150	9	4	15	20	5	830
Tomato	1 cup (8.5 oz)	100	2	2	0	19	1	790

FOOD	PORTION	CALS	PROT	FAT	CHOL	CARB	FIBER	SOD
Tomato Basil	1 cup (8.8 oz)	100	2	2	0	19	1	790
Tomato Vegetable	1 cup (8.5 oz)	90	3	2	0	15	4	990
Tortellini In Chicken Broth	1 cup (8.3 oz)	70	3	2	10	10	2	970
Traditional Chicken & Herb Dumplings	1 cup	110	7	3	30	15	1	750
Traditional Chicken Noodle	1 cup	100	9	2	25	13	1	980
Traditional Hearty Chicken & Rotini	1 cup	100	8	2	15	12	1	940
Turkey Noodle	1 cup	90	7	2	20	11	1	1060
Turkey Rice w/ Vegetables	1 cup (8.5 oz)	110	7	1	15	18	1	1040
Vegetable Classics Green Split Pea	1 cup	170	10	3	5	28	4	870
Vegetable Classics Lentil	1 cup	180	10	2	0	30	5	880
Vegetable Classics Tomato Rotini	1 cup	140	4	1	0	30	2	1000
Vegetable Classics Vegetable	1 cup	80	3	1	0	16	2	940
Vegetables Classics Minestrone	1 cup	110	4	2	0	19	5	980
Vegetable Classics French Onion	1 cup	50	tr	2	<5	9	1	900
Snow's								
Clam Chowder	1 cup	200	5	15	15	13	1	900
Streit's								
Hearty Vegetarian Vegetable	1 cup	90	3	0	0	19	3	520
Mushroom Barley	1 cup	100	3	2	0	17	3	890
Swanson								
Beef Broth 100% Fat Free Lower Sodium	1 cup	15	2	0	<5	1	—	440
Beef Broth 99% Fat Free	1 cup	10	2	1	—	0	0	890

FOOD	PORTION	CALS	PROT	FAT	CHOL	CARB	FIBER	SOD
Beef Broth Onion Seasoned	1 cup (8.4 oz)	20	2	0	0	2	tr	890
Chicken Broth 100% Fat Free 33% Less Sodium	1 cup	15	3	0	0	1	–	570
Chicken Broth 99% Fat Free	1 cup	15	1	1	<5	1	–	960
Vegetable Broth	1 cup	19	1	1	1	3	0	996
Walnut Acres								
Organic Country Corn Chowder	1 cup (8.8 oz)	150	4	3	10	28	2	690
FROZEN								
Brids Eye								
Hearty Spoonfuls Pasta & Chicken	1 bowl (11.2 oz)	140	11	2	20	19	2	1000
Nature's Entree								
Chowder	1 pkg (12 oz)	230	16	6	15	26	5	960
Tortellini Minestone	1 pkg (12 oz)	360	22	9	10	48	5	960
MIX								
asparagus cream of as prep w/ water	1 cup	59	2	2	tr	9	–	801
beef broth	1 pkg (0.2 oz)	14	1	1	1	1	–	1019
beef broth as prep w/ water	1 cup	19	1	1	1	2	–	1368
beef broth cube	1 cube (3.6 g)	6	1	tr	tr	1	–	864
beef broth cube as prep w/ water	1 cup	8	1	tr	tr	1	–	1152
celery cream of as prep w/ water	1 cup	63	3	2	1	10	–	839
chicken broth	1 pkg (0.2 oz)	16	1	1	1	1	–	1116
chicken broth as prep w/ water	1 cup	21	1	1	1	1	–	1484

FOOD	PORTION	CALS	PROT	FAT	CHOL	CARB	FIBER	SOD
chicken broth cube	1 cube (4.8 g)	9	1	tr	1	1	–	1152
chicken broth cube, as prep w/ water	1 cup	13	1	tr	1	2	–	792
chicken cream of as prep w/ water	1 cup	107	2	5	3	13	–	1184
chicken noodle as prep w/ water	1 cup	53	3	1	3	7	–	1284
french onion not prep	1 pkg (1.4 oz)	115	5	2	2	21	–	3493
leek as prep w/ water	1 cup	71	2	2	3	11	–	966
onion as prep w/ water	1 cup	28	1	1	0	5	–	848
tomato as prep w/ water	1 cup	102	2	2	1	19	–	943
Alpine Aire								
Low Carb Bay Shrimp Bisque	1 pkg	150	6	11	35	6	1	500
Low Carb Beefy Vegetable	1 pkg	100	9	4	30	7	1	1260
Low Carb Broccoli Cheddar	1 pkg	140	6	10	35	6	2	640
Low Carb Mushroom & Chicken w/ Roasted Garlic	1 pkg	130	7	8	35	7	1	650
Azumaya								
Thin Cut Noodle	1 cup	120	5	0	0	24	tr	820
Wide Cut Noodle	1 cup	120	5	0	0	24	tr	800
Bean Cuisine								
13 Bean Bouillabasse	1 cup	220	6	0	0	17	5	0
Island Black Bean	1 cup	210	6	0	0	17	7	0
Lots of Lentil	1 cup	230	6	0	0	17	5	5
Mesa Maize	1 cup	160	6	0	0	18	6	10
White Bean Provencal	1 cup	250	10	1	0	32	11	15

FOOD	PORTION	CALS	PROT	FAT	CHOL.	CARB	FIBER	SOD
Fantastic								
Noodle Bowls Mandarin Broccoli	1 pkg (2.2 oz)	220	10	0	0	40	4	1260
Hodgson Mill								
Choice Bean not prep	¼ cup (1.5 oz)	150	9	0	0	27	11	5
MiniCarb								
Miso w/ Tofu & Shitake	1 pkg	33	1	1	0	5	1	420
Szechuan Beef	1 pkg	24	1	1	0	4	0	1325
Thai Coconut Cream	1 pkg	100	3	6	3	9	1	770
Miso-Cup								
Golden Vegetable as prep	1 cup	30	2	1	0	3	tr	780
Miso Reduced Sodium as prep	1 cup	25	2	1	0	3	tr	270
Organic Miso as prep	1 cup	35	2	1	0	4	tr	480
Savory Seaweed as prep	1 cup	30	3	1	0	3	tr	690
Ramen Noodle								
Beef as prep	1 pkg (2.2 oz)	280	6	11	tr	40	3	1236
Beef Low Fat as prep	1 pkg (2.2 oz)	216	6	1	1	45	2	1361
Chicken as prep	1 pkg (2.2 oz)	279	6	11	1	40	6	1360
Chicken Low Fat as prep	1 pkg (2.2 oz)	216	7	1	tr	44	2	1335
Oriental Low Fat as prep	1 pkg (2.2 oz)	217	7	1	0	45	2	1359
Shrimp as prep	1 pkg (2.2 oz)	294	6	13	1	39	3	972
Shrimp Low Fat as prep	1 pkg (2.2 oz)	218	7	1	5	45	3	1111
Tomato as prep	1 pkg (2.2 oz)	295	6	13	tr	39	2	822

FOOD	PORTION	CALS	PROT	FAT	CHOL	CARB	FIBER	SOD
Rapunzel								
Cubes Vegetable Bouillon No Salt Added	½ cube	25	2	2	–	0	0	130
Cubes Vegetable Bouillon w/ Sea Salt	½ cube	15	tr	1	–	0	0	1000
Cubes Vegetable Bouillon w/ Sea Salt & Herbs	½ cube	15	tr	2	–	0	0	950
Slim-Fast								
Creamy Broccoli	1 pkg	210	10	5	20	30	5	890
Creamy Chicken	1 pkg	220	10	5	20	33	5	890
Creamy Potato Cheddar & Chive	1 pkg	220	10	5	15	35	5	890
Steero								
Beef Bouillon Cube	1 (3.5 g)	5	0	0	–	1	–	900
Beef Bouillon Cube Reduced Sodium	1 cube (3.5 oz)	5	0	0	–	1	–	600
Beef Bouillon Instant	1 tsp (3.5 oz)	5	0	0	–	1	–	900
Beef Bouillon Instant Reduced Sodium	1 tsp (3.5 oz)	5	0	0	–	1	–	600
Chicken Bouillon Cube	1 (3.5 g)	5	0	0	–	1	–	900
Chicken Bouillon Cube Reduced Sodium	1 (3.5 g)	5	0	0	–	1	–	600
Chicken Bouillon Instant	1 tsp (3.5 g)	5	0	0	–	1	–	900
Chicken Bouillon Instant Reduced Sodium	1 tsp (3.5 g)	5	0	0	–	1	–	600

FOOD	PORTION	CALS	PROT	FAT	CHOL	CARB	FIBER	SOD
Thai Kitchen								
Instant Rice Noodle Bangkok Curry	1 pkg	192	3	5	0	35	0	400
Rice Noodle Bowl Roasted Garlic	1 bowl	170	3	2	0	35	0	390
Rice Noodle Bowl Spring Onion	1 bowl	170	3	2	0	35	0	400
Wyler's								
Beef Bouillon Cube	1 (3.5 g)	5	0	0	–	1	–	900
Beef Bouillon Cube Reduced Sodium	1 (3.5 g)	5	0	0	–	1	–	600
Beef Bouillon Instant	1 tsp (3.5 g)	5	0	0	–	1	–	900
Beef Bouillon Instant Reduced Sodium	1 tsp (3.5 g)	5	0	0	–	1	–	600
Chicken Bouillon Cube	1 (3.5 g)	5	0	0	–	1	–	900
Chicken Bouillon Cube Reduced Sodium	1 (3.5 g)	5	0	0	–	1	–	600
Chicken Bouillon Instant	1 tsp (3.5)	5	0	0	–	1	–	900
Chicken Bouillon Instant Reduced Sodium	1 tsp (3.5 g)	5	0	0	–	1	–	600
SHELF-STABLE								
Annie Chun's								
Ginger Chicken	1 cup	30	4	0	0	3	0	730
Shiitake Mushroom	1 cup	25	2	0	0	3	0	90
Traditional Miso	1 cup	35	2	1	0	5	1	870
Campbell's								
Soup At Hand Blended Vegetable Medley	1 pkg (10.75 oz)	110	3	2	10	21	4	950

FOOD	PORTION	CALS	PROT	FAT	CHOL	CARB	FIBER	SOD
Lunch Bucket								
Chicken Noodle	1 pkg (7.25 oz)	80	2	2	10	13	0	830
TastyBite								
Tom Yum	½ pkg (5.3 oz)	92	2	7	0	6	1	740
TAKE-OUT								
albondigas meatball soup	1 bowl	318	–	17	71	–	–	1385
beef stew soup	1 cup (8.8 oz)	221	23	5	60	20	–	461
black bean turtle soup	1 cup	241	15	1	0	45	10	6
brunswick stew soup	1 cup (8.5 oz)	232	27	6	71	17	–	438
caldo de res beef soup	1 bowl	327	–	12	50	–	–	1861
chinese velvet corn	1¼ cup	135	–	0	1	–	–	708
corn & cheese chowder	¾ cup	215	9	12	66	21	3	386
egg drop	1 cup	73	–	4	103	–	–	729
gazpacho	1 cup	46	1	tr	0	5	–	63
greek lemon	¾ cup	63	4	2	83	7	2	386
hot & sour	1 serv (14 oz)	173	15	8	87	8	1	475
middle eastern chilled fruit	1 cup	99	–	0	0	–	–	12
middle eastern chilled yogurt & cucumber	1 bowl	85	–	3	6	–	–	66
minestrone	1 cup	154	–	0	5	–	–	790
miso w/ tofu	1 bowl	36	–	0	1	–	–	309
onion soup gratinee	1 serv	492	25	27	77	38	4	1325
oxtail	5 oz	64	4	3	–	7	–	–
pasta e fagioli	1 cup (8.8 oz)	194	9	5	3	30	–	790
ratatouille	1 cup (7.5 oz)	266	2	25	0	12	–	329
thai lemon grass	1 bowl	100	10	4	65	5	–	553

FOOD	PORTION	CALS	PROT	FAT	CHOL	CARB	FIBER	SOD
vietnamese pho beef noodle	1 serv (7.8 oz)	480	15	12	46	78	1	43
wonton soup	1 cup	205	16	3	89	26	1	322
zupa koprowa polish dill soup	1 bowl	54	11	2	55	6	–	524
zuppa toscana	1 bowl	543	–	123	45	–	–	1673

SOUR CREAM

sour cream	1 cup (8 oz)	493	7	48	102	10	–	123
sour cream	1 tbsp (0.4 oz)	26	tr	3	5	1	–	6
Breakstone's								
Sour Cream	2 tbsp (1 oz)	60	tr	5	20	1	0	10
Cabot								
Light	2 tbsp	35	1	3	10	2	0	25
No Fat	2 tbsp	20	1	0	0	3	0	40
Sour Cream	2 tbsp	50	1	5	15	1	0	35
Crowley								
Sour Cream	2 tbsp	60	tr	5	20	1	0	15
Land O Lakes								
Fat Free	2 tbsp (1.1 oz)	25	2	0	<5	4	0	40
Light	2 tbsp (1 oz)	40	1	3	10	3	0	35
Sour Cream	2 tbsp (1 oz)	60	tr	6	15	1	0	30

SOUR CREAM SUBSTITUTES

nondairy	1 cup	479	6	45	0	15	–	235
nondairy	1 oz	59	1	6	0	2	–	29

SOURSOP

fresh	1	416	6	2	0	105	–	87
fresh cut up	1 cup	150	2	1	0	38	–	31

SOY *(see also CHEESE SUBSTITUTES, ICE CREAM AND FROZEN DESSERTS, MILK SUBSTITUTES, MISO, SOY SAUCE, SOYBEANS, TEMPEH, TOFU, YOGURT)*

lecithin	1 tbsp	104	0	14	0	0	0	–
soy milk	1 cup	79	7	5	0	4	–	30
soya cheese	1.4 oz	128	7	11	–	tr	0	–
Bob's Red Mill								
Flour	½ cup	130	11	6	0	11	5	0
Dakota Gourmet								
Soy Nuts	1 oz	129	11	7	0	9	1	217

FOOD	PORTION	CALS	PROT	FAT	CHOL	CARB	FIBER	SOD
Fearn								
Granules	¼ cup	110	22	1	0	13	8	5
Powder	¼ cup	100	10	5	0	7	4	1
GeniSoy								
Soy Nuts Deep Sea Salted	1 oz	120	12	4	0	9	5	150
Soy Nuts Old Hickory Smoked	1 oz	120	12	4	0	9	5	490
Soy Nuts Praline	55 pieces (1 oz)	120	6	3	0	18	2	110
Soy Nuts Unsalted	1 oz	120	12	4	0	9	5	10
Soy Nuts Zesty Barbeque	1 oz	120	12	4	0	9	5	420
Health Trip								
Soynut Butter Honey Sweet	2 tbsp	170	8	13	0	9	1	70
Soynut Butter Original	2 tbsp	180	9	13	0	8	1	70
Soynut Butter Unsalted	2 tbsp	180	9	13	0	8	1	0
I.M. Healthy								
SoyNut Butter Chocolate	2 tbsp (1.1 oz)	190	5	14	0	12	4	50
SoyNut Butter Honey Creamy	2 tbsp (1.1 oz)	170	7	11	0	12	2	150
SoyNut Butter Original Creamy	2 tbsp (1.1 oz)	170	8	11	0	10	1	170
SoyNut Butter Unsweetened Chunky	2 tbsp (1.1 oz)	160	7	13	0	5	5	160
SoyNut Butter Unsweetened Creamy	2 tbsp (1.1 oz)	160	7	13	0	5	5	160
Loma Linda								
Soyagen All Purpose	¼ cup (1 oz)	130	6	6	0	12	3	150
Soyagen Carob	¼ cup (1 oz)	130	6	6	0	13	2	170

FOOD	PORTION	CALS	PROT	FAT	CHOL	CARB	FIBER	SOD
Soyagen No Sucrose	¼ cup (1 oz)	130	6	6	0	12	3	160
Natural Touch								
Roasted Soy Butter	2 tbsp (1.1 oz)	170	6	11	0	10	1	170
Revival								
Shake Chocolate Daydream Frustose	1 pkg	240	20	3	0	36	2	290
Shake Strawberry Smile Unsweetened	1 pkg	130	20	2	0	4	0	200
Shake Strawberry Smile Fructose	1 pkg	225	20	2	0	33	0	250
Shake Strawberry Smile Splenda	1 pkg	130	20	2	0	4	0	200
Soy Shake Plain	1 pkg	110	20	2	0	2	0	360
Soy Shake Vanilla Pleasure	1 pkg	220	20	2	0	31	0	290
Soy Shake Vanilla Pleasure Splenda	1 pkg	120	20	2	0	6	0	290
Soy Shake Vanilla Pleasure Unsweetened	1 pkg	120	20	2	0	6	0	290
Soynuts Chocolate Covered	⅛ cup	70	2	4	2	7	tr	8
Soynuts Hot Jalapeno & Cheddar	⅛ cup	78	5	4	0	5	2	68
Soynuts Unsalted	⅛ cup	78	5	4	0	5	2	2
Soynuts Yogurt Covered	⅛ cup	720	2	4	0	8	tr	12
Soy Juicy								
All Flavors	8 oz	160	7	3	0	25	1	30
Soy Wonder								
Creamy	2 tbsp	170	8	11	0	10	1	170
Crunchy	2 tbsp	170	8	11	0	10	1	170

FOOD	PORTION	CALS	PROT	FAT	CHOL	CARB	FIBER	SOD
SOY SAUCE								
shoyu	1 tbsp	9	1	tr	0	2	–	1029
soy sauce	1 tbsp	7	tr	tr	0	1	–	1024
tamari	1 tbsp	11	2	tr	0	1	–	1005
Chun King								
Lite	1 tbsp (0.5 oz)	15	2	tr	0	2	0	542
Soy Sauce	1 tbsp (0.6 oz)	11	2	tr	0	1	0	1227
Eden								
Organic Shoyu Reduced Sodium	1 tbsp	10	2	0	0	2	0	500
Organic Tamari	1 tbsp	15	2	0	0	2	0	860
Ponzu Sauce	1 tbsp	5	0	0	0	1	0	340
Shoyu	1 tbsp	15	2	0	0	2	0	1010
Just Rite								
Soy Sauce	1 tbsp (0.5 oz)	11	2	tr	0	1	0	1227
Kikkoman								
Lite	1 tbsp (0.5 oz)	10	1	0	0	1	–	575
Soy Sauce	1 tbsp (0.5 oz)	10	2	0	0	0	0	920
La Choy								
Lite	1 tbsp (0.5 oz)	15	2	tr	0	2	0	542
Soy Sauce	1 tbsp (0.6 oz)	11	2	tr	0	1	0	1227
Tree Of Life								
Shoyu	1 tbsp (0.5 oz)	15	2	0	0	1	–	960
Tamari Wheat Free	1 tbsp (0.5 oz)	15	2	0	0	1	–	940
SOYBEANS								
dried cooked	1 cup	298	29	15	0	17	–	1
dry roasted	½ cup	387	34	19	0	28	–	2
green cooked	½ cup	127	11	6	0	10	4	13
roasted	½ cup	405	30	22	0	29	–	140
roasted & toasted	1 cup	490	40	26	0	33	–	4

FOOD	PORTION	CALS	PROT	FAT	CHOL	CARB	FIBER	SOD
roasted & toasted	1 oz	129	11	7	0	9	–	1
roasted & toasted salted	1 oz	129	11	7	0	9	–	54
roasted & toasted salted	1 cup	490	40	26	0	33	–	176
sprouts raw	½ cup	43	5	2	0	3	–	5
sprouts steamed	½ cup	38	4	2	0	3	–	5
sprouts stir fried	1 cup	125	13	7	0	9	–	14
Arrowhead								
Organic not prep	¼ cup	180	15	8	0	14	10	0
Eden								
Organic Black	½ cup (4.6 oz)	120	11	6	0	8	7	30
Seapoint Farms								
Edamame Organic	½ cup (2.6 oz)	100	8	3	0	9	4	30
Edamame In Pods frzn	½ cup (2.6 oz)	100	8	3	0	9	4	30
Edamame Rice Bowl Kung Pao Vegetable	1 pkg (12 oz)	420	15	6	0	72	6	960
Edamame Rice Bowl Szechwan Vegetables	1 pkg (12 oz)	420	13	4	0	80	6	510
Edamame Rice Bowl Teriyaki Vegetable	1 pkg (12 oz)	430	14	5	0	83	5	1130
Edamame Rice Bowl Vegetable Fried Rice	1 pkg (11 oz)	220	11	6	40	31	1	950
Edamame Shelled	½ cup (2.6 oz)	100	8	3	0	9	4	30

SPAGHETTI (see PASTA, PASTA DINNERS, PASTA SALAD, SPAGHETTI SAUCE)

SPAGHETTI SAUCE
JARRED

FOOD	PORTION	CALS	PROT	FAT	CHOL	CARB	FIBER	SOD
marinara sauce	1 cup	171	4	8	0	25	–	1572
spaghetti sauce	1 cup	272	12	12	0	40	–	1236
Amy's								
Family Marinara	½ cup	50	1	1	0	8	3	590

FOOD	PORTION	CALS	PROT	FAT	CHOL	CARB	FIBER	SOD
Garlic Mushroom	½ cup	120	3	7	5	10	3	680
Puttanesca	½ cup	40	1	2	0	5	1	680
Tomato Basil	½ cup	80	2	3	0	11	3	580
Wild Mushroom	½ cup	60	2	3	0	7	2	580
Barilla								
Restaurant Creations Cheese & Tomatoes	¼ cup	110	1	8	3	5	1	400
Restaurant Creations Garlic Herbs & Tomatoes	¼ cup	100	1	8	3	6	2	460
Restaurant Creations Pesto & Tomatoes	¼ cup	150	2	12	3	7	2	400
Classico								
Italian Sausage	½ cup	90	5	2	5	13	2	470
Colavita								
Garden Style	½ cup (4.4 oz)	60	3	3	0	12	3	290
Del Monte								
Chunky Garlic & Herb	½ cup (4.4 oz)	60	2	2	0	11	1	490
Chunky Italian Herb	½ cup (4.4 oz)	60	2	1	0	12	1	520
Tomato & Basil	½ cup (4.4 oz)	70	2	1	0	16	3	600
Traditional	½ cup (4.4 oz)	60	2	1	0	15	3	590
With Garlic & Onion	½ cup (4.4 oz)	80	2	1	0	16	2	490
With Green Peppers & Mushrooms	½ cup (4.4 oz)	80	2	1	0	16	3	490
With Meat	½ cup (4.4 oz)	60	3	1	4	14	3	720
With Mushrooms	½ cup (4.4 oz)	60	2	1	0	14	2	630

FOOD	PORTION	CALS	PROT	FAT	CHOL	CARB	FIBER	SOD
Eden								
Organic Lightly Seasoned	½ cup (4.4 oz)	80	3	3	0	12	3	320
Francesco Rinaldi								
Alfredo	¼ cup (2.1 oz)	70	2	5	15	4	0	410
Chunky Garden Mushroom & Onion	½ cup (4.4 oz)	80	3	2	0	12	3	690
Chunky Garden Tomato Garlic & Onion	½ cup (4.4 oz)	80	3	2	0	12	3	690
Dolce Sweet & Tasty Tomato	½ cup (4.4 oz)	110	2	5	0	15	3	610
Dolce Three Cheese	½ cup (4.4 oz)	90	3	2	0	15	3	490
Dulce Super Mushroom	½ cup (4.4 oz)	110	3	5	0	15	3	490
Hearty Diavolo	½ cup (4.4 oz)	70	2	4	0	7	3	550
Hearty Mushroom Pepper & Onion	½ cup (4.4 oz)	80	3	3	0	10	3	690
Hearty Tomato & Basil	½ cup (4.4 oz)	80	2	3	0	11	4	730
Puttanesca	½ cup (4.3 oz)	70	2	4	0	8	tr	720
Tomato Alfredo	¼ cup (2.1 oz)	60	2	4	10	4	0	290
Traditional Meat Flavored	½ cup (4.4 oz)	90	2	4	4	11	3	700
Traditional Mushroom	1.2 cup (4.4 oz)	90	2	4	0	11	3	700
Traditional No Salt Added	½ cup (4.4 oz)	70	2	3	0	10	tr	25
Traditional Original	½ cup (4.4 oz)	90	2	4	0	11	3	700

FOOD	PORTION	CALS	PROT	FAT	CHOL	CARB	FIBER	SOD
Vodka Sauce	¼ cup (2.1 oz)	60	2	4	10	4	0	290
Healthy Choice								
Chunky Italian Vegetable	½ cup (4.4 oz)	40	2	tr	0	9	2	299
Chunky Mushroom	½ cup (4.4 oz)	42	2	tr	0	9	2	297
Garlic & Herbs	½ cup (4.4 oz)	49	2	tr	0	10	2	337
Garlic Lovers Garlic & Mushroom	½ cup (4.4 oz)	44	2	tr	0	10	2	362
Garlic Lovers Roasted Garlic	½ cup (4.4 oz)	52	2	tr	0	12	3	293
Garlic Lovers Roasted Garlic & Sun Dried Tomato	½ cup (4.4 oz)	52	2	tr	0	11	3	357
Super Chunky Mushroom & Sweet Peppers	½ cup (4.4 oz)	43	2	tr	0	9	2	308
Super Chunky Tomato Mushroom & Garlic	½ cup (4.4 oz)	45	2	tr	0	10	2	372
Super Chunky Vegetable Primavera	½ cup (4.4 oz)	43	2	tr	0	9	2	327
Traditional	½ cup (4.4 oz)	48	2	tr	0	11	2	378
With Mushrooms	½ cup (4.4 oz)	48	2	tr	0	11	2	378
Hunt's								
Basil Garlic & Oregano	½ cup	15	tr	0	0	3	tr	350
Cheese & Garlic	½ cup	50	3	1	0	9	2	600
Chunky Vegetable	½ cup	50	2	1	0	11	3	560
Diced In Tomato Sauce	½ cup	30	tr	0	0	7	1	430
Family Favorites Lasagna	¼ cup	30	1	0	0	6	1	330
Four Cheese	½ cup	50	3	1	0	10	3	600

FOOD	PORTION	CALS	PROT	FAT	CHOL	CARB	FIBER	SOD
Italian Sausage	½ cup	60	2	2	0	10	3	590
Light	½ cup	45	2	0	0	9	3	430
Meat	½ cup	68	3	1	0	11	3	610
No Added Sugar	½ cup	45	2	1	0	9	3	610
Roasted Garlic & Onion	½ cup	50	2	1	0	10	3	540
Traditional	½ cup	50	2	1	0	10	3	580
With Mushrooms	½ cup	50	2	1	0	10	3	600
Muir Glen								
Organic Balsamic Roasted Onion	½ cup (4.4 oz)	50	2	1	0	10	0	320
Organic Cabernet Marinara	½ cup (4.4 oz)	50	2	1	0	10	0	330
Organic Chunky Herb	½ cup (4.4 oz)	50	2	1	0	10	0	320
Organic Garden Vegetable	½ cup (4.4 oz)	50	2	1	0	10	0	120
Organic Garlic & Onion	½ cup (4.4 oz)	55	2	1	0	10	0	320
Organic Garlic Roasted Garlic	½ cup (4.4 oz)	50	2	1	0	10	0	320
Organic Green Olive	½ cup (4.4 oz)	60	2	2	0	10	0	350
Organic Italian Herb	½ cup (4.4 oz)	55	2	1	0	10	0	320
Organic Mushroom Marinara	½ cup (4.4 oz)	45	2	0	0	10	0	120
Organic Portabello Mushroom	½ cup (4.4 oz)	50	2	0	0	10	0	330
Organic Sun Dried Tomato	½ cup (4.4 oz)	55	2	1	0	10	1	170
Organic Tomato Basil	½ cup (4.4 oz)	50	2	1	0	12	0	370
Newman's Own								
Sockarooni	½ cup	60	2	2	0	9	3	590
Prego								
Pasta Bake Sauce Tomato Garlic & Basil	1 serv (3.4 oz)	80	1	4	0	11	2	530

FOOD	PORTION	CALS	PROT	FAT	CHOL	CARB	FIBER	SOD
Traditional	½ cup (4.2 oz)	140	2	5	0	23	2	610
Progresso								
Marinara	½ cup (4.3 oz)	80	2	5	<5	8	2	480
Meat Flavored	½ cup (4.4 oz)	100	4	5	5	12	3	610
Sauce	½ cup (4.4 oz)	100	3	5	<5	12	2	620
Ragu								
Chunky Garden Style Tomato Garlic & Onion	½ cup (4.5 oz)	110	2	3	0	18	2	520
Sara Lee								
Chunky Garden Mushroom & Peppers	½ cup (4.4 oz)	80	3	2	0	12	3	690
Tree Of Life								
Pasta Sauce	½ cup (4 oz)	50	2	2	0	9	–	290
Pasta Sauce Fat Free Classic	½ cup (3.9 oz)	40	2	0	0	8	0	250
Pasta Sauce Fat Free Mushroom & Basil	½ cup (3.9 oz)	30	1	0	0	7	0	300
Pasta Sauce Fat Free Onion & Garlic	½ cup (3.9 oz)	30	1	0	0	7	0	240
Pasta Sauce Fat Free Sweet Pepper	½ cup (3.9 oz)	30	1	0	0	7	0	280
Pasta Sauce No Salt Added	½ cup (3.9 oz)	50	2	2	0	9	–	0
Walden Farms								
Alfredo Sauce Calorie Free	¼ cup	0	0	0	0	0	0	20
Marinara Calorie Free	⅓ cup	0	1	0	0	0	0	350

FOOD	PORTION	CALS	PROT	FAT	CHOL	CARB	FIBER	SOD
MIX								
Durkee								
Spaghetti Sauce as prep	½ cup	15	0	0	0	5	0	390
With Mushrooms as prep	½ cup	15	1	0	0	4	0	520
French's								
Italian as prep	½ cup	16	0	0	0	5	0	390
Mushroom as prep	½ cup	20	1	1	2	4	0	760
Thick as prep	½ cup	10	0	0	0	4	0	630
McCormick								
Alfredo Pasta Blend as prep	½ cup	60	–	2	10	4	0	680
Pasta Rosa Blend	1 tbsp (10 g)	40	1	2	<5	4	0	540
Pesto Pasta Sauce as prep	2 tsp (4 g)	10	tr	0	–	tr	–	480
Primavera Pasta Blend	1 tbsp (7 g)	30	0	1	–	4	–	490
Spaghetti Sauce	1 tbsp (8 g)	25	0	0	–	5	–	490
REFRIGERATED								
Buitoni								
Alfredo Portabello Mushroom	¼ cup	100	2	8	20	5	0	340
Alfredo Light	¼ cup	80	4	5	20	5	0	370
Marinara	½ cup	80	2	3	0	11	2	580
Marinara Portabello Mushroom	½ cup	80	2	3	0	11	2	520
Marinara Roasted Garlic	½ cup	60	2	2	0	9	1	580
Pesto w/ Basil	¼ oz	300	7	26	20	9	2	560
Pesto w/ Basil Reduced Fat	¼ cup	230	7	18	15	9	2	560
Pesto w/ Sun Dried Tomatoes	¼ cup	210	4	18	5	8	2	400
Tomato Herb Parmesan	½ cup	120	0	8	10	9	2	790
TAKE-OUT								
bolognese	5 oz	195	11	15	–	4	tr	–

FOOD	PORTION	CALS	PROT	FAT	CHOL	CARB	FIBER	SOD

SPANISH FOOD
CANNED
Derby

FOOD	PORTION	CALS	PROT	FAT	CHOL	CARB	FIBER	SOD
Tamales	3 (6.5 oz)	253	7	17	23	21	4	1034
Gebhardt								
Enchiladas	2 (5.7 oz)	258	4	19	25	20	3	687
Tamales	2 (5.7 oz)	268	5	21	28	19	3	770
Tamales Jumbo	2 (6.9 oz)	332	6	25	34	24	3	930
Rosarita								
Enchilada Sauce Mild	¼ cup (2.1 oz)	23	1	1	0	3	0	409
Van Camp								
Tamales	2 (5 oz)	210	5	13	20	20	3	610
FROZEN								
Amy's								
Black Bean Vegetable Enchilada	1 (4.75 oz)	130	4	4	0	20	2	390
Bowls Santa Fe Enchilada	1 pkg (10 oz)	340	17	9	5	47	10	780
Burrito Bean & Cheese	1 (6 oz)	280	10	8	10	43	6	540
Burrito Bean & Rice Non-Dairy	1 (6 oz)	270	9	6	0	48	5	550
Burrito Black Bean Vegetable	1 (6 oz)	320	9	8	0	54	4	540
Burrito Breakfast	1 (6 oz)	210	9	6	0	38	5	540
Burrito Especial	1 (6 oz)	260	8	6	5	45	3	620
Cheese Enchilada	1 (4.75 oz)	210	10	12	35	13	2	440
Mexican Tamale Pie	1 (8 oz)	150	5	3	0	27	4	590
Banquet								
Chimichanga Meal	1 meal (9.5 oz)	500	13	24	20	56	9	1180
Enchilada Beef	1 pkg (11 oz)	370	10	12	20	54	6	1330
Enchilada Cheese	1 pkg (11 oz)	360	12	10	20	56	6	1500
Enchilada Chicken	1 pkg (11 oz)	350	12	10	25	54	9	1580

FOOD	PORTION	CALS	PROT	FAT	CHOL	CARB	FIBER	SOD
Enchilada Beef & Tamale Combo	1 pkg (11 oz)	450	10	20	30	50	9	1530
Mexican Style Enchilada Combo	1 meal (11 oz)	360	10	11	20	55	9	1390
Health Is Wealth								
Burrito Munchees	10 (5 oz)	310	11	7	5	53	6	610
Mexican Munchees	2 (1 oz)	49	2	1	0	8	1	110
Healthy Choice								
Chicken Enchilada Supreme	1 meal (11.3 oz)	300	13	7	40	46	4	560
Chicken Enchiladas Suiz	1 meal (10 oz)	280	14	6	40	43	5	440
Chicken Breast Con Queso Burrito	1 meal (10.55 oz)	350	14	6	35	60	6	590
Jose Ole								
Burrito Chicken	1 (5 oz)	260	10	4	10	48	3	600
Lean Cuisine								
Everyday Favorites Chicken Enchilada Suiza	1 pkg (9 oz)	280	11	5	25	48	3	520
Patio								
Beef & Cheese Enchiladas Chili 'N Beans	1 meal (15.5 oz)	670	19	30	60	80	12	2400
Beef Enchiladas Chili 'N Beans	1 meal (15.5 oz)	540	12	27	50	73	12	2690
Burrito Bean & Cheese	1 (5 oz)	300	9	9	15	45	4	690
Burrito Beef & Bean Hot	1 (5 oz)	320	10	12	25	43	4	840
Burrito Beef & Bean Mild	1 (5 oz)	330	10	12	20	45	4	890
Burrito Chicken	1 (5 oz)	290	11	6	20	44	2	740
Burritos Beef & Bean Medium	1 (5 oz)	310	10	10	20	45	4	660
Burritos Beef & Bean Red Chili Pepper Red Hot	1 (5 oz)	320	10	12	20	42	4	850

FOOD	PORTION	CALS	PROT	FAT	CHOL	CARB	FIBER	SOD
Enchilada Beef	1 meal (12 oz)	320	12	12	25	52	9	1700
Enchilada Cheese	1 meal (12 oz)	370	11	12	25	54	7	1570
Enchilada Chicken	1 meal (12 oz)	400	13	12	35	60	8	1470
Fiesta	1 meal (12 oz)	350	11	11	25	53	7	1760
Mexican Style	1 meal (13.25 oz)	470	15	19	20	59	10	2210
MIX								
Gebhardt								
Menudo Mix	¼ tsp (0.4 g)	1	tr	tr	0	tr	tr	52
McCormick								
Burrito Seasoning	1 tbsp (8 g)	25	tr	1	–	5	tr	500
Fajitas Marinade Mix	2 tsp (4 g)	15	0	0	–	2	–	250
Taco Seasoning Hot	2 tsp (6 g)	20	tr	0	–	3	tr	430
Taco Seasoning Mild	2 tsp (7 g)	20	tr	0	–	4	tr	460
READY-TO-EAT								
taco shell baked	1 med (0.5 oz)	61	1	3	0	8	tr	48
taco shell baked w/o salt	1 med (½ oz)	61	1	3	0	8	tr	2
Gebhardt								
Taco Shells	3 (1.1 oz)	155	2	8	0	19	3	1
La Mexicana								
Flour Burritos	1 (1.6 oz)	160	4	5	0	26	2	580
Rosarita								
Taco Shells	3 (1.1 oz)	155	2	8	0	19	3	1
Tostada Shells	2 (1 oz)	125	2	5	37	17	0	20
TAKE-OUT								
burrito w/ apple	1 lg (5.4 oz)	484	5	20	7	73	–	443
burrito w/ apple	1 sm (2.6 oz)	231	3	10	3	35	–	211
burrito w/ beans	2 (7.6 oz)	448	14	14	5	71	–	986

FOOD	PORTION	CALS	PROT	FAT	CHOL	CARB	FIBER	SOD
burrito w/ beans & cheese	2 (6.5 oz)	377	15	12	27	55	–	1166
burrito w/ beans & chili peppers	2 (7.2 oz)	413	16	15	33	58	–	1043
burrito w/ beans & meat	2 (8.1 oz)	508	22	18	48	66	–	1335
burrito w/ beans cheese & beef	2 (7.1 oz)	331	15	13	125	40	–	990
burrito w/ beans cheese & chili peppers	2 (11.8 oz)	663	33	23	158	85	–	2060
burrito w/ beef	2 (7.7 oz)	523	27	21	65	59	–	1492
burrito w/ beef & chili peppers	2 (7.1 oz)	426	22	17	54	49	–	1116
burrito w/ beef cheese & chili peppers	2 (10.7 oz)	634	41	25	170	64	–	2091
burrito w/ cherry	1 sm (2.6 oz)	231	3	10	3	35	–	211
burrito w/ cherry	1 lg (5.4 oz)	484	5	20	7	73	–	443
chimichanga w/ beef	1 (6.1 oz)	425	20	20	9	43	–	910
chimichanga w/ beef & cheese	1 (6.4 oz)	443	20	23	51	39	–	956
chimichanga w/ beef & red chili peppers	1 (6.7 oz)	424	18	19	9	46	–	1169
chimichanga w/ beef cheese & red chili peppers	1 (6.3 oz)	364	15	18	50	38	–	895
enchilada eggplant	1	142	–	5	7	–	–	–
enchilada w/ cheese	1 (5.7 oz)	320	10	19	44	29	–	784
enchilada w/ cheese & beef	1 (6.7 oz)	324	12	18	40	30	–	1320
enchirito w/ cheese beef & beans	1 (6.8 oz)	344	18	16	49	34	–	1251

FOOD	PORTION	CALS	PROT	FAT	CHOL	CARB	FIBER	SOD
frijoles w/ cheese	1 cup (5.9 oz)	226	11	8	36	29	–	882
nachos w/ cheese	6 to 8 (4 oz)	345	9	19	18	36	–	816
nachos w/ cheese & jalapeno peppers	6 to 8 (7.2 oz)	607	17	34	83	60	–	1736
nachos w/ cheese beans ground beef & peppers	6 to 8 (8.9 oz)	568	20	31	21	56	–	1800
nachos w/ cinnamon & sugar	6 to 8 (3.8 oz)	592	7	36	39	63	–	439
quesadilla	1	290	–	16	40	–	–	470
taco	1 sm (6 oz)	370	21	21	57	27	–	802
taco salad	1½ cups	279	13	15	44	24	–	763
taco salad w/ chili con carne	1½ cups	288	17	13	4	27	–	886
tostada w/ beans & cheese	1 (5.1 oz)	223	10	10	30	27	–	543
tostada w/ beans beef & cheese	1 (7.9 oz)	334	16	17	75	30	–	870
tostada w/ beef & cheese	1 (5.7 oz)	315	19	16	41	23	–	896
tostada w/ guacamole	2 (9.2 oz)	360	12	23	39	32	–	789

SPICES (see individual names, HERBS/SPICES)

SPINACH
CANNED
spinach	½ cup	25	3	1	0	4	–	29
Del Monte								
Chopped	½ cup (4 oz)	30	2	0	0	4	2	360
No Salt Added	½ cup (4 oz)	30	2	0	0	4	2	85
Whole Leaf	½ cup (4 oz)	30	2	0	0	4	2	360
S&W								
Spinach	½ cup (4.5 oz)	30	3	0	0	4	2	440
FRESH								
baby raw	2 cups	20	1	0	0	5	3	80
cooked	½ cup	21	3	tr	0	3	2	63

FOOD	PORTION	CALS	PROT	FAT	CHOL	CARB	FIBER	SOD
malabar cooked	1 cup (1.5 oz)	10	1	tr	0	1	1	24
mustard chopped cooked	½ cup	14	2	tr	0	3	–	–
mustard raw chopped	½ cup	17	2	tr	0	3	–	–
new zealand chopped cooked	½ cup	11	1	tr	0	2	–	97
new zealand raw	½ cup	4	tr	tr	0	1	–	36
raw chopped	1 pkg (10 oz)	46	6	1	0	7	–	160
raw chopped	½ cup	6	1	tr	0	1	1	22
Dole								
Baby Spinach	3½ cups (3 oz)	35	2	0	0	9	4	135
Fresh Express								
Baby Spinach	3 cups	20	2	0	0	3	2	65
Ready Pac								
Baby	2 cups	20	1	0	0	5	3	80
Microwave Spinach as prep	½ cup	20	2	0	0	3	tr	60
FROZEN								
cooked	½ cup	27	3	tr	0	5	–	82
Amy's Organic								
Snacks Spinach Feta	5–6 pieces	170	7	6	15	24	2	430
Birds Eye								
Chopped	⅓ cup	20	–	0	0	–	2	80
Creamed	½ cup	100	3	7	35	7	1	660
Cut Leaf	1 cup	20	2	0	0	2	2	110
Fresh Like								
Cut Leaf	3.5 oz	21	3	tr	–	4	1	81
Green Giant								
Creamed Low Fat Sauce	½ cup	80	3	3	0	9	1	510
Health Is Wealth								
Spinach Munchees	2 (1 oz)	60	2	3	0	9	1	105
Spinach Feta Munchees	2 (1 oz)	70	2	3	5	9	1	115
Tree Of Life								
Organic	1 cup (3 oz)	20	2	0	0	2	2	110

FOOD	PORTION	CALS	PROT	FAT	CHOL	CARB	FIBER	SOD
SHELF-STABLE								
TastyBite								
Kashmir Spinach	½ pkg (5 oz)	170	10	10	35	8	3	960
TAKE-OUT								
indian saag	1 serv	28	2	2	0	2	1	44
spanakopita spinach pie	1 cup (6 oz)	196	14	3	30	35	4	590
SPINACH JUICE								
juice	7 oz	14	2	0	—	2	—	146
SPORTS DRINKS *(see ENERGY DRINKS)*								
SPOT								
baked	3 oz	134	20	5	—	0	—	32
SPROUTS								
kidney bean	½ cup	27	4	tr	0	4	—	—
kidney bean cooked	1 lb	152	22	3	0	21	—	—
lentil sprouts	½ cup	40	3	tr	0	8	—	4
mung bean	½ cup	16	2	tr	0	3	—	3
mung bean canned	½ cup	8	1	tr	0	1	—	—
mung bean cooked	½ cup	13	1	tr	0	3	—	6
navy bean	½ cup	35	—	tr	0	—	—	—
navy bean cooked	3½ oz	78	—	1	0	—	—	—
pea	½ cup	77	5	tr	0	17	—	12
pinto bean	3½ oz	62	—	1	0	12	—	—
pinto bean cooked	3½ oz	22	—	tr	0	4	—	—
radish	½ cup	8	1	tr	0	1	—	1
Chun King								
Bean Sprouts	1 cup (3 oz)	11	1	tr	0	1	1	17
Fresh Alternatives								
BroccoSprouts	½ cup (1 oz)	10	1	0	0	1	1	0

FOOD	PORTION	CALS	PROT	FAT	CHOL	CARB	FIBER	SOD
Deli Blend	½ cup (1 oz)	10	1	0	0	1	tr	0
Salad Blend	½ cup (1 oz)	10	1	0	0	2	tr	0
Sandwich Blend	½ cup (1 oz)	5	1	0	0	1	tr	0
La Choy								
Bean Sprouts	1 cup (2.9 oz)	11	1	tr	0	1	1	17
TAKE-OUT								
mung bean stir fried	½ cup	31	3	tr	0	7	–	–
SQUAB								
boneless baked	3.5 oz	175	37	3	75	0	0	100
breast w/o skin raw	1 (3.5 oz)	135	22	5	91	0	–	–
w/o skin raw	1 squab (5.9 oz)	239	29	13	–	0	–	–
SQUASH (see also SQUASH SEEDS, ZUCCHINI)								
CANNED								
crookneck sliced	½ cup	14	1	tr	0	3	–	5
FRESH								
acorn cooked mashed	½ cup	41	1	tr	0	11	3	3
acorn cubed baked	½ cup	57	1	tr	0	15	2	4
butternut baked	½ cup	41	1	tr	0	11	2	4
crookneck raw sliced	½ cup	12	1	tr	0	3	1	1
crookneck sliced cooked	½ cup	18	1	tr	0	4	1	1
hubbard baked	½ cup	51	3	tr	0	11	3	8
hubbard cooked mashed	½ cup	35	2	tr	0	8	3	6
scallop raw sliced	½ cup	12	1	tr	0	3	1	1
scallop sliced cooked	½ cup	14	1	tr	0	3	1	1
spaghetti cooked	½ cup	23	1	tr	0	5	2	14

FOOD	PORTION	CALS	PROT	FAT	CHOL	CARB	FIBER	SOD
Martin Farms								
Butternut Fresh Cut	½ cup	40	1	0	0	10	1	3
FROZEN								
butternut cooked mashed	½ cup	47	1	tr	0	12	3	2
crookneck sliced cooked	½ cup	24	1	tr	0	5	–	6
Birds Eye								
Cooked Squash	½ cup	50	–	0	0	–	4	0
Sliced Yellow	⅔ cup	15	tr	0	0	2	1	15
SQUASH SEEDS								
roasted	1 oz	148	9	12	0	4	–	5
salted & roasted	1 oz	148	9	12	0	4	–	5
seeds dried	1 oz	154	7	13	0	5	–	5
seeds whole roasted	1 oz	127	5	6	0	15	–	5
SQUID								
fried	3 oz	149	15	6	221	7	–	260
raw	3 oz	78	13	1	198	3	–	37
TAKE-OUT								
calamari deep fried	1 serv	451	–	423	25	–	–	546
SQUIRREL								
roasted	3 oz	147	26	4	103	0	–	102
STARFRUIT								
fresh	1	42	1	tr	0	10	–	2
STRAWBERRIES								
CANNED								
in heavy syrup	½ cup	117	1	tr	0	30	–	5
FRESH								
strawberries	1 pint	97	2	1	0	22	–	4
strawberries	1 cup	45	1	1	0	10	4	2
FROZEN								
sweetened sliced	1 pkg (10 oz)	273	2	tr	0	74	–	9

FOOD	PORTION	CALS	PROT	FAT	CHOL	CARB	FIBER	SOD
sweetened sliced	1 cup	245	1	tr	0	66	–	8
unsweetened	1 cup	52	1	tr	0	14	–	3
whole sweetened	1 cup	200	1	tr	0	54	–	3
whole sweetened	1 pkg (10 oz)	223	1	tr	0	60	–	3
Birds Eye								
In Syrup	½ cup	120	1	0	0	31	1	0
Lite Syrup	1 pkg (10 oz)	120	1	0	0	31	1	0
Whole	½ cup	100	tr	0	0	25	1	0
Tree Of Life								
Organic	¾ cup (5 oz)	50	1	0	0	13	2	0

STRAWBERRY JUICE
Ceres

FOOD	PORTION	CALS	PROT	FAT	CHOL	CARB	FIBER	SOD
Strawberry	8 oz	115	0	0	0	28	1	35

STUFFING/DRESSING

FOOD	PORTION	CALS	PROT	FAT	CHOL	CARB	FIBER	SOD
bread as prep w/ water & fat	½ cup	251	5	15	tr	25	–	627
bread as prep w/ water egg & fat	½ cup	107	3	7	75	9	–	319
bread dry as prep	½ cup	178	3	9	–	22	3	543
cornbread as prep	½ cup	179	3	9	0	22	–	455
TAKE-OUT								
bread	½ cup (3½ oz)	195	4	8	0	26	3	534
sausage	½ cup	292	8	11	12	40	1	258

STURGEON

FOOD	PORTION	CALS	PROT	FAT	CHOL	CARB	FIBER	SOD
cooked	3 oz	115	18	4	–	0	–	–
raw	3 oz	90	14	3	–	0	–	–
roe raw	1 oz	59	7	3	–	tr	–	–
smoked	1 oz	48	9	1	–	0	–	–
smoked	3 oz	147	27	4	–	0	–	–

SUCKER

FOOD	PORTION	CALS	PROT	FAT	CHOL	CARB	FIBER	SOD
white baked	3 oz	101	18	3	45	0	–	44

FOOD	PORTION	CALS	PROT	FAT	CHOL	CARB	FIBER	SOD
SUGAR								
brown packed	1 cup (7.7 oz)	828	0	0	0	214	–	86
brown unpacked	1 cup (5.1 oz)	546	0	0	0	141	–	57
maple	1 piece (1 oz)	100	0	tr	0	26	–	3
powdered	1 tbsp (0.3 oz)	31	0	0	0	8	–	0
powdered unsifted	1 cup (4.2 oz)	467	tr	tr	0	119	–	2
sugarcane stem	3 oz	54	1	0	0	14	3	–
white	1 tbsp	45	0	0	0	12	–	tr
white	1 packet (6 g)	25	0	0	0	6	–	tr
white	1 cup (7 oz)	773	0	0	0	200	–	3
white	1 tsp (4 g)	15	0	0	0	4	–	0
Billington's								
Muscovado Light Brown	1 tsp	15	0	0	0	4	–	0
Domino								
Dark Brown	1 tsp	15	0	0	0	4	–	0
Light Brown	1 tsp	15	0	0	0	4	–	0
White	1 tsp	15	0	0	0	4	–	0
Maui Brand								
Raw Sugar	1 tsp	15	0	0	0	4	–	0
Princess Of Yum								
Citrus Lemon	2.5 tsp	40	0	0	0	10	–	0
French Vanilla	2.5 tsp	40	0	0	0	10	–	0
SUGAR SUBSTITUTES								
Equal								
Packet	1 pkg	0	0	0	0	tr	–	0
Fran Gare's								
Miracle Sweet	1 tsp	10	0	0	0	5	0	0
Keto								
Sweet	½ tsp	0	0	0	0	0	0	0

FOOD	PORTION	CALS	PROT	FAT	CHOL	CARB	FIBER	SOD
Lo Han								
Sweet	2 scoops	2	0	0	0	2	tr	0
SomerSweet								
Sweetener	¼ tsp	0	0	0	0	tr	tr	0
Splenda								
Sugar Blend For Baking	½ tsp	10	0	0	0	2	–	0
Sweetener	1 pkg	0	0	0	0	tr	0	0
Steel's								
Brown	1 tsp	10	0	0	0	1	0	0
Sugar Substitute	1 tsp	10	0	0	0	1	0	0
Stevita								
Spoonable	⅓ tsp	0	0	0	0	0	0	0
Sugar Twin								
Packets	1	0	0	0	0	tr	–	0
Spoonable Brown	1 tsp	0	0	0	0	0	0	0
Spoonable White	1 tsp	0	0	0	0	0	0	0
SUGAR-APPLE								
fresh	1	146	3	tr	0	37	–	15
fresh cut up	1 cup	236	5	1	0	59	–	24
SUNCHOKE								
fresh raw sliced	½ cup	57	2	tr	0	13	–	–
SUNFISH								
pumpkinseed baked	3 oz	97	21	1	73	0	–	87
SUNFLOWER								
seeds dried	1 cup	821	33	71	0	27	–	4
seeds dried	1 oz	162	33	14	0	5	–	1
seeds dry roasted	1 cup	745	25	64	0	31	–	4
seeds dry roasted	1 oz	165	5	14	0	7	–	1
seeds dry roasted salted	1 oz	165	5	14	0	7	–	195
seeds dry roasted salted	1 cup	745	25	64	0	31	–	975
seeds oil roasted	1 cup	830	29	78	0	20	–	4
seeds oil roasted salted	1 cup	830	29	78	0	20	–	804

FOOD	PORTION	CALS	PROT	FAT	CHOL	CARB	FIBER	SOD
seeds oil roasted salted	1 oz	175	6	16	0	4	–	201
seeds toasted	1 cup	826	23	76	0	28	–	4
seeds toasted	1 oz	176	5	16	0	6	–	1
seeds toasted salted	1 oz	176	5	16	0	6	–	204
seeds toasted salted	1 cup	826	23	76	0	28	–	817
sunflower butter	1 tbsp	93	3	8	0	4	–	82
sunflower butter w/o salt	1 tbsp	93	3	8	0	4	–	1
Dakota Gourmet								
Honey Roasted Kernels	1 pkg (1 oz)	158	6	12	0	8	1	56
Lightly Salted Kernels	1 pkg (1 oz)	168	6	14	0	5	2	85
Frito Lay								
Seeds	1 oz	180	7	15	0	5	2	25
Maranatha								
Tamari Seeds	¼ cup	160	6	14	0	7	2	140
SunGold								
SunButter	2 tbsp	200	7	16	0	7	4	120

SUSHI
TAKE-OUT

FOOD	PORTION	CALS	PROT	FAT	CHOL	CARB	FIBER	SOD
california roll	1 piece (0.8 oz)	28	1	1	1	4	–	37
fresh salmon rolls	4 pieces	250	11	7	20	37	3	590
sashimi	1 serv (6 oz)	198	24	7	63	4	–	718
tuna roll	1 piece (0.7 oz)	23	2	tr	3	3	–	33
vegetable roll	1 piece (1.2 oz)	27	1	1	0	5	–	47
vinegared ginger	⅓ cup (1.6 oz)	48	1	tr	0	12	–	6
wasabi	2 tsp (0.3 oz)	5	tr	tr	0	1	–	124
yellowtail roll	1 piece (0.6 oz)	25	1	1	0	3		32

FOOD	PORTION	CALS	PROT	FAT	CHOL	CARB	FIBER	SOD
SWAMP CABBAGE								
chopped cooked	½ cup	10	1	tr	0	2	–	60
raw chopped	1 cup	11	1	tr	0	2	–	63
SWEET POTATO (see also YAM)								
baked w/ skin	1 (3½ oz)	118	2	tr	0	28	3	12
canned in syrup	½ cup	106	1	tr	0	25	–	38
canned pieces	1 cup	183	3	tr	0	42	–	107
frzn cooked	½ cup	88	2	tr	0	21	–	7
leaves cooked	½ cup	11	1	tr	0	2	–	4
mashed	½ cup	172	3	tr	0	40	3	21
TAKE-OUT								
candied	3½ oz	144	1	3	0	29	–	73
SWEETBREADS								
beef braised	3 oz	230	23	15	–	0	–	51
lamb braised	3 oz	199	19	13	340	0	–	44
veal braised	3 oz	218	25	12	–	0	–	–
SWISS CHARD								
cooked	½ cup	18	2	tr	0	4	–	158
raw chopped	½ cup	3	tr	tr	0	1	–	38
SWORDFISH								
cooked	3 oz	132	22	4	43	0	–	98
raw	3 oz	103	17	3	33	0	–	76
SYRUP								
corn dark	1 cup (11.5 oz)	925	0	tr	0	251	–	608
corn dark	1 tbsp (0.7 oz)	56	0	0	0	15	–	31
corn light	1 tbsp (0.7 oz)	56	0	0	0	15	–	24
corn light	1 cup (11.5 oz)	925	0	tr	0	251	–	395
date syrup	1 tbsp	63	tr	tr	–	15	0	–
malt	1 cup (13 oz)	1222	24	tr	0	274	–	134
malt	1 tbsp (0.8 oz)	76	2	0	0	17	–	8

FOOD	PORTION	CALS	PROT	FAT	CHOL	CARB	FIBER	SOD
maple	1 tbsp (0.8 oz)	52	0	0	0	13	–	2
maple	1 cup (11.1 oz)	824	tr	1	0	212	–	27
raspberry	1 oz	76	tr	0	0	19	–	1
rose hip	1 oz	9	0	0	–	2	0	–
sorghum	1 tbsp (0.7 oz)	61	0	0	0	16	–	2
sorghum	1 cup (11.6 oz)	957	0	0	0	247	–	28
DaVinci Gourmet								
Sugar Free All Flavors	1 tbsp	0	0	0	0	0	0	5
Eden								
Organic Barley Malt	1 tbsp	60	1	0	0	14	0	0
Hershey's								
Strawberry	2 tbsp	100	0	0	0	26	–	10
Karo								
Corn Syrup Light	2 tbsp (1 oz)	120	0	0	0	31	–	35
Quik								
Strawberry	2 tbsp (1.5 oz)	110	0	0	0	27	0	0
Smucker's								
Apricot	¼ cup	210	0	0	0	52	–	0
Blackberry	¼ cup	210	0	0	0	52	–	0
Plate Scapers Kiwi Lime	2 tbsp (1.3 oz)	100	0	0	0	25	–	10
Plate Scapers Mango Orange	2 tbsp	100	0	0	0	24	–	0
Plate Scapers Raspberry	2 tbsp (1.3 oz)	100	0	0	0	25	–	5

TAHINI *(see SESAME)*

TAMARIND

FOOD	PORTION	CALS	PROT	FAT	CHOL	CARB	FIBER	SOD
fresh	1	5	tr	tr	0	1	–	1
fresh cut up	1 cup	287	3	1	0	75	–	33

FOOD	PORTION	CALS	PROT	FAT	CHOL	CARB	FIBER	SOD
TANGERINE								
CANNED								
in light syrup	½ cup	76	1	tr	0	20	–	8
juice pack	½ cup	46	1	tr	0	12	–	7
FRESH								
sections	1 cup	86	1	tr	0	22	–	3
tangerine	1	37	1	tr	0	9	–	1
Chiquita								
Tangerine	1 med (3.5 oz)	50	1	1	0	15	2	0
TANGERINE JUICE								
canned sweetened	1 cup	125	1	1	0	30	–	2
fresh	1 cup	106	1	tr	0	25	–	2
frzn sweetened as prep	1 cup	110	1	tr	0	27	–	2
frzn sweetened not prep	6 oz	344	3	1	0	83	–	7
Fresh Samantha								
Fresh Juice	1 cup (8 oz)	110	2	0	0	8	0	0
Naked Juice								
Tangerine Scream	8 oz	110	1	0	0	25	0	0
Odwalla								
Juice	8 fl oz	110	1	0	0	25	0	25
TAPIOCA								
pearl dry	½ cup (2.7 oz)	272	tr	tr	0	67	1	1
starch	1 oz	98	17	tr	–	24	–	1
TARO								
chips	1 oz	141	1	7	0	19	–	97
chips	10 (0.8 oz)	115	1	6	0	16	–	79
leaves cooked	½ cup	18	2	tr	0	3	–	2
raw sliced	½ cup	56	1	tr	0	14	–	6
shoots sliced cooked	½ cup	10	1	tr	0	2	–	1
sliced cooked	½ cup (2.3 oz)	94	tr	tr	0	23	–	10
tahitian sliced cooked	½ cup	30	3	tr	0	5	–	37

FOOD	PORTION	CALS	PROT	FAT	CHOL	CARB	FIBER	SOD
TARPON								
fresh	3 oz	87	17	2	–	0	0	70
TARRAGON								
ground	1 tsp	5	tr	tr	0	1	–	1
TEA/HERBAL TEA (see also ICED TEA)								
HERBAL								
chamomile brewed	1 cup	2	0	tr	0	tr	0	2
Celestial Seasonings								
Mandarin Orange Spice	1 tea bag	0	0	0	0	tr	–	0
Eden								
Organic Genmaicha Tea	1 cup	0	0	0	0	0	0	0
Organic Kukicha Tea	1 cup	0	0	0	0	0	0	0
Guayaki								
Yerba Mate Magical Mint	1 tea bag	5	–	0	0	1	–	–
Yerba Mate Organic Chai Spice	1 tea bag	5	–	0	0	1	–	–
Yerba Mate Organic Chocolatte	1 tea bag	5	–	0	0	1	–	–
Yerba Mate Organic Orange Blossom	1 tea bag	5	–	0	0	1	–	–
Yerba Mate Organic Rooiboost	1 tea bag	5	0	0	0	1	–	3
Yerba Mate Organic Traditional	1 tea bag	5	0	0	0	1	–	3
Lipton								
Bedtime Story	1 tea bag	0	0	0	0	1	–	0
Cinnamon Apple	1 tea bag	0	0	0	0	1	–	0
Ginger Twist	1 tea bag	0	0	0	0	0	0	0
Lemon	1 tea bag	0	0	0	0	1	–	0
Orange	1 tea bag	0	0	0	0	1	–	0
Peppermint	1 tea bag	0	0	0	0	1	–	0
Quietly Chamomile	1 tea bag	0	0	0	0	1	–	0

FOOD	PORTION	CALS	PROT	FAT	CHOL	CARB	FIBER	SOD
Silk								
Chai	1 cup	140	6	4	0	19	0	50
REGULAR								
brewed tea	6 oz	2	0	0	0	1	0	5
instant unsweetened as prep w/ water	8 oz	2	tr	0	0	tr	—	8
Activitea								
Green Tea	1 cup	36	0	0	0	3	—	3
Celestial Seasonings								
Green Tea Raspberry Garden as prep	1 cup	0	0	0	0	0	0	0
Green Tea Honey Lemon Ginseng	1 cup	0	0	0	0	0	0	0
Honey Darjeeling as prep	1 cup	0	0	0	0	0	0	0
DaVinci Gourmet								
Sugar Free Tea Concentrate Green	2 tbsp	0	0	0	0	0	0	5
Sugar Free Tea Concentrate Lemon	2 tbsp	0	0	0	0	0	0	5
Sugar Free Tea Concentrate Spiced Chai	1.5 tbsp	0	0	0	0	0	0	15
Guayaki								
Yerba Mate Organic Greener Green Tea	1 tea bag	5	0	0	0	1	—	3
Lipton								
Brisk Tea as prep	1 serv	0	0	0	0	0	0	0
Decaffeinated Brisk Tea as prep	1 serv	0	0	0	0	0	0	0
Green Tea	1 tea bag	0	0	0	0	0	—	0
Low Carb Creations								
Chai as prep	1 cup	25	0	2	0	3	0	50
Pacific Chai								
All Flavors as prep	1 serv	93	2	1	0	18	0	30

FOOD	PORTION	CALS	PROT	FAT	CHOL	CARB	FIBER	SOD
Paradise								
Tropical Tea	8 fl oz	1	0	0	0	tr	0	7
Tropical Tea Decafe	8 fl oz	1	0	0	0	tr	0	7
Tropical Tea Passion Fruit	8 fl oz	1	0	0	0	tr	0	7
Salada								
Green Tea	1 cup	0	0	0	0	0	0	0
Green Tea Decaffeinated	1 tea bag	0	0	0	0	0	–	0
Tetley								
British Blend Round Teabags	1 cup	0	0	0	0	0	0	0
Decaffeinated Tea Bag as prep	1	0	0	0	0	0	0	0
TAKE-OUT								
chai spiced latte decaf	1 cup	130	2	3	0	23	0	45
TEMPEH								
tempeh	½ cup	165	16	6	0	14	–	5
Lightlife								
Garden Vege	4 oz	200	21	8	0	12	6	399
Quinoa Sesame	4 oz	220	21	8	0	15	7	0
Smokey Strips	3 slices (2 oz)	80	8	3	0	6	1	230
Soy	4 oz	210	24	8	0	11	7	0
Three Grain	4 oz	200	20	7	0	13	6	0
Wild Rice	4 oz	190	19	7	0	13	6	0
Turtle Island								
Five Grain	3 oz	190	11	6	0	20	6	10
Low Fat Millet	3 oz	130	8	2	0	20	3	10
Soy	3 oz	160	13	4	0	20	7	15
Wild Rice Rhapsody	3 oz	160	13	4	0	20	7	15
White Wave								
Five Grain	⅓ block	140	12	4	0	15	4	0
Organic Original Soy	⅓ block	150	16	6	0	10	6	0

FOOD	PORTION	CALS	PROT	FAT	CHOL	CARB	FIBER	SOD
Organic Sea Veggie	⅓ block	120	12	3	0	11	8	25
Soy Rice	⅓ block	140	12	5	0	13	5	0
THYME								
ground	1 tsp	4	tr	tr	0	1	–	1
TILEFISH								
cooked	3 oz	125	21	4	–	0	–	50
cooked	½ fillet (5.3 oz)	220	37	7	–	0	–	88
raw	3 oz	81	15	2	–	0	–	45
TOFU								
firm	½ cup	183	20	11	0	5	2	17
firm	¼ block (3 oz)	118	13	7	0	3	1	11
fresh fried	1 piece (0.5 oz)	35	2	3	0	1	tr	2
fuyu salted & fermented	1 block (⅓ oz)	13	1	1	0	1	tr	316
koyadofu dried frozen	1 piece (½ oz)	82	8	5	0	2	tr	1
okara	½ cup	47	2	1	0	8	1	6
regular	½ cup	94	6	6	0	2	1	9
regular	¼ block (4 oz)	88	9	6	0	2	1	8
Azumaya								
Baked Chili Picante	2 pieces	200	20	10	0	9	2	320
Baked Mesquite	2 pieces	100	20	10	0	6	2	480
Baked Spicy Thai Peanut	2 pieces	190	20	10	0	6	2	500
Baked Teriyaki	2 pieces	200	20	10	0	9	2	730
Extra Firm	1 serv (2.8 oz)	70	8	4	0	2	1	0
Firm	1 serv (2.8 oz)	70	7	4	0	2	0	0
Lite Extra Firm	1 serv (2.8 oz)	60	8	2	0	3	1	30

FOOD	PORTION	CALS	PROT	FAT	CHOL	CARB	FIBER	SOD
Lite Silken	1 serv (3.2 oz)	40	5	1	0	3	0	45
Silken	1 serv (3.2 oz)	40	4	2	0	1	—	0
Galaxy								
Slices Hickory Smoked	1 slice (1 oz)	50	2	2	0	5	0	340
Slices Italian Garlic Herb	1 slice (1 oz)	50	2	2	0	5	0	390
Slices Original	1 slice (1 oz)	50	2	2	0	5	0	340
Slices Savory	1 slice (1 oz)	50	2	2	0	5	0	390
Hinoichi								
Firm	1 inch slice (3 oz)	60	6	3	0	2	1	10
Nasoya								
5 Spice	1 serv (3 oz)	70	7	4	0	0	0	220
Baked Mesquite Smoke	2 pieces	220	21	9	0	17	3	560
Baked Teriyaki	2 pieces	230	20	9	0	21	3	700
Baked TexMex	2 pieces	230	21	9	0	21	4	360
Baked Thai Peanut	2 pieces	240	21	10	0	19	3	540
Extra Firm	1 serv (3 oz)	90	8	5	0	3	0	0
Firm	1 serv (3 oz)	70	7	4	0	2	tr	0
Frim Enriched	1 serv (3 oz)	45	7	1	0	0	0	30
Garlic & Onion	1 serv (3 oz)	70	7	4	0	1	0	250
Silken	1 serv (3.2 oz)	45	4	3	0	2	0	5
Soft	1 serv (3 oz)	60	7	4	0	1	0	0
TofuMate Breakfast Scramble	¼ pkg	15	1	0	0	3	—	330
TofuMate Eggless Salad	¼ pkg	15	0	0	0	4	—	310
TofuMate Mandarin Stirfry	¼ pkg	30	1	0	0	6	—	310
TofuMate Mediterranean Herb	¼ pkg	15	1	0	0	3	—	330
TofuMate Szechwan StirFry	¼ pkg	25	1	0	0	4	—	280

FOOD	PORTION	CALS	PROT	FAT	CHOL	CARB	FIBER	SOD
TofuMate Texas Taco	¼ pkg	15	1	0	0	3	0	360
Pete's Tofu								
Dessert Peach Mango	1 serv (6 oz)	120	4	3	0	20	0	5
Dessert Very Berry	1 serv (6 oz)	120	6	3	0	17	0	25
Medium Firm	3 oz	70	6	4	0	2	0	0
Soft	3 oz	56	5	3	0	2	0	1
Super Firm Italian Herb	3 oz	120	13	7	0	1	tr	10
Super Firm	3 oz	130	12	8	0	2	0	5
Tofu 2 Go Lemon Pepper	2 pieces + sauce	160	13	9	0	9	2	400
Tofu 2 Go Santa Fe	2 pieces + sauce	150	14	9	0	6	2	340
Tofu 2 Go Sesame Ginger	2 pieces + sauce	160	13	10	0	7	2	390
Tofu 2 Go Thai Tango	2 pieces + sauce	165	12	10	0	9	2	380
Tree Of Life								
30% Reduced Fat Firm	⅓ block (3.2 oz)	90	10	4	0	4	2	5
Easymeal Pasta Primavera as prep	1 serv	460	20	16	10	54	3	790
Easymeal Southwest Medley as prep	1 serv	380	15	14	0	44	3	790
Easymeal Teriyaki Stir Fry as prep	1 serv	270	13	14	0	24	6	560
Easymeal Thai Stir Fry as prep	1 serv	270	14	14	0	21	6	230
Organic Baked	⅓ block (2.7 oz)	150	16	8	0	5	0	310
Organic Baked Island Spice	⅓ pkg (2.7 oz)	130	15	7	0	3	0	320

FOOD	PORTION	CALS	PROT	FAT	CHOL	CARB	FIBER	SOD
Organic Baked Oriental	⅓ pkg (2.7 oz)	130	15	7	0	5	0	330
Organic Baked Savory	⅓ block (2.7 oz)	140	15	7	0	4	0	310
Organic Firm	⅓ block (3.2 oz)	100	9	5	0	2	0	5
Raw Firm	⅓ block (3.2 oz)	100	9	5	0	2	0	5
White Wave								
Baked Garlic Herb Italian	1 piece	120	13	6	0	3	1	240
Baked Hickory Smoke BBQ	1 piece	75	8	3	0	4	1	140
Baked Roma Italian Basil	1 piece	100	8	6	0	3	2	220
Baked Teriyaki Oriental	1 piece	120	13	6	0	3	1	240
Baked Thai Style	1 piece	120	13	6	0	3	1	240
Baked Zesty Lemon Pepper	1 piece	120	8	8	0	3	1	100
Extra Firm	¼ block	80	10	5	0	1	1	10
Organic Extra Firm	⅓ block	90	10	6	0	1	1	10
Organic Soft	⅓ block	90	10	6	0	1	1	10
Reduced Fat	⅓ block	90	10	4	0	4	2	5
TOMATILLO								
fresh	1 (1.2 oz)	11	tr	tr	0	2	–	0
fresh chopped	½ cup	21	1	1	0	4	–	1
TOMATO								
CANNED								
paste	½ cup	110	5	1	0	25	6	86
puree	1 cup	102	4	tr	0	25	6	532
puree w/o salt	1 cup	102	4	tr	0	25	6	49
red whole	½ cup	24	1	tr	0	5	–	195
sauce	½ cup	37	2	tr	0	9	2	738
sauce spanish style	½ cup	40	2	tr	0	9	2	–
sauce w/ mushrooms	½ cup	42	2	tr	0	10	–	552
sauce w/ onion	½ cup	52	1	tr	0	12	–	672

FOOD	PORTION	CALS	PROT	FAT	CHOL	CARB	FIBER	SOD
stewed	½ cup	34	1	tr	0	8	—	325
w/ green chiles	½ cup	18	1	tr	0	4	—	481
wedges in tomato juice	½ cup	34	1	tr	0	8	—	285
Big R								
Cajun Stewed	½ cup (4.2 oz)	25	1	0	0	4	1	150
Diced w/ Chilies	½ cup (4.2 oz)	25	1	0	0	4	1	340
Mexican Stewed	½ cup (4.2 oz)	25	1	0	0	5	1	190
Stewed	½ cup (4.2 oz)	25	1	0	0	5	1	190
Whole	½ cup (4.2 oz)	25	1	0	0	5	1	190
Cento								
Puree	¼ cup	25	1	0	0	5	1	15
Claussen								
Halves	1 serv (1 oz)	5	0	0	0	1	tr	320
Contadina								
Italian Pasta	2 tbsp	35	1	1	0	7	1	290
Italian Paste Roasted Garlic	2 tbsp	35	1	1	0	6	1	300
Paste	2 tbsp (1.2 oz)	30	2	0	0	6	1	20
Puree	¼ cup (2.2 oz)	20	tr	0	0	4	tr	15
Recipe Ready Diced Roasted Garlic	½ cup (4.3 oz)	45	1	0	0	10	tr	560
Stewed	½ cup	35	1	0	0	9	1	220
Stewed w/ Celery & Green Peppers	½ cup	35	1	0	0	9	1	220
Del Monte								
Chunky Chili Style	½ cup (4.5 oz)	30	1	0	0	8	2	670
Chunky Pasta Style	½ cup (4.5 oz)	45	1	0	0	11	2	560
Crushed Italian Recipe	½ cup (4.4 oz)	45	2	0	0	9	1	390
Crushed Original Recipe	½ cup (4.4 oz)	45	2	0	0	9	1	390
Crushed w/ Garlic	½ cup (4.4 oz)	50	2	0	0	11	1	510
Diced	½ cup (4.4 oz)	25	1	0	0	6	2	160

FOOD	PORTION	CALS	PROT	FAT	CHOL	CARB	FIBER	SOD
Diced No Salt Added	½ cup (4.4 oz)	25	1	0	0	6	2	50
Diced w/ Basil Garlic & Oregano	½ cup	50	2	0	0	11	tr	650
Diced w/ Garlic & Onion	½ cup (4.4 oz)	40	2	1	0	8	1	610
Diced w/ Green Pepper & Onion	½ cup (4.4 oz)	40	1	0	0	9	2	480
Paste	2 tbsp (1.2 oz)	30	1	0	0	7	2	25
Petite Cut Garlic & Olive Oil	½ cup	45	1	1	0	10	1	620
Sauce	¼ cup (2.1 oz)	20	1	0	0	4	1	340
Sauce No Salt Added	¼ cup (2.1 oz)	20	0	0	0	4	1	20
Stewed Cajun Recipe	½ cup (4.4 oz)	35	1	0	0	9	2	460
Stewed Italian Recipe	½ cup (4.4 oz)	30	1	0	0	8	2	420
Stewed Mexican Recipe	½ cup (4.4 oz)	35	1	0	0	9	2	400
Stewed Original	½ cup (4.4 oz)	35	1	0	0	9	2	360
Stewed Original No Salt Added	½ cup (4.4 oz)	35	1	0	0	9	2	50
Wedges	½ cup (4.4 oz)	35	1	0	0	9	2	380
Zesty Diced w/ Mild Green Chilies	½ cup (4.4 oz)	30	1	0	0	6	1	550
Eden								
Organic Diced	½ cup	30	1	0	0	6	2	5
Organic Diced w/ Green Chilies	½ cup	30	2	0	0	5	2	35
Hunt's								
Crushed	½ cup	30	2	0	0	7	2	350
Diced Original	½ cup	20	1	0	0	5	tr	380

FOOD	PORTION	CALS	PROT	FAT	CHOL	CARB	FIBER	SOD
Diced w/ Balsamic Vinegar Basil & Oil	½ cup	60	1	3	0	8	1	460
Diced w/ Basil Garlic & Oregano	½ cup	24	1	0	0	6	1	360
Diced w/ Green Pepper Celery & Onions	½ cup	45	1	0	0	10	1	340
Diced w/ Mild Green Chilies	½ cup	30	2	0	0	6	2	360
Diced w/ Roasted Garlic	½ cup	30	1	0	0	6	1	480
Diced w/ Sweet Onion	½ cup	45	1	0	0	10	tr	460
Family Favorites Meatloaf	¼ cup	30	1	0	0	7	2	390
Paste	2 tbsp	25	1	0	0	6	2	90
Paste No Salt Added	2 tbsp	30	1	0	0	6	2	15
Paste w/ Basil Garlic & Oregano	2 tbsp	25	1	0	0	6	2	260
Petite Diced	½ cup	20	1	0	0	5	1	330
Petite Diced w/ Mushrooms	½ cup	40	1	1	0	6	tr	380
Puree	½ cup	30	1	0	0	7	2	450
Sauce	¼ cup	15	tr	0	0	3	tr	360
Sauce Garlic & Herb	½ cup	40	2	1	0	8	3	610
Sauce No Salt Added	¼ cup	60	2	0	0	14	4	30
Sauce Roasted Garlic	¼ cup	15	tr	0	0	3	tr	380
Stewed	½ cup	35	1	0	0	8	1	390
Stewed No Salt Added	½ cup	40	2	0	0	9	1	30
Whole	½ cup	20	1	0	0	4	1	190
Whole No Salt Added	2 oz	20	tr	0	0	4	1	15

FOOD	PORTION	CALS	PROT	FAT	CHOL	CARB	FIBER	SOD
Muir Glen								
Diced Fire Roasted	¼ cup	30	1	0	0	6	1	290
Diced w/ Green Chilies	½ cup (4.5 oz)	25	1	0	0	4	1	290
Organic Chunky Sauce	¼ cup (2.3 oz)	20	tr	0	0	4	1	160
Organic Crushed Fire Roasted	¼ cup	20	1	0	0	5	1	160
Organic Diced	½ cup (4.5 oz)	25	1	0	0	4	1	290
Organic Diced No Salt Added	½ cup (4.5 oz)	25	1	0	0	4	1	45
Organic Diced w/ Basil & Garlic	½ cup (4.5 oz)	25	1	0	0	4	1	290
Organic Diced w/ Italian Herbs	½ cup (4.4 oz)	25	1	0	0	4	1	290
Organic Ground Peeled	¼ cup (2.3 oz)	10	tr	0	0	2	1	100
Organic Paste	2 tbsp (1.2 oz)	30	2	0	0	6	1	20
Organic Puree	¼ cup (2.2 oz)	20	1	0	0	5	1	20
Organic Sauce	¼ cup (2.2 oz)	20	tr	0	0	5	1	310
Organic Sauce No Salt Added	¼ cup (2.2 oz)	20	tr	0	0	5	1	30
Organic Stewed	½ cup (4.5 oz)	30	1	0	0	7	tr	290
Organic Whole Peeled	½ cup (4.6 oz)	30	1	0	0	5	1	260
Whole Peeled w/ Basil	½ cup (4.6 oz)	30	1	0	0	5	1	260
Progresso								
Crushed w/ Added Puree	¼ cup (2.1 oz)	20	tr	0	0	3	0	95
Italian Style Peeled	½ cup (4.2 oz)	20	1	0	0	4	1	220

FOOD	PORTION	CALS	PROT	FAT	CHOL	CARB	FIBER	SOD
Paste	2 tbsp (1.2 oz)	30	2	0	0	6	1	20
Puree	¼ cup (2.2 oz)	25	1	0	0	5	1	15
Puree Thick Style	¼ cup (2.2 oz)	20	tr	0	0	5	1	15
Sauce	¼ cup (2.1 oz)	20	1	0	0	4	1	260
Whole Peeled	½ cup (4.2 oz)	25	1	0	0	5	1	220
Redpack								
Chunky Style In Puree	½ cup	30	1	0	0	6	1	270
Crushed In Puree	¼ cup	20	0	0	0	4	1	120
Paste	2 tbsp	0	2	0	0	6	1	20
Puree	¼ cup (2.2 oz)	25	1	0	0	5	1	10
Tuttorosso								
Puree	¼ cup	20	1	0	0	4	1	15
DRIED								
sun dried	1 piece	5	tr	tr	0	1	—	42
sun dried	1 cup	140	8	2	0	30	—	1131
sun dried in oil	1 cup (4 oz)	235	6	15	0	26	—	293
sun dried in oil	1 piece (3 g)	6	tr	tr	0	1	—	8
sun-dried	5 pieces (0.5 oz)	40	2	0	0	7	3	90
FRESH								
bruschetta	¼ cup	50	2	3	0	6	tr	360
cooked	½ cup	32	1	1	0	7	—	13
grape tomatoes	20	30	1	0	0	6	1	0
green	1	30	1	tr	0	6	—	16
red	1 (4.5 oz)	26	1	tr	0	6	2	11
red chopped	1 cup	35	2	tr	0	8	2	16
Chiquita								
Tomato	1 med (5.2 oz)	35	1	1	0	7	1	5
Eurofresh								
Tomatoes On The Vine	1 med (5.2 oz)	35	1	1	0	—	1	5

FOOD	PORTION	CALS	PROT	FAT	CHOL	CARB	FIBER	SOD
TAKE-OUT								
bruschetta on toasted italian bread	1 slice	106	4	3	0	18	tr	355
stewed	1 cup	80	2	3	0	13	—	460
TOMATO JUICE								
beef broth & tomato	5½ oz	61	1	tr	—	14	—	220
clam & tomato	1 can (5½ oz)	77	1	tr	—	18	—	664
tomato juice	½ cup	21	1	tr	0	5	—	441
tomato juice	6 oz	32	1	tr	0	8	—	658
Campbell's								
Juice	8 oz	51	2	1	—	10	2	683
Del Monte								
Juice	8 fl oz	50	2	0	0	10	1	760
Snap-E-Tom Chile Cocktail	6 fl oz	40	2	0	0	8	1	500
Dole								
Juice	1 bottle (12 oz)	85	4	0	0	17	2	1000
Hunt's								
Juice	1 can (6 oz)	22	1	tr	0	5	1	452
No Salt Added	8 fl oz	34	2	tr	0	8	2	12
Mott's								
Tomato Juice	8 fl oz	40	2	0	0	9	—	850
Muir Glen								
Organic	5.5 oz	40	1	0	0	8	4	420
TONGUE								
beef simmered	3 oz	241	19	18	91	tr	—	51
lamb braised	3 oz	234	18	17	161	0	—	57
pork braised	3 oz	230	20	16	124	0	0	93
TORTILLA								
corn	1 (6 in diam)	56	1	1	0	12	1	40
corn w/o salt	1–6 in diam (.9 oz)	56	1	1	0	12	1	3

FOOD	PORTION	CALS	PROT	FAT	CHOL	CARB	FIBER	SOD
flour w/o salt	1–8 in diam (1.2 oz)	114	3	3	0	20	1	167
CarbOle								
Low-Carb	1 (2 oz)	100	11	4	0	14	9	310
La Mexicana								
Corn	1 (0.8 oz)	50	1	1	0	10	1	0
Flour	1 (0.8 oz)	80	2	3	0	13	1	260
Tortillas de Trigo	1 (1 oz)	140	2	7	0	18	1	75
La Tortilla Factory								
Low Carb Whole Wheat	1 reg	60	5	2	–	12	9	–
Low Carb Whole Wheat	1 lg	100	8	3	–	21	15	–
Mariachi								
Tortilla	1	112	3	3	–	20	–	174
Old El Paso								
Flour	1 (1.4 oz)	130	3	4	0	21	0	290
Tumaro's								
Low In Carb Green Onion	1 (8 inch)	100	6	3	0	13	8	120
Low In Carb Multi-grain	1 (8 inch)	100	6	3	–	13	8	120
Low In Carb Sour Cream & Salsa	1 (8 inch)	100	6	3	0	13	8	125
Low In Carbs Garden Vegetable	1 (8 inch)	100	6	3	0	13	8	125

TORTILLA CHIPS (see CHIPS)

TREE FERN

chopped cooked	½ cup	28	tr	tr	0	8	–	3

TRITICALE

dry	1 cup (6.7 oz)	645	25	4	0	138	–	10
triticale not prep	1 oz	94	4	tr	–	18	2	1

TROUT

baked	3 oz	162	23	7	63	0	–	57
rainbow cooked	3 oz	129	22	4	62	0	–	29
sea trout baked	3 oz	113	18	4	90	0	–	63

FOOD	PORTION	CALS	PROT	FAT	CHOL	CARB	FIBER	SOD
TRUFFLES								
fresh	0.5 oz	4	2	tr	0	9	2	39
TUNA								
CANNED								
light in oil	3 oz	169	25	7	15	0	—	301
light in oil	1 can (6 oz)	399	50	14	30	0	—	606
light in water	3 oz	99	22	1	25	0	—	287
light in water	1 can (5.8 oz)	192	42	1	49	0	—	558
white in oil	3 oz	158	23	7	26	0	—	336
white in oil	1 can (6.2 oz)	331	47	14	55	0	—	704
white in water	3 oz	116	23	2	35	0	—	333
white in water	1 can (6 oz)	234	46	4	72	0	—	673
Bumble Bee								
Chunk Light In Water	¼ cup (2 oz)	60	13	1	30	0	0	250
Chunk Light In Water Pouch	2 oz	60	13	1	30	0	0	250
Chunk Light In Water Touch Of Lemon	2 oz	60	13	1	30	0	0	250
Solid White Albacore In Water	2 oz	70	15	1	25	0	0	250
Solid White Albacore In Oil	¼ cup	90	14	3	25	0	0	250
Solid White In Water	2 oz	70	15	1	25	0	0	250
Chicken Of The Sea								
Albacore In Spring Water	2 oz	60	13	1	25	0	0	250
Chunk Light In Water	¼ cup (2 oz)	60	13	1	30	0	0	125
Progresso								
In Olive Oil drained	¼ cup (2 oz)	160	13	12	30	0	0	250

FOOD	PORTION	CALS	PROT	FAT	CHOL	CARB	FIBER	SOD
StarKist								
Chunk Light In Water	¼ cup (2 oz)	60	13	1	30	0	0	250
Chunk Light No Drain Package	¼ cup (2 oz)	60	13	1	30	0	0	250
Low Sodium Chunk White In Water	2 oz	60	14	1	25	0	0	35
Solid White Albacore In Water	¼ cup	70	15	1	25	0	0	250
Tuna Fillet In Spring Water	¼ cup (2 oz)	60	13	1	30	0	0	250
FRESH								
bluefin cooked	3 oz	157	25	5	42	0	—	43
bluefin raw	3 oz	122	20	4	32	0	—	33
skipjack baked	3 oz	112	24	1	51	0	—	40
yellowfin baked	3 oz	118	25	1	49	0	—	40
TUNA DISHES								
MIX								
Tuna Helper								
AuGratin 50% Less Fat Recipe as prep	1 cup	240	13	6	15	37	1	840
AuGratin as prep	1 cup	300	13	11	20	37	1	890
Cheesy Broccoli 50% Less Fat Recipe as prep	1 cup	240	15	5	15	38	1	820
Cheesy Broccoli as prep	1 cup	290	15	9	20	38	1	860
Cheesy Pasta 50% Less Fat Recipe as prep	1 cup	230	14	5	15	32	tr	850
Cheesy Pasta as prep	1 cup	280	14	11	20	32	tr	890
Creamy Broccoli 50% Less Fat Recipe as prep	1 cup	240	14	5	15	35	1	820

FOOD	PORTION	CALS	PROT	FAT	CHOL	CARB	FIBER	SOD
Creamy Pasta 50% Less Fat Recipe as prep	1 cup	230	14	6	15	31	1	840
Creamy Pasta as prep	1 cup	300	14	13	20	31	1	910
Fettuccine Alfredo 50% Less Fat Recipe as prep	1 cup	240	14	6	15	32	1	870
Fettuccine Alfredo as prep	1 cup	310	14	14	15	32	1	950
Garden Cheddar 50% Less Fat Recipe as prep	1 cup	240	13	5	15	36	1	980
Garden Cheddar as prep	1 cup	290	13	11	20	36	1	1030
Pasta Salad as prep	⅔ cup	380	10	27	10	26	1	730
Pasta Salad Low Fat Recipe as prep	⅔ cup	230	10	2	10	26	1	790
Tetrazzini 50% Less Fat Recipe as prep	1 cup	230	14	5	20	34	1	980
Tetrazzini as prep	1 cup	300	14	12	20	34	1	1040
Tuna Melt as prep	1 cup	300	12	12	20	34	1	900
Tuna Melt Reduced Fat Recipe as prep	1 cup	240	12	6	15	34	1	850
Tuna Pot Pie as prep	1 cup	440	18	24	110	40	1	1080
Tuna Romanoff 50% Less Fat Recipe as prep	1 cup	240	15	3	20	38	1	740
Tuna Romanoff as prep	1 cup	280	15	8	20	38	1	800
READY-TO-EAT								
Bumble Bee								
Tuna Salad Fat Free	1 pkg (3.5 oz)	190	9	2	15	25	0	510

FOOD	PORTION	CALS	PROT	FAT	CHOL	CARB	FIBER	SOD
Tuna Salad Kit	1 pkg (3.8 oz)	250	17	13	45	15	0	550
StarKist								
Lunch To-Go	1 pkg	310	22	13	40	26	tr	690
Ready-Mixed Tuna Salad Kit	1 pkg (3.5 oz)	190	9	6	5	25	2	420
Tuna Salad Lunch Kit	1 pkg (4.3 oz)	230	20	9	35	17	1	730
Wampler								
Salad	⅓ cup	180	6	12	20	9	–	450
Salad Chunky	⅓ cup	180	8	13	20	8	–	380
TAKE-OUT								
tuna salad	3 oz	159	14	8	11	8	–	342
tuna salad	1 cup	383	33	19	27	19	–	824
TURBOT								
european baked	3 oz	104	17	3	–	0	–	163
TURKEY *(see also TURKEY DISHES, TURKEY SUBSTITUTES)*								
CANNED								
w/ broth	1 can (5 oz)	231	34	10	–	0	–	663
w/ broth	½ can (2.5 oz)	116	17	5	–	0	–	332
FRESH								
back w/ skin roasted	½ back (9 oz)	637	70	38	238	0	–	191
breast w/ skin roasted	4 oz	212	32	8	83	0	–	70
dark meat w/ skin roasted	3.6 oz	230	29	12	93	0	–	79
dark meat w/o skin roasted	3 oz	170	26	7	78	0	–	72
dark meat w/o skin roasted	1 cup (5 oz)	262	40	10	119	0	–	110
ground cooked	3 oz	188	20	11	57	0	–	68
leg w/ skin roasted	2.5 oz	147	20	7	61	0	–	55
leg w/ skin roasted	1 (1.2 lbs)	1133	152	54	466	0	–	420
light meat w/ skin roasted	from ½ turkey (2.3 lbs)	2069	87	87	794	0	–	658

FOOD	PORTION	CALS	PROT	FAT	CHOL	CARB	FIBER	SOD
light meat w/ skin roasted	4.7 oz	268	39	11	103	0	—	85
light meat w/o skin roasted	4 oz	183	35	4	81	0	—	75
neck simmered	1 (5.3 oz)	274	41	11	186	0	—	84
skin roasted	from ½ turkey (9 oz)	1096	49	98	281	0	—	132
skin roasted	1 oz	141	13	13	36	0	—	17
w/ skin roasted	½ turkey (4 lbs)	3857	522	181	1914	0	—	1269
w/ skin roasted	8.4 oz	498	67	23	196	0	—	164
w/ skin neck & giblets roasted	½ turkey (8.8 lbs)	4123	190	190	1920	1	—	1358
w/o skin roasted	1 cup (5 oz)	238	41	7	107	0	—	99
w/o skin roasted	7.3 oz	354	61	10	159	0	—	147
wing w/ skin roasted	1 (6.5 oz)	426	51	23	150	0	—	114
Jennie-O								
Ground	4 oz	160	23	8	80	0	0	80
Perdue								
Breast Tenderloins Butter Garlic	3 oz	100	20	1	45	2	—	830
Burger Cooked	1 (4 oz)	160	20	9	85	0	—	85
Dark Cooked	3 oz	180	20	11	85	0	—	65
Drumsticks Cooked	1 (2.2 oz)	110	14	6	80	0	—	65
Ground Cooked	3 oz	160	20	9	85	0	—	85
Tenderloins Black Pepper Cooked	3 oz	90	20	1	45	1	—	690
Thighs Cooked	1 (3.2 oz)	240	17	19	115	0	—	65
White Cooked	3 oz	150	22	7	65	0	—	45
Shady Brook								
Cutlets	4 oz	110	25	1	60	0	0	240
Ground	4 oz	160	22	8	80	0	0	85
Ground Breast	4 oz	120	28	1	70	0	—	55

FOOD	PORTION	CALS	PROT	FAT	CHOL	CARB	FIBER	SOD
Turkey Store								
Lean Ground Italian Style	4 oz	190	20	10	80	4	—	530
Wampler								
Boneless Breast Roast	4 oz	160	25	6	35	0	—	25
Breast Half	4 oz	160	25	6	35	0	—	25
Breast Steaks	4 oz	120	28	1	70	0	—	55
Drumsticks	4 oz	180	22	10	75	0	—	45
Ground	4 oz	210	18	15	100	0	—	70
Ground Breast	4 oz	130	28	1	70	0	—	55
Ground Lean	4 oz	160	20	8	90	0	—	70
Thighs	4 oz	170	22	10	80	0	—	40
Wings	4 oz	220	23	14	80	0	—	60
Woodfire Grill Burger	1 (3 oz)	180	21	9	65	2	—	360
FROZEN								
roast boneless seasoned light & dark meat roasted	1 pkg (1.7 lbs)	1213	167	45	413	24	—	5320
Wampler								
Burger BBQ	1 (4 oz)	240	19	17	140	3	—	240
Burgers Cracked Peppercorn & Garlic	1 (3 oz)	170	21	9	65	0	—	380
Seasoned Burgers Cracker Peppercorn & Garlic	1 (3 oz)	170	21	9	65	0	—	380
READY-TO-EAT								
bologna	1 oz	57	4	4	28	tr	—	249
breast	1 slice (0.75 oz)	23	5	tr	9	0	—	301
diced light & dark seasoned	½ lb	313	42	14	—	2	—	1928
diced light & dark seasoned	1 oz	39	5	2	—	tr	—	241
ham thigh meat	1 pkg (8 oz)	291	43	12	—	1	—	2260
ham thigh meat	2 oz	73	11	3	—	tr	—	565

FOOD	PORTION	CALS	PROT	FAT	CHOL	CARB	FIBER	SOD
pastrami	2 oz	80	10	4	–	1	–	698
pastrami	1 pkg (8 oz)	320	42	14	–	4	–	2372
patties battered & fried	1 (2.3 oz)	181	9	12	–	10	–	512
patties breaded & fried	1 (3.3 oz)	266	13	17	–	15	–	752
poultry salad sandwich spread	1 oz	238	4	4	9	2	–	107
poultry salad sandwich spread	1 tbsp	109	2	2	4	1	–	49
prebasted breast w/ skin roasted	1 breast (3.8 lbs)	2175	383	60	718	0	–	6868
prebasted breast w/ skin roasted	½ breast (1.9 lbs)	1087	191	30	359	0	–	3434
prebasted thigh w/ skin roasted	1 thigh (11 oz)	494	59	27	194	0	–	1371
roll light & dark meat	1 oz	42	5	2	16	1	–	166
roll light meat	1 oz	42	5	2	12	2	–	139
salami cooked	2 oz	111	9	8	46	tr	–	569
salami cooked	1 pkg (8 oz)	446	37	31	186	1	–	2278
turkey loaf breast meat	1 pkg (6 oz)	187	38	3	69	0	–	2433
turkey loaf breast meat	2 slices (1.5 oz)	47	10	1	17	0	–	608
turkey sticks battered & fried	1 stick (2.3 oz)	178	9	11	–	11	–	536
turkey sticks breaded & fried	1 stick (2.3 oz)	178	9	11	–	11	–	536
Alpine Lace								
Breast Fat Free	2 oz	45	10	0	25	0	0	350
Boar's Head								
Breast Cracked Pepper Smoked	2 oz	60	13	1	30	1	0	460
Breast Golden Skin On	2 oz	60	11	2	25	0	0	340
Breast Golden Skinless	2 oz	60	12	1	25	tr	0	350

FOOD	PORTION	CALS	PROT	FAT	CHOL	CARB	FIBER	SOD
Breast Hickory Smoked	2 oz	70	12	2	25	tr	0	340
Breast Low Sodium Skinless	2 oz	60	12	1	25	tr	0	340
Breast Lower Sodium Skin On	2 oz	60	11	2	25	tr	0	310
Breast Maple Glazed Honey Coat	2 oz	70	14	1	30	2	0	440
Breast Ovengold Skin On	2 oz	60	12	2	35	1	0	360
Breast Ovengold Skinless	2 oz	60	13	1	20	0	0	350
Breast Roasted Mesquite Smoked Skinless	2 oz	60	13	1	25	0	0	440
Breast Roasted Salsalito	2 oz	60	13	1	25	1	0	460
Pastrami Seasoned	2 oz	60	13	1	25	1	0	440
Carl Buddig								
Honey Roasted Turkey Breast	1 pkg (2.5 oz)	120	12	7	40	3	—	780
Lean Slices Honey Roasted Breast	1 pkg (2.5 oz)	70	13	1	30	4	—	980
Lean Slices Oven Roasted Breast	1 pkg (2.5 oz)	70	15	1	30	1	—	980
Lean Slices Smoked Breast	1 pkg (2.5 oz)	70	15	1	30	1	—	880
Oven Roasted Breast	1 pkg (2.5 oz)	110	12	7	40	1	—	780
Smoked Breast	1 pkg (2.5 oz)	110	12	7	40	1	—	780
Turkey Ham	1 pkg (2.5 oz)	100	13	5	40	1	—	1020

FOOD	PORTION	CALS	PROT	FAT	CHOL	CARB	FIBER	SOD
Healthy Choice								
Smoked Breast	4 slices (1.8 oz)	60	9	2	25	2	0	450
Jennie-O								
Turkey Breast Golden Roast	3 oz	100	19	3	35	2	—	740
Jordan's								
Fat Free Turkey Breast	1 slice (1 oz)	25	5	0	10	1	—	250
Oscar Mayer								
Lunchables Turkey Bagels	1 pkg	420	16	10	35	54	2	830
Smoked White	3 slices (3 oz)	90	12	3	30	2	—	950
Smoked White Turkey	3 slices (3 oz)	90	12	3	30	2	—	950
Turkey Bologna	3 slices (3 oz)	160	10	12	55	4	—	810
Turkey Cotto Salami	3 slices (3 oz)	130	13	8	65	tr	—	850
Perdue								
Breast Sliced Cajun Style	2 oz	50	9	1	20	1	—	800
Breast Sliced Honey Smoked	2 oz	50	10	0	20	2	—	510
Breast Sliced Pan Roasted	2 oz	70	14	2	30	0	—	390
Ham Hickory Smoked	2 oz	60	9	3	40	1	—	770
Healthsense Breast Sliced Oven Roasted	2 oz	60	10	0	20	3	—	290
Pastrami Hickory Smoked	2 oz	70	9	3	40	2	—	670
Shady Brook								
Meatballs Italian Style	3 (3 oz)	130	12	7	45	5	1	350
Wampler								
Bologna	2 oz	130	8	11	50	1	—	550
Dark Cured	2 oz	80	8	5	30	2	—	600

FOOD	PORTION	CALS	PROT	FAT	CHOL	CARB	FIBER	SOD
Deli Roast Breast	2 oz	50	12	1	25	0	—	250
Deli Roast Classic Spiced Breast	2 oz	70	16	1	25	1	—	380
Deli Roast Pan Roasted Breast	2 oz	70	13	2	20	1	—	400
Deli Roast Pan Roasted Skinless Breast	2 oz	50	12	0	20	1	—	400
Deli Roast Peppered Breast	2 oz	40	8	0	20	1	—	520
Deli Roast Rotisserie Breast	2 oz	50	9	2	20	1	—	500
Pastrami	2 oz	90	9	5	40	1	—	220
Salami	2 oz	90	9	6	55	1	—	560
Turkey Ham	2 oz	60	10	3	40	0	—	590

TURKEY DISHES
FROZEN

FOOD	PORTION	CALS	PROT	FAT	CHOL	CARB	FIBER	SOD
gravy & turkey	1 cup (8.4 oz)	160	14	6	—	11	—	1328
gravy & turkey	1 pkg (5 oz)	95	8	4	—	7	—	786
Banquet								
Homestyle Gravy & Sliced Turkey	2 slices + gravy	130	8	9	45	3	1	550
Sandwich Toppers Gravy & Sliced Turkey	1 pkg (5 oz)	160	8	11	30	6	0	670

READY-TO-EAT
Jennie-O

FOOD	PORTION	CALS	PROT	FAT	CHOL	CARB	FIBER	SOD
Stuffed Breast Cheddar Cheese & Broccoli	1 serv (6 oz)	240	36	9	85	3	0	1350
Stuffed Turkey Breast Pepper Cheese & Rice	1 piece (6 oz)	250	32	7	70	13	0	1290
Turkey Breast Roast In Homestyle Gravy	1 serv (5 oz)	110	20	1	40	3	0	680

FOOD	PORTION	CALS	PROT	FAT	CHOL	CARB	FIBER	SOD
Mosey's								
Turkey Breast w/ Gravy	1 serv (5 oz)	140	30	1	90	4	0	540
Wampler								
Turkey Ham Salad	⅓ cup	150	7	10	30	9	—	500
TAKE-OUT								
boneless breast w/ cranberry apple stuffing	1 serv (5 oz)	260	32	9	80	10	1	250

TURKEY SUBSTITUTES

FOOD	PORTION	CALS	PROT	FAT	CHOL	CARB	FIBER	SOD
Lightlife								
Smart Deli Turkey	3 slices (1.5 oz)	40	9	0	0	1	0	290
Tofurkey								
Deli Slices Hickory	1.5 oz	120	13	2	0	14	2	286
Deli Slices Original	1.5 oz	120	13	2	0	14	2	286
Deli Slices Peppered	1.5 oz	120	13	2	0	14	2	286
Drummettes	1 (3 oz)	105	11	2	0	11	4	380
Giblet Gravy	1 serv (3.5 oz)	42	4	2	0	5	1	340
Stuffed Tofu Roast	1 serv (4 oz)	193	26	5	0	10	2	310
Yves								
Veggie Turkey Deli Slices	1 serv (2.2 oz)	85	18	0	0	4	1	480

TURMERIC

FOOD	PORTION	CALS	PROT	FAT	CHOL	CARB	FIBER	SOD
ground	1 tsp	8	tr	tr	0	1	—	1

TURNIPS

FOOD	PORTION	CALS	PROT	FAT	CHOL	CARB	FIBER	SOD
canned greens	½ cup	17	2	tr	0	3	—	325
cooked mashed	½ cup (4.2 oz)	47	2	tr	0	10	—	25
cubed cooked	½ cup (3 oz)	33	1	tr	0	7	—	17
frzn greens cooked	½ cup	24	3	tr	0	4	2	12

FOOD	PORTION	CALS	PROT	FAT	CHOL	CARB	FIBER	SOD
greens chopped cooked	½ cup	15	1	tr	0	3	2	21
greens raw chopped	½ cup	7	tr	tr	0	2	1	11
raw cubed	½ cup (2.4 oz)	25	1	tr	0	6	—	14
Birds Eye								
Greens w/ Diced Turnip	1 cup	25	2	0	0	2	2	20
TURTLE								
raw	3.5 oz	85	18	1	—	0	—	—
TUSK FISH								
raw	3.5 oz	79	17	tr	—	0	—	113
VANILLA								
Steel's								
Sugar Free	1 tbsp	24	0	0	0	6	0	0
Virginia Dare								
Extract	1 tsp	10	—	0	0	—	—	—
VEAL *(see also VEAL DISHES)*								
cutlet lean only braised	3 oz	172	31	4	115	0	—	57
cutlet lean only fried	3 oz	156	28	4	91	0	—	65
ground broiled	3 oz	146	21	6	87	0	—	70
loin chop w/ bone lean & fat braised	1 chop (2.8 oz)	227	24	14	94	0	—	64
loin chop w/ bone lean only braised	1 chop (2.4 oz)	155	23	6	86	0	—	58
shoulder w/ bone lean only braised	3 oz	169	29	5	110	0	—	83
sirloin w/ bone lean & fat roasted	3 oz	171	21	9	87	0	—	71
sirloin w/ bone lean only roasted	3 oz	143	22	5	89	0	—	72

FOOD	PORTION	CALS	PROT	FAT	CHOL	CARB	FIBER	SOD
VEAL DISHES								
TAKE-OUT								
parmigiana	4.2 oz	279	22	18	136	6	2	545
scallopini	1 serv (8 oz)	608	–	146	46	–	–	900
VEGETABLE JUICE								
vegetable juice cocktail	½ cup	22	1	tr	0	6	–	442
vegetable juice cocktail	6 fl oz	34	1	tr	0	8	–	664
Dole								
Vegetable Blend	1 bottle (12 oz)	90	4	0	0	19	2	820
Hunt's								
Cocktail	1 can (6 oz)	20	2	0	0	7	2	630
Muir Glen								
Organic	5.5 oz	50	1	0	0	10	2	420
V8								
Lightly Tangy	8 oz	58	2	1	–	11	2	345
Low Sodium	8 oz	53	2	tr	–	11	2	95
Original	8 oz	51	2	1	–	10	2	615
Picante Vegetable	8 oz	51	2	tr	–	10	2	673
Spicy Hot	8 oz	49	2	tr	–	10	2	780
VEGETABLES MIXED								
CANNED								
mixed vegetables	½ cup	39	2	tr	0	8	–	122
peas & carrots	½ cup	48	3	tr	0	11	–	332
peas & carrots low sodium	½ cup	48	3	tr	0	11	–	332
peas & onions	½ cup	30	2	tr	0	5	–	265
succotash	½ cup	102	4	1	0	23	–	325
Chun King								
Chow Mein Vegetables	⅔ cup (3 oz)	14	1	tr	0	3	1	323
Del Monte								
Mixed	½ cup (4.4 oz)	40	2	0	0	8	2	360
Mixed No Salt Added	½ cup (4.4 oz)	40	2	0	0	8	2	25

FOOD	PORTION	CALS	PROT	FAT	CHOL	CARB	FIBER	SOD
Peas And Carrots	½ cup (4.5 oz)	60	2	0	0	11	2	360
La Choy								
Chop Suey Vegetables	½ cup (2.2 oz)	10	1	tr	0	2	1	241
S&W								
Mixed	½ cup (4.4 oz)	35	1	0	0	7	2	370
Peas & Carrots	½ cup (4.5 oz)	60	2	0	0	11	2	360
Peas & Onions	½ cup (4.3 oz)	40	3	0	0	11	3	530
Veg-All								
Cajun Mixed	½ cup	50	2	0	0	10	3	410
FROZEN								
mixed vegetables cooked	½ cup	54	3	tr	0	12	2	32
peas & carrots cooked	½ cup	38	3	tr	0	8	—	55
peas & onions cooked	½ cup	40	2	tr	0	8	—	—
succotash cooked	½ cup	79	4	1	0	17	—	38
Birds Eye								
Baby Sweet Peas & Pearl Onions	⅔ cup	60	4	1	0	12	4	85
Bavarian Vegetables	1 cup (5.5 oz)	150	5	8	30	15	3	460
Broccoli Cauliflower & Carrots	½ cup	25	2	0	0	5	2	30
Broccoli Cauliflower & Carrots In Cheese Sauce	½ cup	70	3	4	5	7	2	460
Broccoli Cauliflower & Red Peppers	½ cup	20	2	0	0	5	2	20
Broccoli & Cauliflower	½ cup	20	2	0	0	4	2	20

FOOD	PORTION	CALS	PROT	FAT	CHOL	CARB	FIBER	SOD
Broccoli Carrots & Water Chestnuts	½ cup	30	2	0	0	7	3	30
Broccoli Corn & Red Peppers	½ cup	50	3	0	0	12	3	15
Broccoli Red Peppers Onions & Mushrooms	½ cup	25	2	0	0	5	2	20
Brussels Sprouts Cauliflower & Carrots	½ cup	30	2	0	0	7	3	20
California Style Vegetables	½ cup	100	3	5	10	9	3	240
Cauliflower Nuggets Corn Carrots & Snow Peaspods	½ cup	30	2	0	0	6	2	25
Gumbo Blend	¾ cup	40	2	0	0	10	2	30
Italian Style Vegetables & Bow Tie Pasta	1 cup	150	3	9	10	13	2	380
Mixed Vegetables	⅓ cup	50	–	0	0	–	3	35
New England Style Vegetables & Pasta Shells	1 pkg (9 oz)	260	6	14	15	29	3	480
Oriental Style Vegetables	½ cup	60	2	4	10	4	2	260
Peas & Pearl Onions	⅔ cup	90	5	1	0	18	5	520
Peas & Potatoes In Real Cream Sauce	½ cup	90	4	3	10	13	2	350
Radiatore Pasta & Vegetables	1 cup	200	6	8	5	27	1	430
Roasted Potatoes & Broccoli	⅔ cup (3.9 oz)	100	3	4	5	15	1	470
Roletti Pasta & Vegetables	1 cup (4.4 oz)	190	5	8	5	11	1	350
Simply Grillin' Garden Herb	1 cup	140	3	6	0	19	4	490

FOOD	PORTION	CALS	PROT	FAT	CHOL	CARB	FIBER	SOD
Stir Fry Asparagus	2 cups	90	5	1	0	16	3	35
Stir Fry Broccoli	1 cup	30	2	0	0	5	2	30
Stir Fry Pepper	1 cup	25	1	0	0	5	2	15
Stir Fry Sugar Snap	¾ cup	35	1	0	0	5	1	20
Stir Fry Whole Green Bean	1¾ cup	100	4	1	0	19	2	25
Stir Fry Style Vegetables	½ cup	60	2	4	10	5	1	270
Vegetables For Soup	⅔ cup	45	–	0	0	–	2	45
Vegetables For Stew	⅔ cup	40	1	0	0	9	1	40
Voila! Italian Pesto Chicken	2 cups	240	15	9	25	24	1	690
Voila! Three Cheese Chicken	1¾ cups	220	14	8	20	24	1	570
Fresh Like								
California Blend	3.5 oz	31	2	tr	–	7	1	21
Midwestern Blend	3.5 oz	42	2	tr	–	9	1	32
Mixed	3.5 oz	69	30	tr	–	14	1	48
Oriental Blend	3.5 oz	26	3	tr	–	5	1	11
Winter Blend	3.5 oz	26	3	tr	–	5	1	26
Green Giant								
Alfredo Vegetables	¾ cup	70	4	2	5	8	2	360
Cheese Sauce Broccoli Cauliflower Carrots	1 cup (4.1 oz)	60	3	3	5	7	2	460
Seasoned Broccoli & Carrots w/ Garlic & Herbs	½ cup	45	2	1	0	8	3	200
Health Is Wealth								
Veggie Munchees	2 (1 oz)	50	2	1	0	9	1	170
La Choy								
Fancy Chinese Mixed Vegetables	½ cup (2.9 oz)	9	1	tr	0	1	1	31

FOOD	PORTION	CALS	PROT	FAT	CHOL	CARB	FIBER	SOD
McKenzie's								
Gumbo Mixture	1 serv (2.9 oz)	35	1	0	0	8	2	30
Tree Of Life								
Mixed	½ cup (3 oz)	65	3	0	0	13	3	60
SHELF-STABLE								
TastyBite								
Curry Bangkok Red	½ pkg (5.3 oz)	88	2	6	0	7	1	825
Curry Patong Yellow	½ pkg (5.3 oz)	118	2	7	0	12	1	489
Curry Siam Green	½ pkg (5.3 oz)	63	2	3	0	6	1	522
Jaipur Vegetables	½ pkg (5 oz)	220	9	15	25	13	7	680
Malabar Mixed	½ pkg (5 oz)	67	1	1	0	15	1	475
TAKE-OUT								
buddha's delight	1 serv (16 oz)	174	17	5	35	17	3	1368
caponata	¼ cup	28	–	1	0	–	–	–
curry	1 serv (7.7 oz)	398	4	33	–	22	–	–
gyoza potstickers vegetable	8 (4.9 oz)	210	8	4	0	34	5	500
pakoras	1 (2 oz)	108	5	5	–	12	3	–
ratatouille	1 serv (3.5 oz)	96	2	7	0	7	4	812
samosa	2 (4 oz)	519	3	46	–	25	3	–
succotash	½ cup	111	5	1	0	23	–	16
tapenade grilled vegetables	¼ cup	40	0	3	0	4	tr	150
VENISON								
roasted	3 oz	134	26	3	95	0	–	46
VINEGAR								
cider	1 tbsp	tr	tr	0	0	1	–	tr
Eden								
Organic Brown Rice	1 tbsp	2	0	0	0	0	0	0
Ume Plum	1 tsp	2	0	0	0	0	0	1050

FOOD	PORTION	CALS	PROT	FAT	CHOL	CARB	FIBER	SOD
Heinz								
White	1 tbsp	2	0	0	0	0	0	0
Progresso								
Balsamic	2 tbsp (0.5 oz)	10	0	0	0	2	0	0
Wild Thyme Farms								
Balsamic Red Raspberry	1 tbsp	13	0	0	0	3	–	0

WAFFLES
FROZEN
buttermilk	1 4 in sq (1.2 oz)	88	2	3	–	14	1	262
plain	1 4 in sq (1.2 oz)	88	2	3	–	14	1	262
Kid Cuisine								
Wave Rider Waffle Sticks	1 meal (6.6 oz)	380	3	8	30	75	3	580

MIX
plain as prep	1 7 in diam (2.6 oz)	218	5	10	39	26	1	458

READY-TO-EAT
Gol D Lite
Low Carb Belgian	1 (0.9 oz)	100	2	5	0	15	5	0
Low Carb Belgian Chocolate Covered	1 (1.1 oz)	130	2	8	0	18	1	0
Kashi								
GoLean Blueberry	2	170	8	3	0	33	6	300
GoLean Original	2	170	8	3	0	33	6	330
Thomas'								
Buttermilk	1 (1.6 oz)	130	3	5	0	18	tr	490
Homestyle	1 (1.6 oz)	140	3	5	0	19	tr	390

TAKE-OUT
plain	1 (7 in diam)	218	6	11	52	25	–	383

WALNUTS
black dried chopped	1 cup	759	30	71	0	15	–	2

FOOD	PORTION	CALS	PROT	FAT	CHOL	CARB	FIBER	SOD
english dried	1 oz	182	4	18	0	5	1	3
english dried chopped	1 cup	770	17	74	0	22	6	12
halves	14 (1 oz)	190	4	19	0	4	2	tr
Sweet Delights								
Walnut Roasters	⅓ pkg (1 oz)	210	5	20	0	3	2	200

WASABI (see HORSERADISH)

WATER

FOOD	PORTION	CALS	PROT	FAT	CHOL	CARB	FIBER	SOD
ice cubes	3	0	0	0	0	0	–	2
tap water	8 oz	0	0	0	0	0	–	7
Absopure								
Natural Spring	8 fl oz	0	0	0	0	0	–	0
Aquafina								
Essentials B-Power Wild Berry	8 fl oz	40	0	0	0	11	–	10
Essentials Calcium + Tangerine Pineapple	8 fl oz	40	0	0	0	11	–	15
Essentials Daily C Citrus	8 fl oz	40	0	0	0	11	–	15
Essentials Multi-V Watermelon	8 fl oz	40	0	0	0	11	–	10
Water	8 fl oz	0	0	0	0	0	–	0
Aquess								
Purified Water w/ Soluble Fiber	1 bottle (18 oz)	30	0	0	0	8	5	0
Base Energy + Water								
All Flavors	8 oz	28	0	0	0	7	–	45
Blu Italy								
Sparkling Lemon	8 oz	0	0	0	0	0	0	25
Calabria								
Mineral	8 oz	0	0	0	0	0	0	0
Castellina								
Sparking Spring	8 fl oz	0	0	0	0	0	0	<5
Clearly Canadian								
Sparkling All Flavors	8 oz	45	0	0	0	10	–	10

FOOD	PORTION	CALS	PROT	FAT	CHOL	CARB	FIBER	SOD
Crystal Geyser								
Spring Water	8 fl oz	0	0	0	0	0	0	0
Dasani								
Purfied Water	8 oz	0	0	0	0	0	–	0
Evamor								
Artesian Water	8 fl oz	0	0	0	0	0	0	12
Evian								
Spring Water	1 bottle (11.5 oz)	0	0	0	0	0	0	<5
Ferrarelle								
Sparkling	8 fl oz	0	0	0	0	0	1	10
FlavH20								
All Flavors	1 can (12.3 oz)	80	0	0	0	21	–	0
Gerolsteiner								
Sparkling Mineral	8 fl oz	0	0	0	0	0	0	30
Glaceau Vitamin Water								
Balance	8 oz	50	0	0	0	13	–	0
Defense	8 oz	40	0	0	0	9	–	0
Endurance	8 oz	50	0	0	0	13	–	0
Energy	8 oz	40	0	0	0	9	–	0
Essential	8 oz	40	0	0	0	9	–	0
Focus	8 oz	40	0	0	0	9	–	0
Multi-V	8 oz	40	0	0	0	9	–	0
Power-C	8 oz	40	0	0	0	9	–	5
Rescue	8 oz	40	0	0	0	9	–	0
Revive	8 oz	50	0	0	0	13	–	0
Stress-B	8 oz	40	0	0	0	9	–	0
Hansen's								
Energy Water Lemon	8 oz	10	0	0	0	3	–	0
Iceland Spring								
Spring Water	1 liter	0	0	0	0	0	0	10
Meridian								
Clear All Flavors	0 oz	100	0	0	0	25	–	0
Metromint								
Peppermint Water	8 oz	0	0	0	0	0	0	0
Paradiso								
Slightly Sparkling	8 oz	0	0	0	0	0	0	1

FOOD	PORTION	CALS	PROT	FAT	CHOL	CARB	FIBER	SOD
Propel								
Fitness Water Berry	8 fl oz	10	0	0	0	3	–	35
Fitness Water Black Cherry	8 fl oz	10	0	0	0	3	–	35
Reebok								
Fitness Water Berry	1 bottle (24 oz)	30	0	0	0	0	0	0
Fitness Water Natural	1 bottle (24 oz)	0	0	0	0	0	0	0
Replenish								
Elements Enhanced Water Orange	8 oz	40	0	0	0	10	–	80
San Benedetto								
Nautral Mineral Water	1 liter	0	0	0	0	0	0	7
San Pellegrino								
Mineral Water	1 liter (33.8 oz)	0	0	0	0	0	–	41
Sanfaustino								
Mineral	8 oz	0	0	0	0	0	0	4
Saratoga								
Spring	8 oz	0	0	0	0	0	–	0
Spa								
Mineral Water Reine	1 bottle (17.5 oz)	0	0	0	0	0	–	2
Speedo Sportswater								
All Flavors	8 oz	10	0	0	0	3	–	40
Ty Nant								
Mineral Water	1 liter	0	0	0	0	0	0	22
Vasa								
Natural Spring	8 oz	0	0	0	0	0	0	0
Veryfine								
Fruit 2 O Lemon	8 oz	0	0	0	0	0	–	5
Fruit 2 O Lemon Lime	8 fl oz	0	0	0	0	0	–	5
Fruit 2 O Orange	8 fl oz	0	0	0	0	0	–	5
Fruit 2 O Raspberry	8 fl oz	0	0	0	0	0	–	5
VitaZest								
All Flavors	8 oz	0	0	0	0	0	0	10

FOOD	PORTION	CALS	PROT	FAT	CHOL	CARB	FIBER	SOD
Vittel								
Mineral Water	1 bottle (18 oz)	0	0	0	0	0	–	5
Volvic								
Spring Water	8 oz	0	0	0	0	0	0	<5
Voss								
Artesian	8 oz	0	0	0	0	0	0	–
WATER CHESTNUTS								
chinese sliced canned	½ cup	35	1	tr	0	9	–	6
fresh sliced	½ cup	66	1	tr	0	15	–	9
Chun King								
Sliced	2 tbsp (0.8 oz)	11	tr	tr	0	3	1	3
Whole	2 (0.7 oz)	10	tr	tr	0	2	1	2
La Choy								
Chopped	2 tbsp (0.6 oz)	9	tr	tr	0	2	1	2
Sliced	2 tbsp (0.8 oz)	11	tr	tr	0	3	1	3
Whole	2 (0.7 oz)	10	tr	tr	0	2	1	2
WATERCRESS								
fresh chopped	½ cup	2	tr	tr	0	tr	tr	7
garden fresh	½ cup	8	tr	tr	0	1	–	4
garden fresh cooked	½ cup	16	1	tr	0	3	–	5
WATERMELON								
cut up	1 cup	50	1	1	0	11	1	3
seeds dried	1 cup	602	8	51	0	17	–	28
seeds dried	1 oz	158	8	13	0	4	–	28
wedge	1/16	152	3	2	0	35	2	10
WATERMELON JUICE								
Snapple								
What-A-Melon	8 oz	90	0	0	0	25	–	40

FOOD	PORTION	CALS	PROT	FAT	CHOL	CARB	FIBER	SOD
WAX BEANS								
CANNED								
Del Monte								
Cut Golden	½ cup (4.2 oz)	20	1	0	0	4	2	360
S&W								
Cut	½ cup (4.2 oz)	20	1	0	0	4	2	360
WHALE								
raw	3.5 oz	134	23	3	—	0	—	100
WHEAT								
sprouted	1 cup (3.8 oz)	214	8	1	0	46	1	17
starch	3.5 oz	348	tr	tr	—	86	—	2
Bob's Red Mill								
Vital Wheat Gluten	¼ cup	120	23	1	0	6	0	9
Lightlife								
Savory Seitan Barbecue	4 oz	160	24	2	0	12	0	360
Savory Seitan Teriyaki	4 oz	160	26	2	0	10	0	320
Near East								
Pilaf Mix Wheat as prep	1 cup	220	7	5	9	40	9	640
Taboule Salad Mix as prep	⅔ cup	110	3	3	0	21	5	270
NOW								
Wheat Gluten Flour	¼ cup	125	23	0	0	5	—	40
WHEAT GERM								
plain toasted	1 cup	431	33	12	0	56	—	4
plain toasted	¼ cup (1 oz)	108	8	3	0	14	4	1
w/ brown sugar & honey toasted	1 cup	426	25	9	—	69	—	3
w/ brown sugar & honey toasted	1 oz	107	6	2	—	17	—	1
Hodgson Mill								
Untoasted	2 tbsp	55	4	1	0	7	4	0
Kretschmer								
Original Toasted	2 tbsp (0.5 oz)	50	4	1	0	6	2	0

FOOD	PORTION	CALS	PROT	FAT	CHOL	CARB	FIBER	SOD
Mother's								
Toasted	2 tbsp	50	4	1	0	6	2	0
WHEY								
acid dry	1 tbsp (3 g)	10	tr	tr	—	2	—	28
acid fluid	1 cup (8 fl oz)	59	25	tr	—	13	—	118
sweet dry	1 tbsp (8 g)	26	1	tr	—	6	—	80
sweet fluid	1 cup (8 fl oz)	66	2	1	—	13	—	132
whey cheese	1 oz	126	4	8	—	9	0	146
WHIPPED TOPPINGS								
cream pressurized	1 tbsp (3 g)	8	tr	tr	2	tr	—	4
cream pressurized	1 cup (2.1 oz)	154	2	13	46	7	—	78
nondairy frzn	1 tbsp	13	tr	1	0	1	—	1
nondairy powdered as prep w/ whole milk	1 cup	151	3	10	8	13	—	53
nondairy powdered as prep w/ whole milk	1 tbsp (4 g)	8	tr	tr	tr	1	—	3
nondairy pressurized	1 cup	184	1	16	0	11	—	43
nondairy pressurized	1 tbsp (4 g)	11	tr	1	0	1	—	2
WHITE BEANS								
canned	1 cup	306	19	1	0	58	—	13
dried regular cooked	1 cup	249	17	1	0	45	—	11
dried small cooked	1 cup	253	16	1	0	46	—	4
Progresso								
Cannellini	½ cup (4.6 oz)	100	5	1	0	18	5	270
WHITEFISH								
baked	3 oz	146	21	6	65	0	—	56
smoked	1 oz	39	7	tr	9	0	—	285
smoked	3 oz	92	20	1	28	0	—	866

FOOD	PORTION	CALS	PROT	FAT	CHOL	CARB	FIBER	SOD
WHITING								
cooked	3 oz	98	20	1	71	0	−	113
raw	3 oz	77	16	1	57	0	−	61
WILD RICE								
cooked	1 cup (5.7 oz)	166	7	1	0	35	3	5
Gourmet House								
Cracked not prep	¼ cup	170	6	0	0	35	2	0
Hand Harvested not prep	¼ cup	170	6	0	0	35	2	0
Quick Cooking not prep	½ cup	170	6	0	0	25	2	0
White & Wild not prep	¼ cup	170	4	0	0	35	1	0
Wild & Rice Garden Blend no prep	¼ cup	190	5	1	0	40	1	15
WINE								
beaujolais	4 oz	95	−	−	−	−	−	−
bordeaux red	4 oz	95	−	−	−	−	−	−
chianti	4 oz	101	−	−	−	−	−	−
haiku	1 serv	93	tr	0	0	3	0	2
japanese plum	3 oz	139	tr	tr	0	16	0	−
japanese sake	1 oz	33	tr	0	0	2	0	1
kir	1 serv	78	tr	0	0	3	0	4
liebfraumilch	4 oz	86	−	−	−	−	−	−
madeira	3.5 oz	169	0	0	−	10	0	−
marsala	4 oz	80	−	−	−	−	−	−
merlot	4 oz	95	−	−	−	−	−	−
muscatel	4 oz	160	−	−	−	−	−	−
port	3.5 oz	156	tr	0	−	11	0	4
red	1 serv (3.5 oz)	74	tr	0	0	2	0	6
rose	1 serv (3.5 oz)	73	tr	0	0	2	0	5
sake screwdriver	1 serv	175	2	tr	0	23	tr	3
sangria	1 serv	88	tr	tr	0	6	tr	4

FOOD	PORTION	CALS	PROT	FAT	CHOL	CARB	FIBER	SOD
sangria blanco	1 serv	155	1	tr	0	24	3	13
sherry	2 oz	84	tr	0	0	5	–	–
sweet dessert	1 serv (3.5 oz)	158	tr	0	0	12	0	9
vermouth dry	3½ oz	105	–	0	0	1	–	–
vermouth sweet	3½ oz	167	–	0	0	12	–	–
wassail wine	1 serv	142	1	tr	0	22	2	6
white	1 serv (3.5 oz)	70	tr	0	0	1	0	5
wine cooler	1 serv	218	1	tr	0	8	0	10
wine spritzer	1 serv	60	tr	0	0	1	0	11
Boone's								
Country Kwencher	4 fl oz	96	0	0	0	12	–	4
Delicious Apple	4 fl oz	84	0	0	0	12	–	4
Sangria	4 fl oz	88	0	0	0	12	–	4
Snow Creek Berry	4 fl oz	72	0	0	0	12	–	tr
Strawberry Hill	4 fl oz	88	0	0	0	12	–	4
Sun Peak Peach	4 fl oz	72	0	0	0	12	–	4
Wild Island	4 fl oz	72	0	0	0	12	–	tr
Carlo Rossi								
Blush	4 fl oz	84	0	0	0	4	–	4
Burgundy	4 fl oz	88	0	0	0	tr	–	4
Chablis	4 fl oz	84	0	0	0	tr	–	4
Paisano	4 fl oz	92	0	0	0	tr	–	12
Red Sangria	4 fl oz	92	0	0	0	8	–	4
Rhine	4 fl oz	84	0	0	0	4	–	4
Vin Rosé	4 fl oz	84	0	0	0	4	–	4
White Grenache	4 fl oz	80	0	0	0	4	–	tr
Eden								
Mirin Rice Cooking Wine	1 tbsp	25	0	0	0	7	0	130
Fairbanks								
Cream Sherry	4 fl oz	168	0	0	0	16	–	4
Port	4 fl oz	176	0	0	0	16	–	4
Sherry	4 fl oz	136	0	0	0	8	–	8
White Port	4 fl oz	136	0	0	0	16	–	4
Gallo								
Blush Chablis	4 fl oz	88	0	0	0	4	–	8
Burgundy	4 fl oz	88	0	0	0	tr	–	4

FOOD	PORTION	CALS	PROT	FAT	CHOL	CARB	FIBER	SOD
Cabernet Sauvignon	4 fl oz	88	0	0	0	0	—	tr
Chablis Blanc	4 fl oz	80	0	0	0	tr	—	4
Chardonnay	4 fl oz	92	0	0	0	tr	—	4
Classic Burgundy	4 fl oz	84	0	0	0	0	—	tr
French Colombard	4 fl oz	84	0	0	0	4	—	4
Hearty Burgundy	4 fl oz	88	0	0	0	tr	—	4
Pink Chablis	4 fl oz	80	0	0	0	4	—	4
Red Rosé	4 fl oz	92	0	0	0	4	—	8
Rhine	4 fl oz	88	0	0	0	4	—	4
Sheffield Cellars								
Sherry	4 fl oz	136	0	0	0	16	—	4
Tawny Port	4 fl oz	180	0	0	0	16	—	8
Vermouth Extra Dry	1 fl oz	28	0	0	0	1	—	1
Vermouth Sweet	1 fl oz	43	0	0	0	4	—	2
Very Dry Sherry	4 fl oz	128	0	0	0	4	—	8

WINGED BEANS

FOOD	PORTION	CALS	PROT	FAT	CHOL	CARB	FIBER	SOD
dried cooked	1 cup	252	18	10	0	26	—	22

WOLFFISH

FOOD	PORTION	CALS	PROT	FAT	CHOL	CARB	FIBER	SOD
atlantic baked	3 oz	105	19	3	50	0	—	93

WRAPS (see BREAD)

XANTHAN GUM
Bob's Red Mill

FOOD	PORTION	CALS	PROT	FAT	CHOL	CARB	FIBER	SOD
Xanthan Gum	1 tbsp	8	0	0	0	9	8	10

YAM (see also SWEET POTATO)
CANNED
S&W

FOOD	PORTION	CALS	PROT	FAT	CHOL	CARB	FIBER	SOD
Candied	½ cup (4.9 oz)	170	2	0	0	46	4	360

FRESH

FOOD	PORTION	CALS	PROT	FAT	CHOL	CARB	FIBER	SOD
mountain yam hawaii cooked	½ cup	59	1	tr	0	14	—	9
yam cubed cooked	½ cup	79	1	tr	0	19	—	6

YAMBEAN

FOOD	PORTION	CALS	PROT	FAT	CHOL	CARB	FIBER	SOD
cooked	¾ cup	38	1	tr	0	9	—	4

FOOD	PORTION	CALS	PROT	FAT	CHOL	CARB	FIBER	SOD
YARDLONG BEANS								
dried cooked	1 cup	202	14	1	0	36	–	9
YAUTIA (TANNIER)								
fresh sliced	1 cup (4.7 oz)	132	2	1	0	32	2	28
root raw	1 (10.7 oz)	299	4	1	0	72	5	64
YEAST								
baker's compressed	1 cake (0.6 oz)	18	1	tr	0	3	2	5
baker's dry	1 tbsp	35	5	1	0	5	3	–
baker's dry	1 pkg (¼ oz)	21	3	tr	0	3	–	–
brewer's dry	1 tbsp	25	3	tr	0	3	–	10
Hodgson Mill								
Fast Rise	1 tsp (9 g)	25	3	0	0	4	1	0
YELLOW BEANS								
canned	½ cup	13	1	tr	0	3	1	170
canned low sodium	½ cup	13	1	tr	0	3	1	1
dried cooked	1 cup	254	16	2	0	45	–	8
fresh cooked	½ cup	22	1	tr	0	5	–	2
fresh raw	½ cup	17	1	tr	0	4	–	3
frozen cooked	½ cup	18	1	tr	0	4	–	9
YELLOWTAIL								
baked	3 oz	159	25	6	–	0	–	42
YOGURT *(see also YOGURT DRINKS, YOGURT FROZEN)*								
coffee lowfat	8 oz	194	11	3	11	31	–	149
fruit lowfat	8 oz	225	9	3	10	42	–	121
fruit lowfat	4 oz	113	5	1	5	21	–	60
plain	8 oz	139	8	7	29	11	–	105
plain lowfat	8 oz	144	12	4	14	16	–	159
plain no fat	8 oz	127	13	tr	4	17	–	174
vanilla lowfat	8 oz	194	11	3	11	31	–	149
Axelrod								
Fat Free Lemon	1 pkg (6 oz)	90	5	0	<5	17	0	95
Fat Free Raspberry	6 oz	90	5	0	<5	17	0	95
Fat Free Vanilla	1 pkg (6 oz)	90	5	0	<5	17	0	95

FOOD	PORTION	CALS	PROT	FAT	CHOL	CARB	FIBER	SOD
Breyers								
Vanilla 98% Fat Free	½ cup	90	2	2	5	21	4	50
Cabot								
Non Fat	8 oz	100	10	0	0	19	0	135
Non Fat Berry Banana	8 oz	130	8	0	5	24	0	120
Non Fat Blueberry	8 oz	130	8	0	5	24	0	115
Non Fat Lemon	8 oz	130	8	0	5	24	0	115
Non Fat Raspberry	8 oz	130	8	0	5	24	0	115
Non Fat Very Berry	8 oz	130	8	0	5	24	0	115
Colombo								
Fat Free Plain	8 oz	100	10	0	10	16	0	160
Fat Free Vanilla	8 oz	160	8	0	5	32	0	140
French Vanilla	8 oz	180	8	2	15	42	0	120
Fruit On The Bottom Strawberry Banana	8 oz	230	7	2	15	47	0	90
Lowfat Plain	8 oz	130	10	3	15	16	0	125
Multipack Blended All Flavors	4 oz	110	3	1	5	22	0	60
Strawberry	8 oz	190	8	3	15	42	–	130
Dannon								
Chunky Fruit Nonfat Apple Cinnamon	6 oz	160	7	0	5	33	0	100
Chunky Fruit Nonfat Blueberry	6 oz	160	7	0	5	32	0	110
Chunky Fruit Nonfat Cherry Vanilla	6 oz	160	7	0	5	31	0	100
Chunky Fruit Nonfat Peach	6 oz	160	7	0	5	33	0	100
Chunky Fruit Nonfat Strawberry	6 oz	160	7	0	5	32	0	105

FOOD	PORTION	CALS	PROT	FAT	CHOL	CARB	FIBER	SOD
Chunky Fruit Nonfat Strawberry Banana	6 oz	160	7	0	5	32	0	105
Creamy Fruit Blends Raspberry	6 oz	170	6	2	10	31	tr	115
Danimals Lowfat Tropical Punch	4.4 oz	130	6	1	5	25	0	95
Danimals Lowfat Blueberry	4.4 oz	130	6	1	5	24	0	100
Danimals Lowfat Grape Lemonade	4.4 oz	120	6	1	5	22	0	90
Danimals Lowfat Lemon Ice	4.4 oz	120	6	1	5	22	0	100
Danimals Lowfat Orange Banana	4.4 oz	130	6	1	5	24	0	90
Danimals Lowfat Strawberry	4.4 oz	130	6	1	5	24	0	90
Danimals Lowfat Vanilla	4.4 oz	120	6	1	5	23	0	90
Danimals Lowfat Wild Raspberry	4.4 oz	120	6	1	5	22	0	90
Double Delights Banana Creme Strawberry	6 oz	160	7	1	10	32	0	100
Double Delights Bavarian Creme Raspberry	6 oz	170	7	1	10	34	0	125
Double Delights Cheesecake Cherry	6 oz	170	7	1	10	34	0	100
Double Delights Cheesecake Strawberry	6 oz	170	7	1	10	33	0	100
Double Delights Chocolate Cheesecake	6 oz	220	8	1	10	45	0	150

FOOD	PORTION	CALS	PROT	FAT	CHOL	CARB	FIBER	SOD
Double Delights Chocolate Dipped Strawberry	6 oz	210	8	1	10	45	0	150
Double Delights Chocolate Eclair	6 oz	220	8	1	10	45	0	150
Double Delights Vanilla Strawberry	6 oz	170	7	1	10	33	0	100
Double Delights Vanilla Peach & Apricot	6 oz	170	7	1	10	33	0	100
Fruit On The Bottom Lowfat Apple Cinnamon	8 oz	240	9	3	15	46	1	140
Fruit On The Bottom Lowfat Blueberry	8 oz	240	9	3	15	46	1	140
Fruit On The Bottom Lowfat Boysenberry	8 oz	240	9	3	15	45	1	150
Fruit On The Bottom Lowfat Cherry	8 oz	240	9	3	15	46	1	135
Fruit On The Bottom Lowfat Minipack Mixed Berry	4.4 oz	130	5	2	10	25	tr	80
Fruit On The Bottom Lowfat Minipack Strawberry	4.4 oz	130	5	2	10	25	tr	75
Fruit On The Bottom Lowfat Mixed Berries	8 oz	240	9	3	15	45	1	150
Fruit On The Bottom Lowfat Orange	8 oz	240	9	3	15	45	0	135
Fruit On The Bottom Lowfat Peach	8 oz	240	9	3	15	45	1	140

FOOD	PORTION	CALS	PROT	FAT	CHOL	CARB	FIBER	SOD
Fruit On The Bottom Lowfat Strawberry	8 oz	240	9	3	15	46	1	135
Fruit On The Bottom Lowfat Strawberry Banana	8 oz	240	9	3	15	43	1	140
La Creme Strawberry	1 pkg (4 oz)	140	5	5	20	21	—	75
La Creme Vanilla	1 pkg (4 oz)	140	5	5	20	20	—	75
Light Duets Cherry Cheesecake	6 oz	90	5	0	0	18	0	70
Light Duets Peaches N' Cream	6 oz	90	5	0	0	18	0	70
Light Duets Raspberry Royale	6 oz	90	5	0	0	17	0	75
Light Duets Strawberry Cheesecake	6 oz	90	5	0	0	18	0	70
Light 'N Crunchy Mint Chocolate Chip	8 oz	140	8	0	5	27	0	150
Light 'N Crunchy Nonfat Caramel Apple Crunch	8 oz	140	8	0	<5	26	0	340
Light 'N Crunchy Nonfat Lemon Blueberry Cobbler	8 oz	140	8	0	<5	25	0	135
Light 'N Crunchy Nonfat Mocha Cappuccino	8 oz	140	8	0	<5	26	0	150
Light 'N Crunchy Nonfat Raspberry w/ Granola	8 oz	140	9	0	<5	26	2	120
Light 'N Crunchy Nonfat Vanilla Chocolate Crunch	8 oz	130	8	0	<5	23	0	140

FOOD	PORTION	CALS	PROT	FAT	CHOL	CARB	FIBER	SOD
Light 'N Fit Vanilla	6 oz	90	6	0	<5	16	–	95
Light Nonfat Banana Cream Pie	8 oz	100	8	0	<5	15	0	120
Light Nonfat Blueberry	8 oz	100	8	0	<5	18	0	115
Light Nonfat Cappuccino	8 oz	100	8	0	5	16	0	120
Light Nonfat Cherry Vanilla	8 oz	100	8	0	<5	18	0	120
Light Nonfat Coconut Cream Pie	8 oz	100	8	0	5	16	0	120
Light Nonfat Creme Caramel	8 oz	100	8	0	<5	15	0	120
Light Nonfat Lemon Chiffon	8 oz	100	8	0	5	15	0	120
Light Nonfat Mint Chocolate Cream Pie	8 oz	100	8	0	<5	17	0	120
Light Nonfat Peach	8 oz	100	8	0	<5	16	0	115
Light Nonfat Raspberry	8 oz	100	8	0	<5	17	0	120
Light Nonfat Strawberry	8 oz	100	8	0	<5	16	0	115
Light Nonfat Strawberry Banana	8 oz	100	8	0	<5	17	0	120
Light Nonfat Strawberry Kiwi	8 oz	100	8	0	5	16	0	120
Light Nonfat Tangerine Chiffon	8 oz	100	8	0	5	15	0	120
Lowfat Coffee	8 oz	210	10	3	15	36	0	160
Lowfat Cranberry Raspberry	8 oz	210	10	3	15	36	0	160
Lowfat Lemon	8 oz	210	10	3	15	36	0	160
Lowfat Vanilla	8 oz	210	10	3	15	36	0	160

FOOD	PORTION	CALS	PROT	FAT	CHOL	CARB	FIBER	SOD
Minipack Blended Nonfat Blueberry	4.4 oz	120	5	0	5	25	0	80
Minipack Blended Nonfat Cherry	4.4 oz	110	5	0	5	24	0	80
Minipack Blended Nonfat Peach	4.4 oz	120	5	0	5	23	0	80
Minipack Blended Nonfat Raspberry	4.4 oz	120	5	0	5	24	0	80
Minipack Blended Nonfat Strawberry	4.4 oz	120	5	0	5	23	0	85
Minipack Blended Nonfat Strawberry Banana	4.4 oz	120	5	0	5	23	0	85
Sprinkl'ins Cherry Vanilla	1 (4.1 oz)	130	5	2	5	24	0	85
Sprinkl'ins Strawberry	1 (4.1 oz)	130	5	2	5	24	0	85
Sprinkl'ins Strawberry Banana	1 (4.1 oz)	130	5	2	5	24	0	80
Sprinkl'ins Vanilla w/ Cherry Crystals	1 (4.1 oz)	110	5	1	5	21	0	85
Sprinkl'ins Vanilla w/ Orange Crystals	1 (4.1 oz)	110	5	1	5	21	0	85
Horizon Organic								
Fat Free Apricot Mango	¾ cup (6 oz)	120	7	0	<5	23	0	100
Fat Free Honey	1 cup (8 oz)	160	9	0	<5	32	0	135
LeCarb								
YoCarb Plain	1 pkg (4 oz)	50	5	3	10	3	—	110

FOOD	PORTION	CALS	PROT	FAT	CHOL	CARB	FIBER	SOD
Oberweis								
Peach	1 pkg (8 oz)	210	10	3	15	39	0	140
Pascual								
Nonfat Cherries & Berries	1 pkg (4.4 oz)	100	4	0	0	19	5	70
Nonfat Peach	1 pkg (4.4 oz)	100	4	0	0	19	5	70
Silk								
Organic Soy Strawberry	1 pkg (6 oz)	160	4	2	0	31	1	20
Soy Apricot Mango	1 pkg	160	4	2	0	30	1	20
Soy Banana Strawberry	1 pkg	160	4	2	0	30	1	20
Soy Black Cherry	1 pkg	160	4	2	0	29	1	20
Soy Blueberry	1 pkg	160	4	2	0	29	1	20
Soy Key Lime	1 pkg	170	4	2	0	30	1	20
Soy Lemon	1 pkg	160	4	2	0	31	1	20
Soy Lemon Kiwi	1 pkg	150	4	2	0	29	1	20
Soy Peach	1 pkg	170	4	2	0	32	1	20
Soy Plain	8 oz	120	5	3	0	22	1	30
Soy Raspberry	1 pkg	160	4	2	0	30	1	20
Soy Vanilla	1 pkg (8 oz)	120	4	2	0	23	1	20
Spega								
La Natura Low Fat	1 pkg (5.2 oz)	80	6	1	5	11	0	70
Stonyfield Farm								
Creamy Maple	1 pkg	160	6	6	25	19	0	90
Mocho-Ccino	1 pkg	170	6	6	20	23	0	95
Nonfat Apricot Mango	1 pkg (8 oz)	160	8	0	0	31	tr	125
Nonfat Black Cherry	1 pkg (8 oz)	160	8	0	0	31	tr	130
Nonfat Cappuccino	1 pkg (8 oz)	160	9	0	0	31	0	135
Nonfat Cherry Vanilla	1 pkg (8 oz)	190	7	0	0	43	tr	120

FOOD	PORTION	CALS	PROT	FAT	CHOL	CARB	FIBER	SOD
Nonfat Chocolate Underground	1 pkg (8 oz)	200	8	0	0	46	tr	135
Nonfat French Vanilla	1 pkg (8 oz)	180	9	0	0	30	0	135
Nonfat Lotsa Lemon	1 pkg (8 oz)	160	9	0	0	30	0	140
Nonfat Peach	1 pkg (8 oz)	150	8	0	0	30	tr	130
Nonfat Plain	1 pkg (8 oz)	100	10	0	<5	15	0	150
Nonfat Raspberry	1 pkg (8 oz)	160	8	0	0	31	tr	130
Nonfat Strawberry	1 pkg (8 oz)	180	8	0	0	32	tr	130
Organic French Vanilla	1 pkg	170	6	6	20	23	0	85
Organic Wild Blueberry	1 pkg	160	5	6	20	22	tr	85
Organic Lowfat Blueberry	1 pkg (6 oz)	130	5	2	5	23	1	90
Organic Lowfat Luscious Lemon	1 pkg (6 oz)	130	5	2	5	23	1	115
Organic Lowfat Maple Vanilla	1 pkg (6 oz)	120	6	2	6	19	0	90
Organic Lowfat Mocha Latte	1 pkg (6 oz)	120	6	2	5	20	0	85
Organic Lowfat Plain	1 cup (8 oz)	110	9	2	10	14	0	135
Organic Lowfat Raspberry	1 pkg (6 oz)	130	6	2	5	23	1	100
Organic Lowfat Strawberry	1 pkg (6 oz)	130	5	2	5	23	1	115
Organic Lowfat Vanilla	1 pkg (6 oz)	120	6	2	5	20	0	100
Strawberries & Cream	1 pkg	160	5	5	20	23	tr	110
Vanilla Truffle	1 pkg	220	7	5	20	37	tr	100
YoSelf Organic Chocolate	1 (4 oz)	110	4	1	0	21	2	65

FOOD	PORTION	CALS	PROT	FAT	CHOL	CARB	FIBER	SOD
YoSelf Organic Creme Carmel	1 (4 oz)	110	4	1	5	21	2	65
Yosqueeze Strawberry	1 tube (2 oz)	60	2	1	5	11	1	30
Total								
Greek Yogurt	1 pkg (5 oz)	180	10	12	25	10	0	180
Greek Yogurt 0% Fat	1 pkg (5 oz)	80	15	0	0	6	0	110
Greek Yogurt 1% Fat	1 pkg (5 oz)	120	8	8	25	8	0	120
Yoplait								
99% Fat Free Blueberry	6 oz	180	6	2	10	34	0	80
99% Fat Free Boysenberry	6 oz	180	6	2	10	34	0	80
99% Fat Free Cherry	6 oz	180	6	2	10	34	0	80
99% Fat Free Harvest Peach	6 oz	180	6	2	10	34	0	80
99% Fat Free Harvest Peach	4 oz	120	4	1	5	23	0	55
99% Fat Free Key Lime Pie	6 oz	180	6	2	10	34	0	80
99% Fat Free Lemon	6 oz	180	6	2	10	34	0	80
99% Fat Free Mixed Berry	6 oz	180	6	2	10	34	0	80
99% Fat Free Mixed Berry	4 oz	120	4	1	5	23	0	55
99% Fat Free Orange	6 oz	180	6	2	10	34	0	80
99% Fat Free Pina Colada	6 oz	180	6	2	10	34	0	80
99% Fat Free Pineapple	6 oz	180	6	2	10	34	0	80
99% Fat Free Raspberry	6 oz	180	6	2	10	34	0	80
99% Fat Free Strawberry	4 oz	120	4	1	5	23	0	55

FOOD	PORTION	CALS	PROT	FAT	CHOL	CARB	FIBER	SOD
99% Fat Free Strawberry	6 oz	180	6	2	10	43	0	80
99% Fat Free Strawberry Banana	4 oz	120	4	1	5	23	0	55
99% Fat Free Strawberry Banana	6 oz	180	6	2	10	34	0	80
99% Fat Free Strawberry Cheesecake	6 oz	180	6	2	10	34	0	80
Custard Style Banana	6 oz	190	7	4	15	32	0	100
Custard Style Blueberry	6 oz	190	7	4	15	32	0	100
Custard Style Cherry Vanilla	6 oz	190	7	4	15	32	0	100
Custard Style Key Lime Pie	6 oz	190	7	4	15	32	0	100
Custard Style Lemon	6 oz	190	7	4	15	32	0	100
Custard Style Peaches'n Cream	6 oz	190	7	4	15	32	0	100
Custard Style Raspberry	6 oz	190	7	4	15	32	0	100
Custard Style Raspberry Cheesecake	6 oz	190	7	4	15	32	0	100
Custard Style Strawberry	6 oz	190	7	4	15	32	0	100
Custard Style Strawberry Banana	6 oz	190	7	4	15	32	0	100
Custard Style Strawberry Vanilla	4 oz	120	5	2	10	21	0	70
Custard Style Vanilla	6 oz	190	8	4	15	32	0	95

FOOD	PORTION	CALS	PROT	FAT	CHOL	CARB	FIBER	SOD
Go-Gurt Strawberry Banana Burst	1 pkg (2.25 oz)	80	2	2	5	12	0	40
Go-Gurt Watermelon Meltdown	1 pkg (2.25 oz)	80	2	2	5	12	0	40
Light Amaretto Cheesecake	6 oz	90	6	0	5	16	0	95
Light Apricot Mango	6 oz	90	5	0	5	16	0	75
Light Banana Cream	6 oz	90	6	0	5	16	0	95
Light Blueberry	6 oz	90	5	0	5	16	0	75
Light Boston Cream Pie	6 oz	90	6	0	5	16	0	95
Light Caramel Apple	6 oz	90	6	0	5	16	0	95
Light Cherry	6 oz	90	5	0	5	16	0	75
Light Key Lime Pie	6 oz	90	6	0	5	16	0	95
Light Lemon Cream Pie	6 oz	90	6	0	5	16	0	95
Light Peach	6 oz	90	5	0	5	16	0	75
Light Peach Melba	6 oz	90	5	0	5	16	0	75
Light Raspberry	6 oz	90	5	0	5	16	0	75
Light Strawberry	6 oz	90	5	0	5	16	0	75
Light Strawberry Banana	6 oz	90	5	0	5	16	0	75
Light White Chocolate Strawberry	6 oz	90	5	0	5	16	0	75
Original Cafe Au Lait	6 oz	170	6	2	10	31	0	80
Original Coconut Cream Pie	6 oz	200	6	4	10	35	0	80
Original French Vanilla	6 oz	180	6	2	10	34	0	90
Trix Rainbow Punch	6 oz	190	6	2	10	36	0	85

FOOD	PORTION	CALS	PROT	FAT	CHOL	CARB	FIBER	SOD
Trix Raspberry Rainbow	6 oz	190	6	2	10	36	0	85
Trix Strawberry Banana Bash	6 oz	190	6	2	10	36	0	85
Trix Strawberry Punch	4 oz	130	4	2	5	24	0	55
Trix Triple Cherry	6 oz	190	6	2	10	36	0	85
Trix Watermelon Burst	4 oz	130	4	2	5	24	0	55
Trix Wild Berry Blue	4 oz	130	4	2	5	24	0	55
Whips! Orange Creme	1 pkg (4 oz)	140	5	3	10	23	–	75
Whips! Raspberry Mousse	1 pkg (4 oz)	140	5	3	10	23	–	75

YOGURT DRINKS
Dannon

FOOD	PORTION	CALS	PROT	FAT	CHOL	CARB	FIBER	SOD
Frusion Smoothie Peach Passion Fruit	1 bottle (10 oz)	270	8	4	15	51	0	180
Frusion Smoothie Tropical Fruit	1 bottle (10 oz)	270	8	4	15	52	0	130

Stonyfield

| Smoothie Lowfat Strawberry | 1 bottle (8.8 oz) | 250 | 10 | 3 | 10 | 46 | 4 | 160 |

Yo-Goat

| Blueberry | 8 oz | 150 | 8 | 8 | 30 | 13 | – | 135 |

Yoplait

| Nouriche All Flavors | 1 bottle (11 oz) | 290 | 10 | 0 | 5 | 60 | 6 | 290 |

YOGURT FROZEN

FOOD	PORTION	CALS	PROT	FAT	CHOL	CARB	FIBER	SOD
chocolate soft serve	½ cup (4 fl oz)	115	3	4	3	18	–	71
vanilla soft serve	½ cup (4 fl oz)	114	3	4	2	17	–	63

Breyers

| Chocolate | ½ cup | 150 | 3 | 5 | 15 | 23 | tr | 50 |
| Vanilla | ½ cup | 140 | 3 | 5 | 15 | 21 | 0 | 45 |

FOOD	PORTION	CALS	PROT	FAT	CHOL	CARB	FIBER	SOD
Vanilla No Sugar Added	½ cup	100	3	5	20	13	0	60
Edy's								
Black Cherry Vanilla Swirl	½ cup	90	3	0	0	20	–	45
Caramel Fudge Cosmo	½ cup	140	2	4	10	23	–	50
Caramel Praline Crunch	½ cup	100	3	0	0	23	–	60
Chocolate Decadence	½ cup	120	2	4	10	20	–	45
Chocolate Fudge	½ cup	100	3	0	0	22	–	55
Coffee Fudge Sundae	½ cup	100	3	0	0	22	–	60
Cookies'N Cream	½ cup	120	2	4	10	19	–	45
Heath Toffee Crunch	½ cup	120	2	4	10	18	–	45
Raspberry	½ cup	90	2	3	10	16	–	25
Ultimate Tin Roof Sundae	½ cup	130	3	4	5	20	–	50
Vanilla	½ cup	90	3	0	0	19	–	45
Vanilla Chocolate Swirl	½ cup	90	3	0	0	19	–	45
Haagen-Dazs								
Lowfat Dulce De Leche	½ cup	190	6	3	5	35	0	75
Nonfat Chocolate	½ cup	140	7	0	<5	28	tr	45
Nonfat Coffee	½ cup	140	7	0	<5	29	0	45
Nonfat Strawberry	½ cup	140	5	0	<5	31	0	40
Nonfat Vanilla	½ cup	140	6	0	<5	29	0	45
Nonfat Vanilla Raspberry Swirl	½ cup	130	4	0	<5	29	tr	30
Nonfat Vanilla Fudge	½ cup	160	6	0	<5	34	0	105
Turkey Hill								
Black Raspberry	½ cup	110	–	3	10	20	–	60
Caramel Cashew Crunch	½ cup	160	–	9	25	18	–	60

FOOD	PORTION	CALS	PROT	FAT	CHOL	CARB	FIBER	SOD
Chocolate Chip Cookie Dough	½ cup	140	3	5	10	23	0	120
Chocolate Chip Cookie Dough	½ cup	190	–	10	30	23	–	80
Clark Bar	½ cup	140	–	5	10	22	–	95
Fat Free Chocolate Cherry Cordial	½ cup	100	4	0	0	24	0	70
Fat Free Chocolate Marshmallow	½ cup	130	3	0	0	30	0	40
Fat Free Mint Cookies 'N Cream	½ cup	110	4	0	0	24	0	80
Fat Free Neapolitan	½ cup	100	3	0	0	22	0	50
Fat Free Orange Swirl	½ cup	100	–	0	0	22	–	40
Fat Free Vanilla Fudge	½ cup	110	3	0	0	24	0	80
Peach Raspberry	½ cup	110	3	2	10	20	0	60
Tin Roof Sundae	½ cup	140	4	5	10	21	0	100
Vanilla & Chocolate	½ cup	110	3	3	10	19	0	70
Vanilla Bean	½ cup	110	4	3	10	17	0	70
ZUCCHINI								
baby raw	1 (0.5 oz)	3	tr	tr	0	1	tr	0
canned italian style	½ cup	33	1	tr	0	8	–	427
frzn cooked	½ cup	19	1	tr	0	4	–	2
raw sliced	½ cup	9	1	tr	0	2	1	2
sliced cooked	½ cup	14	1	tr	0	4	1	2
Progresso								
Italian Style	½ cup (4.2 oz)	50	2	2	0	7	2	400
TAKE-OUT								
indian paalkora	1 serv	46	2	2	1	7	2	141

PART TWO

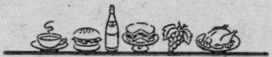

Restaurant Chains

Smart Stuff

Bigger isn't always better.
Supersizing, add-ons, toppings, extras, stuffed, doubles, and "buy one get one free" may cost little, but the extra calories, fat, and sodium you'll be tempted to eat are no bargain.

FOOD	PORTION	CALS	PROT	FAT	CHOL	CARB	FIBER	SOD

APPLEBEE'S
DESSERTS

FOOD	PORTION	CALS	PROT	FAT	CHOL	CARB	FIBER	SOD
Apple Betty Cobbler Ala Mode	1 serv	598	7	22	31	94	2	197
Berry Lemon Cheesecake	1 slice	230	–	7	–	–	2	–
Chocolate Raspberry Cake	1 slice	230	–	3	–	–	3	–
Fudge Brownie Sundae	1 serv	739	9	40	66	87	6	332
Low Fat Bikini Banana Strawberry Shortcake	1 serv	248	6	2	8	48	2	223
Low Fat Brownie Sundae	1 serv	415	11	2	3	82	3	417
Low Fat Marble Cheesecake	1 serv	261	10	2	10	50	4	378

MAIN MENU SELECTIONS

FOOD	PORTION	CALS	PROT	FAT	CHOL	CARB	FIBER	SOD
Applebee's Burger w/ Fries	1 serv	1274	55	79	263	90	7	2713
Baja Chicken Rollup	1 serv	490	–	10	–	–	10	–
Basic Hamburger w/ Fries	1 serv	980	31	58	118	86	6	1814
Beef Fajita Quesadilla	1 serv	1205	51	86	159	58	6	2969
Bourbon Street Steak w/ Fried New Potatoes	1 serv	1115	60	94	168	50	–	3542
Grilled Citrus Chicken Salad	1 serv	240	–	6	–	–	4	–
Grilled Talapia w/ Mango Salsa	1 serv	340	–	8	–	–	4	–
Low Fat Asian Chicken Salad	1 med serv (2.5 oz)	370	19	6	40	64	7	1431
Low Fat Asian Chicken Salad	1 serv (5 oz)	623	35	9	76	107	14	2487
Low Fat Blackened Chicken Salad	1 serv (5 oz)	411	56	5	82	39	11	2188

FOOD	PORTION	CALS	PROT	FAT	CHOL	CARB	FIBER	SOD
Low Fat Blackened Chicken Salad	1 med serv (2.5 oz)	287	40	3	43	27	6	1763
Low Fat Garlic ChickenPasta	1 serv	587	41	8	39	89	9	1551
Low Fat Lemon ChickenPasta	1 serv	528	33	11	50	78	8	2438
Low Fat Quesadilla Chicken Fajita	1 serv	518	42	11	35	63	2	2244
Low Fat Quesadilla Veggie	1 serv	344	27	8	8	46	3	1138
Mesquite Chicken Salad	1 serv	200	–	4	–	–	5	–
Mozzarella Stix	8 pieces	963	41	57	64	74	1	1990
Onion Soup Au Gratin	1 serv	150	–	8	–	–	1	–
Quesadillas	1 serv	684	31	46	99	40	4	2175
Riblet Basket w/ Fries	1 serv	1317	78	92	219	45	7	2697
Salad Dinner w/o Dressing	1 serv	303	22	18	277	13	3	661
Salad Santa Fe Chicken	1 med	724	33	42	96	56	7	2409
Sandwich Bacon Cheese Chicken Grill w/o Fries	1	746	46	46	133	36	1	1722
Sandwich Gyro	1	880	24	69	15	44	3	2015
Sizzling Chicken Skillet	1 serv	360	–	4	–	–	10	–
Stir Fry Chicken	1 serv	566	38	7	76	89	5	2470
Teriyaki Shrimp Skewers	1 serv	260	–	2	–	–	6	–
Tortilla Chicken Melt	1 serv	480	–	13	–	–	6	–

ARBY'S
BEVERAGES

FOOD	PORTION	CALS	PROT	FAT	CHOL	CARB	FIBER	SOD
Chocolate Shake	1 (14 oz)	480	10	16	45	84	0	370
Hot Chocolate	1 serv (8.6 oz)	110	2	1	0	23	0	120
Jamocha Shake	1 (14 oz)	470	10	15	45	82	0	390

FOOD	PORTION	CALS	PROT	FAT	CHOL	CARB	FIBER	SOD
Milk	1 serv (8 oz)	120	8	5	20	12	0	120
Orange Juice	1 serv (10 oz)	140	1	0	0	34	0	0
Strawberry Shake	1 (14 oz)	500	11	13	15	87	0	340
Vanilla Shake	1 (14 oz)	470	10	15	45	83	0	360
BREAKFAST SELECTIONS								
Add Egg	1 serv (2 oz)	110	5	9	175	2	0	170
Add Swiss Cheese Slice	1 slice (0.5 oz)	45	3	3	10	0	0	220
Biscuit w/ Bacon	1 (3.2 oz)	320	7	21	10	27	1	930
Biscuit w/ Butter	1 (2.9 oz)	280	5	17	0	27	1	780
Biscuit w/ Ham	1 (4.3 oz)	330	12	20	30	28	1	1610
Biscuit w/ Sausage	1 (4.2)	460	10	33	30	27	1	1150
Croissant w/ Bacon	1 (2.5 oz)	300	8	20	30	28	0	450
Croissant w/ Ham	1 (3.7 oz)	310	13	19	50	29	0	1130
Croissant w/ Sausage	1 (3.6 oz)	420	11	32	50	28	0	670
French Toast Syrup	1 serv (0.5 oz)	130	0	0	0	32	0	45
Sourdough w/ Bacon	1 (5 oz)	380	14	7	10	29	2	890
Sourdough w/ Ham	1 (4 oz)	220	12	7	30	30	1	1270
Sourdough w/ Sausage	1 (4 oz)	330	10	19	30	29	1	810
Toastix w/o Syrup	1 serv (4.4 oz)	370	7	17	0	48	4	440
DESSERTS								
Apple Turnover Iced	1 (4.5 oz)	420	4	16	0	65	2	230
Cherry Turnover Iced	1 (4.5 oz)	410	4	16	0	63	1	250
MAIN MENU SELECTIONS								
Arby's Sauce	1 serv (0.5 oz)	15	0	0	0	4	0	180
Au Jus Sauce	1 serv (3 oz)	5	tr	1	0	1	tr	386
Baked Potato Broccoli'N Cheddar	1 (14 oz)	540	12	24	50	71	7	680
Baked Potato Deluxe	1 (13 oz)	650	20	34	90	67	6	750

FOOD	PORTION	CALS	PROT	FAT	CHOL	CARB	FIBER	SOD
Baked Potato w/ Butter & Sour Cream	1 (11.2 oz)	500	8	24	55	65	6	170
BBQ Dipping Sauce	1 serv (1 oz)	40	0	0	0	10	0	350
Bronco Berry Sauce	1 serv (1.5 oz)	90	0	0	0	23	0	35
Chicken Finger 4-Pak	1 serv (6.77 oz)	640	31	38	70	42	0	1590
Chicken Finger Snack w/ Curly Fries	1 serv (6.4 oz)	580	19	32	35	55	3	1450
Curly Fries	1 sm (3.8 oz)	310	4	15	0	39	3	770
Curly Fries	1 lg (7 oz)	620	8	30	0	78	7	1540
Curly Fries	1 med (4.5 oz)	400	5	20	0	50	4	990
Curly Fries Cheddar	1 serv (6 oz)	460	6	24	5	54	4	1290
German Mustard	1 pkg (0.25 oz)	5	0	0	0	0	0	60
Homestyle Fries	1 sm (4 oz)	300	3	13	0	42	3	570
Homestyle Fries	1 med (5 oz)	370	4	16	0	53	4	710
Homestyle Fries	1 lg (7.5 oz)	560	6	24	0	79	6	1070
Homestyle Fries Child-Size	1 serv (3 oz)	220	3	10	0	32	3	430
Honey Mustard	1 serv (1 oz)	130	0	12	10	5	0	160
Horsey Sauce	1 pkg (0.5 oz)	60	0	5	5	3	0	150
Jalapeno Bites	1 serv (4 oz)	330	7	21	40	30	2	670
Ketchup	1 pkg (0.3 oz)	10	0	0	0	2	0	100
Marinara Sauce	1 serv (1.5 oz)	35	1	1	0	4	0	260
Mayonnaise	1 pkg (0.4 oz)	90	0	10	10	0	0	65
Mayonnaise Light Cholesterol Free	1 pkg (0.4 oz)	20	0	2	0	1	0	110
Mozzarella Sticks	4 (4.8 oz)	470	18	29	60	34	2	1330
Onion Petals	1 serv (4 oz)	410	4	24	0	43	2	300
Potato Cakes	2 (3.5 oz)	250	2	16	0	26	3	490
Sandwich Chicken Bacon 'N Swiss	1 (7.4 oz)	610	31	33	110	49	2	1550
Sandwich Chicken Breast Fillet	1 (7.2 oz)	540	24	30	90	47	2	1160

FOOD	PORTION	CALS	PROT	FAT	CHOL	CARB	FIBER	SOD
Sandwich Chicken Cordon Bleu	1 (8.4 oz)	630	34	35	120	47	2	1820
Sandwich Grilled Chicken Deluxe	1 (8.7 oz)	450	29	22	110	37	2	1050
Sandwich Hot Ham 'N Swiss	1 (5.9 oz)	340	23	13	90	35	1	1450
Sandwich Market Fresh Roast Beef & Swiss	1 (12.5 oz)	810	37	42	130	73	5	1780
Sandwich Market Fresh Roast Beef Ranch & Bacon	1 (13.5 oz)	880	48	44	155	74	5	2320
Sandwich Market Fresh Roast Chicken Caesar	1 (12.7 oz)	820	43	38	140	75	5	2160
Sandwich Market Fresh Roast Ham & Swiss	1 (12.5 oz)	730	36	34	125	74	5	2180
Sandwich Market Fresh Roast Turkey & Swiss	1 (12.5 oz)	760	43	33	130	75	5	1920
Sandwich Market Fresh Ultimate BLT	1 (10.5 oz)	820	24	49	110	72	5	1480
Sandwich Roast Beef Arby-Q	1 (6.4 oz)	360	16	14	70	40	2	1530
Sandwich Roast Beef Beef'N Cheddar	1 (6.9 oz)	480	23	24	90	43	2	1240
Sandwich Roast Beef Big Montana	1 (11 oz)	630	47	32	155	41	3	2080
Sandwich Roast Beef Giant	1 (7.9 oz)	480	32	23	110	41	3	1440
Sandwich Roast Beef Junior	1 (4.4 oz)	310	16	13	70	34	2	740
Sandwich Roast Beef Melt w/ Cheddar	1 (5.2 oz)	340	16	15	70	36	2	890

FOOD	PORTION	CALS	PROT	FAT	CHOL	CARB	FIBER	SOD
Sandwich Roast Beef Regular	1 (5.4 oz)	350	21	16	85	34	2	950
Sandwich Roast Beef Super	1 (8.5 oz)	470	22	23	85	47	3	1130
Sandwich Roast Chicken Club	1 (8.4 oz)	520	29	28	115	38	2	1440
Sub Sandwich French Dip	1 (10 oz)	440	28	18	100	42	2	1680
Sub Sandwich Hot Ham'N Swiss	1 (9.7 oz)	530	29	27	110	45	3	1860
Sub Sandwich Italian	1 (11 oz)	780	29	53	120	49	3	2440
Sub Sandwich Philly Beef'N Swiss	1 (10.8 oz)	700	36	42	130	46	4	1940
Sub Sandwich Roast Beef	1 (11.6 oz)	760	35	48	130	47	3	2230
Sub Sandwich Roast Beef	1 (11.6 oz)	760	35	48	130	47	3	2230
Sub Sandwich Turkey	1 (10.6 oz)	630	26	37	100	51	2	2170
Tangy Southwest Sauce	1 serv (1.5 oz)	250	0	26	30	3	0	290
SALAD DRESSINGS								
Bleu Cheese	1 serv (2 oz)	300	2	31	45	3	0	580
Buttermilk Ranch	1 serv (2 oz)	290	1	30	25	3	0	580
Buttermilk Ranch Light	1 serv (2 oz)	100	1	6	0	12	1	480
Caesar	1 serv (2 oz)	310	1	34	60	1	0	470
Honey French	1 serv (2 oz)	290	0	24	0	18	tr	410
Italian Reduced Calorie	1 serv (2 oz)	25	0	1	0	3	tr	1030
Italian Parmesan	1 serv (2 oz)	240	1	24	0	4	0	950
Thousand Island	1 serv (2 oz)	290	1	28	35	9	0	480
SALADS AND SALAD BARS								
Caesar Side Salad	1 (5 oz)	45	4	2	5	4	2	95
Caesar Salad w/o Dressing	1 serv (8 oz)	90	7	4	10	8	3	170
Chicken Finger w/o Dressing	1 serv (13 oz)	570	30	34	65	39	3	1300

FOOD	PORTION	CALS	PROT	FAT	CHOL	CARB	FIBER	SOD
Croutons Seasoned	1 serv (0.25 oz)	30	1	1	0	5	1	70
Croutons Cheese & Garlic	1 serv (0.63 oz)	100	3	6	—	10	0	138
Garden Salad	1 (12.3 oz)	70	4	1	0	14	6	45
Grilled Chicken	1 serv (16.3 oz)	210	30	5	65	14	6	800
Grilled Chicken Caesar w/o Dressing	1 serv (12 oz)	230	33	8	80	8	3	920
Roast Chicken	1 serv (14.8 oz)	160	20	3	40	15	6	700
Side Salad	1 (5.7 oz)	25	2	0	0	5	2	20
Turkey Club Salad w/o Dressing	1 serv (12 oz)	350	33	21	90	9	3	920

AU BON PAIN
BAKED SELECTIONS

FOOD	PORTION	CALS	PROT	FAT	CHOL	CARB	FIBER	SOD
Bagel Cinnamon Crisp	1 (6 oz)	540	12	7	0	123	4	470
Baguette	1 loaf (10.6 oz)	680	28	3	0	136	6	1820
Bread Stick	1 (2.3 oz)	200	7	3	0	37	2	610
Cinnamon Roll	1 (4 oz)	300	7	5	20	60	2	280
Cookie Chocolate Chip	1 (2 oz)	230	3	7	20	39	1	125
Cookie Chocolate Chunk Macadamia	1 (2 oz)	250	3	13	25	31	1	230
Cookie Gingerbread Man w/ Raisins & Icing	1 (2.7 oz)	280	4	7	30	52	tr	250
Cookie Oatmeal Raisin	1 (2 oz)	210	3	6	20	38	2	190
Cookie Peanut Butter	1 (2 oz)	240	6	12	20	21	2	250
Cookie Shortbread	1 (2.3 oz)	240	5	7	15	44	1	260
Cookie Walnut Raisin	1 (2 oz)	250	4	13	20	31	2	210

FOOD	PORTION	CALS	PROT	FAT	CHOL	CARB	FIBER	SOD
Cookie English Toffee	1 (2 oz)	230	3	7	35	38	tr	200
Creme De Fleur	1 serv (5.55 oz)	470	12	19	70	69	2	530
Croissant Almond	1 (4.7 oz)	480	12	25	95	58	3	400
Croissant Apple	1 (3.5 oz)	200	5	3	20	40	2	200
Croissant Chocolate	1 (3.1 oz)	330	8	10	20	53	3	250
Croissant Cinnamon Raisin	1 (3.8 oz)	300	8	5	20	60	2	300
Croissant Raspberry Cheese	1 (3.6 oz)	290	8	9	45	47	1	310
Croissant Sweet Cheese	1 (3.6 oz)	320	8	12	60	46	1	350
Danish Cranberry	1 (4.5 oz)	350	7	9	45	59	2	360
Danish Lemon	1 (4.3 oz)	340	8	9	45	59	5	320
Danish Sweet Cheese	1 (4.2 oz)	390	9	16	70	55	1	380
Focaccia	1 piece (5.4 oz)	430	12	16	0	61	3	760
Four Grain Bread	1 serv (4.7 oz)	400	18	4	0	74	3	1110
French Roll	1 (4.2 oz)	260	11	1	0	53	2	710
French Roll Roast Beef	1 (11 oz)	540	39	19	80	58	3	1600
Hearth Roll	1 (3 oz)	210	10	2	0	38	2	430
Holiday Cookie w/ Icing & Sprinkles	1 (1.6 oz)	150	2	3	10	31	0	70
Loaf Multigrain	1 slice (1.8 oz)	130	6	1	0	24	1	360
Muffin Banana Walnut	1 (5.4 oz)	430	8	21	45	57	2	380
Muffin Blueberry	1 (5.6 oz)	470	8	15	90	79	2	450
Muffin Bran Raisin	1 (5.5 oz)	400	9	12	50	77	8	1060
Muffin Carrot	1 (5.8 oz)	520	9	25	55	67	4	780
Muffin Corn	1 (5.7 oz)	390	7	16	60	56	2	500
Muffin Cranberry Walnut	1 (5.4 oz)	500	9	27	50	57	3	430
Muffin Milk Chocolate Chunk	1 (5.3 oz)	530	9	23	65	77	3	390

FOOD	PORTION	CALS	PROT	FAT	CHOL	CARB	FIBER	SOD
Muffin Pumpkin	1 (6 oz)	510	9	18	65	74	3	350
Muffin Low Fat 3 Berry	1 (4.4 oz)	270	4	3	25	58	2	300
Muffin Low Fat Chocolate Cake	1 (4.2 oz)	470	0	0	0	117	0	—
Parisienne Loaf	1 loaf (19 oz)	1210	50	5	0	244	11	3220
Petit Pain	1 (2.9 oz)	180	7	1	0	37	2	490
Roll Braided w/ Topping	1 (10 oz)	430	13	14	40	63	3	730
Roll Pecan	1 (6 oz)	620	11	24	15	94	3	470
Sandwich Loaf Country White	1 serv (1.75 oz)	110	5	1	0	23	1	290
Sandwich Loaf Tomato Herb	1 serv (1.75 oz)	120	5	1	0	27	1	300
Scone Chocolate Walnut	1 (4 oz)	420	8	19	55	56	3	125
Scone Cranberry Orange Almond	1 (4 oz)	400	8	15	77	60	3	190
Scone Maple Oat Pecan Date	1 (4 oz)	410	7	17	60	58	3	170
Scone Orange	1 (4.2 oz)	370	10	13	115	56	2	310
Shortbread Heart ½ Chocolate	1 (2.7 oz)	290	6	10	20	51	1	280
Shortbread Heart w/ Red Sugar	1 (2.5 oz)	270	5	7	15	51	1	260
Sourdough Bagel Asiago Cheese	1 (4.8 oz)	340	16	5	15	57	2	560
Sourdough Bagel Cheddar Scallion	1 (4.1 oz)	310	15	5	10	51	2	610
Sourdough Bagel Cinnamon Crisp	1 (4.6 oz)	360	11	5	0	52	3	430
Sourdough Bagel Cinnamon Raisin	1 (4.5 oz)	300	11	1	0	65	3	440
Sourdough Bagel Cranberry Nut	1 (4.7 oz)	400	12	7	0	73	6	440
Sourdough Bagel Cranberry Nut	1 (4.7 oz)	400	12	7	0	73	6	440

FOOD	PORTION	CALS	PROT	FAT	CHOL	CARB	FIBER	SOD
Sourdough Bagel Double Cheddar Jalpeno	1 serv (4.1 oz)	320	14	6	20	50	2	580
Sourdough Bagel Dutch Apple	1 (4.7 oz)	380	11	3	0	80	4	440
Sourdough Bagel Everything	1 (4.4 oz)	330	13	3	0	54	3	710
Sourdough Bagel Focaccia	1 (4.1 oz)	320	12	5	0	61	3	990
Sourdough Bagel Honey 9 Grain	1 (4.8 oz)	310	12	2	0	66	6	490
Sourdough Bagel Onion	1 (4.4 oz)	320	12	1	0	67	3	480
Sourdough Bagel Plain	1 (4 oz)	300	12	1	0	61	3	480
Sourdough Bagel Poppy Seed	1 (4.4 oz)	330	13	3	0	64	3	480
Sourdough Bagel Sesame	1 (4.4 oz)	340	13	4	0	64	3	480
Sourdough Bagel Wild Blueberry	1 (4.1 oz)	280	10	1	0	58	3	410
Streudel Cherry	1 serv (4 oz)	380	4	23	0	37	tr	90
Streudel Apple	1 serv (4.35 oz)	400	4	23	0	48	tr	110
SALADS AND SALAD BARS								
Caesar w/o Dressing	1 serv (7.8 oz)	240	13	12	30	19	4	370
Chef's	1 serv (10.3 oz)	290	27	15	65	11	3	1290
Chicken Caesar	1 serv (10.2 oz)	380	34	18	85	19	4	420
Chicken Oriental	1 serv (8.6 oz)	220	24	6	60	16	5	75
Chicken Pesto Salad	1 serv (8 oz)	400	40	23	105	7	2	310
Garden	1 serv (9.3 oz)	160	6	5	0	26	5	320
Garden Side	1 serv (5.1 oz)	90	3	2	0	14	3	160

FOOD	PORTION	CALS	PROT	FAT	CHOL	CARB	FIBER	SOD
Gorgonzola & Walnut	1 serv (5 oz)	330	11	28	25	8	5	410
Mozzarella & Red Pepper Salad	1 serv (10.5 oz)	360	23	25	90	10	2	380
Tuna	1 serv (13.2 oz)	440	27	24	35	28	5	710
SANDWICHES AND FILLINGS								
Club Hot Roasted Turkey	1 (11.7 oz)	630	43	28	80	53	3	2290
Cream Cheese Plain	1 serv (2 oz)	190	4	10	55	0	0	210
Cream Cheese Reduced Fat Honey Walnut	1 serv (2 oz)	150	4	10	35	10	0	180
Cream Cheese Reduced Fat Sundried Tomato	1 serv (2 oz)	140	5	12	40	3	0	410
Cream Cheese Reduced Fat Veggie	1 serv (2 oz)	140	6	12	40	3	0	360
Croissant Spinach & Cheese	1 (3.6 oz)	220	9	9	35	29	2	360
Croque Madame	1 (11 oz)	570	40	22	75	53	3	1580
Croque Monsieur	1 (11 oz)	590	39	25	85	53	3	1740
Egg On A Bagel	1 serv (7.1 oz)	500	29	5	120	64	4	880
Egg On A Bagel w/ Bacon	1 serv (7.6 oz)	580	34	12	130	84	4	1110
Egg On A Bagel w/ Cheese	1 serv (7.85 oz)	590	25	12	145	84	4	1020
Egg On A Bagel w/ Cheese & Bacon	1 serv (8.35 oz)	670	39	19	155	84	4	1250
Focaccia Chicken & Mozzarella	1 serv (13.75 oz)	800	93	14	125	73	6	2430
Focaccia Chicken Tarragon w/ Field Greens	1 (12.5 oz)	870	47	47	115	54	4	1080

FOOD	PORTION	CALS	PROT	FAT	CHOL	CARB	FIBER	SOD
Focaccia Garden Vegetable Goat Cheese w/ Artichoke Spread	1 (14.25 oz)	570	20	21	25	75	5	1210
Focaccia Hickory Smoked Ham & Brie	1 (13.3 oz)	620	51	27	100	72	5	2320
Focaccia Smoked Turkey & Swiss w/ Cilantro	1 (13.25 oz)	810	42	40	90	68	4	2280
Fo-Ca-Cha-Cha Chicken	1 serv (11.15 oz)	730	68	17	110	75	9	2030
French Roll Ham	1 (11 oz)	390	32	16	65	58	3	2430
French Roll Hot Grilled Chicken	1 (11 oz)	620	46	23	100	57	3	1220
French Roll Hot Roast Turkey	1 (11 oz)	500	33	15	55	59	3	2020
French Roll Tuna	1 (10.6 oz)	550	33	21	35	58	4	1100
Hot Croissant Spinach & Cheese	1 (4 oz)	290	15	9	45	39	1	630
Pane Bagniate	1 (12 oz)	670	34	28	30	71	6	1220
Sandwich Arizona Chicken	1 (12 oz)	600	61	15	120	56	4	1390
Sandwich Cheese	1 (7.2 oz)	590	35	26	60	54	2	920
Sandwich Fresh Mozzarella Tomato & Pesto	1 (11 oz)	790	38	43	100	60	3	1140
Sandwich Honey Dijon Chicken	1 (13.6 oz)	750	66	24	145	65	3	2410
Sandwich Thai Chicken	1 (11.4 oz)	550	47	12	95	62	3	1080
Wrap Chicken Caesar	1 (10.5 oz)	640	43	26	115	61	5	920
Wrap Fields & Feta	1 (13.5 oz)	620	22	19	15	100	14	950
Wrap Honey Smoked Turkey	1 (15 oz)	520	36	7	35	85	11	1460
Wrap Roast Beef & Brie	1 (14 oz)	570	47	28	125	64	6	1160

FOOD	PORTION	CALS	PROT	FAT	CHOL	CARB	FIBER	SOD
SOUPS								
Autumn Pumpkin	1 serv (8 oz)	170	3	9	20	18	5	770
Black Bean	1 serv (8 oz)	180	11	1	0	33	18	910
Chicken Florentine	1 serv (8 oz)	140	4	8	30	14	1	660
Chicken Noodle	1 serv (8 oz)	100	8	2	15	12	1	760
Clam Chowder	1 serv (8 oz)	220	8	15	35	16	1	780
Corn & Green Chili Bisque	1 serv (8 oz)	200	5	10	30	21	2	1130
Corn Chowder	1 serv (8 oz)	270	6	15	40	28	2	580
Curried Rice & Lentil	1 serv (8 oz)	140	7	2	0	24	5	1220
French Moroccan Tomato Lentil	1 serv (8 oz)	130	7	2	0	22	7	550
Garden Vegetable	1 serv (8 oz)	50	2	1	0	8	2	720
Low Sodium Mediterranean Pepper	1 serv (12 oz)	280	12	6	0	44	10	640
Low Sodium Southwest Vegetable	1 serv (12 oz)	220	8	5	0	34	6	380
Old Fashioned Tomato	1 serv (8 oz)	140	4	6	10	19	2	1080
Pasta E Fagioli	1 serv (8 oz)	240	10	7	5	36	7	780
Potato Cheese	1 serv (8 oz)	190	5	10	5	21	1	910
Potato Leek	1 serv (8 oz)	200	4	13	45	18	2	1060
Red Beans & Rice	1 serv (8 oz)	200	11	5	10	31	12	690
Soup Bread Bowl	1 (9.25 oz)	600	26	3	0	118	5	1700
Southern Black Eyed Pea	1 serv (8 oz)	320	19	2	5	56	20	670
Split Pea	1 serv (8 oz)	160	12	1	5	27	9	800
Tomato Florentine	1 serv (8 oz)	120	5	3	5	17	2	1050
Tuscan Vegetable	1 serv (8 oz)	140	6	4	5	22	3	750
Vegetable Beef Barley	1 serv (8 oz)	110	7	3	10	14	3	1070
Vegetarian Lentil	1 serv (8 oz)	120	7	1	0	21	8	860
Vegetarian Chili	1 serv (8 oz)	170	9	2	0	31	15	940
Wild Mushroom Bisque	1 serv (8 oz)	140	4	7	5	16	2	1190

FOOD	PORTION	CALS	PROT	FAT	CHOL	CARB	FIBER	SOD
AUNTIE ANNE'S								
BEVERAGES								
Dutch Ice Blue Raspberry	1 (14 oz)	165	0	0	0	38	0	20
Dutch Ice Grape	1 (14 oz)	180	0	0	0	43	0	20
Dutch Ice Kiwi Banana	1 (14 oz)	190	0	0	0	44	0	30
Dutch Ice Lemonade	1 (14 oz)	315	0	0	0	77	0	0
Dutch Ice Mocha	1 (14 oz)	400	0	10	0	74	0	100
Dutch Ice Orange Creme	1 (14 oz)	280	0	0	0	64	0	35
Dutch Ice Pina Colada	1 (14 oz)	220	0	0	0	53	0	15
Dutch Ice Strawberry	1 (14 oz)	220	0	0	0	50	0	40
Dutch Ice Wild Cherry	1 (14 oz)	210	0	0	0	48	0	25
Dutch Shake Chocolate	1 (14 oz)	580	10	27	105	75	0	380
Dutch Shake Coffee	1 (14 oz)	590	10	27	105	77	0	304
Dutch Shake Strawberry	1 (14 oz)	610	10	27	105	78	0	304
Dutch Shake Vanilla	1 (14 oz)	510	10	27	105	58	0	300
Dutch Smoothie Blue Raspberry	1 (14 oz)	230	3	8	30	34	0	100
Dutch Smoothie Grape	1 (14 oz)	230	3	8	30	36	0	100
Dutch Smoothie Kiwi Banana	1 (14 oz)	240	3	8	30	38	0	100
Dutch Smoothie Lemonade	1 (14 oz)	300	3	8	30	53	0	80
Dutch Smoothie Mocha	1 (14 oz)	330	3	13	30	50	0	130
Dutch Smoothie Orange Creme	1 (14 oz)	280	3	8	30	46	0	100
Dutch Smoothie Pina Colada	1 (14 oz)	260	3	8	30	44	0	90
Dutch Smoothie Strawberry	1 (14 oz)	250	3	8	30	40	0	100

FOOD	PORTION	CALS	PROT	FAT	CHOL	CARB	FIBER	SOD
Dutch Smoothie Wild Cherry	1 (14 oz)	250	3	8	30	41	0	90
Lemonade	1 (22 oz)	180	0	0	0	43	0	0
Lemonade Strawberry	1 (22 oz)	190	0	0	0	48	0	0
DIPPING SAUCES								
Caramel Dip	1 serv (1.5 oz)	135	1	3	5	27	0	110
Cheese Sauce	1 serv (1.25 oz)	100	3	8	10	4	0	510
Chocolate Dip	1 serv (1.25 oz)	130	1	4	2	24	1	65
Cream Cheese Light	1 serv (1.25 oz)	70	3	6	25	1	0	140
Cream Cheese Strawberry	1 serv (1.25 oz)	110	2	10	35	4	0	105
Hot Salsa Cheese	1 serv (1.25 oz)	100	2	8	10	4	0	550
Marinara Sauce	1 serv (1.25 oz)	10	0	0	0	4	0	180
Sweet Mustard	1 serv (1.25 oz)	60	tr	2	40	8	0	120
PRETZELS								
Almond	1	400	9	8	20	72	2	400
Almond w/o Butter	1	350	9	2	0	72	2	390
Cinnamon Raisin w/o Butter	1	350	9	2	0	74	2	410
Cinnamon Sugar	1	450	8	9	25	83	3	430
Garlic	1	350	9	5	10	68	2	850
Garlic w/o Butter	1	320	9	1	0	66	2	830
Glazin' Raisin	1	510	11	4	10	107	4	480
Glazin' Raisin w/o Butter	1	470	11	1	0	104	3	460
Jalapeno	1	310	8	5	10	59	2	940
Jalapeno w/o Butter	1	270	8	1	0	58	2	780
Maple Crumb	1	550	10	6	10	112	3	550
Maple Crumb w/o Butter	1	520	10	3	0	112	3	550
Original	1	370	10	4	10	72	2	930

FOOD	PORTION	CALS	PROT	FAT	CHOL	CARB	FIBER	SOD
Original w/o Butter	1	340	10	1	0	72	3	900
Parmesan Herb	1	440	10	13	30	72	9	660
Parmesan Herb w/o Butter	1	390	11	5	10	74	4	780
Sesame	1	410	12	12	15	64	7	860
Sesame w/o Butter	1	350	11	6	0	63	3	840
Sour Cream & Onion w/o Butter	1	310	9	1	0	66	2	920
Sour Cream & Onion	1	340	9	5	10	66	2	930
Stixs	4	247	7	3	7	48	2	620
Stixs w/o Butter	4	227	7	1	0	48	2	600
Whole Wheat	1	370	11	5	10	72	7	1120
Whole Wheat w/o Butter	1	350	11	2	0	72	7	1100

BAJA FRESH
MAIN MENU SELECTIONS

FOOD	PORTION	CALS	PROT	FAT	CHOL	CARB	FIBER	SOD
Baja Burrito Chicken	1 serv	820	54	35	130	75	11	—
Baja Burrito Steak	1 serv	920	59	42	155	75	9	—
Black Beans	1 serv	360	23	3	5	61	26	1120
Burrito Bean & Cheese Chicken	1 serv	1000	69	33	145	104	21	2080
Burrito Bean & Cheese Steak	1 serv	1100	74	41	170	104	20	2090
Burrito Bean & Cheese Vegetarian	1 serv	870	41	31	70	104	20	1640
Burrito Dos Manos Chicken	1 full serv	1480	76	40	130	202	28	3680
Burrito Dos Manos Steak	1 full serv	1580	42	48	160	202	26	3680
Burrito Mexicano Chicken	1 serv	830	51	13	75	124	20	2110
Burrito Mexicano Steak	1 serv	920	56	20	100	124	19	2120
Burrito Ultimo Chicken	1 serv	860	55	30	130	90	10	2000
Burrito Ultimo Steak	1 serv	950	59	37	155	90	8	2010

FOOD	PORTION	CALS	PROT	FAT	CHOL	CARB	FIBER	SOD
Cebollitas	1 serv	40	1	2	0	5	3	160
Chips & Salsa Baja	1 serv	1100	17	50	0	134	17	1210
Enchiladas Cheese	1 serv	850	39	37	90	92	19	2310
Enchiladas Chicken	1 serv	780	48	25	100	91	20	2340
Enchiladas Steak	1 serv	890	51	33	125	94	20	2530
Enchiladas Verde Cheese	1 serv	840	39	35	90	91	19	2440
Enchiladas Verde Chicken	1 serv	770	48	23	100	91	20	2630
Enchiladas Verde Vegetarian	1 serv	720	30	22	50	100	21	2450
Fajitas Chicken Corn Tortillas	1 serv	1200	77	29	155	164	36	2780
Fajitas Chicken Flour Tortillas	1 serv	1360	82	37	155	176	32	3310
Fajitas Steak Corn Tortillas	1 serv	1360	87	42	205	164	33	2830
Fajitas Steak Flour Tortillas	1 serv	1530	92	50	205	176	30	3350
Grilled Vegetarian	1 serv	770	32	27	60	100	16	1680
Mini Quesa-Dita Cheese	1 serv	620	27	20	45	81	15	1480
Mini Quesa-Dita Chicken	1 serv	670	37	21	70	81	16	1640
Mini Quesa-Dita Steak	1 serv	700	38	23	80	81	15	1630
Mini Tosta-Dita Chicken	1 serv	570	32	17	55	67	13	1550
Mini Tosta-Dita Steak	1 serv	630	35	22	75	67	12	1560
Nachos Cheese	1 serv	1880	65	103	175	166	33	2590
Nachos Chicken	1 serv	2010	93	105	245	166	34	3030
Nachos Steak	1 serv	2100	98	113	275	166	33	3050
Pinto Beans	1 serv	320	19	1	5	56	21	840
Quesadilla	1 serv	1180	49	70	175	92	12	2330
Quesadilla Cheese	1 serv	1130	48	69	170	80	9	2170
Quesadilla Chicken	1 serv	1260	76	71	245	80	10	2170
Quesadilla Steak	1 serv	1350	81	79	270	80	9	2620
Rice	1 serv	280	5	4	0	55	4	980

FOOD	PORTION	CALS	PROT	FAT	CHOL	CARB	FIBER	SOD
Taco Baja Style Chicken	1 serv	190	13	5	25	26	4	310
Taco Baja Style Steak	1 serv	220	14	7	30	26	3	300
Taco Baja Style Wild Gulf Shrimp	1 serv	190	12	5	90	26	3	350
Taco Chilito Chicken	1 serv	320	20	10	40	38	9	600
Taco Chilito Steak	1 serv	340	21	12	45	38	8	600
Taco Fish	1 serv	270	9	13	15	31	3	480
Taco Mahi Mahi	1 serv	260	13	10	20	32	6	460
Taquitos Chicken w/ Beans	1 serv	750	30	36	85	64	9	—
Taquitos Chicken w/ Rice	1 serv	710	30	36	80	64	9	—
Taquitos Steak w/ Beans	1 serv	820	40	42	105	69	20	—
Taquitos Steak w/ Rice	1 serv	790	32	42	105	67	10	—
Tostada Chicken	1 serv	1140	61	52	120	102	30	2430
Tostada Steak	1 serv	1230	66	60	145	102	28	2440
Tostada Vegetarian	1 serv	1010	33	50	45	102	28	1990
SALAD DRESSINGS								
Fat Free Salsa Verde	1 serv (2.6 oz)	15	0	0	0	3	0	290
Guacamole	2 oz	70	1	6	0	5	4	190
Olive Oil Vinaigrette	1 serv (2.6 oz)	230	0	25	0	1	0	230
Pico De Gallo	1 serv	50	2	1	0	12	3	890
Pronto Guacamole	1 serv	550	8	30	0	61	11	380
Ranch	1 serv (2.6 oz)	220	1	19	15	6	0	440
Salsa Baja	1 serv	70	2	3	0	7	4	970
Salsa Roja	1 serv	70	3	1	0	13	4	1080
Salsa Verde	1 serv	50	2	0	0	11	3	1170
Sour Cream	1 oz	60	1	5	15	2	0	50
SALADS AND SALAD BARS								
Baja Ensalada Chicken	1 serv	310	47	18	110	17	7	1210
Baja Ensalada Fish	1 serv	360	35	15	70	27	10	1030

FOOD	PORTION	CALS	PROT	FAT	CHOL	CARB	FIBER	SOD
Baja Ensalada Steak	1 serv	460	55	18	150	17	5	1250
Side Salad	1 serv	70	4	3	5	10	3	240

BASKIN-ROBBINS
FROZEN YOGURT

FOOD	PORTION	CALS	PROT	FAT	CHOL	CARB	FIBER	SOD
Cafe Mocha Truly Free Soft Serve	1 reg	140	–	1	5	27	–	130
Chocolate Nonfat Soft Serve	1 reg	190	–	1	5	39	–	125
Lowfat Maui Brownie Madness	1 reg	250	38	9	20	34	–	130

ICE CREAM

FOOD	PORTION	CALS	PROT	FAT	CHOL	CARB	FIBER	SOD
Cappuccino Blast w/ Whipped Cream	1 reg	340	–	16	70	44	–	120
Chocolate	1 reg	270	–	16	55	31	–	105
Chocolate Chip	1 reg	270	–	17	60	26	–	80
Espresso'n Cream Lowfat	1 reg	180	–	3	10	31	–	100
Jamoca Almond Fudge	1 reg	280	–	16	45	30	–	70
Peach Crumb Pie No Sugar Added	1 reg	180	–	5	10	27	–	170
Pralines'n Cream	1 reg	280	–	15	50	33	–	160
Shake Chocolate	16 oz	750	–	43	115	80	–	290
Shake Vanilla	16 oz	630	–	35	170	69	–	220
Smoothie Very Strawberry w/ Soft Serve Ice Cream	1 reg	320	–	1	5	70	–	160
Thin Mint No Sugar Added	1 reg	160	–	4	10	27	–	110
Vanilla	1 reg	270	–	16	80	24	–	60

ICES

FOOD	PORTION	CALS	PROT	FAT	CHOL	CARB	FIBER	SOD
Daiquiri Ice	1 reg	130	0	0	0	33	–	10
Sherbet Rainbow	1 reg	160	–	2	10	34	–	35
Sorbet Peachy Keen	1 reg	110	–	0	0	29	–	10

BEAR ROCK CAFE
BAKED SELECTIONS

FOOD	PORTION	CALS	PROT	FAT	CHOL	CARB	FIBER	SOD
Almond French Horn	1	491	8	23	5	68	4	471

FOOD	PORTION	CALS	PROT	FAT	CHOL	CARB	FIBER	SOD
Bear Claw	1	260	8	6	20	43	1	350
Cinnamon Roll w/ Cream Cheese Icing	1	540	9	26	25	68	2	540
English Muffin	1	120	4	1	0	25	1	200
Pecan Sticky Bun	1	555	6	33	25	52	2	500
SALAD DRESSINGS								
Balsamic Vinaigrette	1 serv (1.5 oz)	156	0	17	0	1	0	397
Blue Cheese	1 serv (1.5 oz)	230	1	25	25	2	0	380
Caesar	1 serv (1.5 oz)	198	3	21	21	3	0	595
Creamy Italian	1 serv (1.5 oz)	180	0	18	0	4	0	420
Fat Free Ranch	1 serv (1.5 oz)	40	0	0	0	11	1	560
Fat Free Vidalia Onion	1 serv (1.5 oz)	56	tr	tr	0	12	tr	166
Honey Mustard	1 serv (1.5 oz)	184	0	16	21	10	0	298
Oil & Vinegar	1 serv (1.5 oz)	250	0	28	0	1	0	0
Ranch	1 serv (1.5 oz)	213	0	23	7	3	0	425
Red Wine Vinaigrette	1 serv (1.5 oz)	198	0	21	0	4	0	468
Sesame Oriental	1 serv (1.5 oz)	128	0	6	0	17	0	482
Sweet Vidalia Onion	1 serv (1.5 oz)	170	0	13	0	14	0	106
Thousand Island	1 serv (1.5 oz)	184	0	18	21	6	0	425
SALADS								
Almond Citrus Chicken w/o Dressing	1 serv	443	33	25	85	26	4	967
BLT Chicken w/o Dressing	1 serv	394	44	22	124	9	4	1755

FOOD	PORTION	CALS	PROT	FAT	CHOL	CARB	FIBER	SOD
BLT w/o Dressing	1 sm	146	13	10	34	4	2	530
BLT w/o Dressing	1 lg	285	24	19	68	7	4	1057
Caesar Chicken w/ Dressing	1 serv	580	39	43	107	12	3	2056
Caesar w/ Dressing	1 lg	451	19	40	51	11	3	1380
Caesar w/ Dressing	1 sm	236	10	20	26	7	2	688
Dusk Mountain Blackened Chicken w/o Dressing	1 serv	304	30	19	85	13	3	915
Fruit Salad	1 serv (4 oz)	61	tr	tr	0	15	1	5
Lodge	1 sm	55	2	5	0	7	2	33
Lodge w/o Dressing	1 lg	82	3	7	0	12	3	49
Low Carb BLT	1 serv	721	29	63	92	13	4	2080
Low Carb Side Salad w/ Dressing	1 serv	316	2	31	9	10	2	581
Low Carb w/ Chicken w/ Dressing	1 serv	567	23	49	70	14	3	1662
Low Fat Grilled Chicken w/o Dressing	1 serv	151	23	4	56	9	3	811
Mount Fuji w/ Dressing	1 serv	554	26	31	56	62	4	1893
SANDWICHES								
Bagel & Cream Cheese	1	378	13	11	30	59	2	593
Bear Cristo	1	310	36	32	91	48	6	2026
BLT	1	585	19	42	61	34	2	1147
Coop's Chicken Salad Croissant	1	439	24	31	44	46	5	375
Fajita Chicken	1	659	36	40	95	47	2	1767
Fireside Jack	1	699	36	42	98	53	6	1428
Garden	1	390	12	24	44	35	2	833
Giant Panda Wrap	1	556	31	23	58	68	23	2045
Grilled Cheese	1	480	17	32	52	29	1	1100
Ham & Swiss On Rye	1	394	31	13	76	38	2	2140
Hoot Owl	1	641	34	42	92	32	2	1618

FOOD	PORTION	CALS	PROT	FAT	CHOL	CARB	FIBER	SOD
Italian Asiago Focaccia	1	901	40	60	107	60	3	2360
Low Carb Wrap	1	308	33	11	56	28	19	1232
Low Fat Ham	1	309	24	7	50	39	2	1997
Low Fat Turkey	1	280	29	3	40	35	3	1537
Mountain Bird	1	691	36	38	98	51	6	1284
Peanut Butter & Jelly	1	387	12	15	0	53	3	440
Reuben's Peak	1	540	36	23	76	49	3	3575
Rising Sunflower	1	591	35	41	93	34	2	1619
Roast Turkey & Bacon	1	522	32	30	71	31	2	1665
Rockside Focaccia	1	958	43	52	129	57	3	2546
Sasquash	1	408	14	26	19	41	3	632
The Early Bear Bagel + Bacon	1	530	27	21	254	59	2	1350
The Early Bear English Muffin + Bacon	1	344	19	19	248	26	1	1087
The Early Bear English Muffin + Sausage	1	514	24	34	288	25	1	1407
The Moose	1	976	54	54	142	54	7	2565
Turkey On Whole Wheat	1	602	34	41	102	36	2	1667
SOUPS								
Aztec Black Bean	1 serv	162	9	1	0	28	9	1180
Baked Potato Mountain Chowder	1 serv	352	13	16	27	42	4	1179
Chicken & Dumpling	1 serv	249	16	7	73	28	4	1427
Chicken Gumbo	1 serv	123	8	3	14	10	3	1750
Chicken Noodle	1 serv	165	10	3	28	25	1	1176
Chicken w/ Wild Rice	1 serv	313	14	16	41	29	3	1655
Cream Of Broccoli w/ Cheddar	1 serv	264	8	17	21	21	4	1313
French Onion	1 serv	121	3	5	0	17	2	1556
Grande Chili	1 serv	351	25	12	35	36	19	1714
In Bread Bowl Aztec Black Bean	1 serv	545	23	3	0	105	12	2001

FOOD	PORTION	CALS	PROT	FAT	CHOL	CARB	FIBER	SOD
In Bread Bowl Baked Potato Mountain Chowder	1 serv	735	27	17	27	119	7	2000
In Bread Bowl Chicken & Dumplings	1 serv	632	29	9	73	104	7	2248
In Bread Bowl Chicken Gumbo	1 serv	506	22	4	14	86	5	2571
In Bread Bowl Chicken Noodle	1 serv	548	23	5	28	101	4	1997
In Bread Bowl Chicken w/ Wild Rice	1 serv	696	27	18	41	105	5	2475
In Bread Bowl Cream Of Broccoli w/ Cheddar	1 serv	647	22	18	21	97	7	2133
In Bread Bowl French Onion	1 serv	504	17	7	0	93	4	2377
In Bread Bowl Grande Chili	1 serv	734	39	14	35	113	22	2535
In Bread Bowl New England Clam Chowder	1 serv	653	15	9	15	113	4	2411
In Bread Bowl Normandy Vegetable Cheddar	1 serv	728	30	22	38	102	4	2771
In Bread Bowl Tomato Florentine	1 serv	533	20	4	5	104	4	2066
New England Clam Chowder	1 serv	270	1	8	15	36	1	1590
Normandy Vegetable Cheddar	1 serv	345	17	21	38	26	2	1950
Tomato Florentine	1 serv	150	6	2	5	27	2	1245

BEN & JERRY'S

Sugar Cone	1	48	1	tr	0	10	tr	42

FROZEN YOGURT

Black Raspberry Low Fat	½ cup	140	3	2	15	28	tr	60

FOOD	PORTION	CALS	PROT	FAT	CHOL	CARB	FIBER	SOD
Cherry Garcia	½ cup	170	4	3	20	32	0	80
Chocolate Fudge Brownie	½ cup	190	6	3	15	36	1	105
Half Baked	½ cup	210	5	4	20	30	tr	125
Phish Food	½ cup	230	4	5	15	42	1	110
ICE CREAM								
Brownie Batter	½ cup	310	5	18	70	32	1	115
Butter Pecan	½ cup	290	4	21	70	20	1	80
Cherry Garcia	½ cup	250	4	15	70	26	0	60
Chocolate Chip Cookie Dough	½ cup	280	4	16	70	31	0	90
Chocolate Chocolate Cookie	½ cup	280	4	14	35	34	2	115
Chocolate For A Change	½ cup	270	4	17	55	36	2	50
Chocolate Fudge Brownie	½ cup	280	5	14	40	33	2	85
Chubby Hubby	½ cup	330	7	21	60	32	1	160
Chunky Monkey	½ cup	300	4	19	60	30	1	45
Coffee For A Change	½ cup	240	4	15	75	21	0	55
Coffee Heath Bar Crunch	½ cup	310	4	18	65	32	0	125
Everything But The Fudge Central	½ cup	320	5	19	60	30	1	80
	½ cup	300	4	18	55	31	1	60
Half Baked	½ cup	280	4	14	60	34	1	105
Karamel Sutra	½ cup	290	4	15	55	33	1	75
Makin' Whoopie Pie	½ cup	270	4	14	40	33	2	75
Mint Chocolate Cookie	½ cup	270	4	16	70	26	tr	120
New York Super Fudge Chunk	½ cup	270	5	20	40	30	2	55
Oatmeal Cookie Chunk	½ cup	280	4	16	55	32	1	120
One Sweet Whirled	½ cup	280	4	15	60	33	1	85
Organic Chocolate Fudge Brownie	½ cup	260	4	13	35	30	2	55
Organic Strawberry	½ cup	200	3	12	55	20	0	40

FOOD	PORTION	CALS	PROT	FAT	CHOL	CARB	FIBER	SOD
Organic Sweet Cream & Cookies	½ cup	240	3	15	60 ·	23	0	90
Organic Vanilla	½ cup	220	3	14	65	18	0	50
Peanut Butter Cup	½ cup	380	8	26	70	29	2	140
Peanut Butter Me Up	½ cup	330	6	21	50	28	2	130
Phish Food	½ cup	280	4	13	35	38	2	90
Pistachio Pistachio	½ cup	280	6	19	70	21	0	125
Uncanny Cashew	½ cup	290	4	19	70	27	0	130
Vanilla Heath Bar Crunch	½ cup	300	4	19	70	29	0	120
Vanilla For A Change	½ cup	240	4	16	75	21	0	55
SORBETS								
Berry Berry Extraordinary	½ cup	100	0	0	0	25	tr	5
Mango Lime	½ cup	100	0	0	0	27	0	10
Strawberry Kiwi	½ cup	100	0	0	0	27	tr	10

BLIMPIE
COOKIES

FOOD	PORTION	CALS	PROT	FAT	CHOL	CARB	FIBER	SOD
Chocolate Chunk	1	200	2	10	15	26	1	210
Macadamia White Chunk	1	210	2	10	20	26	1	140
Oatmeal Raisin	1	190	3	8	10	27	1	200
Peanut Butter	1	220	4	12	15	23	1	210
Sugar	1	330	3	17	30	24	0	290
SALAD DRESSINGS AND TOPPINGS								
Caesar Dressing	1 serv (1.5 oz)	208	1	22	10	2	0	504
Cracked Peppercorn Dressing	1 serv (1.5 oz)	237	1	25	15	2	0	386
Frank's Red Hot Buffalo Sauce	1 serv (1 oz)	13	2	tr	0	2	tr	836
French's Honey Mustard	1 tbsp	5	0	0	0	1	0	35
GourMayo Chipotle Chili	1 tbsp	50	0	5	10	1	0	100
GourMayo Sun Dried Tomato	1 tbsp	50	0	5	10	1	0	100

FOOD	PORTION	CALS	PROT	FAT	CHOL	CARB	FIBER	SOD
GourMayo Wasabi Horseradish	1 tbsp	50	0	5	10	1	0	100
Guacamole	1 serv (1.5 oz)	194	2	18	tr	7	1	468
Oil & Vinegar	1 serv	36	0	4	0	1	0	0
Pesto Dressing	1 serv (1 oz)	132	0	13	0	1	0	236
SALADS AND SALAD BARS								
Antipasto	1 reg serv	244	23	13	69	10	3	1217
Chef	1 reg serv	212	20	9	66	9	3	961
Chili Ole	1 reg serv	480	21	27	45	42	3	1240
Grilled Chicken w/ Caesar Dressing	1 reg serv	347	18	27	45	9	3	862
Grilled Chicken w/o Dressing	1 serv	139	17	5	35	7	3	358
Roast Beef 'N Blue	1 reg serv	390	31	16	70	29	0	1550
Seafood	1 reg serv	122	6	4	19	16	3	418
Tuna	1 reg serv	261	16	20	50	8	3	398
Zesto Pesto Turkey	1 reg serv	370	20	19	40	31	0	1410
SANDWICHES								
6 Inch Hot Sub BLT	1	588	28	32	41	49	3	1596
6 Inch Hot Sub Buffalo Chicken	1	400	32	13	61	50	3	2108
6 Inch Hot Sub Buffalo Chicken w/o Cheese	1	320	32	7	61	50	3	2108
6 Inch Hot Sub ChiliMax	1	511	29	13	0	71	8	1287
6 Inch Hot Sub Grilled Chicken	1	373	29	9	35	50	3	836
6 Inch Hot Sub Meatball	1	572	28	27	58	55	2	1145
6 Inch Hot Sub MexiMelt	1	425	23	9	0	65	7	1012
6 Inch Hot Sub Pastrami	1	507	36	17	74	53	3	1658
6 Inch Hot Sub Steak & Onion Melt	1	440	29	16	68	49	3	1056
6 Inch Hot Sub VegiMax	1	395	24	7	0	60	8	982

FOOD	PORTION	CALS	PROT	FAT	CHOL	CARB	FIBER	SOD
6 Inch Sub Blimpie Best	1	476	30	16	69	52	2	1690
6 Inch Sub Club	1	440	28	12	66	51	3	1437
6 Inch Sub Ham & Cheese	1	436	28	13	59	52	3	1302
6 Inch Sub Roast Beef	1	468	37	14	71	49	3	1384
6 Inch Sub Roast Beef w/o Cheese	1	388	30	8	51	49	3	1338
6 Inch Sub Seafood	1	355	14	8	19	58	4	895
6 Inch Sub Tuna	1	493	24	23	50	51	3	876
6 inch Sub Turkey	1	424	25	11	62	49	3	1597
6 Inch Sub Turkey w/o Cheese	1	344	18	5	42	49	3	1551
Cheddar	1 slice	52	3	5	10	0	0	250
Grilled Subs Beef Turkey & Cheddar	1	600	28	31	69	49	3	1836
Grilled Subs Cuban	1	462	30	12	67	50	3	1526
Grilled Subs Pastrami	1	462	32	14	44	52	3	1438
Grilled Subs Reuben	1	630	31	33	46	55	2	1914
Provolone	1 slice	80	6	6	20	0	0	200
Swiss	1 slice	80	7	6	20	0	0	46
Wraps Beef & Cheddar	1	714	34	37	78	57	3	2183
Wraps Chicken Caesar	1	646	25	35	45	56	3	1635
Wraps Southwestern	1	674	26	35	56	54	3	2504
Wraps Steak & Onions	1	716	30	37	78	64	3	1716
Wraps Ultimate BLT	1	831	34	50	78	60	3	2677
Wraps Zesty Italian	1	638	26	33	62	74	3	2374
SIDE ORDERS								
Cole Slaw	1 serv (5 oz)	180	1	13	<5	13	1	230
Macaroni Salad	1 serv (5 oz)	360	4	25	10	25	1	660
Mustard Potato Salad	1 serv (5 oz)	160	2	5	5	21	1	660

FOOD	PORTION	CALS	PROT	FAT	CHOL	CARB	FIBER	SOD
Potato Chips Cheddar & Sour Cream	1 bag	210	3	11	<5	25	1	220
Potato Chips Jalapeno	1 bag	210	2	11	0	25	2	250
Potato Chips Lea & Perrins Barbecue	1 bag	210	3	10	0	25	2	270
Potato Chips Regular	1 bag	210	3	11	0	25	2	190
Potato Chips Romano & Garlic	1 bag	210	3	11	<5	25	2	220
Potato Chips Sour Cream & Onion	1 bag	210	2	11	<5	25	1	250
Potato Salad	1 serv (5 oz)	270	2	19	10	19	1	560
SOUPS								
Chicken w/ White & Wild Rice	1 serv (8 oz)	230	10	12	30	21	2	1210
Cream Of Broccoli & Cheese	1 serv (8 oz)	190	6	12	15	15	3	940
Cream Of Potato	1 serv (8 oz)	190	5	9	<5	24	3	860
Garden Vegetable	1 serv (8 oz)	80	5	1	0	14	3	620
Grande Chili w/ Beans & Beef	1 serv (8 oz)	250	18	7	40	30	18	1230
Homestyle Chicken Noodle	1 serv (8 oz)	120	7	3	20	18	1	850
Tomato Basil w/ Raviolini	1 serv (8 oz)	110	4	1	10	22	tr	720
Vegetable Beef	1 serv (8 oz)	80	4	2	5	13	2	1010

BOB EVANS
BREAKFAST SELECTIONS

FOOD	PORTION	CALS	PROT	FAT	CHOL	CARB	FIBER	SOD
Bacon	1 piece	36	1	4	5	0	—	55
Belgian Waffle	1	351	7	10	0	58	—	834
Canadian Bacon	1 piece	21	4	1	9	0	—	261
Country Biscuit Breakfast	1 serv	841	31	41	267	71	—	2387
Egg Hardboiled	1	60	6	4	190	1	—	55
Egg Over Easy	1	93	6	7	213	1	—	63
Eggs Scrambled	1 serv	170	14	11	482	2	—	142
Eggs Benedict	1 serv	514	41	23	484	37	—	2311

FOOD	PORTION	CALS	PROT	FAT	CHOL	CARB	FIBER	SOD
French Toast	1 slice	135	3	2	25	14	—	175
Fruit Cup	1 serv	164	2	1	0	42	—	11
Grits	1 serv	187	3	7	0	29	—	186
Ham Smoked	1 slice	66	11	2	39	2	—	855
Home Fries	1 serv	193	4	7	0	28	—	577
Hotcake Blueberry	1	192	4	5	0	33	—	419
Hotcake Buttermilk	1	176	3	5	0	29	—	417
Hotcake Cinnamon	1	166	4	5	8	28	—	409
Hotcake Multigrain	1	208	5	6	10	34	—	505
Lite Sausage Breakfast	1 serv	479	32	21	42	50	—	1011
Mush	1 serv	73	1	1	0	14	—	194
Oatmeal Plain	1 serv	185	7	3	0	34	—	301
Omelette Border	1	847	33	60	571	60	—	1551
Omelette Cheese	1	457	25	40	530	3	—	428
Omelette Farmer's Market	1	634	32	49	558	11	—	1986
Pot Roast Hash Breakfast	1 serv	698	45	41	529	36	—	1207
Sausage	1 link	117	5	13	21	0	0	167
Sausage Lite	1 link	100	10	7	37	0	—	278
Strawberry Yogurt	1 serv	145	6	1	5	28	—	85
CHILDREN'S MENU SELECTIONS								
Colorful Cool Cakes	1 serv	542	9	17	1	87	—	1112
Garden Salad	1 kid serv	41	3	2	7	3	—	54
Hot Diggety Dog Plain	1	446	15	33	55	23	—	1214
L'il Homesteader	1 serv	414	16	25	262	34	—	781
Mac & Cheese	1 serv	330	11	12	20	45	—	610
Mini Cheeseburger	1 serv	252	9	14	25	20	—	288
Pizza Pizzazz	1 serv	520	27	20	31	58	—	883
Plenty O Pancakes	1 serv	515	9	17	0	81	—	1114
Quesadilla Chicken	1 serv	542	28	31	73	39	—	1238
Smiley Face Potatoes	1 serv	335	5	13	0	49	—	786
Spaghetti & Meatballs	1 serv	523	27	21	51	57	—	999
Sundae Fudge Blast	1 serv	254	3	10	30	37	—	92
Sundae Oreo Cookies 'n' Cream	1 serv	315	3	13	21	64	—	200

FOOD	PORTION	CALS	PROT	FAT	CHOL	CARB	FIBER	SOD
Sundae Rainbow	1 serv	320	4	14	30	46	—	92
Sundae Reese's I'm Smiling	1 serv	325	5	15	31	42	—	130
MAIN MENU SELECTIONS								
Catfish Grilled New Orleans	1 piece	255	22	19	58	4	—	896
Cheeseburger Bacon Plain	1	1005	45	76	153	31	—	1367
Cheeseburger Plain	1	691	38	46	104	31	—	792
Chicken Quesadilla	1 serv	502	25	36	61	50	—	1674
Chicken & Broccoli Alfredo	1 serv	826	58	29	112	90	—	1105
Chicken Fried	1 piece	291	31	30	154	9	—	1332
Chicken Grilled	1 piece	229	38	10	98	0	—	632
Chicken Pot Pie	1 serv	758	32	49	209	46	—	1754
Chicken Tenders Grilled	1 piece	103	12	7	33	0	—	220
Chicken-N-Noodle	1 serv	407	20	22	115	32	—	658
Country Fried Steak w/ Gravy	1 serv	535	20	37	60	31	—	1763
Country Fried Steak w/o Gravy	1 serv	481	20	33	60	26	—	1217
Fish Market Halibut	1 piece	209	12	12	32	13	—	327
Hamburger Patty	1	388	28	30	82	0	—	64
Hamburger Plain	1	585	34	36	82	30	—	407
Hamburger Shroomin' Onion Plain	1	695	38	44	104	32	—	938
Meat Loaf	1 serv	626	42	44	157	14	—	1006
Open Faced Roast Beef Dinner	1 serv	633	37	29	118	31	—	1331
Pork Chop Dinner	1 serv	466	48	28	129	2	—	829
Pork Chop Dinner w/ Garlic Herb Butter	1 serv	624	50	39	130	16	—	1227
Pork Chop Dinner w/ Wildfire Barbecue Sauce	1 serv	645	49	35	129	29	—	1099
Salmon	1 serv	334	43	18	109	0	—	109

FOOD	PORTION	CALS	PROT	FAT	CHOL	CARB	FIBER	SOD
Salmon w/ Garlic Herb Butter	1 serv	491	45	29	110	14	—	506
Salmon w/ Wildfire Barbecue Sauce	1 serv	512	44	25	109	27	—	379
Sandwich Bob's BLT	1	795	25	54	276	55	—	1435
Sandwich Chicken Salad	1	694	21	43	62	55	—	1329
Sandwich Fish Market Haddock	1	570	21	25	32	65	—	944
Sandwich Fried Chicken	1	508	36	23	77	39	—	1032
Sandwich Fried Chicken Club	1	994	49	70	155	40	—	2002
Sandwich Grilled Cheese	1	391	9	17	30	25	—	776
Sandwich Grilled Chicken	1	447	44	18	98	30	—	998
Sandwich Grilled Chicken Club	1	993	59	70	194	32	—	2259
Sandwich Pot Roast	1	728	38	35	113	68	—	1614
Sandwich Turkey Bacon Melt	1	872	47	52	166	55	—	1794
Seniors Chicken & Broccoli Alfredo	1 serv	513	37	21	77	49	—	935
Seniors Chicken Pot Pie	1 serv	758	32	49	209	46	—	1754
Seniors Spaghetti & Meatballs	1 serv	617	31	29	69	59	—	1166
Seniors Steak Tips & Noodles	1 serv	550	38	25	134	46	—	1654
Seniors Stir-Fry Grilled Chicken	1 serv	479	31	18	66	54	—	1292
Spaghetti & Marinara Sauce	1 serv	619	34	7	15	104	—	1128
Spaghetti w/ Meatballs	1 serv	1087	54	45	107	116	—	1964
Steak Monterey	1 serv	584	44	41	126	7	—	1671
Steak Tips & Noodles	1 serv	985	76	37	266	90	—	2972

FOOD	PORTION	CALS	PROT	FAT	CHOL	CARB	FIBER	SOD
Stir-Fry Grilled Chicken	1 serv	728	46	28	98	31	—	2048
Stir-Fry Grilled Shrimp	1 serv	713	52	17	334	98	—	1798
Stir-Fry Vegetable	1 serv	497	15	7	0	98	—	1413
T-Bone Steak Plain	1 serv	1335	111	92	261	7	—	4944
T-Bone Steak w/ Garlic Herb Butter	1 serv	1492	113	102	262	21	—	5342
Turkey & Dressing	1 serv	542	37	24	105	41	—	1400
SALAD DRESSINGS AND TOPPINGS								
Dressing Bleu Cheese	1 serv (1.5 oz)	220	1	23	22	3	—	337
Dressing Colonial	1 serv (1.5 oz)	232	0	21	0	12	—	193
Dressing French	1 serv (1.5 oz)	219	0	21	14	10	—	247
Dressing Honey Mustard	1 serv (1.5 oz)	192	0	18	21	8	—	247
Dressing Hot Bacon	1 serv (1.5 oz)	106	0	3	4	18	—	189
Dressing Lite Italian	1 serv (1.5 oz)	82	0	7	0	4	—	590
Dressing Oriental	1 serv (1.5 oz)	194	0	16	0	12	—	253
Dressing Ranch	1 serv (1.5 oz)	156	1	16	14	1	—	312
Dressing Ranch Lite	1 serv (1.5 oz)	103	1	10	11	2	—	377
Dressing Raspberry Vinaigrette	1 serv (1.5 oz)	155	0	13	0	12	—	90
Dressing Thousand Island	1 serv (1.5 oz)	212	0	20	21	7	—	354
Dressing Wildfire Ranch	1 serv (1.5 oz)	212	1	9	8	9	—	307
SALADS								
Chicken Salad Plate	1 serv	789	23	46	87	78	—	1137
Cobb Salad w/ Grilled Chicken	1 serv	778	68	54	373	14	—	1852

FOOD	PORTION	CALS	PROT	FAT	CHOL	CARB	FIBER	SOD
Country Spinach w/ Grilled Chicken	1 serv	532	43	38	282	11	—	1128
Frisco Salad w/ Fried Chicken	1 serv	672	40	40	98	39	—	1685
Frisco Salad w/ Grilled Chicken	1 serv	599	54	40	154	13	—	1380
Fruit & Yogurt	1 serv	414	9	2	5	96	—	106
Raspberry Grilled Chicken	1 serv	637	55	42	155	18	—	1657
Speciality Side	1 serv	174	9	9	22	16	—	449
Wildfire Fried Chicken Salad	1 serv	806	36	31	66	100	—	1237
Wildfried Grilled Chicken Salad	1 serv	733	50	30	123	74	—	932

BOJANGLES

FOOD	PORTION	CALS	PROT	FAT	CHOL	CARB	FIBER	SOD
Biscuit	1	243	4	12	2	29	2	663
Biscuit + Bacon	1	290	8	17	10	26	1	810
Biscuit + Bacon Egg Cheese	1	550	17	42	160	27	1	1250
Biscuit + Cajun Fillet	1	454	20	21	41	46	1	949
Biscuit + Country Ham	1	270	9	15	20	26	1	1010
Biscuit + Egg	1	400	8	30	120	26	1	630
Biscuit + Sausage	1	350	9	23	20	26	1	810
Biscuit + Smoked Sausage	1	380	10	26	20	27	1	940
Biscuit + Steak	1	649	14	49	34	37	1	1126
Botato Rounds	1 serv	235	3	11	13	31	3	328
Buffalo Bites	1 serv	180	27	5	105	5	0	720
Cajun Pintos	1 serv	110	6	0	0	18	6	480
Cajun Spiced Breast	1 serv	278	18	17	75	12	tr	565
Cajun Spiced Leg	1 serv	284	19	19	96	11	tr	530
Cajun Spiced Thigh	1 serv	310	15	23	67	11	tr	465
Cajun Spiced Wing	1 serv	355	21	25	94	11	tr	630
Chicken Supremes	1 serv	337	21	16	58	26	1	629
Corn On The Cob	1 serv	140	5	2	0	34	2	20
Dirty Rice	1 serv	166	5	6	10	24	1	762
Green Beans	1 serv	25	0	0	0	5	2	710

FOOD	PORTION	CALS	PROT	FAT	CHOL	CARB	FIBER	SOD
Macaroni & Cheese	1 serv	198	7	14	26	12	tr	418
Marinated Cole Slaw	1 serv	136	1	3	0	26	3	454
Potatoes w/o Gravy	1 serv	80	2	1	0	16	1	380
Sandwich Cajun Filet w/o Mayo	1	337	22	11	45	41	3	401
Sandwich Cajun Filet w/ Mayo	1	437	22	22	55	41	3	506
Sandwich Grilled Filet w/ Mayo	1	335	23	16	61	25	2	645
Sandwich Grilled Filet w/o Mayo	1 serv	235	23	5	51	25	2	540
Seasoned Fries	1 serv	344	5	19	13	39	4	480
Southern Style Breast	1 serv	261	16	16	76	12	tr	702
Southern Style Leg	1 serv	254	19	15	94	11	tr	446
Southern Style Thigh	1 serv	308	16	21	78	14	tr	630
Southern Style Wing	1 serv	337	17	21	86	19	tr	684
Sweet Biscuit Bo Berry	1	220	3	10	tr	29	1	410
Sweet Biscuit Cinnamon	1	320	4	18	tr	37	1	560

BOSTON MARKET
BAKED SELECTIONS

FOOD	PORTION	CALS	PROT	FAT	CHOL	CARB	FIBER	SOD
Brownie	1 (3.3 oz)	450	6	27	80	47	3	190
Cinnamon Apple Pie	⅛ pie (4.8 oz)	390	2	23	0	46	2	250
Cookie Chocolate Chip	1 (2.8 oz)	340	4	17	25	48	1	240

MAIN MENU SELECTIONS

FOOD	PORTION	CALS	PROT	FAT	CHOL	CARB	FIBER	SOD
½ Chicken w/ Skin	1 serv (9.7 oz)	590	70	33	280	4	0	1010
¼ Dark Meat Chicken No Skin	1 serv (3.3 oz)	190	22	10	115	1	0	440
¼ Dark Meat Chicken w/ Skin	1 serv (4.4 oz)	320	30	21	155	2	0	500
¼ White Meat Chicken No Skin Or Wing	1 serv (4.9 oz)	170	23	4	85	2	0	480

FOOD	PORTION	CALS	PROT	FAT	CHOL	CARB	FIBER	SOD
¼ White Meat Chicken w/ Skin And Wing	1 serv (5.3 oz)	280	40	12	135	2	0	510
Baked Sweet Potato Low Fat	1 (12.5 oz)	460	6	7	0	94	10	510
BBQ Baked Beans	¾ cup (7.1 oz)	270	8	5	0	48	12	540
BBQ Chicken Sandwich	1 (9.9 oz)	540	30	9	75	84	3	1690
Black Beans And Rice	1 cup (8 oz)	300	8	10	0	45	5	1050
Boston Hearth Ham Lean	1 serv (5 oz)	210	25	9	75	9	0	1490
Broccoli Cauliflower Au Gratin	¾ cup (6.1 oz)	200	9	11	20	14	3	600
Broccoli Rice Casserole	¾ cup (6 oz)	240	5	12	40	26	2	800
Broccoli With Red Peppers	¾ cup (3.4 oz)	60	3	4	0	5	3	130
Butternut Squash Low Fat	¾ cup (6.8 oz)	160	2	6	15	25	3	580
Chicken Gravy	1 serv (1 oz)	15	0	1	0	2	0	170
Chicken Salad Sandwich	1 (11.5 oz)	680	39	30	120	63	4	1360
Chicken Sandwich w/ Cheese & Sauce	1 (12.4 oz)	750	41	33	135	72	5	1860
Chicken Sandwich w/o Cheese & Sauce Low Fat	1 (10 oz)	430	34	5	65	62	4	910
Chunky Chicken Salad	¾ cup (5.5 oz)	370	28	27	120	3	1	800
Chunky Cinnamon Apple Sauce No Fat	¾ cup (6.4 oz)	250	1	0	0	62	2	30
Cole Slaw	¾ cup (6.5 oz)	300	2	19	20	30	3	540
Corn Bread	1 (2.4 oz)	200	3	6	25	33	1	390

FOOD	PORTION	CALS	PROT	FAT	CHOL	CARB	FIBER	SOD
Coyote Bean Salad	¾ cup (5.3 oz)	190	4	9	0	24	9	210
Cranberry Relish Low Fat	¾ cup (7.9 oz)	370	2	5	0	84	5	5
Creamed Spinach	¾ cup (6.4 oz)	260	9	20	55	11	2	740
Fruit Salad Low Fat	¾ cup (5.5 oz)	70	1	1	0	15	1	10
Green Bean Casserole	¾ cup (6 oz)	130	2	9	20	10	2	440
Green Beans	¾ cup (3 oz)	80	1	6	0	5	3	200
Ham Sandwich w/ Cheese & Sauce	1 (11.8 oz)	760	38	34	100	72	5	1730
Ham Sandwich w/o Cheese & Sauce	1 (9.3 oz)	440	25	8	45	66	4	1450
Homestyle Mashed Potatoes & Gravy	¾ cup (6.6 oz)	210	4	10	25	26	1	740
Honey Glazed Carrots	¾ cup (5.4 oz)	280	1	15	0	35	4	80
Hot Cinnamon Apples	¾ cup (6.4 oz)	250	0	5	0	56	3	45
Macaroni & Cheese	¾ cup (6.7 oz)	280	13	11	30	32	1	830
Mashed Potatoes	⅔ cup (5.6 oz)	190	3	9	25	24	1	570
Meat Loaf & Brown Gravy	1 serv (7 oz)	390	30	22	120	19	1	1040
Meat Loaf & Chunky Tomato Sauce	1 serv (8 oz)	370	30	18	120	22	2	1170
Meat Loaf Sandwich w/ Cheese	1 (13.8 oz)	860	46	33	165	95	6	2270
Meat Loaf Sandwich w/o Cheese	1 (12.3 oz)	690	40	21	120	86	6	1610
New Potatoes Low Fat	¾ cup (4.6 oz)	130	3	3	0	25	2	150
Old Fashioned Potato Salad	¾ cup (6.2 oz)	340	2	24	30	30	2	870
Open Face Turkey Sandwich	1 (13.4 oz)	500	37	12	80	61	3	2170

FOOD	PORTION	CALS	PROT	FAT	CHOL	CARB	FIBER	SOD
Original Chicken Pot Pie	1 pie (14.9 oz)	780	32	46	135	61	4	1480
Oven Roasted Potato Planks Low Fat	5 pieces (5.8 oz)	180	3	5	0	32	3	370
Pastry Sandwich BBQ Chicken	1 (7.2 oz)	640	17	39	60	56	1	1260
Pastry Sandwich Broccoli Chicken Cheddar	1 (7.2 oz)	690	21	47	85	45	2	1050
Pastry Sandwich Ham & Cheddar	1 (6.6 oz)	640	19	41	60	47	1	1560
Pastry Sandwich Italian Chicken	1 (7.2 oz)	630	21	41	60	43	2	910
Red Beans And Rice Low Fat	1 cup (8 oz)	260	8	5	5	45	4	1050
Rice Pilaf	⅔ cup (5.1 oz)	180	5	5	0	32	2	600
Rotisserie Turkey Breast Skinless Low Fat	1 serv (5 oz)	170	36	1	100	1	0	850
Savory Stuffing	¾ cup (6.1 oz)	310	6	12	0	44	3	1140
Southwest Savory Chicken	1 serv (9.6 oz)	400	40	15	100	26	4	1670
Squash Casserole	¾ cup (6.6 oz)	330	7	24	70	20	3	1110
Steamed Vegetables Low Fat	⅔ cup (3.7 oz)	35	2	1	0	7	3	35
Sweet Potato Casserole	¾ cup (6.4 oz)	280	3	18	10	39	2	190
Tabasco BBQ Drumstick	1 (2.4 oz)	130	14	6	50	4	0	190
Tabasco BBQ Wing	1 (1.8 oz)	110	9	7	30	4	0	170
Teriyaki Chicken ¼ w/ Skin	1 serv (5.9 oz)	380	30	21	155	17	0	870
Teriyaki Chicken White w/ Skin	1 serv (6.8 oz)	340	40	12	135	17	0	890

FOOD	PORTION	CALS	PROT	FAT	CHOL	CARB	FIBER	SOD
Triple Topped Chicken	1 serv (9.2 oz)	470	50	22	155	20	1	1350
Turkey Club Sandwich	1 (11.1 oz)	650	39	26	105	64	4	1590
Turkey Sandwich w/ Cheese & Sauce	1 (11.8 oz)	710	45	28	110	68	4	1390
Turkey Sandwich w/o Cheese & Sauce	1 (9.3 oz)	400	45	4	60	61	4	1070
Whole Kernel Corn	¾ cup (5.8 oz)	180	5	4	0	30	2	170
Zucchini Marinara Low Fat	¾ cup (6.6 oz)	60	1	3	0	7	2	330
SALADS AND SALAD BARS								
Caesar Salad Entree	1 serv (10 oz)	510	17	42	35	17	3	1130
Caesar Salad w/o Dressing	1 serv (8 oz)	230	16	12	20	14	3	500
Caesar Side Salad	1 (4 oz)	200	7	17	15	7	1	450
Chicken Caesar Salad	1 serv (13 oz)	650	43	45	105	17	3	1580
Tossed Salad w/ Caesar Dressing	1 serv (8 oz)	380	5	31	15	18	3	810
Tossed Salad w/ Fat Free Ranch	1 serv (8 oz)	160	5	3	0	29	4	940
Tossed Salad w/ Old Venice Dressing	1 serv (8 oz)	340	4	27	0	20	3	1110
SOUPS								
Chicken Chili	1 cup (8.7 oz)	220	18	7	40	21	6	1000
Chicken Noodle	1 cup (8.4 oz)	130	11	5	40	12	2	1310
Chicken Tortilla	1 cup (8.4 oz)	220	10	11	35	19	2	1410
Potato	1 cup (8 oz)	270	8	16	40	24	2	1020
Tomato Bisque	1 cup (8 oz)	280	4	23	50	16	2	1280

FOOD	PORTION	CALS	PROT	FAT	CHOL	CARB	FIBER	SOD

BOSTON PIZZA
CHILDREN'S MENU SELECTIONS

FOOD	PORTION	CALS	PROT	FAT	CHOL	CARB	FIBER	SOD
Corkscrews n' Cheese	1 serv	870	30	33	–	112	–	760
Dino Fingers & Fries w/ Ketchup	1 serv	680	22	35	–	87	–	1270
Grill Cheese Sandwich w/ Fries & Ketchup	1 serv	770	25	32	–	103	–	1450
Mini Lasagna	1 serv	400	19	14	–	48	–	630
Pint Sized Ham Pizza	1 serv	430	22	8	–	66	–	850
Potato Smiles	1 serv	580	8	30	–	84	–	1470
Stuffed Pizza w/ Fries & Ketchup	1 serv	850	30	31	–	124	–	1520
Super Spaghetti	1 serv	340	10	6	–	61	–	660

MAIN MENU SELECTIONS

FOOD	PORTION	CALS	PROT	FAT	CHOL	CARB	FIBER	SOD
Baked Onion Soup	1 serv	210	11	7	–	28	–	1130
Bayou Chicken Strips w/ Dipping Sauce	1 serv	370	43	16	–	6	–	3740
BBQ Ribs w/ Fries	1 serv	2220	71	148	–	140	–	2420
BBQ Ribs w/ Garlic Mashed Potatoes	1 serv	1760	65	122	–	94	–	3090
BBQ Ribs w/ Spaghetti	1 serv	1870	74	121	–	113	–	2570
Boston's Extreme Double Order	1 serv	1660	159	107	–	15	–	7990
Boston's Extreme Starter Order	1 serv	940	90	61	–	10	–	5400
Bruschetta	1 serv	640	17	39	–	55	–	1590
Buffalo Chicken Fingers w/ Caesar Salad	1 serv	650	37	38	–	42	–	2790
Buffalo Chicken Fingers w/ Fries	1 serv	1430	45	82	–	122	–	3440
Buffalo Chicken Fingers w/ Light Ranch	1 serv	600	35	34	–	40	–	3260
Cactus Cuts & Dip	1 serv	1380	21	83	–	136	–	1110
Carne Amore	1 full order	1250	50	50	–	144	–	2970

FOOD	PORTION	CALS	PROT	FAT	CHOL	CARB	FIBER	SOD
Cheese Toast	1 serv	400	18	21	–	32	–	670
Cheese Toast	1 basket	800	36	41	–	64	–	1310
Chicken & Rib Combo	1 serv	1470	68	90	–	94	–	2910
Chicken & Rib Combo w/ Fries	1 serv	1920	74	116	–	140	–	2250
Chicken & Rib Combo w/ Spaghetti	1 serv	1590	78	90	–	113	–	2440
Chicken Fingers w/ Caesar Salad	1 serv	640	37	38	–	38	–	980
Chicken Fingers w/ Fries	1 serv	1420	45	82	–	118	–	1630
Chicken Fingers w/ Light Ranch	1 serv	590	34	34	–	36	–	1440
Chips & Salsa	1 serv	830	11	41	–	109	–	1620
Deluxe Cheese Bread	1 basket	890	37	42	–	84	–	6450
Deluxe Cheese Toast	1 serv	420	19	21	–	35	–	1140
Fettuccini Cajun Shrimp	1 full order	1200	53	43	–	144	–	3260
Fettuccini Four Cheese	1 full order	1370	54	64	–	140	–	2280
Fettuccini Jambalaya	1 full order	1360	68	50	–	151	–	5640
Fettuccini Spicy Chicken & Spinach	1 full order	1330	53	53	–	146	–	4520
Fries	1 serv	700	10	33	–	87	–	450
Garlic Toast w/ Garlic Margarine	1 slice	170	4	6	–	22	–	240
Garlic Twist Bread	1 basket	1080	33	30	–	168	–	1180
Garlic Twist Bread	1 serv	540	17	15	–	84	–	590
Homestyle Macaroni	1 full order	1490	62	83	–	119	–	2490
Italian Pizza Bread w/ Dip	1 serv	1000	32	53	–	98	–	830
Ketchup	1 serv (2 oz)	20	1	1	–	16	–	490
Lasagna Boston's	1 full order	820	40	30	–	95	–	1610

FOOD	PORTION	CALS	PROT	FAT	CHOL	CARB	FIBER	SOD
Lasagna Mediterranean	1 full order	870	41	35	–	97	–	2050
Lasagna Seafood	1 full order	970	41	45	–	95	–	1750
Linguini Chicken & Mushroom	1 full order	1320	59	53	–	144	–	2430
Mashed Potatoes	1 serv	240	4	8	–	41	–	1110
Mexican Beef w/ Sour Cream	1 serv	970	49	57	–	66	–	1820
Mini Tortellini	1 serv	490	17	15	–	73	–	850
Nachos	1 full order	1540	52	95	–	127	–	2370
Nachos Beef	1 full order	1760	73	106	–	129	–	2720
Nachos Chicken	1 full order	1630	68	96	–	129	–	3720
NY Steak Sandwich w/ Fries	1 serv	1580	54	96	–	118	–	970
Penne Baked 3 Cheese	1 full order	990	43	37	–	118	–	1860
Penne Italiano	1 full order	1160	50	46	–	137	–	3820
Penne Pisa Pesto	1 full order	1270	49	63	–	110	–	2260
Penne Roast Veggie	1 full order	900	25	31	–	146	–	2330
Pizza Bread w/o Meat Sauce	1 serv	520	15	14	–	84	–	520
Plain Pasta w/ Alfredo Sauce	1 full order	1200	36	52	–	141	–	1940
Plain Pasta w/ Creamy Tomato Sauce	1 full order	1070	33	38	–	142	–	1850
Plain Pasta w/ Marinara Sauce	1 full order	870	26	20	–	144	–	1730
Plain Pasta w/ Meatsauce	1 full order	910	33	22	–	142	–	1600
Plain Pasta w/ Seafood Sauce	1 full order	1050	34	36	–	141	–	1650
Plain Pasta w/ Spicy Tomato Sauce	1 full order	880	27	20	–	145	–	1770
Plain Pasta w/ Tex Mex Sauce	1 full order	940	37	23	–	141	–	1790
Potato Skins	1 full order	860	28	53	–	70	–	610
Quesadilla Chicken w/ Sour Cream	1 serv	770	36	40	–	67	–	1890

FOOD	PORTION	CALS	PROT	FAT	CHOL	CARB	FIBER	SOD
Quesadilla Garden Veggie w/ Sour Cream	1 serv	750	29	40	—	70	—	1560
Quesadilla Sundried Tomato w/ Sour Cream	1 serv	890	67	50	—	39	—	1870
Shrimp Dinner w/ Fries	1 serv	1510	51	82	—	135	—	1330
Shrimp Dinner w/ Garlic Mashed Potatoes	1 serv	1050	45	57	—	89	—	1990
Shrimp Dinner w/ Spaghetti	1 serv	1180	55	56	—	108	—	1520
Side Tossed Salad w/ House Dressing	1 serv	170	2	14	—	10	—	340
Sirloin Steak Dinner w/ Fries	1 serv	1910	95	113	—	117	—	790
Sirloin Steak Dinner w/ Garlic Mashed Potatoes	1 serv	1450	89	88	—	71	—	1450
Sirloin Steak Dinner w/ Spaghetti	1 serv	1580	100	87	—	90	—	980
Smokey Mountain Spaghetti	1 full order	1860	83	71	—	211	—	2590
Spaghetti w/ Meatsauce	1 serv	370	14	8	—	60	—	650
Spinach & Artichoke Dip w/ Tortilla Chips	1 serv	890	21	57	—	81	—	1290
Steak & Shrimp Dinner w/ Fries	1 serv	1760	65	108	—	129	—	1550
Steak & Shrimp Dinner w/ Garlic Mashed Potatoes	1 serv	1310	59	83	—	83	—	2210
Steak & Shrimp Dinner w/ Spaghetti	1 serv	1430	69	82	—	102	—	1740
The Ribber w/ Fries	1 serv	1470	46	85	—	121	—	1650
The Ribber w/ Garlic Mashed Potatoes	1 serv	1010	40	60	—	74	—	2310

FOOD	PORTION	CALS	PROT	FAT	CHOL	CARB	FIBER	SOD
The Ribber w/ Spaghetti	1 serv	1140	50	60	–	94	–	1850
Tortellini w/ Alfredo Sauce	1 full order	1220	46	40	–	165	–	1820
Tortellini w/ Creamy Tomato Sauce	1 full order	1370	46	57	–	166	–	2070
Tortellini w/ Marinara Sauce	1 full order	1180	40	39	–	167	–	1950
Tortellini w/ Meatsauce	1 full order	1500	50	71	–	164	–	2150
Tortellini w/ Seafood Sauce	1 full order	1360	48	55	–	164	–	1860
Tortellini w/ Spicy Tomato Sauce	1 full order	1180	40	39	–	168	–	1990
Tortellini w/ Tex Mex Sauce	1 full order	1240	51	42	–	164	–	2010
Veal Parmigan w/ Fries	1 serv	1550	46	88	–	138	–	1430
Veal Parmigan w/ Garlic Mashed Potatoes	1 serv	1090	40	63	–	92	–	2100
Veal Parmigan w/ Spaghetti	1 serv	1220	50	62	–	112	–	1450
Wings BBQ Double Order	1 serv	1700	159	107	–	26	–	3200
Wings BBQ Starter Size	1 serv	960	90	61	–	13	–	1810
Wings Cajun Double Order	1 serv	1610	158	107	–	5	–	4940
Wings Cajun Starter Size	1 serv	910	89	60	–	3	–	2680
Wings Honey Garlic Double Order	1 serv	1720	158	107	–	32	–	3370
Wings Honey Garlic Starter Size	1 serv	970	89	60	–	17	–	1890
Wings Screamin' Hot Double Order	1 serv	1630	158	107	–	10	–	5620
Wings Screamin' Hot Starter Size	1 serv	920	89	60	–	5	–	3020

FOOD	PORTION	CALS	PROT	FAT	CHOL	CARB	FIBER	SOD
Wings Teriyaki Double Order	1 serv	1690	159	107	–	21	–	4660
Wings Teriyaki Starter Size	1 serv	950	90	60	–	11	–	2540
Wings Thai Double Order	1 serv	1870	164	123	–	27	–	3200
Wings Thai Starter Size	1 serv	1040	92	69	–	14	–	1810
PIZZA								
Bacon Double Cheeseburger Individual	1 pie	1210	77	56	–	94	–	2170
Bacon Double Cheeseburger Large	1 slice	350	23	15	–	30	–	650
Bacon Double Cheeseburger Medium	1 slice	300	19	13	–	25	–	550
Boston Royal Individual	1 pie	770	45	23	–	96	–	1980
Boston Royal Large	1 slice	230	13	6	–	31	–	590
Boston Royal Medium	1 slice	200	11	6	–	26	–	540
Cajun Chicken Individual	1 pie	780	41	25	–	99	–	2140
Cajun Chicken Large	1 slice	250	13	8	–	31	–	610
Cajun Chicken Medium	1 slice	200	10	7	–	26	–	530
Californian Individual	1 pie	580	23	8	–	109	–	960
Californian Large	1 slice	190	8	3	–	35	–	320
Californian Medium	1 slice	160	6	2	–	30	–	290
Four Cheese Individual	1 pie	800	45	29	–	89	–	1580
Four Cheese Large	1 slice	260	14	10	–	29	–	540
Four Cheese Medium	1 slice	240	14	10	–	24	–	510
Great White Individual	1 pie	880	53	34	–	89	–	1820

FOOD	PORTION	CALS	PROT	FAT	CHOL	CARB	FIBER	SOD
Great White Large	1 slice	260	16	9	–	29	–	560
Great White Medium	1 slice	220	13	8	–	24	–	490
Hawaiian Individual	1 pie	690	39	16	–	97	–	1460
Hawaiian Large	1 slice	220	13	5	–	31	–	490
Hawaiian Medium	1 slice	180	10	4	–	26	–	420
Meat Lovers Individual	1 pie	1120	64	55	–	89	–	2450
Meat Lovers Large	1 slice	330	19	15	–	28	–	680
Meat Lovers Medium	1 slice	280	15	14	–	24	–	600
Pepperoni Individual	1 pie	760	39	27	–	89	–	1500
Pepperoni Large	1 slice	240	13	9	–	28	–	490
Pepperoni Medium	1 slice	200	10	7	–	24	–	430
Pepperoni & Mushroom Individual	1 pie	760	90	27	–	40	–	1500
Pepperoni & Mushroom Large	1 slice	250	13	9	–	29	–	490
Pepperoni & Mushroom Medium	1 slice	200	10	7	–	24	–	430
Perogy Individual	1 pie	1010	50	45	–	102	–	1020
Perogy Large	1 slice	330	16	15	–	33	–	340
Perogy Medium	1 slice	280	13	13	–	28	–	280
Popeye Individual	1 pie	730	41	21	–	94	–	1390
Popeye Large	1 slice	240	14	7	–	30	–	490
Popeye Medium	1 slice	200	11	6	–	26	–	420
Rustic Italian Individual	1 pie	940	50	37	–	102	–	4250
Rustic Italian Large	1 slice	310	16	12	–	33	–	1420
Rustic Italian Medium	1 slice	250	13	10	–	28	–	1250
Sante Fe Chicken Individual	1 pie	800	47	27	–	94	–	1650
Sante Fe Chicken Large	1 slice	260	15	9	–	30	–	550
Sante Fe Chicken Medium	1 slice	220	12	7	–	25	–	470

FOOD	PORTION	CALS	PROT	FAT	CHOL	CARB	FIBER	SOD
Super Veggie Individual	1 pie	850	42	29	–	108	–	2020
Super Veggie Large	1 slice	280	14	10	–	35	–	670
Super Veggie Medium	1 slice	230	11	7	–	30	–	580
Thai Chicken Individual	1 pie	870	45	29	–	106	–	850
Thai Chicken Large	1 slice	280	15	10	–	34	–	280
Thai Chicken Medium	1 slice	240	12	8	–	29	–	230
The Basic Individual	1 pie	620	34	15	–	89	–	1050
The Basic Large	1 slice	200	11	5	–	28	–	350
The Basic Medium	1 slice	160	9	4	–	24	–	290
The Deluxe Individual	1 pie	780	43	26	–	92	–	1830
The Deluxe Large	1 slice	240	14	7	–	30	–	540
The Deluxe Medium	1 slice	190	11	6	–	25	–	460
Tropical Chicken Individual	1 pie	1060	57	50	–	94	–	1930
Tropical Chicken Large	1 slice	340	18	16	–	30	–	610
Tropical Chicken Medium	1 slice	280	15	13	–	25	–	520
Tuscan Individual	1 pie	900	49	32	–	108	–	2060
Tuscan Large	1 slice	290	16	11	–	35	–	690
Tuscan Medium	1 slice	240	13	8	–	30	–	590
Vegetarian Individual	1 pie	670	36	15	–	100	–	1060
Vegetarian Large	1 slice	220	12	5	–	31	–	350
Vegetarian Medium	1 slice	170	9	4	–	26	–	300
Zorba The Greek Individual	1 pie	810	43	27	–	99	–	1780
Zorba The Greek Large	1 slice	270	14	9	–	32	–	610
Zorba The Greek Medium	1 slice	220	11	7	–	27	–	510
SALADS AND SALAD BARS								
Boston's Cobb Salad	1 serv	1100	25	80	–	66	–	2280
Caesar Salad	1 reg	260	5	21	–	15	–	410

FOOD	PORTION	CALS	PROT	FAT	CHOL	CARB	FIBER	SOD
Caesar Salad Meal Sized	1 serv	690	13	48	–	52	–	1060
Greek Salad	1 serv	500	10	44	–	19	–	2380
Greek Salad Meal Sized	1 serv	1110	22	90	–	53	–	3680
House Dressing	1 serv (2 oz)	136	tr	13	–	4	–	340
Spinach Salad	1 serv	190	10	14	–	6	–	470
Spinach Salad Meal Sized	1 serv	500	20	31	–	32	–	1050
Taco Salad Beef w/ Sour Cream & Salsa	1 serv	640	33	41	–	40	–	1130
Taco Salad Chicken w/ Sour Cream & Salsa	1 serv	520	28	28	–	39	–	2130
Thai Chicken Salad	1 serv	730	44	21	–	90	–	1150
Tossed Garden Greens w/ House Dressing	1 serv	170	2	14	–	10	–	350
Veggie Plate w/ Low Fat Ranch Dressing	1 serv	180	6	7	–	26	–	115
SANDWICHES								
BBQ Beef w/ Fries	1 serv	1580	66	62	–	179	–	2220
Beef Dip w/ Fries & Au Jus	1 serv	1560	64	72	–	151	–	1360
Boston Cheesesteak w/ Fries & Au Jus	1 serv	1790	80	87	–	172	–	2200
Boston Brute w/ Fries	1 serv	1420	48	60	–	163	–	3260
Buffalo Chicken w/ Fries	1 serv	1720	85	80	–	187	–	4470
Chicken Foccacia w/ Fries	1 serv	1350	45	65	–	140	–	1320
Spicy Italian Sausage w/ Caesar Salad	1 serv	1070	47	51	–	104	–	1580
Stromboli Chicken w/ Caesar Salad	1 serv	1020	53	44	–	101	–	1490
Stromboli Perogy w/ Caesar Salad	1 serv	1120	41	58	–	109	–	1550

FOOD	PORTION	CALS	PROT	FAT	CHOL	CARB	FIBER	SOD
Stromboli Santa Fe w/ Caesar Salad	1 serv	1000	44	45	–	104	–	2000
Super Ham & Cheese w/ Fries	1 serv	1370	39	71	–	137	–	2130
Tango Chicken Wrap w/ Caesar Salad	1 serv	740	37	42	–	55	–	1460

BRUEGGER'S BAGELS
BAGELS

FOOD	PORTION	CALS	PROT	FAT	CHOL	CARB	FIBER	SOD
Blueberry	1	330	11	2	0	68	4	530
Chocolate Chip	1	310	11	5	0	69	4	500
Cinnamon Raisin	1	320	11	2	0	68	4	510
Cinnamon Sugar	1	340	12	2	0	71	6	540
Everything	1	310	12	2	0	62	4	710
Garlic	1	310	12	2	0	62	4	540
Honey Grain	1	330	13	3	0	64	5	500
Jalapeno Bagel	1	310	12	2	0	63	4	550
Onion	1	310	12	2	0	62	4	540
Orange Cranberry	1	330	11	2	0	68	4	510
Plain	1	300	12	2	0	61	4	540
Poppy Seed	1	310	12	3	0	61	4	540
Pumpernickel	1	320	12	3	0	64	5	600
Rosemary Olive Oil	1	350	11	6	0	62	4	530
Salt	1	300	12	2	0	61	4	1540
Sesame	1	320	12	2	0	61	4	540
Sun Dried Tomato	1	320	11	2	0	65	4	630

DESSERTS

FOOD	PORTION	CALS	PROT	FAT	CHOL	CARB	FIBER	SOD
Blondies	1	370	5	23	25	42	2	220
Brownie Chocolate Chunk	1	330	4	19	55	39	2	150
Brownie Mint	1	300	3	17	40	34	0	95
Bruegger Bar	1	420	6	24	15	47	3	240
Cappuccino Bar	1	420	5	25	60	45	1	125
Luscious Lemon Bar	1	350	4	20	85	39	0	260
Oatmeal Cranberry Mountains	1	430	7	24	60	49	3	320
Raspberry Sammies	1	270	3	13	35	36	1	130

SANDWICH FILLINGS

FOOD	PORTION	CALS	PROT	FAT	CHOL	CARB	FIBER	SOD
Atlantic Smoked Salmon	2 oz	90	15	3	30	tr	0	840

FOOD	PORTION	CALS	PROT	FAT	CHOL	CARB	FIBER	SOD
Cream Cheese Bacon Scallion	2 tbsp	100	2	8	30	4	0	105
Cream Cheese Chive	2 tbsp	100	2	9	30	2	0	90
Cream Cheese Garden Veggie	2 tbsp	90	2	8	25	3	0	95
Cream Cheese Garden Veggie Light	2 tbsp	60	4	4	15	2	0	75
Cream Cheese Herb Garlic Light	2 tbsp	70	4	5	15	3	0	85
Cream Cheese Honey Walnut	2 tbsp	110	2	8	25	5	0	85
Cream Cheese Jalapeno	2 tbsp	100	2	9	30	3	0	100
Cream Cheese Light Strawberry	2 tbsp	70	4	4	15	4	0	85
Cream Cheese Olive Pimento	2 tbsp	100	2	9	30	2	0	90
Cream Cheese Plain	2 tbsp	90	2	8	25	4	0	85
Cream Cheese Plain Light	2 tbsp	70	2	5	15	3	0	90
Cream Cheese Smoked Salmon	2 tbsp	100	2	9	25	2	0	105
Cream Cheese Wildberry	2 tbsp	100	2	9	25	4	0	85
Hummus	2 tbsp	60	2	4	0	4	2	85
Tuna Salad	1 serv (2.5 oz)	180	8	14	20	6	0	440
SANDWICHES								
Atlantic Smoked Salmon	1	470	26	12	55	66	4	590
Chicken Breast	1	440	37	6	60	62	4	1230
Chicken Fajita	1	500	28	12	85	74	5	970
Chicken Salad w/ Mayo	1	460	24	12	55	67	4	820
Deli-Style Ham w/ Honey Mustard	1	440	24	5	30	77	4	1440
Egg Cheese	1	480	22	15	190	66	4	840
Egg Cheese Sausage	1	680	33	33	235	66	4	1570

FOOD	PORTION	CALS	PROT	FAT	CHOL	CARB	FIBER	SOD
Egg Cheese Bacon	1	560	26	22	200	66	4	1070
Egg Cheese Ham	1	520	28	17	205	66	4	1350
Garden Veggie	1	390	16	3	0	80	7	610
Herby Turkey	1	530	28	14	55	73	4	1180
Leonardo Da Veggie	1	460	19	11	40	69	4	740
Santa Fe Turkey	1	480	29	10	55	71	4	1630
Turkey w/ Mayo	1	480	25	14	35	65	4	1220

BURGER KING
BEVERAGES

FOOD	PORTION	CALS	PROT	FAT	CHOL	CARB	FIBER	SOD
Aquafina Water	1 bottle	0	0	0	0	0	0	0
Coffee Black	1 sm	0	0	0	0	1	0	0
Coffee Black	1 lg	10	0	0	0	2	0	10
Coke Classic	1 lg	330	0	0	0	82	0	–
Coke Classic	1 sm	160	0	0	0	41	0	–
Coke Classic frzn	1 sm	370	0	0	0	92	0	–
Diet Coke	1 sm	0	0	0	0	0	0	–
Dr Pepper	1 sm	160	0	0	0	39	0	–
Dr Pepper	1 lg	410	0	0	0	104	0	–
Milk 1%	1	100	8	3	10	12	0	125
Minute Maid Cherry frzn	1 sm	370	0	0	0	92	0	–
Minute Maid Orange Juice	1 serv	140	2	0	0	33	0	25
Shake Chocolate	1 sm	620	12	32	95	72	2	310
Shake Strawberry	1 sm	620	11	32	95	71	1	230
Shake Vanilla	1 sm	560	11	32	95	56	1	220
Sprite	1 lg	320	0	0	0	80	0	–
Sprite	1 sm	160	0	0	0	40	0	–

BREAKFAST SELECTIONS

FOOD	PORTION	CALS	PROT	FAT	CHOL	CARB	FIBER	SOD
Croissan'wich Bacon Egg & Cheese	1	360	15	22	195	25	tr	950
Croissan'wich Egg & Cheese	1	320	12	19	185	24	tr	730
Croissan'wich Ham Egg & Cheese	1	360	18	20	200	25	tr	1500
Croissan'wich Sausage Egg & Cheese	1	520	19	39	210	24	1	1090

FOOD	PORTION	CALS	PROT	FAT	CHOL	CARB	FIBER	SOD
Croissan'wich w/ Sausage & Cheese	1	420	14	31	45	23	tr	840
French Toast Sticks	5 pieces	390	7	20	0	46	2	440
Hash Browns	1 lg	390	3	25	0	38	4	760
Hash Browns	1 sm	230	2	15	0	23	2	450
Sourdough Breakfast Sandwich Bacon Egg & Cheese	1	380	16	22	190	30	2	990
Sourdough Breakfast Sandwich Ham Egg & Cheese	1	380	19	20	195	30	2	1560
Sourdough Breakfast Sandwich Sausage Egg & Cheese	1	540	20	39	210	30	2	1140
DESSERTS								
Chocolate Chip Cookies	2	440	5	16	20	68	0	360
Hershey Sundae Pie	1	300	3	18	10	31	1	190
MAIN MENU SELECTIONS								
Bacon Cheeseburger	1	400	22	20	60	32	2	1010
Bacon Double Cheeseburger	1	580	35	34	110	32	2	1270
Baguette Santa Fe Fire Grilled Chicken	1	350	29	5	45	47	4	1220
Baguette Savory Mustard Fire Grilled Chicken	1	350	28	5	45	47	3	1110
Baguette Smokey BBQ Fire Grilled Chicken	1	350	29	5	45	48	4	1450
Baja BBQ Sauce	1 serv	14	tr	tr	0	3	tr	351
BK Veggie Burger	1	340	14	10	0	47	4	950
Cheeseburger	1	360	19	17	50	31	2	790
Chicken Tenders	8 pieces	340	22	19	50	20	tr	840
Chicken Tenders	5 pieces	210	14	12	30	13	tr	530
Chili	1 serv	190	13	8	25	17	5	1040

FOOD	PORTION	CALS	PROT	FAT	CHOL	CARB	FIBER	SOD
Dipping Sauce Sweet And Sour	1 serv	40	0	0	0	10	0	65
Double Cheeseburger	1	540	32	31	100	32	2	1050
Double Hamburger	1	450	28	24	75	31	2	620
Double Whopper	1	980	52	62	160	52	4	1070
Double Whopper w/ Cheese	1	1070	57	70	185	53	4	1500
Dutch Apple Pie	1 serv	340	2	14	0	52	1	470
French Fries No Salt Added	1 lg	500	6	25	0	63	5	510
French Fries No Salt Added	1 sm	230	3	11	0	29	2	240
French Fries Salted	1 sm	230	3	11	0	29	2	410
French Fries Salted	1 lg	500	6	25	0	63	5	880
Hamburger	1	310	17	14	40	31	2	580
Onion Rings	1 sm	180	2	9	0	22	2	280
Onion Rings	1 lg	480	7	23	<5	60	5	690
Sandwich BK Fish Filet	1	520	18	30	55	44	2	840
Sandwich Grilled Chicken Caesar Club	1	540	34	27	65	40	3	1510
Sandwich Original Chicken	1	560	25	28	60	52	3	1270
Sandwich Whopper	1	580	39	26	75	48	4	1370
Whopper	1	710	31	43	85	52	4	980
Whopper Jr.	1	390	17	22	45	32	2	570
Whopper Jr. w/ Cheese	1	440	19	26	55	32	2	790
Whopper w/ Cheese	1	800	36	50	110	53	4	1420
SALAD DRESSINGS AND TOPPINGS								
Breakfast Syrup	1 serv	80	0	0	0	21	0	20
Dipping Sauce Barbecue	1 serv	35	0	0	0	9	0	390
Dipping Sauce Honey	1 serv	90	0	0	0	23	0	0
Dipping Sauce Honey Mustard	1 serv	90	0	6	10	9	0	150

FOOD	PORTION	CALS	PROT	FAT	CHOL	CARB	FIBER	SOD
Dipping Sauce Ranch	1 serv	140	tr	15	<5	tr	–	95
Dipping Sauce Zesty Onion Ring	1 serv	150	0	15	15	3	tr	210
Dressing Kraft Catalina	1 serv	180	0	16	0	10	0	530
Dressing Kraft Fat Free Ranch	1 serv	60	0	0	0	6	0	430
Dressing Kraft Ranch	1 serv	220	0	23	10	2	0	410
Dressing Light Done Right Light Italian	1 serv	50	0	5	0	4	0	360
Dressing Signature Creamy Caesar	1 serv	140	tr	13	10	4	0	340
Fire Roasted Sauce	1 serv	9	tr	tr	0	2	tr	129
Grape Jam	1 serv	30	0	0	0	7	0	0
Peppers & Onions Flame Roasted	1 serv	18	tr	tr	0	3	2	81
Savory Mustard Sauce	1 serv	21	tr	tr	2	4	tr	92
Strawberry Jam	1 serv	30	0	0	0	7	0	0
SALADS								
Chicken Caesar w/o Dressing And Croutons	1 serv	230	36	7	60	5	3	1040
Side Salad w/o Dressing	1 srv	25	1	0	0	5	2	15

BURGERVILLE

FOOD	PORTION	CALS	PROT	FAT	CHOL	CARB	FIBER	SOD
BEVERAGES								
Milkshake Black Forest	1 (16 oz)	600	9	20	75	103	–	170
Milkshake Blackberry	1 (16 oz)	610	9	25	100	95	–	180
Milkshake Caramel Apple	1 (16 oz)	540	9	26	110	69	–	230
Milkshake Chocolate	1 (16 oz)	520	9	23	95	73	–	220

FOOD	PORTION	CALS	PROT	FAT	CHOL	CARB	FIBER	SOD
Milkshake Fresh Strawberry	1 (16 oz)	560	8	21	85	88	–	160
Milkshake Mocha Perk	1 (16 oz)	590	11	25	100	83	–	210
Milkshake Pumpkin	1 (16 oz)	460	10	22	90	60	–	170
Milkshake Vanilla	1 (16 oz)	500	8	20	85	74	–	180
Smoothies Chocolate Monkey	1 (16 oz)	470	9	1	0	105	–	180
Smoothies Fresh Blackberry	1 (16 oz)	420	9	0	0	94	–	200
Smoothies Fresh Raspberry	1 (16 oz)	470	9	0	0	103	–	220
Smoothies Fresh Strawberry	1 (16 oz)	390	9	0	0	86	–	170
Smoothies Strawberry Splash	1 (16 oz)	310	7	1	0	70	–	125
Smoothies Triple Berry Blast	1 (16 oz)	360	8	0	0	77	–	160
BREAKFAST SELECTIONS								
American Cheese	2 slices	90	5	7	20	0	–	450
Bagel Bacon Egg	1	450	23	11	250	64	–	1070
Bagel Cheese	1	290	12	6	10	53	–	580
Bagel Ham Egg	1	450	28	8	260	65	–	1380
Bagel Plain	1	310	12	1	0	63	–	700
Bagel Sausage Egg	1	640	29	29	280	65	–	1210
Biscuit Bacon Egg	1	400	16	23	250	32	–	580
Biscuit Ham Egg	1	400	21	20	260	33	–	890
Biscuit Sausage Egg	1	590	22	41	280	33	–	720
Tillamook Cheese	1 slice	120	7	10	40	1	–	170
MAIN MENU SELECTIONS								
Cheeseburger	1	370	17	20	45	29	–	720
Cheeseburger Double Beef	1	470	27	27	75	29	–	760
Cheeseburger Pepper Bacon	1	680	38	45	75	28	–	1120
Cheeseburger Tillamook	1	630	34	40	65	32	–	970
Cheeseburger Walla Walla Onion	1	679	31	44	80	39	–	1660

FOOD	PORTION	CALS	PROT	FAT	CHOL	CARB	FIBER	SOD
Chicken Strips	5 pieces	550	33	30	20	36	—	1330
Colossal	1	530	30	30	35	31	—	1050
French Fries	1 kid size	220	3	12	—	24	—	240
French Fries	1 reg	390	5	22	—	44	—	440
Gardenburger	1	460	18	19	30	53	—	1500
Gardenburger Spicy Black Bean	1	550	24	32	40	45	—	1140
Halibut	3 pieces	230	17	14	15	10	—	300
Hamburger	1	320	15	16	35	29	—	490
Onion Rings Walla Walla	3 pieces	485	7	29	0	50	—	758
Roasted Turkey Salad w/o Hazelnuts	1 serv	375	30	19	65	22	—	880
Rogue River Blue Cheese Bacon Burger	1	510	36	56	70	29	—	1160
Sandwich Crispy Chicken	1	450	20	18	40	55	—	1050
Sandwich Deluxe Crispy Chicken	1	610	30	30	85	56	—	1380
Sandwich Grilled Chicken	1	350	37	3	5	45	—	1100
Sandwich Halibut	1	490	20	30	35	35	—	680
Sandwich Turkey Club	1	490	25	32	55	27	—	910
Side Salad w/o Dressing	1 serv	70	5	4	10	5	—	100
Smoked Salmon Salad w/o Hazelnuts	1 serv	370	31	18	55	21	—	1250
Sweet Potato Fries	1 serv	530	4	29	0	60	—	510
Turkey Burger	1	470	35	21	75	32	—	850
CARIBOU COFFEE								
Black Forest Mocha	1 med	553	12	19	—	83	—	—
Black Forest Wild Drink	1 med	553	12	19	—	86	—	—

FOOD	PORTION	CALS	PROT	FAT	CHOL	CARB	FIBER	SOD
Cappuccino	1 med (16 oz)	113	11	1	–	15	–	–
Cappuccino 2%	1 med (16 oz)	162	11	7	–	17	–	–
Caramel Hirise	1 med (16 oz)	414	11	13	–	59	–	–
Chai Latte 2%	1 med (16 oz)	286	8	5	–	50	–	–
Chai Skim	1 med (16 oz)	236	8	–	–	48	–	–
Cooler Caramel	1 med (12 oz)	450	3	10	–	83	–	–
Cooler Chocolate	1 med (12 oz)	257	4	3	–	54	–	–
Cooler Coffee	1 med (16 oz)	230	4	3	–	48	–	–
Cooler Espresso	1 med (16 oz)	193	3	2	–	40	–	–
Cooler Mint Oreo	1 med (12 oz)	614	10	19	–	108	–	–
Cooler Vanilla	1 med (16 oz)	257	3	4	–	52	–	–
Glacier Gum	2 pieces	5	0	0	0	2	–	–
Hot Apple Blast	1 med	379	–	8	–	76	–	–
Latte 2%	1 med (16 oz)	171	11	6	–	17	–	–
Latte Skim	1 med (16 oz)	121	12	1	–	17	–	–
Latte Skinny Bou Low Cal	1 med	120	12	1	–	17	–	–
Lite White Berry	1 med (16 oz)	311	9	5	–	57	–	–
Mint Condition	1 med (16 oz)	520	10	19	–	75	–	–
Mints All Flavors	3 pieces	5	0	0	0	1	–	–
Mocha 2%	1 med (16 oz)	347	10	16	–	41	–	–
Mocha Skim	1 med (16 oz)	302	13	12	–	34	–	–

FOOD	PORTION	CALS	PROT	FAT	CHOL	CARB	FIBER	SOD
Mocha Turtle	1 med (16 oz)	559	10	19	–	82	–	–
Smoothie Passion Green Tea	1 med (16 oz)	252	2	tr	–	61	–	–
Smoothie Raspberry	1 med (12 oz)	293	2	tr	–	70	–	–
Smoothie Strawberry Banana	1 med (16 oz)	253	2	tr	–	61	–	–
Smoothie Wild Berry	1 med (16 oz)	235	2	tr	–	56	–	–

CARL'S JR.
BAKED SELECTIONS

FOOD	PORTION	CALS	PROT	FAT	CHOL	CARB	FIBER	SOD
Cheese Danish	1	400	5	23	15	49	1	390
Cheesecake Strawberry Swirl	1 serv	290	6	17	55	30	2	230
Chocolate Cake	1 serv	300	3	12	30	48	1	350
Chocolate Chip Cookie	1	350	3	18	20	46	1	330
Muffin Blueberry	1	340	5	14	40	49	1	340
Muffin Bran Raisin	1	370	6	13	45	61	6	410

BEVERAGES

FOOD	PORTION	CALS	PROT	FAT	CHOL	CARB	FIBER	SOD
Coca-Cola Classic	1 reg (21 oz)	220	0	0	0	54	0	30
Coffee	1 reg (12 oz)	2	0	tr	0	tr	0	<5
Diet Coke	1 reg (21 oz)	tr	0	0	0	tr	0	40
Dr. Pepper	1 reg (21 oz)	200	0	0	0	53	0	95
Hot Chocolate	1 serv (12 oz)	120	2	2	0	22	1	125
Iced Tea	1 reg (12 oz)	5	0	0	0	0	0	0
Lemonade Minute Maid Orange	1 reg (21 oz)	200	0	0	0	52	0	100
Milk 1%	1 (10 fl oz)	150	14	3	15	18	0	180
Minute Maid Orange Soda	1 reg (21 oz)	200	0	0	0	52	0	100
Nestea Raspberry	1 reg (21 oz)	160	0	0	0	42	0	40
Orange Juice	1 (10 oz)	150	1	0	0	37	0	0
Ramblin' Root Beer	1 reg (21 oz)	220	0	0	0	60	0	70
Shake Chocolate	1 reg (32 oz)	770	21	15	65	140	tr	520

FOOD	PORTION	CALS	PROT	FAT	CHOL	CARB	FIBER	SOD
Shake Strawberry	1 reg (32 oz)	750	20	15	65	133	0	490
Shake Vanilla	1 reg (32 oz)	700	22	16	70	115	0	530
Sprite	1 reg (21 oz)	200	0	0	0	52	0	65
BREAKFAST SELECTIONS								
Bacon	2 strips	45	3	4	10	0	0	150
Breakfast Burrito	1	560	29	32	495	36	1	980
Breakfast Quesadilla	1	370	16	17	240	36	1	910
English Muffin w/ Margarine	1	210	5	9	0	28	2	300
French Toast Dips w/o Syrup	1 serv	370	6	20	0	42	1	430
Grape Jelly	1 serv (0.5 oz)	40	0	0	0	9	0	15
Hash Brown Nuggets	1 serv	330	3	21	0	32	2	470
Sausage	1 patty	190	7	18	40	2	0	480
Scrambled Eggs	1 serv	180	13	14	455	1	0	110
Sourdough Breakfast	1 serv	410	26	20	275	33	1	930
Strawberry Jam	1 serv (0.5 oz)	40	0	0	0	9	0	15
Sunrise Sandwich w/o Meat	1	360	13	21	245	28	tr	470
Table Syrup	1 serv (1 oz)	90	0	0	0	21	0	0
MAIN MENU SELECTIONS								
American Cheese	1 sm	50	3	4	10	1	0	200
BBQ Sauce	1 serv (1.1 oz)	50	1	0	0	11	0	270
Breadstick	1 (0.3 oz)	35	1	1	0	7	tr	60
Carl's Famous Star	1	590	24	32	70	50	3	910
Chicken Stars	6 pieces	260	13	16	40	14	tr	480
CrissCut Fries	1 serv	410	5	24	0	43	4	950
Croutons	1 serv (0.5 oz)	30	1	1	0	5	0	105
Double Sourdough Bacon Cheeseburger	1	880	50	59	165	37	2	1010
Double Western Bacon Cheeseburger	1	920	51	50	155	65	3	1770
Famous Bacon Cheeseburger	1	700	31	41	95	51	3	1310
French Fries	1 kid size	250	4	12	0	32	2	150
French Fries	1 med	460	7	22	0	59	5	280
Hamburger	1	280	14	9	35	36	1	480

FOOD	PORTION	CALS	PROT	FAT	CHOL	CARB	FIBER	SOD
Honey Sauce	1 serv (1 oz)	90	0	0	0	22	0	0
Mustard Sauce	1 serv (1 oz)	50	0	0	0	11	0	210
Onion Rings	1 serv	430	7	22	0	53	3	700
Potato Bacon & Cheese	1	640	21	29	40	75	6	1660
Potato Broccoli & Cheese	1 serv	530	11	21	15	76	6	940
Potato Plain w/o Margarine	1	290	6	0	0	68	6	20
Potato Sour Cream & Chives	1	430	7	14	10	70	6	180
Salsa	1 serv (0.9 oz)	10	0	0	0	2	0	160
Sandwich Bacon Swiss Crispy Chicken	1	760	31	38	90	72	3	1550
Sandwich Carl's Catch Fish	1	530	18	28	80	55	2	1030
Sandwich Charbroiled Sirloin Stead	1	550	30	24	80	52	2	1080
Sandwich Chargrilled Chicken Club	1	470	31	23	95	37	2	1110
Sandwich Chargrilled Santa Fe Chicken	1	540	28	31	95	37	2	1210
Sandwich Chargrilled BBQ Chicken	1	290	25	4	60	41	2	840
Sandwich Ranch Crispy Chicken	1	660	24	31	70	71	3	1180
Sandwich Southwest Spicy Chicken	1	620	16	41	65	48	2	1640
Sandwich Spicy Chicken	1	480	14	26	40	47	2	1220
Sandwich Western Bacon Crispy Chicken	1	750	31	28	80	91	3	1900

FOOD	PORTION	CALS	PROT	FAT	CHOL	CARB	FIBER	SOD
Sourdough Bacon Cheeseburger	1	640	30	41	95	37	2	690
Sourdough Ranch Bacon Cheeseburger	1	720	33	46	95	43	3	800
Super Star	1	790	41	47	130	51	3	980
Sweet N'Sour Sauce	1 serv (1 oz)	50	0	0	0	12	0	80
Swiss Cheese	1 serv	50	4	4	15	0	0	230
Western Bacon Cheeseburger	1	660	31	30	85	64	3	1410
Zucchini	1 serv	320	6	19	0	31	2	860
SALAD DRESSINGS								
1000 Island	1 serv (2 oz)	230	tr	23	20	5	0	420
Blue Cheese	1 serv (2 oz)	320	2	35	25	1	0	370
French Fat Free	1 serv (2 oz)	60	0	0	0	16	tr	660
House	1 serv (2 oz)	220	1	22	25	1	0	450
Italian Fat Free	1 serv (2 oz)	15	0	0	0	4	0	770
SALADS AND SALAD BARS								
Salad-To-Go Charbroiled Chicken	1 serv	200	25	7	75	12	4	440
Salad-To-Go Garden	1	50	3	3	5	4	2	60

CARVEL
BEVERAGES

FOOD	PORTION	CALS	PROT	FAT	CHOL	CARB	FIBER	SOD
Carvelanche w/ Topping	1 (16 oz)	600	21	30	95	71	tr	280
Regular Fizzlers	1 (16 oz)	340	2	5	10	75	1	105
Thick Shake Chocolate	1 (16 oz)	720	18	31	115	96	0	420
Thick Shake Reduced Fat Chocolate	1 (16 oz)	520	17	8	35	100	tr	350
Thick Shake Reduced Fat Vanilla	1 (16 oz)	460	16	7	35	81	tr	280
ICE CREAM								
Cake Butterscotch Dream	1 slice (4 oz)	260	5	10	25	37	0	180

FOOD	PORTION	CALS	PROT	FAT	CHOL	CARB	FIBER	SOD
Cake Celebration	1 slice (4 oz)	200	4	10	25	24	tr	115
Cake Cookies & Cream	1 serv (4 oz)	240	4	12	25	29	1	140
Cake Fudge Drizzle	1 slice (4 oz)	240	4	11	20	32	1	160
Cake Game Ball	1 slice (4 oz)	330	5	17	40	41	1	170
Cake Holiday	1 slice (4 oz)	200	4	10	25	24	tr	115
Cake Lil'Love	1 piece (4 oz)	200	4	10	25	24	tr	115
Cake Lil'Love All Vanilla	1 piece (4.4 oz)	330	6	16	35	41	tr	200
Cake Sinfully Chocolate	1 slice (4 oz)	240	5	10	20	34	1	170
Cake Strawberries & Cream	1 slice (4 oz)	270	5	10	30	40	1	160
Chocolate	4 oz	190	4	10	25	22	0	100
Chocolate No Fat	4 oz	120	2	0	0	28	0	40
Flying Saucer 98% Fat Free Black Raspberry	1	170	4	2	5	40	tr	170
Flying Saucer 98% Fat Free Chocolate	1	170	4	2	0	34	1	170
Flying Saucer 98% Fat Free Coffee	1	190	5	2	5	40	tr	170
Flying Saucer 98% Fat Free Maple	1	190	5	2	5	40	tr	170
Flying Saucer 98% Fat Free Mint	1	190	5	2	5	40	tr	170
Flying Saucer 98% Fat Free Pistachio	1	190	5	2	5	40	tr	170
Flying Saucer 98% Fat Free Strawberry	1	190	5	2	5	40	1	170

FOOD	PORTION	CALS	PROT	FAT	CHOL	CARB	FIBER	SOD
Flying Saucer 98% Fat Free Vanilla	1	190	5	2	5	40	tr	170
Flying Saucer Chocolate	1	230	5	9	30	33	2	140
Flying Saucer Vanilla	1	240	5	10	30	33	tr	180
Vanilla	4 oz	200	5	10	40	21	0	110
Vanilla No Fat	4 oz	120	4	0	0	25	0	55
Vanilla No Sugar Added	4 oz	130	5	3	15	25	0	85
ICES								
Italian Ice Blue Raspberry	4 oz	70	0	0	0	19	0	0
Italian Ice Bubble Gum	4 oz	70	0	0	0	19	0	0
Italian Ice Cherry	4 oz	100	0	0	0	25	0	0
Italian Ice Chocolate Ice Cream	4 oz	90	1	1	7	20	0	20
Italian Ice Cotton Candy	4 oz	70	0	0	0	19	0	0
Italian Ice Lemon	4 oz	70	0	0	0	19	0	0
Italian Ice Mango	4 oz	70	0	0	0	27	0	0
Italian Ice Orange	4 oz	70	0	0	0	19	0	0
Italian Ice Vanilla Ice Cream	4 oz	90	tr	2	7	20	0	20
Italian Ice Watermelon	4 oz	70	0	0	0	19	0	0
Sherbet All Flavors	4 oz	140	2	1	5	31	0	45

CHICKEN OUT ROTISSERIE
MAIN MENU SELECTIONS

FOOD	PORTION	CALS	PROT	FAT	CHOL	CARB	FIBER	SOD
Apple Cornbread Stuffing	1 serv (6 oz)	215	6	2	–	42	–	–
Baked Potato Wedges	1 serv (6 oz)	110	2	tr	–	26	–	–
Biscuit	1	150	4	4	–	29	–	–
Chicken Breast Skinless	1 serv (6 oz)	210	35	4	–	0	0	–

FOOD	PORTION	CALS	PROT	FAT	CHOL	CARB	FIBER	SOD
Chicken Burger w/o Cheese	1	285	50	7	–	36	–	–
Chunky Cinnamon Applesauce	1 serv (6 oz)	60	0	0	–	25	–	–
Creamed Spinach w/ Artichokes	1 serv (6 oz)	160	8	6	–	20	–	–
Farm Fresh Cole Slaw	1 serv (6 oz)	55	2	0	–	10	–	–
French Baguette	1	80	6	1	–	28	–	–
Fresh Fruit Salad	1 serv (6 oz)	77	1	tr	–	56	–	–
Mandarin Walnut Cranberry Relish	1 serv (6 oz)	240	0	1	–	66	–	–
Mashed Sweet Potatoes	1 serv (6 oz)	120	0	tr	–	40	–	–
Oriental Green Beans	1 serv (6 oz)	34	2	0	–	8	–	–
Pulled White Meat	1 serv (6 oz)	180	25	4	–	0	0	–
Real Cheese & Macaroni	1 serv (6 oz)	311	4	12	–	39	–	–
Red Skin Mashed Potatoes	1 serv (6 oz)	181	3	6	–	26	–	–
Rice Pilaf	1 serv (6 oz)	140	4	1	–	28	–	–
Roasted Peas Corn & Carrots	1 serv (6 oz)	120	8	tr	–	22	–	–
Rotisserie Chicken Quarter Dark No Skin	1 serv	232	31	6	–	0	0	–
Rotisserie Chicken Quarter White No Skin	1 serv	196	35	4	–	0	–	–
Sandwich BBQ Pulled Chicken	1	406	47	8	–	42	–	–
Sandwich Grilled Chicken Breast	1	350	42	6	–	28	–	–
Sandwich Open Faced Pulled Chicken	1	682	37	18	–	80	–	–
Sandwich Pulled Chicken	1	320	32	6	–	28	–	–

FOOD	PORTION	CALS	PROT	FAT	CHOL	CARB	FIBER	SOD
Sandwich Signature Chicken Salad	1	370	42	5	–	31	–	–
Steamed Broccoli & Carrots	1 serv (6 oz)	30	9	0	–	6	–	–
Vegetarian Baked Beans	1 serv (6 oz)	150	7	1	–	26	–	–
Wrap Chinese Chicken Salad w/o Dressing	1	330	41	9	–	36	–	–
Wrap Fajita	1	360	43	10	–	38	–	–
Wrap Fresh Vegetable Salad w/o Dressing	1	170	5	4	–	32	–	–
Wrap Grilled Chicken Caesar	1	355	8	11	–	31	–	–
Wrap Pesto Chicken	1	405	39	11	–	25	–	–
Wrap Pulled Chicken	1	300	28	7	–	24	–	–
Wrap Skinless Grilled Chicken	1	330	38	7	–	24	–	–
SALAD DRESSINGS								
Balsamic Vinaigrette	1 oz	18	0	0	–	4	–	–
Caesar	1 oz	55	0	5	–	1	–	–
Chinese	1 oz	72	0	7	–	2	–	–
Low Fat Honey Mustard	1 oz	23	1	1	–	5	–	–
Ranch	1 oz	90	1	6	–	1	–	–
Southwestern	1 oz	85	1	7	–	3	–	–
SALADS								
Caesar w/ Grilled Chicken w/o Dressing	½ serv	235	5	8	–	7	–	–
Caesar w/o Dressing	½ serv	140	3	4	–	9	–	–
Chicken Salad Apricot	1 serv (6 oz)	300	39	8	–	1	–	–
Chicken Salad BBQ Pulled	1 serv (6 oz)	263	44	5	–	8	–	–

FOOD	PORTION	CALS	PROT	FAT	CHOL	CARB	FIBER	SOD
Chicken Salad Chinese w/o Dressing	½ serv	210	38	6	—	12	—	—
Chicken Salad Pesto	1 serv (6 oz)	285	36	8	—	1	—	—
Chicken Salad Pulled w/o Dressing	½ serv	204	37	4	—	5	—	—
Chicken Salad Santa Fe w/o Dressing	½ serv	240	40	7	—	14	—	—
Chicken Salad Signature	1 serv (6 oz)	230	37	5	—	1	—	—
Garden w/ Grilled Chicken w/o Dressing	½ serv	200	40	4	—	5	—	—
Garden w/o Dressing	½ serv	25	1	1	—	4	—	—
Young Spinach w/ Grilled Chicken w/o Dressing	½ serv	270	35	4	—	19	—	—
Young Spinach w/o Dressing	½ serv	180	5	2	—	19	—	—
SOUPS								
Chicken Noodle	1 serv (6 oz)	130	11	3	—	8	—	—
Vegetable Minestrone	1 serv (6 oz)	96	3	2	—	12	—	—

CHICK-FIL-A
BEVERAGES

FOOD	PORTION	CALS	PROT	FAT	CHOL	CARB	FIBER	SOD
Coca-Cola Classic	1 sm	110	0	0	0	28	0	10
Diet Coke	1 sm	0	0	0	0	0	0	10
Diet Lemonade	1 sm	25	0	0	0	5	0	5
Ice Tea Sweetened	1 sm	80	0	0	0	19	0	0
Iced Tea Unsweetened	1 serv	0	0	0	0	0	0	0
Lemonade	1 sm	170	0	1	0	41	0	10
DESSERTS								
Cheesecake w/ Blueberry Topping	1 slice	370	6	21	90	39	2	280

FOOD	PORTION	CALS	PROT	FAT	CHOL	CARB	FIBER	SOD
Cheesecake w/ Strawberry Topping	1 slice	360	6	21	90	38	2	290
Fudge Nut Brownie	1	330	4	15	20	45	2	210
IceDream Cone	1 sm	160	4	4	15	28	0	80
IceDream Cup	1 sm	230	5	6	25	39	0	100
Lemon Pie	1 slice	320	7	10	110	51	3	220
MAIN MENU SELECTIONS								
Barbecue Sauce	1 pkg	45	0	0	0	11	0	180
Carrot & Raisin Salad	1 sm	130	1	6	0	22	2	90
Chargrilled Chicken Caesar Salad	1 serv	240	31	10	85	6	2	1170
Chargrilled Chicken Club Sandwich w/o Sauce	1	360	30	13	80	31	2	1370
Chargrilled Chicken Deluxe Sandwich	1	280	26	7	60	30	2	1010
Chargrilled Chicken Filet	1	100	20	2	60	1	0	690
Chargrilled Chicken Sandwich	1	280	25	7	60	29	1	1000
Chargrilled Chicken Sandwich w/o Butter	1	240	25	4	60	28	1	1000
Chicken Deluxe Sandwich	1	420	28	16	60	39	2	1300
Chicken Sandwich	1	410	28	16	60	38	1	1300
Chicken Sandwich w/o Butter	1	380	28	13	60	37	1	1290
Chicken Filet	1	230	23	11	60	10	0	990
Chicken Salad Sandwich On Whole Wheat	1	350	20	15	65	32	5	880
Chick-N-Strips	4	250	25	11	70	12	0	570
Cole Slaw	1 sm	210	1	17	20	14	2	180
Cool Wrap Chargrilled Chicken	1	390	31	7	70	53	3	1120
Cool Wrap Chicken Caesar	1	460	38	11	85	51	3	1540

FOOD	PORTION	CALS	PROT	FAT	CHOL	CARB	FIBER	SOD
Cool Wrap Spicy Chicken	1	390	31	7	70	51	3	1150
Dijon Honey Mustard Sauce	1 pkg	50	0	5	5	2	0	65
Hearty Breast of Chicken Soup	1 cup	100	9	2	50	13	1	940
Honey Mustard Sauce	1 pkg	45	0	0	0	10	0	150
Nuggets	8	260	26	12	70	12	tr	1090
Polynesian Sauce	1 pkg	110	0	6	0	13	0	210
Waffle Fries w/o Salt	1 sm	280	3	14	15	36	4	40
Waffle Potato Fries	1 sm	280	3	14	15	37	5	105
SALAD DRESSINGS								
Basil Vinaigrette	1 pkg	210	0	21	0	4	0	160
Blue Cheese	1 pkg	190	1	20	20	2	0	370
Buttermilk Ranch	1 pkg	190	1	20	10	2	0	350
Caesar	1 pkg	200	1	21	45	1	0	300
Fat Free Dijon Honey Mustard	1 pkg	60	0	0	0	14	0	200
Light Italian	1 pkg	20	0	1	0	3	0	640
Spicy	1 pkg	210	0	22	10	2	0	170
Thousand Island	1 pkg	170	0	16	10	6	0	300
SALADS AND SALAD BARS								
Chargrilled Chicken Garden Salad	1 serv	180	23	6	70	8	3	730
Chick-N-Strips Salad	1 serv	340	30	16	85	19	3	680
Croutons Garlic & Butter	1 pkg	90	2	4	0	11	0	140
Roasted Sunflower Kernels Unsalted	1 pkg	80	3	7	0	3	tr	0
Side Salad	1 serv	80	5	5	15	6	2	110
CHIPOTLE								
Barbacoa	1 serv (5 oz)	285	43	16	74	1	—	680
Black Beans	1 serv (4 oz)	130	9	1	0	22	—	318
Carnitas	1 serv (4 oz)	227	29	12	66	0	—	873
Cheese	1 serv (4 oz)	110	7	9	30	tr	0	180
Chicken	1 serv (4 oz)	219	29	11	96	0	—	431

FOOD	PORTION	CALS	PROT	FAT	CHOL	CARB	FIBER	SOD
Chips	1 serv (4 oz)	490	7	19	0	71	5	130
Crispy Taco Shells	4	240	4	9	0	34	2	40
Fajita Vegetables	1 serv (3 oz)	100	1	8	0	6	1	640
Flour Tortilla	1 (13 inch)	340	9	9	0	54	2	860
Flour Tortilla	1 (6 inch)	300	9	8	0	45	2	720
Guacamole	1 serv (4 oz)	170	2	15	0	8	5	370
Lettuce	1 serv (1 oz)	5	tr	0	0	tr	tr	0
Pinto Beans	1 serv (4 oz)	138	9	1	0	23	—	374
Rice	1 serv (5 oz)	240	4	7	0	40	tr	610
Salsa Corn	1 serv (4 oz)	100	3	1	0	22	3	540
Salsa Tomato	1 serv (4 oz)	25	1	0	0	6	1	560
Sour Cream	1 serv (2 oz)	120	2	10	40	2	0	30
Steak	1 serv (4 oz)	230	29	12	51	2	—	306
Tomatillo Green	1 serv (2 oz)	15	1	tr	0	3	—	227
Tomatillo Red	1 serv (2 oz)	28	1	1	0	4	—	493

CHURCH'S CHICKEN

DESSERTS

FOOD	PORTION	CALS	PROT	FAT	CHOL	CARB	FIBER	SOD
Apple Pie	1 pie	280	2	12	<5	41	1	340
Edward's Double Lemon Pie	1 pie	300	5	14	25	39	0	160
Edward's Strawberry Cream Cheese Pie	1 pie	280	4	15	15	32	2	130

MAIN MENU SELECTIONS

FOOD	PORTION	CALS	PROT	FAT	CHOL	CARB	FIBER	SOD
Breast	1 serv	200	19	12	65	4	0	510
Cajun Rice	1 reg	130	1	7	5	16	tr	260
Chicken Fried Steak w/ White Gravy	1 serv	470	21	28	65	36	1	1615
Cole Slaw	1 reg	92	4	6	0	8	2	230
Collard Greens	1 reg	25	2	0	0	5	2	170
Corn On The Cob	1 ear	139	4	3	0	24	9	15
French Fries	1 reg	210	3	11	0	29	2	60
Honey Butter Biscuit	1	250	2	16	<5	26	1	640
Jalapeno Cheese Bombers	4 pieces	240	8	10	28	29	3	968
Krispy Tender Strips	1 piece	137	11	5	25	11	tr	431
Leg	1 serv	140	13	9	45	2	0	160
Macaroni & Cheese	1 reg	210	8	11	15	23	1	690

FOOD	PORTION	CALS	PROT	FAT	CHOL	CARB	FIBER	SOD
Mashed Potatoes & Gravy	1 reg	90	1	3	0	14	1	520
Okra	1 reg	210	3	16	0	19	4	520
Sweet Corn Nuggets	1 reg	250	3	12	0	30	2	530
Tender Crunchers	6–8 pieces	411	34	15	74	32	1	1294
Thigh	1 serv	230	16	16	80	5	0	520
Whole Jalapeno Peppers	2	10	0	0	0	2	1	390
Wing	1 serv	250	19	16	60	8	0	540
SAUCES								
BBQ	1 pkg	29	0	0	0	7	0	181
Creamy Jalapeno	1 pkg	102	0	11	10	1	0	137
Honey Mustard	1 pkg	111	0	11	10	4	0	130
Purple Pepper	1 pkg	21	0	0	0	12	0	26
Sweet & Sour	1 pkg	31	0	0	0	8	0	116

CINNABON

FOOD	PORTION	CALS	PROT	FAT	CHOL	CARB	FIBER	SOD
Caramel Pecanbon	1	890	—	41	—	—	—	—
Cinnabon	1 reg	670	—	34	—	—	—	—

COLOMBO FROZEN YOGURT

FOOD	PORTION	CALS	PROT	FAT	CHOL	CARB	FIBER	SOD
Strawberry Lowfat	½ cup	110	3	2	10	21	0	55
Strawberry Nonfat	½ cup	100	3	0	<5	20	0	55

DAIRY QUEEN
FOOD SELECTIONS

FOOD	PORTION	CALS	PROT	FAT	CHOL	CARB	FIBER	SOD
Chicken Breast Fillet Sandwich	1 (6.7 oz)	430	24	20	55	37	2	760
Chicken Strip Basket	1 serv (14.5 oz)	1000	35	50	55	102	5	2510
Chili 'n' Cheese Dog	1 (5 oz)	330	14	21	45	22	2	1090
DQ Homestyle Bacon Double Cheeseburger	1 (8.9 oz)	610	41	36	130	31	2	1380
DQ Homestyle Cheeseburger	1 (5.3 oz)	340	20	17	55	29	2	850
DQ Homestyle Double Cheeseburger	1 (7.7 oz)	540	35	31	115	30	2	1130

FOOD	PORTION	CALS	PROT	FAT	CHOL	CARB	FIBER	SOD
DQ Homestyle Hamburger	1 (4.8 oz)	290	17	12	45	29	2	630
DQ Ultimate Burger	1 (9.4 oz)	670	40	43	135	29	2	1210
French Fries	1 med (3.9 oz)	440	5	23	0	53	4	1110
French Fries	1 sm (4 oz)	350	4	18	0	42	3	880
Grilled Chicken Sandwich	1 (6.5 oz)	310	24	10	50	30	3	1040
Hot Dog	1 (3.5 oz)	240	9	14	25	19	1	730
Onion Rings	1 serv (4 oz)	320	5	16	0	39	3	180
The Great Steakmelt Basket	1 serv (13.2 oz)	770	32	38	75	72	5	2290
ICE CREAM								
Banana Split	1 (12.9 oz)	510	8	12	30	96	3	180
Blizzard Chocolate Sandwich Cookie	1 sm (12 oz)	520	10	18	40	79	1	380
Blizzard Chocolate Sandwich Cookie	1 med (11.4 oz)	640	12	23	45	97	1	500
Blizzard Chocolate Chip Cookie Dough	1 sm (12 oz)	660	12	24	55	99	1	440
Blizzard Chocolate Chip Cookie Dough	1 med (15.4 oz)	950	17	36	75	143	2	660
Breeze Heath	1 sm (10.2 oz)	470	11	10	10	85	1	380
Breeze Heath	1 med (14.2 oz)	710	15	18	20	123	1	580
Breeze Strawberry	1 sm (12 oz)	320	10	1	5	68	1	190
Breeze Strawberry	1 med (13.4 oz)	460	13	1	10	99	1	270
Buster Bar	1 (5.2 oz)	450	10	28	15	41	2	280
Chocolate Malt	1 sm (14.7 oz)	650	15	16	55	111	0	370
Chocolate Malt	1 med (19.9 oz)	880	19	22	70	153	0	500
Cone Chocolate	1 sm (5 oz)	240	6	8	20	37	0	115
Cone Chocolate	1 med (6.9 oz)	340	8	11	30	53	0	160

FOOD	PORTION	CALS	PROT	FAT	CHOL	CARB	FIBER	SOD
Cone Vanilla	1 med (6.9 oz)	330	8	9	30	53	0	160
Cone Vanilla	1 sm (5 oz)	230	6	7	20	38	0	115
Cone Vanilla	1 lg (8.9 oz)	410	10	12	40	65	0	200
Cone Yogurt	1 med (6.9 oz)	260	9	1	5	56	0	160
Cone Dipped	1 med (7.7 oz)	490	9	24	30	59	1	190
Cone Dipped	1 sm (5.5 oz)	340	6	17	20	42	1	130
Cup Of Yogurt	1 med (6.7 oz)	230	8	1	5	48	0	150
Dilly Bar Chocolate	1 (3 oz)	210	3	13	10	21	0	75
DQ 8 Inch Round Cake Undecorated	⅛ of cake (6.2 oz)	340	7	13	25	56	1	280
DQ Fudge Bar No Sugar Added	1 (2.3 oz)	50	4	0	0	13	0	70
DQ Lemon Freez'r	½ cup (3.2 oz)	80	0	0	0	20	0	10
DQ Nonfat Frozen Yogurt	½ cup (3 oz)	100	3	0	<5	21	0	70
DQ Sandwich	1 (2.1 oz)	200	4	6	10	31	1	140
DQ Soft Serve Chocolate	½ cup (3.3 oz)	150	4	5	15	22	0	75
DQ Soft Serve Vanilla	½ cup (3.3 oz)	140	3	5	15	22	0	70
DQ Treatzza Pizza Heath	⅛ of pie (2.3 oz)	180	3	7	5	28	1	160
DQ Treatzza Pizza M&M	⅛ of pie (2.4 oz)	190	3	7	5	29	1	160
DQ Vanilla Orange Bar No Sugar Added	1 (2.3 oz)	60	2	0	0	17	0	40
Frozen Hot Chocolate	1 (20.9 oz)	860	14	35	50	127	3	350
Misty Slush	1 sm (15.9 oz)	220	0	0	0	56	0	20
Misty Slush	1 med (20.9 oz)	290	0	0	0	74	0	30

FOOD	PORTION	CALS	PROT	FAT	CHOL	CARB	FIBER	SOD
Peanut Buster Parfait	1 (10.7 oz)	730	16	31	35	99	2	400
Pecan Mudslide Treat	1 (4.6 oz)	650	11	30	35	85	2	420
Shake Chocolate	1 med (18.9 oz)	770	17	20	70	130	0	420
Shake Chocolate	1 sm (13.9 oz)	560	13	15	50	94	0	310
S'more Galore Parfait	1 (10.7 oz)	730	11	30	30	111	3	340
Starkiss	1 (3 oz)	80	0	0	0	21	0	10
Strawberry Shortcake	1 (8.5 oz)	430	7	14	60	70	1	360
Sundae Chocolate	1 med (8.2 oz)	400	8	10	30	71	0	210
Sundae Chocolate	1 sm (5.7 oz)	280	5	7	20	49	0	140
Yogurt Sundae Strawberry	1 med (8.2 oz)	280	8	1	5	61	1	160

D'ANGELO'S SANDWICH SHOP
CHILDREN'S MENU SELECTIONS

FOOD	PORTION	CALS	PROT	FAT	CHOL	CARB	FIBER	SOD
D'Lite Turkey	1 kidz	217	19	3	14	30	3	369
Sub Cheeseburger	1 kidz	294	15	13	43	28	3	459
Sub Ham & Cheese	1 kidz	214	13	4	27	31	1	963
Sub Meatball	1 kidz	330	15	15	37	37	4	812
Sub Tuna	1 kidz	450	15	30	35	30	1	611

SALAD DRESSINGS AND TOPPINGS

FOOD	PORTION	CALS	PROT	FAT	CHOL	CARB	FIBER	SOD
Bacon	1 serv	64	5	5	15	0	0	247
Bleu Cheese	1 serv (1 oz)	152	1	15	15	3	0	283
Buffalo Sauce	1 serv (1 oz)	10	0	0	0	2	0	960
Caesar	1 serv (1 oz)	140	2	15	15	2	0	420
Caesar Fat Free	1 serv (1 oz)	20	0	0	0	3	0	590
Creamy Italian	1 serv (1 oz)	122	0	13	0	3	0	304
Cucumbers	3 slices	2	0	0	0	0	tr	0
Greek Dressing w/ Feta	1 serv (3 oz)	227	0	26	14	6	0	765
Honey Mustard Dressing	1 serv (1 oz)	150	0	142	0	7	0	210

FOOD	PORTION	CALS	PROT	FAT	CHOL	CARB	FIBER	SOD
Hot Peppers	1 serv	0	0	0	0	1	0	397
Mayonnaise	2 tbsp	236	0	26	21	0	0	141
Mayonnaise Fat Free	1 pkg	10	0	0	0	2	0	95
Mustard Honey Dijon	2 tbsp	60	0	0	0	18	0	180
Mustard Yellow	2 tbsp	20	1	1	0	2	1	336
Olive Oil Vinaigrette	1 serv (3 oz)	170	0	17	0	9	0	652
Olive Oil Blend	2 tbsp	239	0	27	0	0	0	0
Ranch Lite	1 serv (3 oz)	240	2	19	20	6	1	961
Sesame Ginger	1 serv (1 oz)	170	0	7	0	10	0	420
SALADS								
Antipasto Salad w/o Dressing	1 serv	275	16	16	38	15	6	1102
Asian Chicken w/o Dressing	1 serv	224	27	4	59	23	6	584
Caesar w/ Dressing	1 serv	474	14	39	29	20	3	1051
Chef w/o Dressing	1 serv	273	25	12	48	17	4	621
Chicken Caesar w/ Dressing	1 serv	532	34	38	86	13	3	1497
Chicken Stir Fry w/o Dressing	1 serv	166	25	3	59	10	4	588
Cobb w/o Dressing	1 serv	289	27	17	76	9	4	651
Greek w/o Dressing	1 serv	298	11	23	50	16	4	1099
Lobster w/o Dressing	1 serv	385	26	27	101	11	4	587
Roast Beef w/o Dressing	1 serv	146	23	3	49	9	4	243
Tossed Garden w/o Dressing	1 serv	47	3	1	0	9	4	21
Turkey w/o Dressing	1 serv	157	26	2	22	9	4	87
SANDWICHES								
D'Lite Chicken Stir Fry	1 sm	426	37	6	73	57	7	1240
D'Lite Fresh Veggie	1	348	13	7	13	62	7	650
D'Lite Grilled Chicken Breast	1 sm	387	31	7	67	52	6	952
D'Lite Ham & Cheese	1 sm	351	24	6	46	52	2	1666

FOOD	PORTION	CALS	PROT	FAT	CHOL	CARB	FIBER	SOD
D'Lite Roast Beef	1 sm	353	28	5	49	51	6	761
D'Lite Turkey	1 sm	364	32	4	22	51	6	605
D'Lite Turkey Cranberry	1 sm	460	32	4	22	75	6	605
Pokket Caesar Salad	1 sm	643	20	40	29	55	2	1473
Pokket Capacola & Cheese	1 sm	426	25	14	50	52	6	1522
Pokket Cheeseburger	1 sm	481	28	25	85	37	1	711
Pokket Chicken Caesar Salad	1 sm	701	40	39	88	48	2	1919
Pokket Chicken Club	1 sm	559	35	28	97	47	1	1197
Pokket Chicken Honey Dijon	1 sm	527	41	20	108	45	1	1285
Pokket Chicken Salad	1 sm	705	41	42	129	39	1	758
Pokket Chicken Stir Fry	1 sm	425	40	10	88	45	1	1474
Pokket Classic Veggie No Cheese	1 sm	238	10	2	0	50	4	439
Pokket Greek	1 sm	812	18	61	50	54	3	2003
Pokket Grilled Chicken	1 sm	328	30	5	67	41	1	851
Pokket Ham & Cheese	1 sm	349	26	9	60	41	1	1891
Pokket Ham & Salami	1 sm	412	26	17	60	39	1	1557
Pokket Hamburger	1 sm	422	25	21	72	35	1	442
Pokket Italian	1 sm	574	30	33	88	42	1	1925
Pokket Lobster	1 sm	568	29	32	102	39	1	1004
Pokket Meatball	1 sm	600	27	31	73	56	3	1877
Pokket Mortadella & Cheese	1 sm	505	26	28	73	42	1	1488
Pokket Seafood Salad	1 sm	532	15	28	29	56	2	1320
Pokket Steak	1 sm	335	27	13	59	29	0	411

FOOD	PORTION	CALS	PROT	FAT	CHOL	CARB	FIBER	SOD
Pokket Steak & Cheese	1 sm	407	31	18	74	31	0	751
Pokket Tuna	1 sm	791	—	58	71	28	1	1013
Sub Cheeseburger	1 sm	542	29	27	86	47	5	811
Sub Chicken Club	1 sm	619	36	30	97	52	6	1299
Sub Chicken Honey Dijon	1 sm	587	42	22	108	56	6	1287
Sub Chicken Salad	1 sm	769	42	44	130	50	6	862
Sub Chicken Stir Fry	1 sm	487	41	11	88	57	6	1578
Sub Classic Veggie	1 sm	465	22	15	34	64	8	1161
Sub Grilled Chicken	1 sm	387	31	7	67	52	6	952
Sub Ham & Cheese	1 sm	412	27	11	60	53	2	1995
Sub Ham & Salami	1 sm	474	27	19	60	51	2	1661
Sub Hamburger	1 sm	482	26	22	73	45	5	540
Sub Italian	1 sm	637	31	34	88	54	3	2028
Sub Lobster	1 sm	628	30	33	102	50	5	1107
Sub Meatball	1 sm	663	28	33	73	70	8	1980
Sub Mortadella & Cheese	1 sm	568	27	29	73	54	6	1591
Sub Number 9	1 sm	475	33	19	74	44	5	834
Sub Pastrami	1 sm	526	26	27	91	51	5	1858
Sub Pepperoni	1 sm	614	27	34	76	53	6	1901
Sub Roast Beef	1 sm	350	28	5	49	50	5	780
Sub Salad	1 sm	298	11	3	0	60	9	561
Sub Salami & Cheese	1 sm	597	27	32	75	51	6	1805
Sub Seafood Salad	1	595	16	29	29	67	7	1424
Sub Steak	1 sm	383	28	14	59	37	4	491
Sub Steak & Cheese	1 sm	455	32	19	74	40	4	832
Sub Steak Tip	1 sm	486	28	14	57	63	3	1229
Sub Stuffed Turkey	1 sm	1036	41	37	36	136	10	2717
Sub Tuna	1 sm	853	29	59	71	49	2	1115
Sub Turkey	1 sm	361	32	4	22	50	5	604
Sub Turkey Club	1 sm	360	34	8	54	37	3	692
Wrap Asian Chicken Salad	1	914	36	24	59	105	9	1930
Wrap BLT & Cheese	1	500	26	18	50	58	3	1249

FOOD	PORTION	CALS	PROT	FAT	CHOL	CARB	FIBER	SOD
Wrap Buffalo Chicken Salad	1	778	42	36	101	71	3	2624
Wrap Caesar Salad	1	669	21	37	29	64	4	1230
Wrap Capacola & Cheese	1	451	27	12	50	57	3	1297
Wrap Cheese	1	631	33	27	74	63	3	1754
Wrap Cheeseburger	1	569	32	26	86	52	3	611
Wrap Chef	1	832	34	40	72	82	5	1319
Wrap Chicken Caesar Salad	1	788	43	39	88	65	4	1798
Wrap Chicken Cobb	1	855	38	46	102	69	4	1469
Wrap Chicken Filet & Bacon	1	643	38	28	97	57	3	1074
Wrap Chicken Honey Dijon	1	619	45	20	106	63	4	1167
Wrap Chicken Salad	1	780	44	41	128	55	3	629
Wrap Chicken Stir Fry	1	511	43	10	88	61	3	1352
Wrap Classic Veggie	1	490	24	14	34	69	6	935
Wrap Greek	1	761	16	61	50	43	4	1722
Wrap Grilled Chicken	1	420	34	5	67	56	4	732
Wrap Ham & Cheese	1	436	29	9	60	58	3	1770
Wrap Ham & Salami	1	499	29	17	60	56	3	1435
Wrap Hamburger	1	509	28	21	74	50	3	340
Wrap Italian	1	654	33	32	88	59	3	1803
Wrap Lobster	1	766	32	44	112	56	2	949
Wrap Meatball	1	687	31	31	73	75	5	1755
Wrap Mortadella & Cheese	1	592	29	28	73	58	3	1366
Wrap Number 9	1	494	35	18	74	48	3	659
Wrap Pastrami	1	550	28	25	91	55	2	1632
Wrap Pepperoni	1	638	29	33	76	58	3	1675
Wrap Roast Beef	1	374	31	4	49	55	3	535
Wrap Salad	1	322	13	2	0	65	6	336
Wrap Salami & Cheese	1	605	29	29	72	56	3	1509
Wrap Steak	1	402	29	13	59	41	2	316

FOOD	PORTION	CALS	PROT	FAT	CHOL	CARB	FIBER	SOD
Wrap Steak & Cheese	1	474	34	18	74	43	2	657
Wrap Steak Tip	1	374	25	12	57	40	2	845
Wrap Tuna	1	881	31	58	71	55	3	891
Wrap Turkey	1	385	34	3	22	55	3	379
Wrap Turkey Club	1	435	38	8	54	52	3	603
SOUPS								
#9 Steak & Cheese	1 sm	280	12	21	65	11	1	739
Chicken Noodle	1 sm	130	19	2	50	8	1	839
Hearty Vegetable	1 sm	40	2	0	0	7	2	270
Lobster Bisque	1 sm	360	8	29	105	16	0	849
New England Clam Chowder	1 sm	270	8	20	70	15	1	699
Santa Fe Chipolte Vegetable	1 sm	130	7	1	0	22	8	579
Shrimp & Roasted Corn	1 sm	250	7	16	65	23	2	669
Thanksgiving Everyday	1 sm	250	7	17	55	18	2	999
DEL TACO								
BEVERAGES								
Coffee	1 serv (8 oz)	0	0	0	0	1	0	5
Coke Classic	1 lg (20 oz)	230	0	0	0	59	0	25
Coke Classic	1 med (12 oz)	150	0	0	0	37	0	15
Coke Classic	1 sm (10 oz)	120	0	0	0	29	0	10
Coke Classic Best Value	1 serv (27 oz)	320	0	0	0	81	0	30
Diet Coke	1 sm (10 oz)	0	0	0	0	0	0	15
Diet Coke	1 med (12 oz)	0	0	0	0	0	0	15
Diet Coke	1 lg (20 oz)	5	1	0	0	1	0	35
Diet Coke Best Value	1 serv (27 oz)	10	1	0	0	1	0	45
Iced Tea	1 lg (20 oz)	5	0	0	0	2	0	15
Iced Tea	1 sm (10 oz)	0	0	0	0	0	0	10

FOOD	PORTION	CALS	PROT	FAT	CHOL	CARB	FIBER	SOD
Iced Tea	1 med (12 oz)	0	0	0	0	1	0	10
Iced Tea Best Value	1 serv (27 oz)	10	0	0	0	2	0	25
Milk 1% Lowfat	1 serv (11 oz)	130	10	3	10	15	0	150
Mr Pibb	1 lg (20 oz)	230	0	0	0	59	0	55
Mr Pibb	1 med (12 oz)	150	0	0	0	37	0	10
Mr Pibb	1 sm (10 oz)	120	0	0	0	29	0	30
Mr Pibb Best Value	1 serv (27 oz)	320	0	0	0	81	0	80
Orange Juice	1 serv (11 oz)	140	2	0	0	34	1	0
Shake Chocolate	1 sm (11.4 oz)	520	12	12	35	89	1	270
Shake Chocolate	1 lg (15 oz)	680	16	16	45	117	1	350
Shake Strawberry	1 sm (11.4 oz)	410	11	6	30	76	1	220
Shake Strawberry	1 lg (15 oz)	540	14	8	40	100	1	280
Shake Vanilla	1 sm (11.4 oz)	420	12	7	35	75	0	250
Shake Vanilla	1 lg (15 oz)	550	16	10	50	97	0	320
Sprite	1 sm (10 oz)	110	0	0	0	29	0	30
Sprite	1 med (12 oz)	140	0	0	0	37	0	40
Sprite	1 lg (20 oz)	230	0	0	0	59	0	60
Sprite Best Value	1 serv (27 oz)	310	0	0	0	81	0	85
BREAKFAST SELECTIONS								
Burrito Breakfast	1 (3.8 oz)	250	10	11	160	24	1	520
Burrito Egg & Cheese	1 (7.5 oz)	450	23	24	530	39	3	740
Burrito Macho Bacon & Egg	1 (15.9 oz)	1030	40	60	790	82	6	1760
Burrito Steak & Egg	1 (9 oz)	580	33	34	560	41	3	1270
Quesadilla Bacon & Egg	1 (6.1 oz)	450	21	23	260	40	2	920
Side of Bacon	2 strips (0.3 oz)	50	3	4	10	0	0	170

FOOD	PORTION	CALS	PROT	FAT	CHOL	CARB	FIBER	SOD
MAIN MENU SELECTIONS								
Beans 'n Cheese Cup	1 serv (7.7 oz)	260	16	3	5	44	16	1810
Burrito Combo	1 (8.2 oz)	490	26	21	55	53	8	1380
Burrito Del Beef	1 (8 oz)	550	31	30	90	42	3	1090
Burrito Del Classic Chicken	1 (8.5 oz)	580	24	38	70	42	3	1100
Burrito Deluxe Combo	1 (10.7 oz)	530	27	25	60	56	9	1390
Burrito Deluxe Del Beef	1 (10.5 oz)	590	32	33	95	45	4	1110
Burrito Green	1 (5 oz)	280	11	8	15	38	6	1030
Burrito Macho Beef	1 (18.9 oz)	1170	60	62	190	89	7	2190
Burrito Macho Combo	1 (19.4 oz)	1050	49	44	115	113	17	2760
Burrito Red	1 (5 oz)	270	11	8	15	38	6	1020
Burrito Red Regular	1 (7.5 oz)	390	18	12	20	59	11	1439
Burrito Regular Green	1 (7.5 oz)	400	18	12	10	59	10	1450
Burrito Spicy Chicken	1 (8.7 oz)	480	23	16	40	65	8	1620
Burrito The Works	1 (10.2 oz)	480	18	18	25	69	9	1500
Cheeseburger	1 (4.6 oz)	330	16	13	35	37	3	870
Del Cheeseburger	1 (5.6 oz)	430	16	25	45	35	4	710
Double Del Cheeseburger	1 (7.1 oz)	560	26	35	85	35	4	960
Fries	1 reg (5 oz)	350	3	23	0	34	3	270
Fries	1 sm (3 oz)	210	2	14	0	20	2	160
Fries Best Value	1 serv (7 oz)	490	5	32	0	47	5	380
Fries Chili Cheese	1 serv (10.5 oz)	670	17	46	45	51	5	880
Fries Deluxe Chili Cheese	1 serv (11.9 oz)	710	17	49	50	53	6	880
Get A Lot Meals #1 Combo Burrito Fries Drink	1 meal	980	29	44	55	124	11	1670

FOOD	PORTION	CALS	PROT	FAT	CHOL	CARB	FIBER	SOD
Get A Lot Meals #2 Del Classic Chicken Burrito Fries Drink	1 meal	1080	28	61	70	113	7	1390
Get A Lot Meals #3 Regular Red Burrito Fries Drink	1 meal	890	21	35	20	130	14	1710
Get A Lot Meals #4 Two Chicken Soft Tacos Fries Drink	1 meal	910	25	46	60	102	5	1330
Get A Lot Meals #5 Taco Combo Burrito Drink	1 meal	790	32	31	75	101	9	1540
Get A Lot Meals #6 Two Tacos Quesadilla Drink	1 meal	960	37	47	115	98	3	1170
Get A Lot Meals #7 Macho Combo Burrito Fries Drink	1 meal	1530	52	67	115	183	20	3050
Get A Lot Meals #8 Two Big Fat Tacos Fries Drink	1 meal	802	35	45	70	148	10	1640
Get A Lot Meals #9 Double Del Cheeseburger Fries Drink	1 meal	1050	29	58	85	106	7	1250
Nachos	1 serv (4 oz)	380	5	24	5	40	2	630
Nachos Macho	1 serv (17 oz)	1200	33	66	55	130	16	2720
Quesadilla Chicken	1 (6.8 oz)	580	33	31	104	41	2	1240
Quesadilla Regular	1 (5.3 oz)	500	23	27	75	39	2	860
Quesadilla Spicy Jack Chicken	1 (6.0 oz)	570	32	30	105	40	2	1300
Quesadilla Spicy Jack Regular	1 (5.3 oz)	490	23	26	75	38	2	920
Rice Cup	1 serv (4 oz)	150	3	2	2	28	1	600
Soft Taco	1 (2.8 oz)	160	8	8	20	16	1	330
Soft Taco Chicken	1 (3.3 oz)	210	11	12	30	16	1	520

FOOD	PORTION	CALS	PROT	FAT	CHOL	CARB	FIBER	SOD
Taco	1 (2.2 oz)	160	7	10	20	11	1	150
Taco Big Fat	1 (5.4 oz)	320	16	11	35	39	3	680
Taco Big Fat Chicken	1 (5.4 oz)	340	18	13	45	38	3	840
Taco Big Fat Steak	1 (5.4 oz)	390	18	19	45	38	3	960
Taco Salad Deluxe	1 (18.8 oz)	760	31	37	70	76	14	2010
Tostada Salad	1 (4.5 oz)	210	9	9	15	24	6	640

DENNY'S
BEVERAGES

FOOD	PORTION	CALS	PROT	FAT	CHOL	CARB	FIBER	SOD
2% Milk	10 oz	151	10	6	22	15	0	152
Apple Juice	1 reg	126	0	0	0	33	0	24
Cappuccino French Vanilla	8 oz	100	3	2	0	28	1	220
Cappuccino Original	8 oz	100	2	3	0	17	0	100
Chocolate Milk	10 oz	235	9	9	37	30	0	189
Grapefruit	1 serv (10 oz)	162	0	0	0	41	0	43
Hot Chocolate	8 oz	100	3	2	0	28	1	219
Lemonade	16 oz	150	0	0	0	35	0	38
Malted Milk Shake Chocolate Or Vanilla	12 oz	583	12	26	100	82	tr	278
Orange Juice	10 oz	126	2	0	0	31	0	31
Raspberry Ice Tea	16 oz	78	0	0	0	21	0	0
Tomato Juice	1 serv (10 oz)	56	2	0	0	11	2	921

BREAKFAST SELECTIONS

FOOD	PORTION	CALS	PROT	FAT	CHOL	CARB	FIBER	SOD
All American Slam	1 serv	816	45	67	828	3	1	1826
Applesauce	1 serv	60	0	0	0	15	1	13
Bacon	4 strips	162	12	18	36	1	0	640
Bagel Dry	1	235	9	1	0	46	0	495
Banana	1	110	1	0	0	29	4	0
Belgian Waffle	1	619	22	45	274	28	0	1638
Breakfast Dagwood	1 serv	1446	82	90	765	81	1	4003
Buttermilk Hotcakes	3	466	20	23	47	47	2	2077
Cantaloup	¼	32	1	0	0	8	1	16

FOOD	PORTION	CALS	PROT	FAT	CHOL	CARB	FIBER	SOD
Chicken Fajita Skillet	1 serv	855	26	49	515	30	11	1863
Corned Beef Hash Slam	1 serv	668	32	55	535	11	1	816
Country Fish Potatoes	1 serv	394	3	20	9	23	10	938
Egg	1	120	6	10	210	tr	0	120
English Muffin Dry	1	125	5	1	0	24	1	198
Fabulous French Toast	1 serv	1146	26	71	297	104	3	2441
Farmer's Slam	1 serv	1200	51	80	704	82	3	3204
French Slam	1 serv	1119	45	77	705	71	3	2265
Fruit Mix	1 serv	36	1	0	0	9	1	16
Grand Slam Slugger	1 serv	927	34	55	476	74	3	2399
Grapefruit	½	60	1	0	0	16	6	0
Grapes	1 serv	55	1	1	0	15	1	0
Grits	1 serv	80	2	0	0	18	0	520
Ham & Cheddar Omelette	1 serv	595	41	47	783	5	0	1200
Ham & Cheese Omelette w/ Eggbeaters	1 serv	468	37	32	58	5	0	1351
Ham Slice	1	94	15	3	23	2	0	761
Hashed Browns	1 serv	197	2	12	0	20	2	446
Hashed Browns Covered	1 serv	280	7	19	23	21	2	583
Hashed Browns Covered & Smothered	1 serv	493	14	25	29	54	3	3534
Honeydew	¼	31	1	0	0	8	1	22
Lumberjack Slam w/ Hash Browns	1 serv	1035	51	58	589	73	3	4462
Meat Lover's Skillet	1 serv	1031	39	74	528	27	10	2374
Moon Over My Hammy	1 serv	841	54	51	580	42	2	2699
Oatmeal	1 serv	100	5	2	0	18	3	175
Oatmeal Deluxe	1 serv	460	13	6	11	95	7	87
Original Grand Slam	1 serv	665	26	49	515	33	2	1106
Ready To Eat Cereal	1 serv	100	2	0	0	23	1	276
Sausage	4 links	354	16	32	64	0	0	944

FOOD	PORTION	CALS	PROT	FAT	CHOL	CARB	FIBER	SOD
Scram Slam	1 serv	827	45	68	801	8	1	1937
Senior Belgian Waffle Slam	1 serv	399	16	33	302	12	0	612
Senior Omelette	1 serv	429	25	20	515	8	2	755
Sirloin Steak & Eggs	1 serv	675	52	45	643	1	1	368
Slim Slam	1 serv	438	32	6	50	56	2	2417
T-Bone Steak & Eggs	1 serv	991	73	77	657	1	1	1003
Toast Dry	1 slice	92	3	1	0	17	1	166
Two Egg Breakfast w/ Hash Browns	1 serv	825	31	67	538	24	2	1765
Ultimate Omelette	1 serv	611	34	50	756	11	3	1007
Veggie-Cheese Omelette	1 serv	494	30	39	747	11	2	719
CHILDREN'S MENU SELECTIONS								
Burgerlicious	1 serv	296	13	17	28	24	1	368
Burgerlicious w/ Cheese	1 serv	341	15	20	40	24	1	560
Dennysaur Chicken Nuggets	1 serv	190	9	13	30	9	0	340
Frenchtastic Slam	1 serv	452	19	33	311	22	1	664
Junior Grand Slam	1 serv	397	17	25	230	33	1	1118
Junior Shrimps Ahoy!	1 serv	411	13	18	66	50	4	792
Oreo Blender Blaster	1 serv	580	11	29	87	72	1	194
Pizza Party	1 serv	400	18	15	10	47	7	1090
Smiley-Face Hotcakes w/ Meat	1 serv	463	14	22	38	63	2	1410
Smiley-Face Hotcakes w/o Meat	1 serv	344	7	9	13	62	2	1014
The Big Cheese	1 serv	334	9	20	24	28	2	828
DESSERTS								
Apple Pie	1 serv	470	3	24	0	64	1	470
Banana Split	1	894	15	43	78	121	6	177
Carrot Cake	1 serv	799	9	45	125	99	2	630
Cheesecake	1 serv	580	8	38	174	51	0	380
Chocolate Topping	1 serv	317	2	25	0	27	0	83
Chocolate Peanut Butter Pie	1 serv	653	15	39	27	64	3	319

FOOD	PORTION	CALS	PROT	FAT	CHOL	CARB	FIBER	SOD
Double Scoop Sundae	1 serv	375	6	27	74	29	0	86
Float Rootbeer or Coke	12 oz	280	3	10	39	47	0	109
Hot Fudge Brownie A La Mode	1 serv	997	12	42	14	147	6	82
Milkshake Vanilla Or Chocolate	12 oz	560	11	26	100	76	tr	272
Oreo Blender Blaster	1 serv	895	16	46	135	112	2	280
Single Scoop Sundae	1 serv	188	3	14	37	14	0	43
MAIN MENU SELECTIONS								
Albacore Tuna Melt	1 serv	640	30	39	109	42	3	1436
Applesauce	1 serv	60	0	0	0	15	1	13
Bacon Lettuce & Tomato	1	610	15	38	35	50	2	862
Baked Potato Plain	1	220	5	0	0	51	5	16
BBQ Chicken Sandwich	1 serv	1089	48	62	103	86	5	1872
Bread Stuffing Plain	1 serv	100	3	1	0	19	1	405
Buffalo Chicken Sandwich	1 serv	708	37	28	74	80	5	1733
Buffalo Chicken Strips	5 pieces	734	48	42	96	43	0	1673
Buffalo Wings	12 pieces	856	92	54	500	1	1	5552
Burger Bacon Cheddar	1	875	53	52	163	58	5	1672
Burger BBQ	1 serv	953	52	52	136	72	4	2130
Burger Boca	1 serv	601	32	27	14	64	9	1446
Burger Classic	1	694	40	35	100	56	4	785
Burger Classic w/ Cheese	1	852	49	48	140	57	4	1385
Burger Mushroom Swiss	1 serv	880	51	49	137	63	5	1619
Carrots In Honey Glaze	1 serv	80	1	3	0	12	3	220
Chicken Strips	5 pieces	720	47	33	95	56	0	1666
Chicken Ranch Melt	1 serv	758	44	45	105	44	3	2195

FOOD	PORTION	CALS	PROT	FAT	CHOL	CARB	FIBER	SOD
Chicken Strips	1 serv	635	47	25	95	55	0	1510
Club Sandwich	1	718	32	38	75	62	3	1666
Coleslaw	1 serv	274	2	30	37	14	2	568
Corn In Butter Sauce	1 serv	120	3	4	5	19	5	260
Cottage Cheese	1 serv	72	9	3	10	2	0	281
Country Fried Steak	1 serv	644	28	48	89	30	11	2149
Fish & Chips Dinner	1 serv	955	34	57	97	77	6	1497
French Fries Unsalted	1 serv	423	6	20	0	57	5	221
Fried Shrimp Dinner	1 serv	219	17	10	133	18	1	774
Fried Shrimp & Shrimp Scampi	1 serv	346	27	20	241	15	1	1104
Green Beans w/ Bacon	1 serv	60	1	4	5	6	3	390
Grilled Cheese Sandwich	1	510	19	30	54	40	3	1360
Grilled Chicken Dinner	1 serv	130	24	4	67	0	0	560
Grilled Chicken Sandwich	1	469	35	14	77	53	4	1392
Ham & Swiss On Rye	1	417	32	16	57	39	5	1763
Herb Toast	1 serv	170	2	11	tr	15	1	325
Hoagie Chicken Melt	1	751	46	44	93	43	2	1834
Hoagie Philly Melt	1 serv	874	47	50	114	58	5	2444
Mashed Potatoes Plain	1 serv	168	3	7	8	23	2	498
Mozzarella Sticks	8 pieces	710	36	41	48	49	6	5220
Onion Rings	1 serv	381	5	23	6	38	1	1003
Patty Melt	1	798	45	51	127	37	4	1285
Pot Roast Dinner w/ Gravy	1 serv	292	42	11	87	5	0	927
Roast Turkey & Stuffing w/ Gravy	1 serv	388	46	3	116	38	2	2467
Sampler	1 serv	1405	47	80	75	124	4	5305
Seasoned Fries	1 serv	261	5	12	0	35	0	556
Senior Chicken Strip Dinner	1 serv	285	19	10	37	31	0	969

FOOD	PORTION	CALS	PROT	FAT	CHOL	CARB	FIBER	SOD
Senior Club	1 serv	540	29	31	89	34	3	1499
Senior Country Fried Steak	1 serv	341	14	23	44	18	6	1464
Senior Fish & Chips	1 serv	756	20	47	67	64	6	1116
Senior French Slam	1 serv	820	28	65	432	40	1	777
Senior Fried Shrimp Dinner	1 serv	129	12	5	66	13	1	645
Senior Grilled Chicken Breast	1 serv	200	25	5	67	15	1	824
Senior Pot Roast	1 serv	160	25	6	48	3	0	512
Senior Starter	1 serv	544	16	42	245	23	2	631
Senior Turkey & Stuffing	1 serv	220	25	2	60	25	1	1378
Shrimp Scampi Skillet Dinner	1 serv	289	25	19	192	3	tr	766
Sirloin Steak Dinner	1 serv	337	18	28	687	1	1	344
Sliced Tomatoes	3 slices	13	1	0	0	3	1	6
Smoothered Cheese Fries	1 serv	767	27	48	78	69	0	875
Steak & Shrimp Dinner	1 serv	645	36	42	150	31	2	1143
T-Bone Steak Dinner	1 serv	860	65	65	196	0	0	867
The Super Bird Sandwich	1	620	35	32	60	48	2	1880
Turkey Breast On Multigrain w/o Mayo	1	277	23	4	15	41	5	1607
SALAD DRESSINGS AND TOPPINGS								
BBQ Sauce	1.5 oz	47	0	1	0	11	0	595
Bleu Cheese	1 oz	163	1	18	20	1	0	205
Blueberry Topping	1 serv	71	0	0	0	17	0	10
Caesar	1 oz	133	1	14	2	1	0	380
Cherry Topping	1 serv	57	0	0	0	14	0	3
Cream Cheese	1 oz	100	2	10	31	1	0	6
French	1 oz	106	0	10	7	3	0	274
Fudge Topping	1 serv	201	1	10	3	30	1	96
Gravy Brown	1 serv	13	0	0	0	2	0	184
Gravy Chicken	1 serv	14	0	1	2	2	0	139
Gravy Country	1 serv	17	0	1	0	2	0	93

FOOD	PORTION	CALS	PROT	FAT	CHOL	CARB	FIBER	SOD
Honey Mustard	1 serv	160	0	15	20	20	0	123
Low Calorie Italian	1 oz	15	0	1	0	3	0	390
Marinara Sauce	1 serv	48	1	2	0	7	1	206
Ranch	1 oz	129	0	14	8	1	0	189
Ranch Fat Free	1 serv	25	0	tr	0	6	0	300
Sour Cream	1.5 oz	91	1	9	19	2	0	23
Strawberry Topping	1 serv	77	1	1	0	17	1	8
Syrup	3 tbsp	143	0	0	0	36	0	26
Syrup Sugar Free	1 serv	23	0	0	0	9	0	71
Tartar Sauce	1 serv	225	0	23	15	3	0	157
Thousand Island	2 tbsp	170	0	18	15	2	0	110
Thousand Island	1 oz	118	0	11	15	5	0	170
Whipped Margarine	1 serv	87	0	10	0	0	0	117
Whipped Cream	2 tbsp	23	0	2	7	2	0	3
SALADS								
Garden Salad w/ Albacore Tuna	1 serv	444	35	29	81	12	4	824
Garden Salad w/ Fried Chicken Strips	1 serv	438	33	26	78	26	4	1030
Garden Salad w/ Grilled Chicken Breast	1 serv	264	32	11	89	10	4	714
Grilled Chicken Caesar Salad w/ Dressing	1 serv	600	37	41	101	19	4	1792
Side Caesar w/ Dressing	1 serv	362	11	26	23	20	3	913
Side Garden Salad w/o Dressing	1 serv	113	3	4	0	16	3	147
SOUPS								
Chicken Noodle	1 serv	60	2	2	10	8	0	640
Clam Chowder	1 serv	624	7	42	5	55	4	1474
Cream Of Broccoli	1 serv	574	6	43	0	41	2	1174
Vegetable Beef	1 serv	79	6	1	5	11	2	820

FOOD	PORTION	CALS	PROT	FAT	CHOL	CARB	FIBER	SOD
DOMINO'S PIZZA								
12 INCH MEDIUM PIZZAS								
Deep Dish Cheese Only	2 slices	482	19	22	30	56	3	1123
Hand Tossed America's Favorite Feast	1 serv	508	22	22	49	57	4	1221
Hand Tossed Bacon Cheeseburger Feast	2 slices	549	25	26	60	55	3	1274
Hand Tossed Barbeque Feast	2 slices	506	22	20	46	62	3	1206
Hand Tossed Cheese Only	2 slices	375	15	11	23	55	3	776
Hand Tossed Deluxe Feast	2 slices	465	20	18	40	57	3	1063
Hand Tossed ExtravaganZZa Feast	2 slices	576	27	27	64	59	4	1511
Hand Tossed Hawaiian Feast	2 slices	450	21	16	41	58	3	1102
Hand Tossed MeatZZa Feast	2 slices	560	26	26	64	57	3	1463
Hand Tossed Pepperoni Feast	2 slices	534	24	25	57	56	3	1349
Hand Tossed Vegi Feast	2 slices	439	19	16	34	57	4	987
Thin Crust Cheese	¼ pie	273	12	12	23	31	2	835
Toppings Pineapple	1 serv	12	tr	0	0	3	tr	1
DESSERTS								
Cinna Stix	1 serv	111	2	5	0	15	1	105
Sweet Icing	1 serv	283	0	5	0	60	0	4
MAIN MENU SELECTIONS								
Breadstick	1	116	3	4	0	18	1	152
Buffalo Chicken Kickers	1 piece	47	4	2	9	3	tr	163
Buffalo Wings Barbeque	1 piece	50	6	2	25	2	tr	175

FOOD	PORTION	CALS	PROT	FAT	CHOL	CARB	FIBER	SOD
Buffalo Wings Hot	1 piece	45	5	2	26	1	tr	354
Cheesy Bread	1 piece	142	4	6	6	18	1	183
TOPPINGS								
Blue Cheese	1 serv	223	1	23	20	2	tr	417
Hot Sauce	1 serv	14	tr	tr	0	4	tr	1816
Medium Pizza Anchovies	1 serv	34	6	1	14	0	0	593
Medium Pizza Bacon	1 serv	102	5	9	15	tr	0	283
Medium Pizza Banana Peppers	1 serv	5	tr	tr	0	1	0	137
Medium Pizza Cheddar Cheese	1 serv	57	4	5	15	tr	0	88
Medium Pizza Extra Cheese	1 serv	49	3	4	11	1	tr	163
Medium Pizza Green Olives	1 serv	19	tr	2	0	tr	tr	283
Medium Pizza Green Peppers	1 serv	4	tr	tr	0	1	tr	tr
Medium Pizza Ham	1 serv	23	3	1	9	tr	0	215
Medium Pizza Italian Sausage	1 serv	77	3	6	16	2	tr	239
Medium Pizza Mushrooms	1 serv	6	1	tr	0	1	tr	1
Medium Pizza Onion	1 serv	5	tr	tr	0	1	tr	tr
Medium Pizza Pepperoni	1 serv	74	3	7	15	tr	tr	273
Medium Pizza Ripe Olives	1 serv	21	tr	2	0	1	1	107
Ranch	1 serv	197	1	20	9	2	tr	380

DONATOS PIZZA

PIZZA

FOOD	PORTION	CALS	PROT	FAT	CHOL	CARB	FIBER	SOD
Dessert Apple	¼ pie	722	12	20	21	137	15	926
Dessert Cherry	¼ pie	818	12	20	20	149	13	924
Original	¼ pie	660	30	33	54	58	6	1770
Original Chicken Vegy Medley	¼ pie	500	28	19	80	56	11	1768

FOOD	PORTION	CALS	PROT	FAT	CHOL	CARB	FIBER	SOD
Original Chicken Vegy Medley No Cheese	¼ pie	392	21	10	56	54	11	1536
Original Founders	¼ pie	737	38	42	134	71	10	2954
Original Hawaiian	¼ pie	620	30	30	60	58	4	1780
Original Hawaiian No Cheese	¼ pie	411	17	13	46	58	11	1379
Original Mariachi Beef	¼ pie	613	31	30	81	56	11	2324
Original Mariachi Chicken	¼ pie	580	35	25	94	56	11	2480
Original Serious Cheese	¼ pie	640	34	28	140	62	6	1640
Original Serious Meat	¼ pie	817	45	47	136	68	10	2535
Original Vegy	¼ pie	564	26	24	60	60	12	1674
Original Vegy No Cheese	¼ pie	370	12	9	21	59	12	1207
Original Works	¼ pie	729	35	41	106	75	12	2179
Traditional Chicken Vegy Medley	¼ pie	647	37	17	62	90	4	1997
Traditional Founders	¼ pie	900	48	40	112	107	3	3206
Traditional Hawaiian	¼ pie	794	42	30	74	98	4	2316
Traditional Mariachi Beef	¼ pie	797	41	31	68	95	4	2773
Traditional Mariachi Chicken	¼ pie	770	45	26	79	95	4	2911
Traditional Original	¼ pie	928	40	39	121	89	9	2076
Traditional Serious Cheese	¼ pie	830	40	36	123	123	12	1889
Traditional Serious Meat	¼ pie	977	54	46	118	104	3	2881
Traditional Vegy	¼ pie	752	37	26	49	98	5	2104
Traditional Works	¼ pie	892	45	39	90	111	5	2536
SALAD DRESSINGS								
Italian	1 serv (1.5 oz)	230	0	24	0	1	0	460

FOOD	PORTION	CALS	PROT	FAT	CHOL	CARB	FIBER	SOD
Italian Lite	1 serv (1.5 oz)	20	0	1	0	2	0	780
SALADS								
Grilled Chicken w/o Dressing	1 serv	314	28	18	71	12	5	903
Italian Chef w/o Dressing	1 serv	338	20	23	72	13	5	1856
Side w/o Dressing	1 serv	106	6	7	16	6	2	370
SIDE ORDERS								
Breadsticks	2	220	5	5	0	29	0	330
Chicken Wings Hot	5	449	41	29	286	6	tr	1766
Chicken Wings Mild	5	451	41	29	286	6	tr	1781
Three Cheese Garlic Bread	1 bun	605	24	28	38	66	3	689
SUBS								
Big Don Italian	1 serv	705	34	33	85	68	3	1982
Big Don Lite Italian	1 serv	631	34	25	84	69	3	2069
Grilled Chicken	1 serv	786	31	43	71	68	3	1184
Ham & Cheese Italian	1 serv	609	32	22	86	70	3	1659
Ham & Cheese Lite Italian	1 serv	534	32	14	85	70	3	1745
Southwest Turkey	1 serv	710	33	33	70	74	3	1519
Steak & Cheese	1 serv	929	43	52	111	107	3	907
Vegy Italian	1 serv	730	26	36	38	75	6	1267
Vegy Lite Italian	1 serv	661	26	28	38	78	6	1487

DUNKIN' DONUTS
BAGELS AND CREAM CHEESE

FOOD	PORTION	CALS	PROT	FAT	CHOL	CARB	FIBER	SOD
Bagel Blueberry	1	340	10	1	0	75	tr	670
Bagel Cinnamon Raisin	1	340	10	1	0	74	1	480
Bagel Egg	1	350	11	2	25	72	0	610
Bagel Everything	1	360	11	2	0	74	0	710
Bagel Garlic	1	360	11	1	0	76	0	720
Bagel Onion	1	330	10	1	0	70	0	660
Bagel Plain	1	340	10	1	0	73	0	710
Bagel Poppyseed	1	360	11	3	0	74	tr	710

FOOD	PORTION	CALS	PROT	FAT	CHOL	CARB	FIBER	SOD
Bagel Pumpernickel	1	350	11	2	0	75	2	560
Bagel Salt	1	340	10	1	0	73	0	3030
Bagel Sesame	1	380	12	5	0	74	0	720
Bagel Wheat	1	330	12	2	0	73	4	670
Cream Cheese Chive	1 pkg	190	3	19	55	3	tr	220
Cream Cheese Garden Vegetable	1 pkg	180	3	17	45	3	tr	310
Cream Cheese Lite	1 pkg	130	5	11	30	3	0	250
Cream Cheese Plain	1 pkg	200	4	19	60	3	0	230
Cream Cheese Salmon	1 pkg	180	5	17	50	2	0	150
BAKED SELECTIONS								
Bow Tie Donut	1	300	4	17	0	34	tr	340
Cake Donut Blueberry	1	290	3	16	10	35	tr	400
Cake Donut Butternut	1	300	3	16	0	36	tr	360
Cake Donut Chocolate Coconut	1	300	4	19	0	31	1	370
Cake Donut Chocolate Frosted	1	300	3	16	0	38	tr	370
Cake Donut Chocolate Glazed	1	290	3	16	0	33	1	370
Cake Donut Cinnamon	1	270	3	15	0	31	tr	360
Cake Donut Coconut	1	290	3	17	0	33	tr	360
Cake Donut Double Chocolate	1	310	3	17	0	37	2	370
Cake Donut Glazed	1	270	3	15	0	33	tr	360
Cake Donut Old Fashioned	1	250	3	15	0	26	tr	360
Cake Donut Powdered	1	270	3	15	0	32	tr	350
Cake Donut Toasted Coconut	1	300	3	17	0	35	tr	370

FOOD	PORTION	CALS	PROT	FAT	CHOL	CARB	FIBER	SOD
Cake Donut Whole Wheat Glazed	1	310	4	19	0	32	2	380
Chocolate Frosted Donut	1	200	3	9	0	29	tr	260
Chocolate Kreme Filled Donut	1	270	3	13	0	35	tr	260
Cinnamon Bun	1	510	8	15	10	85	0	420
Coffee Roll	1	270	4	14	0	33	1	340
Coffee Roll Chocolate Frosted	1	290	4	15	0	36	1	340
Coffee Roll Maple Frosted	1	290	4	14	0	36	1	340
Coffee Roll Vanilla Frosted	1	290	4	14	0	36	1	340
Cookie Chocolate Chocolate Chunk	1	210	3	11	35	26	2	110
Cookie Chocolate Chunk	1	220	3	11	35	28	1	105
Cookie Chocolate Chunk w/ Nut	1	230	3	12	35	27	1	110
Cookie Chocolate White Chocolate Chunk	1	230	3	12	35	28	1	160
Cookie Oatmeal Raisin Pecan	1	220	3	10	30	29	1	110
Cookie Peanut Butter Chocolate Chunk w/ Nuts	1	240	4	14	25	24	2	125
Cookie Peanut Butter w/ Nuts	1	240	5	14	30	24	1	150
Croissant Almond	1	350	6	22	5	34	2	270
Croissant Chocolate	1	400	5	25	5	37	2	240
Croissant Plain	1	290	5	18	5	26	tr	270
Cruller Glazed	1	290	3	15	0	37	tr	350
Cruller Glazed Chocolate	1	280	3	15	0	35	1	360
Cruller Plain	1	240	3	15	0	25	tr	340
Cruller Powdered	1	270	3	15	0	30	tr	340
Cruller Sugar	1	250	3	15	0	27	tr	340

FOOD	PORTION	CALS	PROT	FAT	CHOL	CARB	FIBER	SOD
Donut Apple Crumb	1	230	3	10	0	34	tr	270
Donut Apple N' Spice	1	200	3	8	0	29	tr	270
Donut Bavarian Kreme	1	210	3	9	0	30	tr	270
Donut Black Raspberry	1	210	3	8	0	32	tr	280
Donut Blueberry Crumb	1	240	3	10	0	36	tr	260
Donut Boston Kreme	1	240	3	9	0	36	tr	280
Donut Chocolate Iced Bismark	1	340	3	15	0	50	tr	290
Dunkin' Donut	1	240	3	15	0	25	tr	340
Eclair Donut	1	270	3	11	0	39	tr	290
Fritter Glazed	1	260	4	14	0	31	1	330
Glazed Donut	1	180	3	8	0	25	tr	250
Jelly Filled Donut	1	210	3	8	0	32	tr	280
Jelly Stick	1	290	3	12	0	44	tr	390
Lemon Donut	1	200	3	9	0	28	tr	270
Maple Frosted Donut	1	210	3	9	0	30	tr	260
Marble Frosted Donut	1	200	3	9	0	29	tr	260
Muffin Apple Cinnamon Pecan	1	510	8	21	70	74	1	590
Muffin Apple N'Spice	1	350	5	12	35	57	2	390
Muffin Banana Nut	1	360	7	15	35	52	3	490
Muffin Blueberry	1 (4 oz)	320	6	12	35	49	3	480
Muffin Blueberry	1 (6 oz)	490	8	17	75	78	2	610
Muffin Bran	1	390	11	12	20	60	3	620
Muffin Cherry	1	340	6	12	40	53	2	510
Muffin Chocolate Hazelnut	1	610	10	26	70	87	3	610
Muffin Chocolate Chip	1 (6 oz)	590	8	24	75	88	3	560
Muffin Chocolate Chip	1 (4 oz)	400	6	17	35	58	4	440

FOOD	PORTION	CALS	PROT	FAT	CHOL	CARB	FIBER	SOD
Muffin Corn	1 (4 oz)	390	8	15	55	57	2	590
Muffin Corn	1 (6 oz)	500	10	16	80	78	1	920
Muffin Cranberry Orange	1	470	8	15	75	76	2	600
Muffin Cranberry Orange Nut	1	350	6	15	35	52	3	500
Muffin Lemon Poppyseed	1	360	5	13	35	56	1	530
Muffin Oat Bran	1	370	11	13	20	55	3	620
Muffin Lowfat Apple & Spice	1	240	4	2	0	54	tr	460
Muffin Lowfat Banana	1	250	4	2	0	57	tr	430
Muffin Lowfat Blueberry	1	250	4	2	0	55	1	430
Muffin Lowfat Bran	1	240	4	1	0	57	4	430
Muffin Lowfat Cherry	1	250	4	2	0	56	tr	430
Muffin Lowfat Chocolate	1	250	4	3	0	53	2	470
Muffin Lowfat Corn	1	240	3	3	45	52	0	480
Muffin Lowfat Cranberry Orange	1	240	4	2	0	55	1	430
Muffin Reduced Fat Blueberry	1	450	8	12	65	77	2	590
Muffin Reduced Fat Corn	1	460	10	11	75	79	1	900
Munchkins Chocolate Cake Glazed	3	200	2	10	0	26	tr	250
Munchkins Cake Butternut	3	200	2	11	0	25	tr	240
Munchkins Cake Cinnamon	4	250	3	14	0	29	tr	350
Munchkins Cake Coconut	3	200	2	12	0	23	tr	240
Munchkins Cake Glazed	3	200	2	10	0	27	0	250

FOOD	PORTION	CALS	PROT	FAT	CHOL	CARB	FIBER	SOD
Munchkins Cake Plain	4	220	2	14	0	22	tr	310
Munchkins Cake Powdered	4	250	2	14	0	29	tr	310
Munchkins Cake Sugared	4	240	2	14	0	28	tr	310
Munchkins Cake Toasted Coconut	3	200	2	11	0	24	tr	—
Munchkins Yeast Glazed	5	200	3	9	0	27	tr	220
Munchkins Yeast Jelly Filled	5	210	3	9	0	30	tr	240
Munchkins Yeast Lemon Filled	4	170	2	8	0	23	0	190
Munchkins Yeast Sugar Raised	7	220	4	12	0	26	tr	290
Strawberry Frosted Donut	1	210	3	9	0	30	tr	260
Strawberry Donut	1	210	3	8	0	32	tr	260
Sugar Raised Donut	1	170	3	8	0	22	tr	250
Sugared Cake Donut	1	250	3	15	0	27	tr	350
Vanilla Frosted Donut	1	210	3	9	0	30	tr	260
Vanilla Kreme Filled Donut	1	270	3	13	0	36	tr	250
BEVERAGES								
Coffee Coolatta w/ 2% Milk	1 (16 oz)	240	4	2	10	52	0	80
Coffee Coolatta w/ Cream	1 (16 oz)	410	3	22	75	51	0	65
Coffee Coolatta w/ Milk	1 (16 oz)	260	4	4	15	52	0	75
Coffee Coolatta w/ Skim Milk	1 (16 oz)	230	4	0	<5	52	0	80
Coolatta Orange Mango Fruit	1 (16 oz)	290	tr	0	0	71	tr	30

FOOD	PORTION	CALS	PROT	FAT	CHOL	CARB	FIBER	SOD
Coolatta Pink Lemonade Fruit	1 (16 oz)	350	0	0	0	88	0	30
Coolatta Raspberry Lemonade	1 (16 oz)	280	0	0	0	68	0	35
Coolatta Strawberry Fruit	1 (16 oz)	280	0	0	0	70	1	30
Coolatta Vanilla	1 (16 oz)	450	1	7	0	94	0	170
Dunkaccino	1 (14 oz)	360	3	17	15	51	1	360
Dunkaccino	1 (10 oz)	250	2	11	10	34	tr	240
Dunkaccino	1 (20 oz)	510	4	23	20	71	1	500
Dunkaccino	1 (18.75 oz)	480	4	22	20	67	1	470
Hot Cocoa	1 (14 oz)	330	3	11	0	57	2	460
Hot Cocoa	1 (10 oz)	230	2	8	0	38	2	310
Hot Cocoa	1 (18.75 oz)	440	4	15	0	75	3	610
Hot Cocoa	1 (20 oz)	470	5	16	0	79	3	640
SANDWICHES								
Breakfast Sandwich Ham Egg Cheese	1	320	22	12	195	31	2	1340
Omwich Bagel Bacon Cheddar	1	600	26	21	295	79	tr	1630
Omwich Bagel Spanish Cheese	1	570	24	18	280	79	tr	1370
Omwich Bagel Three Cheese	1	610	25	22	305	78	tr	1630
Omwich Croissant Spanish Cheese	1	530	19	36	285	33	1	930
Omwich Croissant Bacon Cheddar	1	560	21	38	295	33	1	1190
Omwich Croissant Three Cheese	1	560	20	39	305	33	1	1200
Omwich English Muffin Bacon Cheddar	1	400	21	21	295	33	2	1440
Omwich English Muffin Spanish Cheese	1	370	18	18	280	34	2	1180
Omwich English Muffin Three Cheese	1	400	19	22	305	33	2	1450

FOOD	PORTION	CALS	PROT	FAT	CHOL	CARB	FIBER	SOD

EINSTEIN BROS BAGELS
BAGELS AND BREADS

FOOD	PORTION	CALS	PROT	FAT	CHOL	CARB	FIBER	SOD
Bagel Asiago Cheese	1	360	13	3	5	71	2	570
Bagel Cranberry Special	1	350	10	1	0	78	3	490
Bagel Egg	1	340	11	3	35	69	2	510
Bagel Honey Whole Wheat	1	320	10	1	0	71	3	470
Bagel Jalapeno	1	330	11	1	0	71	2	510
Bagel Lucky Gree	1	320	11	1	0	71	2	520
Bagel Mango	1	360	10	1	0	80	2	490
Bagel Marble Rye	1	340	11	2	0	73	3	690
Bagel Potato	1	350	10	5	0	69	2	590
Bagel Power	1	410	13	5	0	81	4	310
Bagel Power w/ Peanut Butter	1	750	27	34	0	92	7	780
Bagel Pumpkin	1	330	10	2	0	72	3	470
Bagel Roasted Red Pepper & Pesto	1	410	17	7	15	73	2	710
Bagel Six Cheese	1	390	16	6	15	72	2	650
Bagel Spicy Nacho	1	450	17	9	20	77	3	890
Bagel Spinach Florentine	1	410	17	7	20	72	3	620
Bagel Croutons	¼ cup	25	1	1	0	4	0	75
Bagel Twist	1	220	8	4	5	39	1	510
Bread Ciabatta	1 serv	320	12	3	0	64	3	460
Chocolate Chip	1	370	11	3	0	76	3	500
Chopped Garlic	1	380	13	3	0	79	4	600
Chopped Onion	1	330	11	1	0	71	2	500
Cinnamon Raisin Swirl	1	350	11	1	0	78	2	490
Cinnamon Sugar	1	330	10	1	0	74	2	490
Dark Pumpernickel	1	320	11	1	0	68	3	730
Everything	1	340	13	2	0	75	2	820
Focaccia Cheese Pizza	1 serv	500	25	11	35	75	3	1010
Focaccia Margherita	1 serv	400	14	17	5	76	3	580
Focaccia Pepperoni Pizza	1 serv	590	29	19	55	76	3	1380

FOOD	PORTION	CALS	PROT	FAT	CHOL	CARB	FIBER	SOD
Nutty Banana	1	360	11	3	0	74	2	510
Plain	1	320	11	1	0	71	2	520
Poppy Dip'd	1	350	12	2	0	74	2	680
Roll Challah	1	300	11	5	40	55	2	270
Salt	1	330	11	1	0	73	2	1790
Sesame Dip'd	1	380	11	5	0	75	3	680
Sun Dried Tomato	1	320	11	1	0	69	3	520
Wild Blueberry	1	350	11	1	0	77	3	510
BEVERAGES								
Americano	1 reg	1	0	0	0	0	0	0
Cafe Latte	1 reg	140	9	5	20	13	0	140
Cafe Latte Nonfat	1 reg	100	9	0	5	14	0	140
Cappuccino	1 reg	90	6	4	15	9	0	95
Cappuccino Nonfat	1 reg	60	6	0	5	9	0	95
Chai 2% Milk	1 reg	210	4	2	10	41	0	75
Chai Skim Milk	1 reg	190	4	0	0	41	0	75
Coffee	1 reg	0	0	0	0	0	0	0
Espresso	1 reg	1	0	0	0	0	0	0
Half & Half	2 tbsp	40	1	3	15	1	—	25
Hot Chocolate	1 reg	290	9	11	20	39	0	160
Hot Chocolate Lower Fat	1 reg	260	9	7	5	39	0	160
Hot Tea All Flavors	1 cup	0	0	0	0	0	0	0
Iced Americano	1 serv	1	0	0	0	0	0	0
Iced Coffee	1 serv	0	0	0	0	0	0	0
Iced Latte	1 serv	120	8	5	20	12	0	125
Iced Latte Nonfat	1 serv	90	8	0	5	12	0	130
Iced Mocha	1 serv	210	7	6	15	33	0	120
Iced Mocha Low Fat	1 serv	180	7	3	5	32	0	115
Mocha	1 reg	230	8	6	15	34	0	135
Mocha Low Fat	1 reg	190	8	3	5	34	0	130
DESSERTS								
Brownie Iced	1	550	5	24	35	81	3	310
Brownie Iced w/ Walnuts	1	600	6	29	35	82	4	310
Cherry Figure 8	1	400	7	18	40	51	1	380
Cinnamon Roll	1	810	13	32	45	118	4	580
Cookie Chocolate Chunk	1	640	7	31	50	87	3	350

FOOD	PORTION	CALS	PROT	FAT	CHOL	CARB	FIBER	SOD
Cookie Oatmeal Raisin	1	600	7	27	50	82	2	640
Cookie Peanut Butter	1	640	11	34	55	75	3	490
Muffin Banana Nut	1	640	10	32	80	81	2	430
Muffin Blueberry	1	540	8	22	95	80	1	510
Muffin Chocolate Chip	1	620	8	27	90	89	3	460
Pound Cake Lemon Iced	1 slice	540	7	25	155	74	0	420
Pound Cake Marble	1 slice	460	7	24	150	57	1	430
Rice Krispy Bar	1	420	5	8	0	83	1	610
Scone Blueberry w/ Icing	1	450	7	18	55	64	2	460
Scone Lemon Currant	1	430	7	15	40	69	4	450
Strudel Cinnamon Walnut	1 piece	550	7	31	30	63	3	380
Sweetie Pie	1	620	4	20	5	106	1	220
SALAD DRESSINGS								
Asian Sesame	2 tbsp	80	1	2	0	16	0	600
Caesar	2 tbsp	150	1	16	10	1	0	360
Chipotle Vinaigrette	2 tbsp	110	0	10	0	5	0	440
Horseradish Sauce	2 tbsp	170	0	18	20	1	0	190
Raspberry Vinaigrette	2 tbsp	160	0	14	0	8	0	80
Thousand Island	2 tbsp	110	0	9	10	5	0	210
SALADS								
Asian Chicken Salad	1 serv (14.5 oz)	550	29	9	55	88	5	1610
Bros Bistro	1 serv (9.5 oz)	520	10	43	25	25	2	480
Chicken Caesar	1 serv (12.5 oz)	750	33	53	90	26	2	1850
Chicken Chipotle Salad	1 serv	710	34	43	80	48	13	1890
Chicken Salad On Greens	1 serv (10.5 oz)	210	19	9	55	11	3	640
Egg Salad	1 serv (4 oz)	200	9	17	310	5	0	340

FOOD	PORTION	CALS	PROT	FAT	CHOL	CARB	FIBER	SOD
Fresh Fruit Cup	1 serv (8 oz)	110	1	1	0	25	2	10
Mixed Greens	1 serv (3.5 oz)	228	2	18	0	13	1	380
Potato	½ cup	290	3	21	15	21	2	600
Tuna Salad On Greens	1 serv (10.5 oz)	170	20	5	35	10	3	520
SANDWICHES								
12 Grain Bread Deli Chicken Salad	1	440	26	13	55	55	6	1090
12 Grain Bread Deli Egg Salad	1	490	18	21	315	57	5	800
12 Grain Bread Deli Ham	1	560	29	25	75	55	5	1680
12 Grain Bread Deli Roast Beef	1	560	34	24	80	56	5	1170
12 Grain Bread Deli Smoked Turkey	1	530	31	21	70	56	5	1700
12 Grain Bread Deli Tuna Salad	1	440	26	13	55	56	6	1090
12 Grain Bread Deli Turkey Pastrami	1	540	34	21	70	55	5	1900
12 Grain Bread Ultimate Toasted Cheese w/ Tomato	1	870	36	50	110	77	2	1530
Bagel Chicken Salad	1	500	28	10	55	78	4	1160
Bagel Egg Bacon	1	580	29	19	285	74	2	970
Bagel Egg Ham	1	530	31	13	295	74	2	1120
Bagel Egg Salad	1	560	20	18	315	79	3	860
Bagel Egg Sausage	1	550	33	14	295	74	2	1000
Bagel Ham	1	450	26	6	45	74	3	1390
Bagel Holey Cow	1	900	36	50	105	77	3	1450
Bagel Hummus & Feta	1	540	18	13	15	89	5	880
Bagel New York Lox	1	660	26	27	85	79	3	1150
Bagel Original	1	480	23	10	270	74	2	680
Bagel Roast Beef	1	460	31	4	45	76	3	880
Bagel Rueben Deli	1	660	39	19	65	83	4	2590
Bagel Salmon & Shmear	1	650	31	22	310	82	2	1040

FOOD	PORTION	CALS	PROT	FAT	CHOL	CARB	FIBER	SOD
Bagel Santa Fe	1	650	30	24	300	78	2	1210
Bagel Smoked Turkey	1	420	25	2	30	75	3	1270
Bagel Tasty Turkey	1	570	31	15	80	83	4	1420
Bagel The Veg Out	1	490	17	13	30	77	3	850
Bagel Tuna Salad	1	470	29	6	35	77	4	1040
Bagel Turkey Pastrami	1	440	31	2	40	76	3	1610
Challah Club Mex	1	750	39	45	135	47	2	2290
Challah Cobbie	1	630	37	33	110	45	4	1920
Challah Deli Chicken Salad	1	480	29	14	95	62	4	920
Challah Deli Egg Salad	1	430	18	20	345	45	2	540
Challah Deli Pastrami	1	480	34	21	100	43	2	1650
Challah Deli Roast Beef	1	500	34	23	110	44	2	920
Challah Deli Smoked Turkey	1	470	31	21	100	44	2	1450
Challah Deli Tuna Salad	1	370	30	10	60	42	2	740
Challah Deli Turkey Ham	1	500	29	25	105	43	2	1430
Challah EBBQ Chicken	1	380	27	8	80	52	2	1000
Challah Roasted Chicken & Smoked Gouda	1	440	36	13	110	47	2	1010
Chicago Bagel Dog Asiago	1	740	29	34	80	78	2	1360
Chicago Bagel Dog Chili Cheese	1	810	33	38	105	83	4	1550
Chicago Bagel Dog Everything	1	730	26	34	70	80	3	1850
Chicago Bagel Dog Onion w/o Cheese	1	680	25	30	70	78	2	1220
Country White Deli Chicken Salad	1	540	30	15	55	75	4	1570

FOOD	PORTION	CALS	PROT	FAT	CHOL	CARB	FIBER	SOD
Country White Deli Egg Salad	1	590	22	23	315	77	3	1280
Country White Deli Ham	1	660	33	27	15	75	3	2160
Country White Deli Roast Beef	1	660	38	26	80	76	3	1650
Country White Deli Smoked Turkey	1	630	35	23	70	76	3	2180
Country White Deli Tuna Salad	1	510	30	11	35	74	4	1440
Country White Deli Turkey Pastrami	1	640	38	23	70	75	3	2380
Country White Ultimate Toasted Cheese w/ Tomato	1	870	36	51	110	73	2	1610
Panini Cali Club	1	730	47	24	75	90	9	2340
Panini Cuban Ham	1	700	40	31	90	68	4	2010
Panini Denver Omelet Breakfast	1	740	42	33	310	70	3	1380
Panini Italian Chicken	1	770	44	36	85	69	4	1840
Panini Taos Turkey	1	740	45	25	80	93	9	2140
Panini Ultimate Toasted Cheese	1	900	39	44	110	96	7	1910
Roll Ups Albuquerque Turkey	1	790	31	39	85	81	5	2040
Roll Ups Thai Vegetable w/ Chicken	1	670	27	18	40	99	4	1850
Roll Ups Thai Vegetables	1	630	24	21	0	97	5	1310
SOUPS								
Broccoli Sharp Cheddar	1 cup	230	11	15	40	13	1	490
Chicken & Wild Rice	1 cup	190	10	4	15	29	2	1440
Chicken Noodle	1 cup	220	16	9	60	17	2	980
Clam Chowda	1 cup	160	5	11	35	11	0	480

FOOD	PORTION	CALS	PROT	FAT	CHOL	CARB	FIBER	SOD
Minestrone Low Fat	1 cup	180	8	3	0	32	5	1410
Tomato Bisque	1 cup	190	5	10	15	23	3	1390
Tortilla	1 cup	90	2	3	0	14	2	1530
Turkey Chili	1 cup	140	10	5	20	14	2	930
SPREADS								
Butter	1 tbsp	100	0	11	30	0	0	115
Butter & Margarine Blend	1 tbsp	60	0	7	0	0	0	75
Cream Cheese Blueberry	1 tbsp	70	1	5	15	6	0	50
Cream Cheese Cappuccino	2 tbsp	70	1	5	15	4	0	50
Cream Cheese Garden Vegetable	2 tbsp	60	1	5	15	2	0	105
Cream Cheese Honey Almond Reduced Fat	2 tbsp	70	1	5	15	5	0	40
Cream Cheese Jalapeno Salsa	1 tbsp	60	1	5	15	3	0	95
Cream Cheese Maple Walnut Raisin	2 tbsp	60	1	5	15	4	0	45
Cream Cheese Onion & Chive	2 tbsp	70	4	6	20	3	0	55
Cream Cheese Plain	2 tbsp	60	1	7	20	1	0	65
Cream Cheese Plain Reduced Fat	2 tbsp	60	1	5	15	2	0	85
Cream Cheese Pumpkin	2 tbsp	100	1	8	25	6	0	80
Cream Cheese Smoked Salmon	2 tbsp	60	1	5	15	3	0	115
Cream Cheese Strawberry	2 tbsp	70	1	5	15	5	0	50
Cream Cheese Sun Dried Tomato & Basil	2 tbsp	60	1	5	15	2	0	50
Fruit Spread Apricot	1 serv	75	0	0	0	19	0	8

FOOD	PORTION	CALS	PROT	FAT	CHOL	CARB	FIBER	SOD
Fruit Spread Grape	1 serv (1 oz)	75	0	0	0	19	0	3
Fruit Spread Strawberry	1 serv (1 oz)	75	0	0	0	19	0	17
Honey Butter	1 tbsp	90	0	8	15	4	0	35
Hummus	1 serv	110	3	7	0	9	2	390
Mayo Ancho Lime	1 tbsp	50	0	5	5	1	0	160
Mustard French Dijon	1 tsp	10	0	0	0	0	0	130
Mustard Grain Dijon	1 tsp	5	0	0	0	0	0	105
Mustard Honey	1 tsp	15	0	0	0	2	0	45
Mustard Raspberry	2 tbsp	50	1	2	2	7	0	190
Mustard Yellow	1 tbsp	5	0	0	0	0	0	80
Peanut Butter	2 tbsp	190	7	15	0	8	2	140
Salsa Ancho Lime	¼ cup	20	0	1	0	3	0	670

EL POLLO LOCO

DESSERTS

FOOD	PORTION	CALS	PROT	FAT	CHOL	CARB	FIBER	SOD
Churro	1	179	3	11	5	18	1	221
Fosters Freeze Soft Serve	1 cup	180	4	5	20	30	0	100

MAIN MENU SELECTIONS

FOOD	PORTION	CALS	PROT	FAT	CHOL	CARB	FIBER	SOD
Bowl Chicken Caesar	1 serv	535	25	28	50	46	4	1450
Bowl Pollo	1 serv	545	31	10	40	84	12	2160
Bowl Veggie	1 serv	570	20	16	10	91	16	1705
Bowl Veggie w/o Cheese	1 serv	529	17	12	0	91	16	1608
Burrito Classic Chicken	1	580	17	22	108	66	6	1595
Burrito Twice Grilled	1 serv	835	59	39	150	60	2	2880
Burrito BRC	1 serv	530	17	15	15	79	6	1395
Burrito Caesar	1 serv	895	48	45	100	76	4	2680
Burrito Chicken Lover's	1 serv	525	34	18	100	55	2	1810
Burrito Spicy	1 serv	555	31	19	70	64	9	1980
Burrito Ultimate Chicken	1 serv	685	35	23	65	84	6	2250
Chicken Breast	1 piece	153	29	4	95	0	0	540
Chicken Leg	1 piece	86	14	3	80	0	0	206

FOOD	PORTION	CALS	PROT	FAT	CHOL	CARB	FIBER	SOD
Chicken Thigh	1 piece	120	14	7	82	0	0	225
Chicken Wing	1	83	13	3	58	0	0	334
Cole Slaw	1 serv	206	2	16	11	12	2	358
Corn Cobbette	1 serv	80	3	1	0	18	1	10
French Fries	1 serv	444	6	19	0	61	0	605
Fresh Vegetables	1 serv	70	3	4	0	6	4	80
Gravy	1 serv (1 oz)	107	3	4	8	15	0	1344
Mashed Potatoes	1 serv	97	3	1	0	21	2	369
Nachos Chicken	1 serv	1420	47	91	161	105	15	1506
Pinto Beans	1 serv	165	8	4	0	26	10	715
Popcorn Chicken	1 serv	226	17	12	53	15	0	787
Potato Salad	1 serv	256	3	14	15	30	3	527
Quesadilla Cheese	1 serv	495	22	25	53	45	2	1008
Quesadilla Chicken	1 serv	593	36	29	107	48	0	1329
Smokey Black Beans	1 serv	306	7	16	13	35	5	731
Spanish Rice	1 serv	165	3	1	0	34	1	425
Taco Al Carbon Chicken	1 serv	135	9	3	30	18	1	225
Taco Soft Chicken	1	237	17	12	74	15	0	629
Taquitos Chicken	2	370	15	17	25	43	3	690
Tortilla Chips	1 serv	426	5	24	0	48	4	166
Tortilla Corn	1 (6 inches)	70	1	1	0	14	1	35
Tortilla Corn	1 (4.5 inch)	40	1	1	0	8	1	<5
Tortilla Flour	1 (12 inches)	325	8	8	0	51	2	815
Tortilla Flour	1 (6.5 inch)	110	3	4	0	13	0	16
Tortilla Spicy Tomato	1 (12 inches	270	8	7	0	43	2	670
Tostada Salad	1 serv	700	32	32	65	76	10	1725
SALAD DRESSINGS AND TOPPINGS								
Bleu Cheese	1 serv (1.5 oz)	230	2	24	30	2	0	450
Buttermilk Ranch	1 serv (1.5 oz)	220	1	24	10	2	0	420
Creamy Chipolte	1 (0.5 oz)	75	0	8	5	1	0	100
Creamy Cilantro	1 serv (0.5 oz)	80	0	8	5	0	0	85
Guacamole	1 serv (1 oz)	30	0	2	0	3	0	160
Hot Sauce Jalapeno	1 pkg (0.5 oz)	5	0	0	0	1	0	110
Light Italian	1 serv (1.5 oz)	20	0	1	0	2	0	780

FOOD	PORTION	CALS	PROT	FAT	CHOL	CARB	FIBER	SOD
Salsa Avocado	1 serv (1 oz)	20	0	1	0	1	0	225
Salsa House	1 serv (1 oz)	6	0	tr	0	1	0	85
Salsa Pico De Gallo	1 serv (1 oz)	10	0	tr	0	1	0	135
Salsa Spicy Chipotle	1 serv (1 oz)	7	0	0	0	1	0	180
Sour Cream	1 serv (1 oz)	60	1	5	20	1	0	15
Thousand Island	1 serv (1.5 oz)	220	0	21	30	7	0	360
SALADS								
Caesar	1 serv	565	24	45	70	18	3	1305
Caesar w/o Dressing	1 serv	250	22	11	55	16	3	975
Fiesta Salad	1 serv	755	32	58	105	28	4	1680
Fiesta Salad w/o Dressing	1 serv	450	31	26	95	25	4	1275
Garden Salad	1 serv	110	5	7	15	8	2	270
Macaroni & Cheese	1 serv	381	11	26	65	25	2	891
Tostada Salad w/o Shell	1 serv	360	28	14	65	34	6	1365
FAZOLI'S								
DESSERTS								
Cheesecake	1 slice	290	6	22	950	17	0	220
Cheesecake Turtle	1 slice	420	8	34	100	24	2	220
Cookie Milk Chocolate Chunk	1	360	6	15	30	54	0	350
Lemon Ice	1 serv	190	0	0	0	45	0	95
Specialty Cheesecake	1 serv	300	7	22	85	22	1	200
Strawberry Topping	1 serv	35	0	0	0	8	0	95
MAIN MENU SELECTIONS								
Baked Chicken Parmesan	1 serv	740	42	20	65	99	6	900
Baked Spaghetti Parmesan	1 serv	700	38	25	60	76	5	700
Baked Ziti	1 reg	750	36	26	55	87	6	860
Baked Ziti	1 sm	490	23	17	35	56	4	570
Breadstick	1	140	4	6	0	18	1	510
Breadstick Dry	1	90	4	1	0	17	1	170
Broccoli Fettuccine Alfredo	1 reg	830	27	23	20	125	6	250

FOOD	PORTION	CALS	PROT	FAT	CHOL	CARB	FIBER	SOD
Broccoli Fettuccine Alfredo	1 sm	560	19	15	15	85	6	190
Cheese Ravioli w/ Marinara Sauce	1 serv	480	21	15	65	65	4	530
Cheese Ravioli w/ Meat Sauce	1 serv	510	20	17	70	65	4	800
Classic Sampler	1 serv	710	26	21	85	97	6	710
Fettuccine Alfredo	1 reg	800	25	22	20	119	5	230
Fettuccine Alfredo	1 sm	530	17	15	15	80	3	170
Fettuccine w/ Shrimp & Scallop	1 serv	590	32	16	95	81	3	590
Homestyle Lasagna	1 serv	440	22	19	145	41	4	970
Homestyle Lasagna w/ Broccoli	1 serv	420	21	18	140	45	5	750
Minestrone Soup	1 serv	120	1	1	0	23	8	910
Peppery Chicken Alfredo	1 serv	610	31	16	50	80	3	410
Pizza Cheese	1 serv	460	24	15	40	58	2	970
Pizza Combination Double Slice	1 serv	570	29	25	60	63	3	1360
Pizza Pepperoni	1 serv	530	27	22	53	61	2	1230
Pizza Baked Spaghetti	1 serv	750	40	31	75	78	5	1000
Spaghetti w/ Marinara Sauce	1 reg	620	21	8	0	111	7	140
Spaghetti w/ Marinara Sauce	1 sm	420	15	6	0	74	5	105
Spaghetti w/ Meat Sauce	1 reg	670	21	11	10	111	8	530
Spaghetti w/ Meat Sauce	1 sm	450	14	8	10	74	5	370
Spaghetti w/ Meatballs	1 sm	730	28	31	60	80	6	730
Spaghetti w/ Meatballs	1 reg	1020	39	42	80	119	8	970
SALAD DRESSINGS								
Honey French	1 serv	150	0	12	0	9	0	210
House Italian	1 serv	110	0	9	0	5	0	510
Ranch	1 serv	150	0	17	3	1	0	210

FOOD	PORTION	CALS	PROT	FAT	CHOL	CARB	FIBER	SOD
Reduced Calorie Italian	1 serv	50	0	5	0	3	0	390
Thousand Island	1 serv	130	0	13	15	4	0	220
SALADS AND SALAD BARS								
Caesar Side Salad	1	220	7	17	5	13	3	690
Chicken & Pasta Caesar Salad	1	500	28	27	55	35	4	1430
Chicken Caesar Salad	1	420	22	29	45	17	4	1350
Chicken Finger Salad	1	190	20	9	45	8	2	540
Chicken Finger Salad w/ Bacon & Honey Mustard	1	400	20	28	50	17	2	950
Garden Salad	1	25	2	0	0	4	1	15
Garden Salad w/ Balsamic Vinaigrette	1	120	2	9	0	10	1	150
Italian Chef Salad	1	260	15	21	45	13	3	1450
Pasta Salad	1 serv	590	18	25	20	70	5	2010
SANDWICHES								
Panini Chicken Caesar Club	1	660	39	35	110	51	3	1670
Panini Chicken Pesto	1	510	33	20	60	51	3	1350
Panini Four Cheese & Tomato	1	720	28	43	75	55	3	1450
Panini Ham & Swiss	1	600	31	30	70	53	2	2000
Panini Italian Club	1	670	30	37	85	54	3	1970
Panini Italian Deli	1	660	34	35	90	61	4	2450
Panini Smoked Turkey	1	710	32	38	110	57	3	2110
Submarinos Club	half	1100	51	44	120	121	7	2890
Submarinos Ham & Swiss	half	1000	44	37	75	120	7	2350
Submarinos Meatball	half	1260	55	59	125	128	8	2340
Submarinos Original	half	1160	45	55	105	124	8	2530

FOOD	PORTION	CALS	PROT	FAT	CHOL	CARB	FIBER	SOD
Submarinos Pepperoni Pizza	half	1060	55	40	95	133	6	2700
Submarinos Turkey	half	990	43	34	90	121	7	2440

FRULLATI CAFE
BEVERAGES

FOOD	PORTION	CALS	PROT	FAT	CHOL	CARB	FIBER	SOD
Smoothie	1 serv (14 oz)	195	1	3	0	41	tr	154

GREAT STEAK & POTATO COMPANY

FOOD	PORTION	CALS	PROT	FAT	CHOL	CARB	FIBER	SOD
Baked Potato w/ Broccoli & Cheese	1 serv (12 oz)	340	–	5	–	–	–	340
Chicken Philadelpia	1 serv (10 oz)	640	–	27	–	–	–	620
Chicken Teriyaki	1 serv (11 oz)	580	–	17	–	–	–	1470
Fresh Cut Fries	1 reg	540	–	29	–	–	–	440
Fresh Cut Fries	1 sm	460	–	24	–	–	–	380
Fresh Cut Fries	1 serv	920	–	48	–	–	–	760
Great Potato w/ Steak	1 serv (14 oz)	600	–	32	–	–	–	600
Great Potato w/ Turkey	1 serv (14 oz)	610	–	28	–	–	–	620
Great Salad Experience w/ Chicken w/o Dressing	1 serv (15 oz)	260	–	9	–	–	–	490
Great Steak	1 lg (18 oz)	1070	–	55	–	–	–	610
Great Steak	1 serv (11 oz)	660	–	34	–	–	–	400
Ham Delight	1 serv (11 oz)	710	–	33	–	–	–	1590
Turkey Philadelphia	1 serv (10 oz)	690	–	28	–	–	–	290
Veggi Delight	1 serv (7 oz)	570	–	29	–	–	–	440

HAAGEN-DAZS
FROZEN YOGURT

FOOD	PORTION	CALS	PROT	FAT	CHOL	CARB	FIBER	SOD
Pinapple Coconut	½ cup	230	4	13	90	25	0	55
Soft Serve Nonfat Chocolate	½ cup	110	4	0	0	23	0	65

FOOD	PORTION	CALS	PROT	FAT	CHOL	CARB	FIBER	SOD
Soft Serve Nonfat Chocolate Mousse	½ cup	80	5	0	0	24	1	65
Soft Serve Nonfat Coffee	½ cup	110	5	0	<5	22	0	70
Soft Serve Nonfat Strawberry	½ cup	110	4	0	0	24	0	60
Soft Serve Nonfat Vanilla	½ cup	110	5	0	<5	22	0	75
Soft Serve Nonfat Vanilla Mousse	½ cup	70	4	0	<5	23	0	65
Soft Serve Nonfat White Chocolate	½ cup	110	5	0	<5	22	0	75
Vanilla Fudge	½ cup	160	6	0	<5	34	0	100
Vanilla Raspberry Swirl	½ cup	130	4	0	<5	29	tr	30
ICE CREAM								
Bailey's Irish Cream	½ cup	270	5	17	115	23	0	70
Bar Chocolate	1 (2.7 oz)	200	4	12	85	16	tr	55
Bar Chocolate & Dark Chocolate	1 (3.6 oz)	350	5	24	85	28	2	45
Bar Coffee	1 (2.7 oz)	190	3	13	85	15	0	65
Bar Coffee & Almond Crunch	1 (3.7 oz)	370	5	27	90	27	tr	80
Bar Vanilla	1 (2.7 oz)	190	3	13	85	15	0	50
Bar Vanilla & Almonds	1 (3.7 oz)	380	6	28	90	26	1	70
Bar Vanilla & Milk Chocolate	1 (3.5 oz)	340	5	24	90	25	tr	65
Belgian Chocolate Chocolate	½ cup	330	5	21	85	29	2	85
Brownies A La Mode	½ cup	280	5	16	90	28	tr	135
Butter Pecan	½ cup	300	5	22	105	20	tr	110
Cappuccino Commotion	½ cup	310	5	21	100	25	1	90
Chocolate	½ cup	269	5	17	110	21	1	60
Chocolate Chocolate Chip	½ cup	300	5	19	100	26	2	55
Chocolate Chocolate Mint	½ cup	300	5	20	95	25	1	50

FOOD	PORTION	CALS	PROT	FAT	CHOL	CARB	FIBER	SOD
Chocolate Swiss Almond	½ cup	300	5	20	100	24	2	55
Coffee	½ cup	250	5	17	115	20	0	65
Coffee Mocha Chip	½ cup	270	4	19	105	24	tr	75
Cookie Dough Dynamo	½ cup	310	4	20	95	29	0	125
Cookies & Cream	½ cup	270	5	17	105	23	0	95
Cookies & Fudge	½ cup	180	7	3	15	33	tr	115
Deep Chocolate Peanut Butter	½ cup	350	8	24	80	26	4	85
Dulce De Leche Caramel	½ cup	270	5	16	95	27	0	90
Lowfat Coffee Fudge	½ cup	170	5	3	25	32	0	95
Macadamia Brittle	½ cup	280	4	19	105	24	0	105
Macadamia Nut	½ cup	320	5	24	110	20	0	100
Mint Chip	½ cup	280	4	18	105	25	tr	85
Pistachio	½ cup	280	5	19	110	21	tr	80
Pralines & Cream	½ cup	280	4	17	95	28	0	160
Rum Raisin	½ cup	260	4	17	105	21	0	55
Strawberry	½ cup	250	4	16	90	22	tr	90
Vanilla	½ cup	250	4	17	115	20	0	65
Vanilla Chocolate Chip	⅓ cup	290	5	19	100	25	tr	70
Vanilla Swiss Almond	½ cup	290	5	20	100	23	tr	70
SORBET								
Bar Raspberry & Vanilla	1 (2.5 oz)	90	2	0	0	21	tr	15
Mango	½ cup	120	0	0	0	31	tr	0
Orange	½ cup	120	0	0	0	30	tr	0
Raspberry	½ cup	120	0	0	0	30	2	0
Soft Serve Raspberry	½ cup	110	0	0	0	28	2	0
Strawberry	½ cup	120	0	0	0	30	1	0
Zesty Lemon	½ cup	120	0	0	0	31	tr	0

HUNGRY HOWIE'S
MAIN MENU SELECTIONS

FOOD	PORTION	CALS	PROT	FAT	CHOL	CARB	FIBER	SOD
Howie Wings	6 (3 oz)	180	12	14	70	0	0	760

FOOD	PORTION	CALS	PROT	FAT	CHOL	CARB	FIBER	SOD
Three Cheeser Bread	1 serv	370	15	14	17	47	1	384
PIZZA								
Large Cheese	1 slice	175	10	4	11	24	1	387
Large Cheese + Bacon	1 slice	208	17	5	13	25	1	388
Large Cheese + Beef	1 slice	197	11	6	16	24	1	464
Large Cheese + Black Olives	1 slice	181	10	5	12	24	1	436
Large Cheese + Green Olives	1 slice	181	10	5	12	24	1	436
Large Cheese + Green Peppers	1 slice	175	10	4	11	24	1	387
Large Cheese + Ham	1 slice	179	11	6	14	24	1	452
Large Cheese + Mushrooms	1 slice	175	10	4	11	24	1	387
Large Cheese + Onions	1 slice	175	10	5	12	24	1	388
Large Cheese + Pepperoni	1 slice	191	11	4	16	24	1	450
Large Cheese + Pineapple	1 slice	388	11	5	12	25	1	388
Large Cheese + Sausage	1 slice	195	12	6	14	24	1	484
Medium Cheese	1 slice	153	9	5	9	21	1	350
Medium Cheese + Bacon	1 slice	179	14	5	10	21	1	351
Medium Cheese + Beef	1 slice	177	10	6	14	21	1	427
Medium Cheese + Black Olives	1 slice	159	9	5	11	21	1	388
Medium Cheese + Green Olives	1 slice	159	9	4	11	21	1	388
Medium Cheese + Green Peppers	1 slice	155	9	5	10	21	1	351
Medium Cheese + Ham	1 slice	159	10	6	12	21	1	415
Medium Cheese + Mushrooms	1 slice	155	9	5	9	21	1	350

FOOD	PORTION	CALS	PROT	FAT	CHOL	CARB	FIBER	SOD
Medium Cheese + Onions	1 slice	155	9	5	10	21	1	351
Medium Cheese + Pepperoni	1 slice	171	10	6	14	21	1	410
Medium Cheese + Pineapple	1 slice	158	9	5	10	22	1	351
Medium Cheese + Sausage	1 slice	175	10	6	12	21	1	447
Small Cheese	1 slice	121	7	3	8	37	1	278
Small Cheese + Bacon	1 slice	138	10	3	9	17	1	278
Small Cheese + Beef	1 slice	137	8	4	12	17	1	328
Small Cheese + Black Olives	1 slice	125	7	3	9	17	1	303
Small Cheese + Green Olives	1 slice	125	7	3	9	17	1	303
Small Cheese + Green Peppers	1 slice	122	7	3	8	17	1	278
Small Cheese + Ham	1 slice	126	8	3	11	17	1	331
Small Cheese + Mushrooms	1 slice	123	7	3	8	17	1	279
Small Cheese + Onions	1 slice	122	7	3	8	17	1	278
Small Cheese + Pepperoni	1 slice	136	8	4	12	17	1	329
Small Cheese + Pineapple	1 slice	124	7	3	8	18	1	278
Small Cheese + Sausage	1 slice	136	8	3	11	17	1	343
SALADS AND SALAD BARS								
Antipasto Salad w/o Dressing	1 lg	101	8	7	24	3	1	477
Chef Salad w/o Dressing	1 lg	99	8	6	24	4	2	341
Garden Salad w/o Dressing	1 lg	17	1	tr	0	3	2	9
Greek Salad w/o Dressing	1 lg	109	6	7	25	7	2	501

FOOD	PORTION	CALS	PROT	FAT	CHOL	CARB	FIBER	SOD
SANDWICHES								
Sub Deluxe Italian	½ sub	506	24	18	44	61	2	1005
Sub Ham & Cheese	½ sub	475	26	15	44	61	2	1020
Sub Pizza	½ sub	689	30	34	86	67	3	1722
Sub Pizza Special	½ sub	606	29	24	65	68	3	1584
Sub Steak Cheese Mushroom	½ sub	491	27	15	47	64	2	914
Sub Turkey	½ sub	466	25	13	38	63	2	1108
Sub Turkey Club	½ sub	556	42	18	44	62	2	1065
Sub Vegetarian	½ sub	530	22	21	39	64	3	895
IHOP								
Pancake Buckwheat	1 (1.7 oz)	110	3	4	50	15	1	280
Pancake Buttermilk	1 (1.7 oz)	110	3	3	30	17	tr	450
Pancake Country Griddle	1 (2 oz)	120	3	4	35	19	tr	440
Pancake Harvest Grain 'N Nut	1 (2.25 oz)	180	5	9	40	20	2	410
JACK IN THE BOX								
BEVERAGES								
Barq's Root Beer	1 serv (20 oz)	180	0	0	0	50	0	40
Coca-Cola Classic	1 serv (20 oz)	170	0	0	0	46	0	8
Coffee	1 serv (12 oz)	5	0	0	0	1	0	5
Diet Coke	1 serv (20 oz)	0	0	0	0	0	0	15
Dr Pepper	1 serv (20 oz)	190	0	0	0	50	0	25
Ice Cream Shake Caramel	1 serv (16 oz)	660	11	30	115	86	0	280
Ice Cream Shake Chocolate	1 (16 oz)	660	11	29	110	89	1	270
Ice Cream Shake Oreo	1 serv (16 oz)	670	11	33	110	81	1	350
Ice Cream Shake Strawberry	1 serv (16 oz)	640	10	28	110	84	0	220

FOOD	PORTION	CALS	PROT	FAT	CHOL	CARB	FIBER	SOD
Ice Cream Shake Strawberry Banana	1 serv (16 oz)	700	10	28	110	100	0	230
Ice Cream Shake Vanilla	1 (16 oz)	570	11	29	115	65	0	220
Iced Tea	1 serv (20 oz)	0	0	0	0	0	0	0
Lowfat Milk 2%	1 serv (8 oz)	140	10	5	20	14	0	140
Orange Juice	1 serv (10 oz)	140	2	0	0	32	2	25
Sprite	1 serv (20 oz)	160	0	0	0	41	0	40
BREAKFAST SELECTIONS								
Breakfast Sandwich Sourdough	1	440	17	26	215	36	2	880
Breakfast Sandwich Ultimate	1	730	30	40	440	66	2	1870
Breakfast Jack	1	310	13	14	205	33	1	720
Croissant Sausage	1	680	18	50	250	41	2	760
Croissant Supreme	1	570	19	37	240	41	1	1040
French Toast Sticks	4 pieces	430	8	18	10	57	2	460
Hash Brown	1 serv	150	1	10	0	13	2	230
Sandwich Extreme Sausage	1	720	25	53	280	35	2	1180
DESSERTS								
Cheesecake	1 serv	310	7	16	55	34	0	220
Double Fudge Cake	1 serv	310	3	11	25	49	4	270
MAIN MENU SELECTIONS								
American Cheese	1 slice	45	2	4	10	1	0	180
Bacon Cheddar Potato Wedges	1 serv	770	21	53	45	52	4	1330
Cheeseburger Bacon Bacon	1	910	38	59	100	58	3	1780
Cheeseburger Bacon Ultimate	1	1120	52	75	160	59	2	2260
Cheeseburger Junior Bacon	1	540	22	36	75	31	1	940

FOOD	PORTION	CALS	PROT	FAT	CHOL	CARB	FIBER	SOD
Cheeseburger Ultimate	1	990	41	66	130	59	2	1620
Chicken Breast Pieces	4	360	27	17	80	24	1	970
Chicken Breast Strips	1 serv	500	35	25	80	36	3	1260
Chicken Fajita Pita	1	330	24	11	55	35	3	910
Chicken Sandwich	1	410	15	21	35	39	2	740
Dipping Sauce Barbeque	1 serv (1.6 oz)	45	0	0	0	11	0	330
Egg Rolls	1	130	5	6	5	15	2	310
Fish & Chips	1 serv	610	18	31	40	66	5	1240
French Fries	1 med	410	4	20	0	55	4	690
French Fries	1 lg	580	6	28	0	77	6	960
French Fries	1 sm	330	3	16	0	44	3	550
Hamburger	1	310	17	14	45	30	1	600
Hamburger w/ Cheese	1	360	19	18	60	31	1	740
Jumbo Jack	1	600	22	31	45	58	3	980
Jumbo Jack w/ Cheese	1	690	27	38	70	61	3	1360
Onion Rings	1 serv	500	6	30	0	51	3	420
Philly Cheesesteak	1	580	35	22	90	55	3	1660
Salsa	1 serv (1 oz)	10	0	0	0	2	0	220
Sandwich Roasted Turkey	1	580	34	25	110	50	3	1600
Sandwich Ultimate Club	1	640	37	30	105	51	3	2000
Seasoned Curly Fries	1 serv	400	6	23	0	45	5	690
Sour Cream	1 serv (1 oz)	60	1	5	15	2	0	20
Sourdough Grilled Chicken Club	1	520	33	28	85	33	3	1330
Sourdough Jack	1	700	30	49	80	36	3	1220
Spicy Crispy Chicken	1	730	30	37	70	69	4	1480
Stuffed Jalapeno	3 pieces	230	7	13	20	22	2	690
Swiss Style Cheese	1 slice	40	2	3	10	1	0	150
Taco	1	170	6	9	20	15	2	210

FOOD	PORTION	CALS	PROT	FAT	CHOL	CARB	FIBER	SOD
Taco Monster	1	260	9	15	30	21	3	340
Turkey Jack	1	700	38	32	115	69	4	1930
SALAD DRESSINGS AND TOPPINGS								
Almonds Roasted Slivered	1 serv (0.7 oz)	130	5	11	0	4	2	5
Asian Sesame	1 serv (2.5 oz)	230	1	17	0	20	0	780
Bacon Ranch	1 serv (2.5 oz)	320	2	33	30	5	0	820
Balsamic Vinaigrette Low Fat	1 serv (2.5 oz)	40	0	2	0	6	0	600
Country Crock Spread	1 pkg	25	0	3	0	0	0	45
Creamy Southwest Dressing	1 serv (2.5 oz)	270	2	26	30	7	0	1080
Croutons	1 serv (0.5 oz)	60	2	2	0	10	0	130
Dipping Sauce Buttermilk House	1 serv (0.9 oz)	130	0	13	10	3	0	210
Dipping Sauce Frank's Red Hot Buffalo	1 serv (1 oz)	10	0	0	0	2	0	840
Dipping Sauce Sweet & Sour	1 serv (1 oz)	45	0	0	0	11	0	160
Grape Jelly	1 serv (0.5 oz)	35	0	0	0	9	0	10
Herb Mayo Sauce Low Fat	1 serv (1.5 oz)	45	1	4	0	3	1	370
Ketchup	1 pkg (0.3 oz)	10	0	0	0	2	0	105
Marinara Sauce	1 serv (0.9 oz)	15	0	0	0	3	0	210
Mustard	1 pkg	0	0	0	0	0	0	50
Ranch	1 serv (2.5 oz)	390	1	41	30	4	0	590
Ranch Lite	1 serv (2.5 oz)	190	1	18	25	3	0	700
Soy Sauce	1 serv (0.3 oz)	5	1	0	0	1	0	480
Syrup	1 serv (1.5 oz)	130	0	0	0	32	0	30
Taco Sauce	1 serv (0.3 oz)	0	0	0	0	0	0	80
Tartar Sauce	1 serv (1.5 oz)	210	0	22	20	2	0	370

FOOD	PORTION	CALS	PROT	FAT	CHOL	CARB	FIBER	SOD
Thousand Island	1 serv (2 oz)	160	0	12	15	12	0	490
Vinegar	1 serv	0	0	0	0	0	0	20
Wonton Strips	1 serv (0.7 oz)	110	2	6	0	13	2	45

SALADS

FOOD	PORTION	CALS	PROT	FAT	CHOL	CARB	FIBER	SOD
Asian Salad	1 serv	140	15	2	25	18	6	470
Chicken Club Salad	1 serv	290	28	16	65	12	5	890
Side Salad	1 serv	50	3	3	10	4	2	65
Southwest Chicken	1 serv	320	28	13	60	28	8	920

JAMBA JUICE

FOOD	PORTION	CALS	PROT	FAT	CHOL	CARB	FIBER	SOD
Mango-A-Go-Go	1 reg (24 oz)	460	2	2	–	–	3	–
Orchard Oasis	1 reg (24 oz)	440	2	2	–	–	4	–
Protein Berry Pizazz	1 reg (24 oz)	470	25	1	–	–	6	–
Razzmatazz	1 reg (24 oz)	440	3	2	–	–	4	–

JERSEY MIKE'S

FOOD	PORTION	CALS	PROT	FAT	CHOL	CARB	FIBER	SOD
Ham On Wheat	1	240	20	4	35	31	2	1130
Ham On White	1	240	20	5	35	31	1	1230
Ham/Turkey Wheat	1	230	21	3	30	32	1	1130
Ham/Turkey White	1	240	20	4	30	32	2	960
Roast Beef Wheat	1	290	30	5	60	30	2	330
Roast Beef White	1	280	29	5	55	30	0	310
Turkey On Wheat	1	230	23	2	30	30	2	910
Turkey On White	1	230	32	3	30	18	1	860
Veggie On Wheat	1	170	7	2	0	32	2	340
Veggie On White	1	170	7	2	0	31	2	290

KFC
BEVERAGES

FOOD	PORTION	CALS	PROT	FAT	CHOL	CARB	FIBER	SOD
Diet Pepsi	1 sm	0	0	0	0	0	0	35
Mt. Dew	1 sm	150	0	0	0	43	0	50
Pepsi	1 sm (11 oz)	140	0	0	0	37	0	35

DESSERTS

FOOD	PORTION	CALS	PROT	FAT	CHOL	CARB	FIBER	SOD
Cake Double Chocolate Chip	1 slice	400	4	29	45	31	2	230

FOOD	PORTION	CALS	PROT	FAT	CHOL	CARB	FIBER	SOD
Cherry Cheesecake Parfait	1 serv	300	3	11	4	46	2	130
Lil' Bucket Chocolate Creme	1 serv	270	2	13	0	37	2	190
Lil' Bucket Fudge Brownie	1	270	2	9	30	44	1	170
Lil' Bucket Lemon Creme	1 serv	400	4	14	5	65	2	210
Lil' Bucket Strawberry Shortcake	1 serv	200	2	6	20	34	0	110
Pie Apple	1 slice	270	3	9	0	45	4	200
Pie Lemon Meringue	1 slice	310	5	11	40	47	3	160
Pie Pecan	1 slice	370	4	15	40	55	2	190
Pie Strawberry Creme	1 slice	270	3	12	10	37	0	200
MAIN MENU SELECTIONS								
BBQ Beans	1 serv	230	8	1	0	46	7	720
Biscuit	1	190	2	10	2	23	0	580
Boneless Wings HBBQ Sauced	7 pieces	600	35	28	75	40	2	1950
Chicken Pot Pie	1 serv	770	33	40	115	70	5	1680
Cole Slaw	1 serv	190	1	11	5	22	3	300
Corn On The Cob	1 ear (3 inch)	70	2	2	0	13	3	5
Crispy Strips	3	400	29	24	75	17	0	1250
Extra Crispy Breast	1 serv	490	34	28	135	19	0	1230
Extra Crispy Drumstick	1	160	12	10	70	5	0	420
Extra Crispy Thigh	1	370	21	26	120	12	0	710
Extra Crispy Whole Wing	1	190	10	12	55	10	0	390
Green Beans	1 serv	50	5	2	5	5	2	480
Hot & Spicy Breast	1 serv	460	33	27	130	20	0	1450
Hot & Spicy Drumstick	1	150	13	9	65	4	0	380
Hot & Spicy Thigh	1	400	22	28	125	14	0	1240
Hot & Spicy Whole Wing	1	180	11	11	60	9	0	420

FOOD	PORTION	CALS	PROT	FAT	CHOL	CARB	FIBER	SOD
Hot Wings	6 pieces	450	24	29	145	23	1	1120
Mac & Cheese	1 serv	130	5	8	5	15	1	810
Mashed Potatoes w/o Gravy	1 serv	110	2	4	0	16	1	260
Mashed Potatoes With Gravy	1 serv	120	2	5	0	18	1	380
Original Recipe Breast	1 serv	380	40	19	145	11	0	1150
Original Recipe Breast w/o Skin Or Breading	1 serv	140	29	3	95	0	0	410
Original Recipe Drumstick	1	140	14	8	75	4	0	440
Original Recipe Thigh	1	360	22	25	165	12	0	1060
Original Recipe Whole Wing	1	150	11	9	60	5	0	370
Popcorn Chicken	1 reg serv	450	19	30	50	25	0	1030
Potato Salad	1 serv	180	2	9	5	22	1	470
Potato Wedges	1 sm	240	4	12	0	30	3	830
Sandwich HBBQ	1	300	21	8	50	41	4	640
Sandwich Original Recipe w/ Sauce	1	450	29	27	65	22	0	1010
Sandwich Original Recipe w/o Sauce	1	320	29	13	60	21	0	890
Sandwich Tender Roast w/ Sauce	1	390	31	19	70	24	1	810
Sandwich Tender Roast w/o Sauce	1	260	31	5	65	23	1	690
Sandwich Twister	1	670	27	38	60	55	3	1650
Sandwich Zinger w/ Sauce	1	680	35	41	90	42	1	1850
Sandwich Zinger w/o Sauce	1	540	35	26	75	41	1	1510
Wings HBBQ Sauced	6 pieces	540	25	33	150	36	1	1130

KOO-KOO-ROO

FOOD	PORTION	CALS	PROT	FAT	CHOL	CARB	FIBER	SOD
Original Breast	1 piece	187	34	6	117	tr	0	422

FOOD	PORTION	CALS	PROT	FAT	CHOL	CARB	FIBER	SOD
Original Chicken Dark	3 pieces	320	39	16	101	5	0	659
Rotisserie Chicken Breast & Wing	1 serv	355	49	16	140	1	tr	675
Rotisserie Chicken Leg & Thigh	1 serv	300	31	18	114	1	tr	513
Rotisserie Half Chicken	1 serv	655	80	34	254	2	tr	1188
Sandwich BBQ Chicken	1	562	45	12	113	71	3	1398
Sandwich Chicken Caesar	1	781	56	36	138	63	2	1775
Sandwich Original Chicken	1	661	41	29	116	63	3	1144
Traditional Turkey Dinner	1 serv	692	42	29	127	67	8	3719
Turkey Pot Pie	1 serv	883	37	44	98	83	6	1287
Turkey Sandwich Hand Carved	1	599	46	32	122	31	5	786
Wrap Caesar Chicken	1	757	42	39	97	59	4	1890
Wrap Chipotle Chicken	1	924	42	43	123	89	6	2449

KRISPY KREME

FOOD	PORTION	CALS	PROT	FAT	CHOL	CARB	FIBER	SOD
Apple Fritter	1	380	4	21	5	46	2	290
Caramel Kreme Crunch	1	350	4	19	5	43	tr	170
Chocolate Iced Glazed w/ Sprinkles	1	260	3	12	3	38	tr	100
Chocolate Malted Kreme	1	390	4	21	5	49	tr	180
Chocolate Iced	1	250	3	12	5	33	tr	100
Chocolate Iced Cake	1	270	3	14	20	36	tr	320
Chocolate Iced Creme Filled	1	350	3	21	5	39	tr	140

FOOD	PORTION	CALS	PROT	FAT	CHOL	CARB	FIBER	SOD
Chocolate Iced Cruller	1	290	2	15	15	37	tr	240
Chocolate Iced Custard Filled	1	300	3	17	5	35	tr	150
Chocolated Iced w/ Sprinkles	1	290	3	14	20	40	tr	320
Cinnamon Apple Filled	1	290	3	16	5	32	tr	150
Cinnamon Bun	1	260	3	16	5	28	tr	125
Cinnamon Sugar Cake	1	280	3	14	20	37	1	340
Cinnamon Twist	1	230	3	9	5	33	tr	85
Coffee & Kreme	1	360	3	20	5	43	tr	150
Dulce De Leche	1	290	3	18	5	30	tr	160
Glazed Blueberry	1	340	3	18	20	42	tr	310
Glazed Creme Filled	1	340	3	20	5	39	tr	140
Glazed Devil's Food	1	340	3	18	20	42	tr	310
Glazed Lemon Filled	1	290	3	16	5	34	tr	135
Glazed Raspberry Filled	1	300	3	16	5	39	tr	125
Glazed Sour Cream	1	340	3	18	20	42	tr	310
Glazed Strawberry Filled	1	290	3	16	5	35	tr	135
Glazed Cinnamon	1	210	2	12	5	24	tr	100
Glazed Cruller	1	240	2	14	15	26	tr	240
Glazed Custard Filled	1	290	3	16	5	34	tr	160
Glazed Filled Blueberry	1	290	3	16	5	35	tr	140
Glazed Twist	1	210	3	9	5	28	tr	80
Honey & Oat	1	340	3	18	20	42	tr	310
Key Lime Pie	1	330	3	18	5	40	tr	160
Maple Iced	1	240	2	12	5	32	tr	100
Maple Iced Cake	1	270	3	13	20	35	tr	320
New York Cheesecake	1	330	4	19	10	36	1	190
Original Glazed	1	200	2	12	5	22	tr	95
Powdered Blueberry Filled	1	290	3	16	5	32	tr	140

FOOD	PORTION	CALS	PROT	FAT	CHOL	CARB	FIBER	SOD
Powdered Strawberry Filled	1	260	3	16	5	26	tr	130
Powdered Cake	1	280	3	14	20	37	tr	320
Powdered Creme Filled	1	340	3	21	5	36	tr	140
Powdered Raspberry	1	300	3	16	5	36	tr	125
Pumpkin Spice Cake	1	340	3	18	20	42	tr	310
Sugar Coated	1	200	2	12	5	21	0	95
Traditional Cake	1	230	3	13	20	25	tr	320
Vanilla Iced Creme Fill	1	340	3	20	5	38	tr	135
Vanilla Iced Glazed	1	240	2	12	5	32	tr	95
Vanilla Iced Cake w/ Sprinkles	1	270	3	13	20	35	tr	320
Vanilla Iced Custard Filled	1	290	3	16	5	33	tr	150
Vanilla Iced Raspberry Glazed	1	350	3	16	5	50	tr	125

KRYSTAL
BEVERAGES

FOOD	PORTION	CALS	PROT	FAT	CHOL	CARB	FIBER	SOD
Coca-Cola Classic frzn	1 (16 oz)	130	0	0	0	36	0	12
Coca-Cola Classic	1 sm (16 oz)	129	0	0	0	40	0	9
Diet Coke	1 sm (16 oz)	tr	0	0	0	tr	0	15
Sprite	1 sm (16 oz)	126	0	0	0	39	0	33

BREAKFAST SELECTIONS

FOOD	PORTION	CALS	PROT	FAT	CHOL	CARB	FIBER	SOD
Biscuit	1	270	5	13	0	33	0	660
Biscuit And Gravy	1	280	5	14	0	34	0	710
Biscuit Bacon Egg & Cheese	1	390	11	23	40	33	0	1090
Biscuit Chik	1	360	13	15	20	40	0	1030
Biscuit Sausage	1	480	12	33	40	33	0	980
Country Breakfast	1 serv	660	24	42	590	46	8	1450
Kryspers	1 serv	190	1	13	10	17	2	340
Krystal Sunriser	1	240	12	14	255	14	2	460
Scrambler	1 serv	440	20	26	255	33	3	840

FOOD	PORTION	CALS	PROT	FAT	CHOL	CARB	FIBER	SOD
DESSERTS								
Fried Apple Turnover	1	220	3	10	<5	31	2	300
Lemon Icebox Pie	1 serv	260	5	9	25	41	2	180
MAIN MENU SELECTIONS								
Chik'n Bites	1 sm	310	17	19	55	16	1	790
Chik'n Bites Salad	1 serv	290	20	20	66	12	4	490
Fries	1 med	470	4	20	20	53	7	90
Fries Chili Cheese	1 serv	540	13	28	45	59	5	800
Krystal	1	160	7	7	20	17	1	260
Krystal Bacon Cheese	1	190	10	10	25	16	2	430
Krystal Cheese	1	180	9	9	25	17	2	430
Krystal Chik	1	240	11	11	25	24	2	640
Krystal Chili	1 serv	200	13	7	25	22	7	1130
Krystal Double	1	260	13	13	40	24	2	550
Krystal Double Cheese	1	310	16	16	65	26	tr	800
Pup	1	170	6	9	25	15	1	500
Pup Chili Cheese	1	210	9	12	40	17	2	510
Pup Corn	1	260	6	19	50	19	1	490
LITTLE CAESARS								
MAIN MENU SELECTIONS								
Baby Pan! Pan!	1 piece	360	17	16	30	34	2	630
Crazy Bread	1 piece	90	3	3	tr	15	0	140
Crazy Bread Cinnamon	2 pieces	100	3	2	tr	19	0	95
Crazy Sauce	1 serv (4 oz)	45	0	0	0	9	3	380
Deli Sandwich Italian	1	800	35	45	90	66	3	1950
Deli Sandwich Veggie	1	600	24	28	30	67	3	980
Deli Sandwich Ham & Cheese	1	640	32	29	50	66	3	1540
Italian Cheese Bread	1 piece	130	7	6	10	13	0	310
PIZZA								
14 Inch Round Meatsa	⅒ pie	280	15	13	30	26	2	630

FOOD	PORTION	CALS	PROT	FAT	CHOL	CARB	FIBER	SOD
14 Inch Round Supreme	1/10 pie	270	13	10	25	31	3	510
14 Inch Round Veggie	1/10 pie	240	12	8	15	32	3	710
14 Inch Thin Crust Cheese	1/10 pie	160	8	7	15	14	0	210
16 Inch Round Cheese	1/12 pie	220	11	7	15	27	1	340
18 Inch Round Cheese	1/14 pie	230	12	7	15	30	1	350
Deep Dish Large	1/8 pie	320	15	12	20	37	2	460
Deep Dish Medium	1/8 pie	230	11	9	15	27	1	340
SALAD DRESSINGS								
Caesar	1 serv (1.5 oz)	230	1	25	55	1	0	360
Greek	1 serv (1.5 oz)	270	0	29	0	0	0	200
Italian	1 serv (1.5 oz)	220	0	23	0	2	0	370
Italian Fat Free	1 serv (1.5 oz)	25	0	0	0	5	0	390
Ranch	1 serv (1.5 oz)	230	1	24	10	2	0	380
SALADS								
Antipasto	1 serv	140	9	8	20	6	2	560
Caesar	1 serv	90	4	3	0	12	3	190
Greek	1 serv	128	6	7	25	11	3	590
Tossed Salad	1 serv	100	2	3	0	15	3	190
TOPPINGS PER SLICE								
Bacon	1 serv	41	2	4	7	tr	tr	125
Beef	1 serv	20	1	2	2	tr	tr	55
Black Olives	1 serv	12	tr	2	—	tr	tr	47
Extra Cheese	1 serv	26	2	2	6	tr	—	48
Green Peppers	1 serv	2	tr	tr	—	tr	tr	tr
Ham	1 serv	5	1	tr	2	tr	tr	66
Italian Sausage	1 serv	22	1	2	5	tr	tr	68
Mushrooms	1 serv	2	tr	tr	—	tr	tr	40
Onion	1 serv	3	tr	tr	—	1	tr	tr
Pepperoni	1 serv	26	1	2	4	tr	—	110

FOOD	PORTION	CALS	PROT	FAT	CHOL	CARB	FIBER	SOD
Pineapple	1 serv	7	tr	–	–	2	tr	tr
Tomato	1 serv	2	tr	tr	–	tr	tr	1

MAGGIE MOO'S

FOOD	PORTION	CALS	PROT	FAT	CHOL	CARB	FIBER	SOD
Ice Cream Udderly Cream	½ cup	180	3	11	45	18	0	40
Ice Cream Fat Free	½ cup	80	3	0	0	18	0	50
Ice Cream Low Carb Sugar Added	½ cup	100	2	6	30	11	0	60
Sorbet	½ cup	90	0	0	0	22	0	5

MANHATTAN BAGEL

FOOD	PORTION	CALS	PROT	FAT	CHOL	CARB	FIBER	SOD
Blueberry	1	260	9	tr	0	54	2	560
Cheddar Cheese	1	270	11	4	10	48	2	560
Chocolate Chip	1	290	9	3	0	56	2	530
Cinnamon Raisin	1	280	10	tr	0	57	3	560
Cranberry Orange	1	270	10	1	0	55	2	520
Egg	1	270	10	2	0	53	2	710
Everything	1	290	11	3	0	54	3	2000
Garlic	1	270	10	tr	0	55	2	560
Jalapeno Cheddar	1	260	16	2	0	53	2	310
Marble	1	260	10	tr	0	52	3	540
Oat Bran	1	260	10	1	0	53	3	470
Oat Bran Raisin Walnut	1	270	10	3	0	54	3	450
Onion	1	270	10	tr	0	55	2	560
Plain	1	260	10	tr	0	52	2	560
Poppy	1	300	11	4	0	54	5	560
Pumpernickel	1	250	10	1	0	52	3	530
Rye	1	260	10	1	0	52	3	560
Salt	1	260	10	tr	0	53	2	7100
Sesame	1	310	11	5	0	55	3	560
Spinach	1	270	10	tr	0	54	3	580
Sun-Dried Tomato	1	260	10	1	0	53	3	340
Whole Wheat	1	260	10	tr	0	52	3	470

MARBLE SLAB CREAMERY

FOOD	PORTION	CALS	PROT	FAT	CHOL	CARB	FIBER	SOD
Cone Honey Wheat	1	130	3	3	15	24	tr	10
Cone Sugar	1	130	2	3	15	23	0	10

FOOD	PORTION	CALS	PROT	FAT	CHOL	CARB	FIBER	SOD
Cone Vanilla Cinnamon	1	130	2	3	15	24	tr	10
Frozen Yogurt Nonfat	½ cup	100	3	1	0	22	1	55
Frozen Yogurt Nonfat No Sugar Added	½ cup	90	4	1	0	17	1	85
Ice Cream Reduced Fat	1 serv (6.75 oz)	390	6	20	80	47	0	130
Ice Cream Superpremium	1 serv (6.75 oz)	450	8	28	115	44	0	135
Sorbet	½ cup	90	0	0	0	22	0	5

MAUI WOWI

FOOD	PORTION	CALS	PROT	FAT	CHOL	CARB	FIBER	SOD
Smoothie Rip Sticks All Flavors	1	88	2	0	0	22	0	25

MAX & ERMA'S

FOOD	PORTION	CALS	PROT	FAT	CHOL	CARB	FIBER	SOD
Black Bean Roll Up	1 serv	401	—	8	13	71	8	534
Black Bean Salsa	½ cup	215	—	15	0	17	5	338
Fruit Smoothie	1 serv	124	—	tr	0	29	1	4
Garden Grill Sandwich w/ Tex Mex Dressing	1	569	—	7	19	101	14	983
Garlic Breadstick	1	156	—	6	0	21	0	293
Hula Bowl w/ Fat Free Honey Mustard Dressing w/o Breadsticks	1 serv	583	—	10	111	73	5	1580
Salad Dressing Fat Free French	2 tbsp	126	—	tr	0	31	2	1034
Salad Dressing Fat Free Honey Mustard	2 tbsp	60	—	0	0	14	0	360
Salad Dressing Tex Mex	2 tbsp	33	—	tr	5	2	tr	262
Sugar Snap Peas w/ Lemon Pepper Butter	1 serv (4 oz)	106	—	6	15	8	3	100

FOOD	PORTION	CALS	PROT	FAT	CHOL	CARB	FIBER	SOD
MCDONALD'S								
BAKED SELECTIONS								
Apple Pie Baked	1 (2.7 oz)	260	3	13	0	34	tr	200
Cinnamon Roll	1 (3.5 oz)	340	5	15	35	52	3	250
Cookie Chocolate Chip	1 (1.4 oz)	170	2	9	5	23	tr	150
McDonaldland Cookies	1 pkg (2 oz)	230	3	8	0	38	1	250
BEVERAGES								
Coca-Cola Classic	1 sm (16 oz)	150	0	0	0	40	0	15
Coca-Cola Classic	1 lg (32 oz)	310	0	0	0	86	0	30
Coffee	1 sm (8 oz)	0	0	0	0	tr	0	0
Coffee	1 lg (16 oz)	10	0	0	0	2	0	10
Diet Coke	1 sm (16 oz)	0	0	0	0	0	0	30
Diet Coke	1 lg (32 oz)	0	0	0	0	0	0	60
Half & Half Creamer	1 pkg	15	0	2	5	0	0	0
Hi-C Orange	1 sm (16 oz)	160	0	0	0	44	0	30
Hi-C Orange	1 lg (32 oz)	350	0	0	0	94	0	60
Iced Tea	1 lg (32 oz)	0	0	0	0	tr	0	20
Iced Tea	1 sm (16 oz)	0	0	0	0	0	0	0
Milk Lowfat 1%	1 serv (8 oz)	100	8	3	10	13	0	115
Orange Juice	1 (12 oz)	140	2	0	0	33	0	5
Shake Strawberry	1 (12 oz)	420	11	12	50	67	tr	140
Sprite	1 lg (32 oz)	310	0	0	0	83	—	115
Sprite	1 sm (16 oz)	150	0	0	0	39	0	55
Triple Shake Chocolate	1 (12 oz)	430	11	12	50	70	1	210
Triple Shake Vanilla	1 (12 oz)	430	11	12	50	67	0	300
BREAKFAST SELECTIONS								
Bagel Ham Egg Cheese	1 (7.7 oz)	550	26	23	255	58	2	1500
Bagel Spanish Omelet	1 (9.1 oz)	710	27	40	275	59	3	1520
Bagel Steak Egg Cheese	1 (8.5 oz)	640	31	31	265	57	2	1540
Big Breakfast	1 serv (9.4 oz)	710	24	48	455	45	3	1430
Biscuit	1 (2.4 oz)	240	4	11	0	30	1	640

FOOD	PORTION	CALS	PROT	FAT	CHOL	CARB	FIBER	SOD
Biscuit Bacon Egg Cheese	1 (5.4 oz)	480	21	31	250	31	1	1360
Biscuit Sausage	1 (4 oz)	410	10	28	35	30	1	930
Biscuit Sausage w/ Egg	1 (5.7 oz)	490	16	33	245	31	1	1010
Breakfast Burrito Sausage	1 (4 oz)	290	13	16	170	24	2	680
English Muffin	1 (2 oz)	150	5	2	0	27	2	270
Hash Browns	1 serv (1.9 oz)	130	1	8	0	14	1	330
Hotcakes Margarine & Syrup	1 serv (8 oz)	600	9	17	20	104	0	770
McGriddles Bacon Egg & Cheese	1 (5.9 oz)	450	19	23	240	43	1	1270
McGriddles Sausage Egg Cheese	1 (7 oz)	550	20	33	260	43	1	1290
McMuffin Sausage	1 (4 oz)	370	14	23	50	28	2	790
McMuffin Sausage w/ Egg	1 (5.8 oz)	450	20	28	260	29	2	930
McMuffin Egg	1 (4.9 oz)	300	18	12	235	29	2	840
Sausage	1 (1.5 oz)	170	6	16	35	0	0	290
Scrambled Eggs	2 (3.6 oz)	160	13	11	425	1	0	170
DESSERTS								
Fruit 'n Yogurt Parfait	1 snack size (5.3 oz)	160	4	2	5	30	tr	85
Fruit 'n Yogurt Parfait	1 serv (11.9 oz)	380	10	5	15	76	2	240
Fruit 'n Yogurt Parfait w/o Granola	1 serv (10.9 oz)	280	8	4	15	53	tr	115
Fruit 'n Yogurt Parfait w/o Granola	1 serv (5 oz)	130	4	2	5	25	0	55
Kiddo Cone	1 (1 oz)	45	1	2	5	7	0	20
McDonaldland Chocolate Chip Cookies	1 pkg (2 oz)	280	3	14	40	37	1	170
McFlurry Butterfinger	1 (12 oz)	620	16	22	70	90	tr	260

FOOD	PORTION	CALS	PROT	FAT	CHOL	CARB	FIBER	SOD
McFlurry M&M	1 (12 oz)	630	16	23	75	90	1	210
McFlurry Nestle Crunch	1 (12 oz)	630	16	24	75	89	tr	230
McFlurry Oreo	1 (12 oz)	570	15	20	70	82	tr	280
Nuts For Sundaes	1 serv (7 g)	40	2	4	0	2	tr	55
Reduced Fat Ice Cream Cone Vanilla	1 (3.2 oz)	150	4	5	20	23	0	75
Sundae Hot Caramel	1 (6.4 oz)	360	7	10	35	61	0	180
Sundae Hot Fudge	1 (6.3 oz)	340	8	12	30	52	1	170
Sundae Strawberry	1 (6.3 oz)	290	7	7	30	50	tr	95
Triple Shake Chocolate	1 (32 oz)	1150	30	33	125	187	3	550
Triple Shake Raspberry	1 (12 oz)	420	11	12	50	67	tr	150
Triple Shake Raspberry	1 (32 oz)	1120	28	32	135	179	2	390
Triple Shake Strawberry	1 (32 oz)	1120	28	32	135	178	2	380
Triple Shake Vanilla	1 (32 oz)	1140	28	32	125	178	tr	810

MAIN MENU SELECTIONS

FOOD	PORTION	CALS	PROT	FAT	CHOL	CARB	FIBER	SOD
Barbeque Sauce	1 pkg (1 oz)	45	0	0	0	10	0	250
Big Mac	1 (7.6 oz)	560	24	33	85	47	3	1050
Big N' Tasty	1 (8.2 oz)	530	24	32	80	37	2	790
Big N' Tasty w/ Cheese	1 (8.7 oz)	580	28	37	95	38	2	1030
Cheeseburger	1 (4.2 oz)	330	15	14	45	35	2	800
Cheeseburger Double	1 (6.1 oz)	480	25	27	85	37	2	1220
Chicken McNuggets	6 pieces (3.8 oz)	310	15	20	50	18	2	680
Chicken McNuggets	4 pieces (2.5 oz)	210	10	13	35	12	1	400
Chicken McNuggets	10 pieces (6.3 oz)	510	25	33	85	30	3	1140
Chicken McNuggets	20 pieces (12.7 oz)	1030	49	65	170	61	5	2280

FOOD	PORTION	CALS	PROT	FAT	CHOL	CARB	FIBER	SOD
Chicken McGrill	1 (7.5 oz)	400	25	17	60	37	2	890
Crispy Chicken	1 serv (7.7 oz)	500	22	26	50	46	2	1100
Filet-O-Fish	1 (5.5 oz)	470	15	26	50	45	1	730
French Fries	1 lg (6.2 oz)	540	8	26	0	68	6	350
French Fries	1 sm (2.4 oz)	210	3	10	0	26	2	135
French Fries	1 McValue (3.7 oz)	320	5	16	0	40	4	210
French Fries	1 med (5.2 oz)	450	6	22	0	57	5	290
Hamburger	1 (3.7 oz)	280	12	10	30	35	2	560
Honey	1 pkg (0.5 oz)	45	0	0	0	12	0	0
Honey Mustard	1 pkg (0.5 oz)	50	0	5	10	3	0	95
Hot Mustard	1 pkg (1 oz)	60	tr	4	5	7	tr	240
Light Mayonnaise	1 pkg (0.4 oz)	40	0	5	10	tr	0	100
McChicken	1 (5.2 oz)	430	14	23	45	41	3	840
McChicken Hot 'n Spicy	1 (5.1 oz)	450	15	26	45	39	1	830
Quarter Pounder	1 (6.1 oz)	420	23	21	70	36	2	780
Quarter Pounder Double w/ Cheese	1 (9.9 oz)	760	46	48	165	38	2	1450
Quarter Pounder w/ Cheese	1 (7 oz)	530	28	30	95	38	2	1250
Sweet 'N Sour Sauce	1 pkg (1 oz)	50	0	0	0	11	0	140
SALAD DRESSINGS								
Newman's Own Cobb	1 pkg (2 oz)	120	1	9	10	9	0	440
Newman's Own Creamy Caesar	1 pkg (2 oz)	190	2	18	20	4	0	500
Newman's Own Low Fat Balsamic Vinaigrette	1 pkg (1.5 oz)	40	0	0	0	4	0	730
Newman's Own Ranch	1 pkg (2 oz)	290	1	30	20	4	0	530
SALADS AND SALAD BARS								
Bacon Ranch w/o Chicken	1 serv (7.1 oz)	140	9	10	25	7	3	310
Caesar w/o Chicken	1 serv (6.7 oz)	90	7	4	10	7	3	170

FOOD	PORTION	CALS	PROT	FAT	CHOL	CARB	FIBER	SOD
California Cobb w/o Chicken	1 serv (7.6 oz)	160	11	11	85	7	3	450
Crispy Chicken Bacon Ranch	1 serv (10.4 oz)	370	28	21	65	20	3	1040
Crispy Chicken Caesar	1 serv (10 oz)	310	23	16	50	20	3	890
Crispy Chicken California Cobb	1 serv (10.9 oz)	380	27	23	125	20	3	1170
Croutons Butter Garlic	1 pkg (0.5 oz)	50	1	2	0	8	0	140
Grilled Chicken Bacon Ranch	1 serv (10.2 oz)	270	28	13	75	11	3	830
Grilled Chicken Caesar	1 serv (9.8 oz)	210	28	7	60	11	3	680
Grilled Chicken California Cobb	1 serv (10.7 oz)	280	30	14	130	11	3	960
Side Salad	1 (3.1 oz)	15	1	0	0	3	1	10

MIAMI SUBS

FOOD	PORTION	CALS	PROT	FAT	CHOL	CARB	FIBER	SOD
Burger Deluxe	1	784	28	59	30	31	1	532
Cheeseburger Deluxe	1	859	34	65	47	32	1	736
Cheeseburger Deluxe Bacon	1	919	34	70	61	32	1	963
Cheesesteak Classic	1 (6 inch)	420	32	11	77	48	2	993
Cheesesteak Original	1 (6 inch)	409	31	11	77	45	1	925
Cheesesteak Works	1 (6 inch)	532	34	23	87	51	2	1063
Chicken Philly Classic	1 (6 inch)	551	30	27	92	47	2	1033
Mozzarella Sticks	1 serv	757	25	57	60	34	1	1607
Onion Rings	1 serv	869	5	68	0	56	2	895
Pita Chicken	1	392	34	13	75	34	5	546
Pita Gyros	1	662	32	39	84	47	5	1998
Platter Chicken Breast	1 serv	743	34	41	80	57	5	186
Platter Gyros	1 serv	1420	61	93	186	81	5	4055
Salad Caesar w/ Dressing	1 serv	459	12	34	14	26	4	1089

FOOD	PORTION	CALS	PROT	FAT	CHOL	CARB	FIBER	SOD
Salad Chicken Caesar w/ Dressing	1 serv	609	35	39	74	28	4	1929
Salad Chicken Club	1 serv	490	42	25	210	23	5	1433
Salad Garden	1 serv	310	16	18	136	21	5	477
Salad Greek	1 serv	284	14	15	123	24	5	906
Salad Greek Side w/ Dressing	1 serv	78	3	5	8	4	1	349
Spicy Fries	1 reg	532	4	39	19	39	4	575
Subs 6 Inch Ham And Cheese	1	452	23	18	59	49	2	2051
Subs 6 Inch Italian Deli	1	516	24	25	69	49	2	2151
Subs 6 Inch Meatball	1	491	28	22	76	49	4	1319
Subs 6 Inch Tuna	1	468	34	18	67	44	2	1068
Subs 6 Inch Turkey	1	484	29	18	68	51	2	2009
Wings w/ Fries Celery & Blue Cheese	1 serv	1020	48	67	179	50	4	2840

MR. HERO
DESSERTS

FOOD	PORTION	CALS	PROT	FAT	CHOL	CARB	FIBER	SOD
Cheesecake	1 serv	350	6	27	—	26	—	—
Cheesecake w/ Cherries	1 serv	385	6	25	—	35	—	—

MAIN MENU SELECTIONS

FOOD	PORTION	CALS	PROT	FAT	CHOL	CARB	FIBER	SOD
Breadsticks w/ Sauce	1 serv	291	8	9	—	47	—	—
Cheddar Cheese Sauce	1 serv	60	2	5	—	5	—	—
Onion Rings	1 serv	564	8	32	—	64	—	—
Potato Wafers	1 serv	334	4	18	—	42	—	—
Spaghetti Dinner	1 serv	606	22	8	—	112	—	—
Spaghetti w/ Meatballs	1 serv	846	37	26	—	116	—	—

SALAD DRESSINGS

FOOD	PORTION	CALS	PROT	FAT	CHOL	CARB	FIBER	SOD
Buttermilk	1 serv (2 oz)	290	tr	29	—	6	—	—

FOOD	PORTION	CALS	PROT	FAT	CHOL	CARB	FIBER	SOD
Creamy Italian	1 serv (2 oz)	190	tr	17	—	11	—	—
Fat Free French	1 serv (2 oz)	70	tr	0	—	18	—	—
Fat Free Ranch	1 serv (2 oz)	70	tr	0	—	16	—	—
SALADS AND SALAD BARS								
Croutons	1 serv	59	2	2	—	9	—	—
Garden Salad	1 serv	36	2	tr	—	7	—	—
Grilled Chicken	1 serv	225	27	10	—	7	—	—
Seafood Crab	1 serv	452	13	37	—	18	—	—
Side Salad	1 serv	27	1	tr	—	6	—	—
Tuna	1 serv	745	21	69	—	8	—	—
SANDWICHES								
Cheesesteaks Grilled Steak Philly	7 inch	450	37	14	—	48	—	—
Cheesesteaks Hot Buttered Deluxe	7 inch	566	25	33	—	48	—	—
Cold Subs Classic Italian	7 inch	586	21	36	—	50	—	—
Cold Subs Tuna & Cheese	7 inch	666	19	47	—	47	—	—
Cold Subs Turkey & Cheese	7 inch	453	25	21	—	46	—	—
Cold Subs Ultimate Italian	7 inch	608	31	33	—	51	—	—
Hot Subs Grilled Chicken Philly	7 inch	438	34	14	—	48	—	—
Hot Subs Meatball	7 inch	620	35	32	—	53	—	—
Hot Subs Romanburger	7 inch	717	30	47	—	49	—	—
Round Bacon Cheeseburger	1	352	14	23	—	23	—	—
Round Chicken	1	420	31	23	—	23	—	—
Round Fish	1	412	21	23	—	31	—	—
Round Tuna	1	302	11	34	—	23	—	—

FOOD	PORTION	CALS	PROT	FAT	CHOL	CARB	FIBER	SOD
MR. PITA								
Cranberry Turkey	1 reg	424	25	1	45	77	3	1099
Grilled Raspberry Chicken	1 reg	342	22	3	34	56	1	1426
Grilled Chicken & Broccoli	1 reg	373	24	4	41	57	2	878
Grilled Chicken Caesar	1 reg	353	24	4	42	50	1	986
Grilled Hawaiian Chicken	1 reg	375	25	4	41	57	1	1784
Ultra Combo	1 reg	354	24	3	43	56	2	1058
Ultra Grilled Chicken	1 reg	367	23	4	41	56	2	1080
Ultra Supreme	1 reg	350	23	3	37	56	1	1314
Ultra Turkey	1 reg	343	25	1	45	56	2	1099
MRS. FIELDS								
Brownie Double Fudge	1 (2.7 oz)	360	4	19	80	59	2	240
Brownie Frosted Fudge	1 (3.7 oz)	440	4	21	80	62	2	265
Brownie Pecan Fudge	1 (2.7 oz)	340	4	21	70	40	2	220
Brownie Pecan Pie	1 (2.7 oz)	340	5	20	70	40	2	220
Brownie Walnut Fudge	1 (2.7 oz)	380	5	23	80	45	tr	240
Bundt Cake Banana Walnut	1 piece (2.9 oz)	350	6	21	40	35	3	300
Bundt Cake Banana Walnut w/ Chocolate Chips	1 piece (2.9 oz)	370	6	22	35	39	3	240
Bundt Cake Blueberry	1 piece (2.9 oz)	270	4	12	50	36	1	330
Bundt Cake Raspberry	1 piece (2.9 oz)	270	4	12	50	36	tr	330
Bundt Cake White w/ Chocolate Chips	1 piece (2.9 oz)	350	4	17	50	45	tr	330
Cookie Butter Toffee	1 (2.3 oz)	290	3	13	55	40	tr	190

FOOD	PORTION	CALS	PROT	FAT	CHOL	CARB	FIBER	SOD
Cookie Cinnamon Sugar	1 (2.3 oz)	300	3	12	50	41	tr	250
Cookie Coconut Macadamia	1 (2.3 oz)	280	3	13	20	39	tr	220
Cookie Debra's Special	1 (2.3 oz)	280	4	12	40	39	2	180
Cookie Milk Chocolate	1 (2.3 oz)	280	3	13	40	38	tr	180
Cookie Milk Chocolate & Walnuts	1 (2.3 oz)	320	4	17	40	37	1	180
Cookie Milk Chocolate Macadamia	1 (2.3 oz)	320	4	18	40	36	tr	180
Cookie Oatmeal Chocolate Chip	1 (2.3 oz)	280	3	13	35	40	1	140
Cookie Oatmeal Raisin & Walnuts	1 (2.3 oz)	280	4	12	40	39	2	180
Cookie Peanut Butter	1 (2.3 oz)	310	5	16	45	34	tr	260
Cookie Peanut Butter w/ Milk Chocolate Chips	1 (2.3 oz)	300	5	17	40	35	tr	160
Cookie Semi-Sweet Chocolate	1 (2.3 oz)	280	2	14	30	40	1	160
Cookie Semi-Sweet Chocolate & Walnuts	1 (2.3 oz)	310	3	16	35	38	2	170
Cookie White Chunk Macadamia	1 (2.3 oz)	310	4	17	35	37	tr	170
Jumbo Cookie Snickerdoodle	1 (5 oz)	640	7	29	110	90	2	540
Nibbler Cookies	2 (0.9 oz)	110	1	5	15	15	0	90
Nibbler Cookies Chewy Chocolate Fudge	2 (0.9 oz)	110	1	5	10	15	tr	130
Nibbler Cookies Cinnamon Sugar	2 (0.9 oz)	120	1	5	15	17	0	90

FOOD	PORTION	CALS	PROT	FAT	CHOL	CARB	FIBER	SOD
Nibbler Cookies Debra's Special	2 (0.9 oz)	100	1	5	10	13	0	80
Nibbler Cookies M&M	2 (0.9 oz)	110	1	5	15	16	0	55
Nibbler Cookies Milk Chocolate	2 (0.9 oz)	110	1	5	15	15	tr	70
Nibbler Cookies Milk Chocolate w/ Walnuts	2 (0.9 oz)	120	1	6	10	14	tr	65
Nibbler Cookies Peanut Butter	2 (0.9 oz)	110	2	6	15	13	0	95
Nibbler Cookies Semi-Sweet Chocolate	2 (0.9 oz)	110	1	5	10	15	tr	60
Nibbler Cookies Triple Chocolate	2 (0.9 oz)	110	1	6	15	15	tr	65
Nibbler Cookies White Chunk Macadamia	2 (0.9 oz)	120	1	7	10	13	tr	60
NATHAN'S								
¼ Pound Burger	1	537	25	30	90	42	2	813
¼ Pound Burger w/ Cheese	1	850	30	61	136	45	2	1239
Bacon Cheeseburger	1	707	32	44	128	43	2	1340
Cheesesteak Chicken	1 serv	565	38	19	81	62	5	1786
Cheesesteak Original	1	741	44	43	124	50	4	1239
Cheesesteak Supreme	1 serv	786	45	43	124	61	5	1525
Chicken Tender Pita	1	610	22	38	65	45	2	1009
Chicken Tenders	3 pieces	512	21	37	30	24	3	900
Cole Slaw	1 serv	213	1	9	7	34	3	326
Corn Muffin	1	163	2	6	0	25	1	244
Famous Hot Dog	1	309	11	20	35	23	1	684
Fish N Chips	1 serv	1538	31	101	111	132	9	2152
French Fries	1 reg	547	6	38	0	46	6	200

FOOD	PORTION	CALS	PROT	FAT	CHOL	CARB	FIBER	SOD
Hot Dog Nuggets	6 pieces	351	5	28	20	20	0	400
Hush Puppy	2 pieces	277	5	10	5	42	2	967
Onion Rings	1 sm	559	3	44	0	36	2	576
Platter Chicken Breast	1 serv	943	28	54	84	89	9	978
Platter Chicken Tender	1 serv	1301	33	83	105	109	9	1059
Sandwich Chicken Tender	1	725	22	47	65	56	2	1008
Sandwich Fish	1	469	14	20	34	42	13	750
Sandwich Grilled Chicken	1	524	25	29	67	42	2	1179
Seafood Sampler	1 serv	3379	56	270	156	227	15	3553
Shrimp N Chips	1 serv	2051	51	124	222	225	12	3433
Super Burger	1	864	30	62	136	42	3	1245

OLD SPAGHETTI FACTORY
MAIN MENU SELECTIONS

FOOD	PORTION	CALS	PROT	FAT	CHOL	CARB	FIBER	SOD
Caesar Salad	1 sm	330	9	30	30	8	2	610
Caesar Salad Dinner Chicken	1 serv	1280	87	85	250	42	4	2170
Pot Pourri	1 dinner serv	710	26	30	95	84	6	1240
Sandwich Meatball	1	860	49	41	140	74	4	2800
Sandwich Sausage	1	730	40	40	105	53	4	2450
Sandwich Tuscan Chicken	1	1060	76	60	175	53	4	1110
Seafood Cheddar Melt	1 serv	790	40	42	165	65	4	1850
Spaghetti w/ Clam Sauce	1 dinner serv	690	22	28	125	84	5	850
Spaghetti w/ Meat Sauce	1 dinner serv	470	21	5	15	83	6	1110
Spaghetti w/ Meat Sauce & Sausage	1 dinner serv	830	43	35	105	85	6	2150
Spaghetti w/ Meatballs	1 dinner serv	840	47	33	130	86	5	1430
Spaghetti w/ Mizithra	1 dinner serv	1010	37	64	180	74	4	1150

FOOD	PORTION	CALS	PROT	FAT	CHOL	CARB	FIBER	SOD
Spaghetti w/ Mushroom Sauce	1 dinner serv	460	14	7	0	83	6	810
Spaghetti w/ Tomato Sauce	1 dinner serv	440	14	5	0	84	7	1020
Spaghetti w/ Tomato Sauce & Clam Sauce	1 dinner serv	560	18	17	65	84	6	940
Starter Garlic Cheese Bread	1 serv	1220	17	85	0	105	5	2230
Starter Meatballs	1 serv	910	65	61	245	23	1	2450
Starter Sausage	1 serv	690	31	56	140	7	tr	1790
Starter Tortellini	1 serv	930	25	56	205	82	2	1420
SOUPS								
Chicken Mulligatawny	1 serv	250	10	14	60	20	2	990
Chicken Orzo	1 serv	90	8	3	20	9	tr	830
Clam Chowder	1 serv	380	6	29	95	25	–	850
Cream Of Broccoli	1 serv	220	9	12	40	19	2	1110
Mediterranean White Bean	1 serv	150	6	6	0	19	6	470
Minestrone	1 serv	120	5	5	5	15	3	890

P.J. CHANG'S CHINA BISTRO

FOOD	PORTION	CALS	PROT	FAT	CHOL	CARB	FIBER	SOD
Cantonese Scallops	1 serv	305	42	8	–	15	–	–
Chicken w/ Black Bean Sauce	1 serv	426	63	11	–	19	–	–
Pin Rice Noodles	1 serv	270	12	2	–	55	–	–
Vegetable Chow Fun	1 serv	677	16	18	–	112	–	–

PANDA EXPRESS

FOOD	PORTION	CALS	PROT	FAT	CHOL	CARB	FIBER	SOD
Beef & Broccoli	1 serv (5 oz)	180	–	9	–	–	–	910
Black Pepper Chicken	1 serv (5 oz)	210	–	9	–	–	–	570
Chicken w/ Mushrooms	1 serv (5 oz)	170	–	3	–	–	–	570
Chicken w/ String Beans	1 serv (5 oz)	180	–	9	–	–	–	620
Egg Flower Soup	1½ cups	80	–	0	–	–	–	640
Egg Rolls	2 (3 oz)	190	–	6	–	–	–	490

FOOD	PORTION	CALS	PROT	FAT	CHOL	CARB	FIBER	SOD
Hot & Sour Soup	1½ cups	110	–	4	–	–	–	890
Lo Mein	1 serv (8 oz)	300	–	10	–	–	–	1090
Mixed Vegetables	1 serv (5 oz)	80	–	3	0	–	–	450
Orange Chicken	1 serv (5 oz)	310	–	13	–	–	–	420
Spicy Chicken w/ Peanuts	1 serv (5 oz)	510	–	29	–	–	–	1250
Steamed Rice	1 serv (8 oz)	220	–	0	0	–	–	0
Sweet & Sour Pork	1 serv (4 oz)	310	–	20	–	–	–	250
Sweet & Sour Sauce	1 serv (2 oz)	60	–	0	0	–	–	150
Vegetable Chow Mein	1 serv (8 oz)	300	–	10	–	–	–	610
Vegetable Fried Rice	1 serv (8 oz)	410	–	19	–	–	–	440

PANERA BREAD
BAGELS AND SPREADS

FOOD	PORTION	CALS	PROT	FAT	CHOL	CARB	FIBER	SOD
Bagel Asiago Cheese	1	330	15	5	15	58	2	480
Bagel Blueberry	1	320	12	2	0	67	3	490
Bagel Cinnamon Crunch	1	490	12	9	0	91	3	500
Bagel Dutch Apple & Raisin	1	340	10	3	0	70	3	410
Bagel Everything	1	290	11	2	0	58	2	540
Bagel French Toast	1	340	10	5	0	65	2	610
Bagel Mochachip Swirl	1	340	12	4	0	68	3	460
Bagel Nine Grain	1	290	11	1	0	58	3	390
Bagel Peanut Butter Crunch	1	400	11	6	0	77	3	480
Bagel Plain	1	280	11	1	0	57	2	450
Bagel Sesame	1	310	12	3	0	60	3	460

FOOD	PORTION	CALS	PROT	FAT	CHOL	CARB	FIBER	SOD
Cream Cheese Hazelnut Reduced Fat	1 serv (2 oz)	150	5	11	35	6	tr	210
Cream Cheese Honey Walnut Reduced Fat	1 serv (2 oz)	150	4	11	30	9	tr	200
Cream Cheese Mocha Reduced Fat	1 serv (2 oz)	160	5	11	7	10	1	180
Cream Cheese Plain	1 serv (2 oz)	190	3	18	55	2	0	210
Cream Cheese Plain Reduced Fat	1 serv (2 oz)	130	5	12	35	2	tr	230
Cream Cheese Raspberry Reduced Fat	1 serv (2 oz)	120	4	10	30	3	0	200
Cream Cheese Smoked Salmon Reduced Fat	1 serv (2 oz)	120	7	10	35	2	0	180
Cream Cheese Sun Dried Tomato Reduced Fat	1 serv (2 oz)	140	5	11	35	4	tr	220
Cream Cheese Veggie Reduced Fat	1 serv (2 oz)	130	5	11	35	4	1	230
Hummus Roasted Garlic	1 serv (2 oz)	100	3	5	0	11	4	260
BEVERAGES								
Caffe Mocha	1 serv (11.5 oz)	360	11	16	10	47	2	190
Homestyle Lemonade	1 serv (16 oz)	80	0	0	0	19	0	10
Hot Chocolate	1 serv (11 oz)	350	11	15	50	45	2	190
IC Cappuccino Chip	1 serv (16 oz)	590	5	35	70	64	0	125
IC Caramel	1 serv (16 oz)	550	6	24	80	76	0	400

FOOD	PORTION	CALS	PROT	FAT	CHOL	CARB	FIBER	SOD
IC Honeydew Green Tea	1 serv (16 oz)	270	2	13	30	36	0	140
IC Mocha	1 serv (16 oz)	520	7	24	75	70	2	140
IC Spice	1 serv (16 oz)	470	4	22	70	66	0	80
Iced Green Tea	1 serv (16 oz)	60	0	0	0	15	0	5
Latte Caffe	1 serv (8.5 oz)	120	7	5	20	12	0	120
Latte Caramel	1 serv (11 oz)	400	9	16	55	54	0	450
Latte Chai Tea	1 serv (10 oz)	210	7	5	15	37	0	115
Latte House	1 serv (10.8 oz)	320	8	13	50	43	0	135
Sierra Turkey	1	950	40	55	40	71	4	2380
BREADS								
Artisan Country	1 slice	120	5	0	0	25	1	290
Artisan French	1 slice (2 oz)	110	4	0	0	23	tr	310
Artisan Kalamata Olive	1 slice (2 oz)	140	5	2	0	26	1	270
Artisan Multigrain	1 slice (2 oz)	120	4	1	0	24	1	230
Artisan Raisin Pecan	1 slice (2 oz)	140	4	3	0	25	1	280
Artisan Sesame Semolina	1 slice (2 oz)	120	4	0	0	24	4	300
Artisan Stone Milled Rye	1 slice (2 oz)	110	4	0	0	22	2	320
Artisan Three Cheese	1 slice (2 oz)	120	5	2	5	21	tr	270
Artisan Three Seed	1 slice	130	5	2	0	23	1	250
Ciabatta	1 (6 oz)	430	14	10	0	70	3	990
Cinnamon Raisin	1 slice (2 oz)	160	4	3	0	31	1	300
Focaccia Asiago Cheese	1 slice (2 oz)	150	5	6	5	19	1	300
Focaccia Basil Pesto	1 slice (2 oz)	150	4	6	5	19	1	300
Focaccia Rosemary & Onion	1 slice (2 oz)	140	4	5	5	19	1	280
French	1 slice (2 oz)	130	5	1	0	24	1	270

FOOD	PORTION	CALS	PROT	FAT	CHOL	CARB	FIBER	SOD
French Roll	1 (2.25 oz)	140	6	1	0	28	1	310
Holiday	1 slice (2 oz)	150	2	1	5	33	tr	135
Honey Wheat	1 slice (2 oz)	140	5	3	0	25	1	260
Nine Grain	1 slice (2 oz)	150	5	3	0	26	2	270
Rye	1 slice (2 oz)	140	5	3	0	25	1	290
Sourdough	1 slice (2 oz)	120	5	0	0	25	1	270
Sourdough Roll	1 (2.5 oz)	160	6	0	0	32	1	340
Sourdough Soup Bowl	1 serv (8 oz)	500	20	2	0	102	4	1090
Sunflower	1 slice (2 oz)	160	6	5	0	24	1	320
Tomato Basil	1 slice (2 oz)	130	5	1	0	27	1	350
DESSERTS								
Bear Claw	1	380	7	21	70	37	1	310
Brownie Caramel Pecan	1	470	5	24	80	60	2	150
Brownie Chocolate Raspberry	1	370	2	18	75	47	2	130
Brownie Very Chocolate	1	460	5	22	80	62	2	150
Cinnamon Roll	1	560	12	26	90	64	3	480
Cobblestone	1	560	8	9	0	100	4	620
Coffee Cake Cherry Cheese	1	190	3	10	30	21	1	130
Cookie Chocolate Chipper	1	420	5	22	60	51	2	320
Cookie Chocolate Duet w/ Walnuts	1	410	6	25	60	47	3	320
Cookie Nutty Chocolate Chipper	1	440	6	26	55	46	3	300
Cookie Nutty Oatmeal Raisin	1	350	5	14	45	51	5	260
Cookie Shortbread	1	340	3	21	60	36	1	160
Croissant Apple	1	260	4	11	30	34	1	230
Croissant Cheese	1	300	6	16	45	34	1	220
Croissant Chocolate	1	440	7	23	35	56	4	180
Croissant French	1	265	5	15	40	28	1	190
Croissant Raspberry Cheese	1	280	5	13	35	37	1	190
Danish Apple	1	510	9	30	85	50	2	350

FOOD	PORTION	CALS	PROT	FAT	CHOL	CARB	FIBER	SOD
Danish Cheese	1	590	10	35	110	55	1	430
Danish Cherry	1	520	8	26	85	60	1	340
Danish Georgia Peach	1	580	9	30	85	67	2	390
Danish German Chocolate	1	770	10	46	85	83	4	570
Macaroon Chocolate Hazelnut	1	270	3	15	0	30	3	90
Mini Bundt Cake Carrot Walnut	1	430	6	21	75	51	2	340
Mini Bundt Cake Lemon Poppyseed	1	460	6	20	90	62	1	430
Mini Bundt Cake Pineapple Upside Down	1	450	5	20	70	64	2	490
Muffie Banana Nut	1	260	5	12	15	34	3	250
Muffie Chocolate Chip	1	240	4	10	15	36	2	240
Muffie Pumpkin	1	270	3	6	30	43	1	270
Muffin Banana Nut	1	470	9	20	30	57	5	500
Muffin Blueberry	1	450	8	15	35	73	4	570
Muffin Chocolate Chip	1	540	8	22	30	83	5	550
Muffin Pumpkin	1	510	6	12	60	80	1	530
Muffin Low Fat Tripleberry	1	300	6	3	30	63	3	320
Pecan Roll	1	520	6	31	40	60	2	260
Scone Cinnamon Chip	1	560	10	27	150	70	2	440
Scone Orange	1	530	10	25	140	67	3	370
Strudel Apple Raisin	1	390	4	22	0	40	1	330
Strudel Cherry	1	400	5	24	0	38	1	290
SALADS								
Asian Sesame Chicken	1 serv	370	25	19	60	45	5	1280
Caesar	1 serv	350	11	26	110	15	3	1010
Caesar Grilled Chicken	1 serv	470	31	27	165	22	3	1550

FOOD	PORTION	CALS	PROT	FAT	CHOL	CARB	FIBER	SOD
Classic Cafe	1 serv	380	3	36	0	15	4	340
Fandango	1 serv	400	7	28	25	21	6	480
Greek	1 serv	520	9	48	20	17	5	1560
SANDWICHES								
Asiago Roast Beef	1	730	50	35	115	54	2	1620
Bacon Turkey Bravo	1	770	47	28	45	84	5	2850
Chicken Salad On Artisan Sesame Semolina	1	730	39	26	90	80	6	1750
Chicken Salad On Nine Grain	1	640	35	29	90	56	4	1340
Garden Veggie	1	570	15	23	15	74	5	1490
Italian Combo	1	1050	60	54	165	80	5	3570
Panini Coronado Carnitas	1	810	47	35	95	77	3	2210
Panini Portabello & Mozzarella	1	650	25	29	40	73	8	1100
Panini Turkey Artichoke	1	810	41	38	25	76	6	2470
Peanut Butter & Jelly On French	1	450	15	15	0	63	3	580
Panini Frontega Chicken	1	860	49	42	110	71	5	2260
Smoked Ham On Artisan Stone Milled Rye	1	930	52	31	110	106	6	3000
Smoked Ham On Rye	1	650	42	34	110	47	4	2350
Smoked Turkey Breast On Artisan Country	1	590	34	16	10	73	5	2320
Smoked Turkey On Sourdough	1	440	29	15	10	44	3	1950
Tuna Salad On Artisan Multigrain	1	830	32	41	65	78	5	1790
Tuna Salad On Honey Wheat	1	720	28	43	65	50	4	1570
Turkey Fresco	1	580	35	17	0	74	4	2430
Tuscan Chicken	1	950	35	56	80	76	6	2130

FOOD	PORTION	CALS	PROT	FAT	CHOL	CARB	FIBER	SOD
SOUPS								
Baked Potato	1 serv	260	6	16	35	23	1	750
Boston Clam Chowder	1 serv	210	6	11	40	19	tr	990
Broccoli Cheddar	1 serv	230	8	16	45	13	1	1000
Cream Of Chicken & Wild Rice	1 serv	200	5	12	35	19	tr	970
Forest Mushroom	1 serv	140	4	7	15	15	2	920
French Onion	1 serv	220	9	10	20	23	2	1810
Low Fat Chicken Noodle	1 serv	100	5	2	15	15	1	1080
Low Fat Vegetarian Garden Vegetable	1 serv	90	4	1	0	17	2	860
Low Fat Vegetarian Black Bean	1 serv	100	10	1	0	29	17	840
Vegetarian Santa Fe Roasted Corn	1 serv	130	4	4	0	22	3	940
PAPA JOHN'S								
OTHER MENU SELECTIONS								
Bread Sticks	1 serv	140	4	2	0	26	1	260
Cheese Sticks	1 serv	180	8	8	13	20	1	380
Chickenstrips	1	83	6	4	13	5	tr	178
Cinnapie	1 serv	114	1	6	0	14	0	145
PIZZA 14 INCH								
Original All The Meats	⅛ pie	405	18	20	41	39	2	1114
Original BBQ Chicken & Bacon	⅛ pie	369	17	14	31	44	2	929
Original Cheese	⅛ pie	290	12	10	17	39	2	699
Original Chicken Alfredo	⅛ pie	310	15	12	31	37	2	743
Original Garden Fresh	⅛ pie	287	12	9	14	40	3	685
Original Hawaiian BBQ Chicken	⅛ pie	376	17	14	31	46	2	1029
Original Pepperoni	⅛ pie	343	14	15	27	39	2	913
Original Sausage	⅛ pie	336	14	14	28	38	2	894

FOOD	PORTION	CALS	PROT	FAT	CHOL	CARB	FIBER	SOD
Original Spinach Alfredo	⅛ pie	303	13	12	25	37	2	694
Original The Works	⅛ pie	370	17	16	34	40	3	1013
Thin Crust All The Meat	⅛ pie	371	17	24	44	24	2	945
Thin Crust BBQ Chicken & Bacon	⅛ pie	336	15	18	34	30	1	759
Thin Crust Cheese	⅛ pie	238	10	13	17	23	1	490
Thin Crust Chicken Alfredo	⅛ pie	276	14	15	35	22	1	573
Thin Crust Garden Fresh	⅛ pie	228	9	11	14	24	2	447
Thin Crust Hawaiian BBQ Chicken	⅛ pie	324	14	17	31	31	1	805
Thin Crust Pepperoni	⅛ pie	294	12	18	28	23	2	675
Thin Crust Sausage	⅛ pie	303	13	18	31	24	2	724
Thin Crust Spinach Alfredo	⅛ pie	251	10	15	26	22	1	470
Thin Crust The Works	⅛ pie	315	14	18	32	25	2	809
SALAD DRESSINGS AND SAUCES								
BBQ Sauce	1 serv	48	0	0	0	10	0	310
Buffalo Sauce	1 serv	25	0	1	0	3	0	1470
Cheese Sauce	1 serv	60	4	5	19	0	0	300
Garlic Sauce	1 serv	235	0	26	0	0	0	300
Honey Mustard Dressing	1 serv	170	0	19	10	6	0	150
Pizza Sauce	1 serv	25	0	2	0	3	2	125
Ranch Dressing	1 serv	140	1	14	15	2	0	280
PAPA MURPHY'S PIZZA								
Deeper Dish Traditional	⅛ pie	440	23	24	40	34	2	900
Delite Large Cheese	⅟₁₀ pie	130	8	6	15	11	0	240
Delite Large Hawaiian	⅟₁₀ pie	140	9	7	15	14	1	300

FOOD	PORTION	CALS	PROT	FAT	CHOL	CARB	FIBER	SOD
Delite Large Meat	1/10 pie	190	11	12	25	11	0	430
Delite Large Pepperoni	1/10 pie	160	9	9	20	11	0	350
Delite Large Veggie	1/10 pie	150	8	8	15	11	0	200
Family Size Cheese	1/12 pie	270	14	10	20	29	2	470
Gourmet Family Size Chicken Garlic	1/12 pie	320	18	15	35	30	1	600
Gourmet Family Size Classic Italian	1/12 pie	360	18	19	35	30	2	730
Gourmet Family Size Veggie	1/12 pie	300	15	14	25	31	2	570
Papa's Family Size All Meat	1/12 pie	370	20	19	40	31	2	860
Papa's Family Size Cheese	1/12 pie	270	14	10	20	29	2	470
Papa's Family Size Cowboy	1/12 pie	370	18	19	35	31	2	850
Papa's Family Size Favorite	1/12 pie	380	18	20	35	32	2	860
Papa's Family Size Hawaiian	1/12 pie	290	16	11	25	34	2	580
Papa's Family Size Murphy's Combo	1/12 pie	480	18	20	35	32	2	910
Papa's Family Size Pepperoni	1/12 pie	310	16	15	30	29	2	650
Papa's Family Size Perfect	1/12 pie	300	16	13	25	32	2	620
Papa's Family Size Rancher	1/12 pie	330	18	15	30	31	2	720
Papa's Family Size Specialty	1/12 pie	340	17	17	30	31	2	740
Papa's Family Size Veggie Combo	1/12 pie	300	14	13	20	32	2	570
Stuffed Big Murphy	1/8 pie	380	18	17	30	39	2	800
Stuffed Chicago Style	1/8 pie	370	17	16	30	39	2	770

FOOD	PORTION	CALS	PROT	FAT	CHOL	CARB	FIBER	SOD
SALADS								
Club	1 serv	190	21	21	50	11	4	930
Garden	1 serv	160	11	11	20	9	4	270
Italian	1 serv	220	13	17	30	7	3	510

PICCADILLY CAFETERIA
DESSERTS

FOOD	PORTION	CALS	PROT	FAT	CHOL	CARB	FIBER	SOD
Gelatin Sugar Free	1 serv	0	0	0	0	0	0	5
Sugar Free Blueberry Pie	1 serv	314	5	17	0	42	3	253
Sugar Free Cherry Pie	1 serv	334	5	17	0	45	1	253
Sugar Free Chocolate Almond Pie	1 serv	611	5	44	1	49	2	564

MAIN MENU SELECTIONS

FOOD	PORTION	CALS	PROT	FAT	CHOL	CARB	FIBER	SOD
Bass Blackened	1 serv	408	26	32	28	2	1	616
Bass Cajun Baked	1 serv	260	27	15	28	4	1	600
Bass Stuffed	1 serv	447	34	30	64	8	1	1007
Beef Chopped Steak	1 serv	382	21	31	74	4	0	160
Beef Chopped Steak Fried	1 serv	225	26	12	59	2	0	1604
Beef Roast Leg	1 sm serv	353	35	22	103	2	1	213
Broccoli Florets	1 serv	90	3	7	0	5	3	174
Broccoli w/ Cheese Sauce	1 serv	55	3	1	4	9	3	284
Brussels Sprouts	1 serv	92	3	6	0	8	4	119
Cabbage Steamed Bacon Seasoned	1 serv	108	2	8	9	6	2	191
Cabbage Steamed Buttered	1 serv	68	1	5	0	6	2	132
Catfish Filet Blackened	1 serv	523	29	43	87	2	1	647
Catfish Filet Cajun Baked	1 serv	401	30	28	87	5	1	927
Catfish Filet Stuffed	1 serv	561	37	41	123	8	1	1036
Cauliflower Buttered	1 serv	73	1	4	0	5	1	153
Chicken Barbecued Quarters	1 serv	472	65	52	255	9	1	871

FOOD	PORTION	CALS	PROT	FAT	CHOL	CARB	FIBER	SOD
Chicken Grilled Breast	1 serv	345	34	21	136	2	1	512
Chicken Rotisserie Herb Dark Meat	1 serv	823	57	63	276	3	1	877
Chicken Rotisserie Herb White Meat	1 serv	602	71	32	218	3	1	843
Chicken Baked Cajun Boneless Breast	1 serv	428	35	27	136	9	1	1597
Chicken Baked Quarters	1 serv	828	64	59	255	5	1	972
Chicken Breast Italian Boneless Breast	1 serv	371	34	41	139	7	1	1773
Chicken Breast Mesquite Smoke	1 serv	212	34	8	86	1	1	1215
Chicken Breast Mesquite w/ BBQ Sauce	1 serv	240	35	9	86	6	0	1462
Chicken Breast Southwestern	1 serv	315	44	35	133	8	1	1837
Chicken Half Rotisserie Herb	1 serv	833	146	21	478	4	2	1781
Corn	1 serv	125	3	6	0	18	1	128
Cottage Cheese	1 serv	117	14	5	17	3	0	813
Filet Mignon	1 (6 oz)	184	36	20	105	1	0	286
Green Beans	1 serv	136	3	11	12	8	4	291
Greens Collard Mustard Turnip	1 serv	135	4	10	12	3	2	224
Greens Turnip w/ Diced Turnips	1 serv	150	4	12	14	4	2	242
Grouper Filet Baked	1 piece (6 oz)	305	46	9	84	8	1	424
New York Strip	1 (10 oz)	871	55	71	190	1	0	360
Okra Creole	1 serv	77	2	4	5	8	3	205
Okra Fried	1 serv	240	4	13	0	26	4	473
Peas & Sugar Snapped Mixed	1 serv	102	3	5	0	10	3	115

FOOD	PORTION	CALS	PROT	FAT	CHOL	CARB	FIBER	SOD
Pork Loin Marinated Boneless	1 serv	365	34	24	102	1	0	529
Pork Loin Roast Bone In	1 serv	373	49	13	120	10	1	335
Ribeye	1 (10 oz)	1038	50	91	193	2	1	542
Roast Beef	1 serv	481	46	30	141	3	1	292
Roll Parker House	1	147	3	5	0	22	1	198
Roll Whole Wheat	1	231	6	8	0	37	5	376
Shrimp Fried	1 serv	499	26	22	277	45	0	907
Tilapia Baked	1 serv	210	17	11	0	10	1	560
Tilapia Cajun Baked	1 serv	263	17	19	0	6	1	1039
Trout Almondine Baked	1 lg serv	457	60	18	167	10	1	398
Trout Cajun Baked	1 lg serv	517	59	27	167	6	1	1082
Trout Filet Baked	1 lg serv	464	59	19	167	10	1	594
Turkey Breast Carved	1 serv	302	45	11	123	2	0	2605
Vegetables Mixed	1 serv	95	1	6	0	8	3	137
SALAD DRESSINGS AND TOPPINGS								
Au Jus	1 serv	6	0	0	0	1	0	457
Blue Cheese	2 tbsp	160	1	18	20	1	0	210
Cheese Sauce	2 oz	35	1	1	4	5	0	274
French	2 tbsp	130	0	13	0	5	0	240
Italian	2 tbsp	140	0	14	0	3	0	421
Ranch	2 tbsp	150	1	17	15	1	0	210
Ranch Fat Free	2 tbsp	36	1	0	0	7	1	352
SALADS								
Asparagus & Tomato	1 serv	86	2	5	4	10	2	118
Caesar	1 serv	141	4	11	12	7	1	317
Cauilflower	1 serv	118	4	8	33	9	2	361
Chef	1 sm serv	146	13	9	150	4	1	475
Cole Slaw Kosher Style	1 serv	140	1	13	0	7	2	76
Coleslaw Italian	1 serv	163	1	16	0	5	2	645
Combination	1 serv	63	5	3	125	4	2	48
Cucumber & Celery	1 serv	74	1	4	0	9	1	141
Cucumber & Tomato	1 serv	41	1	0	0	10	1	109
Cucumber Mix	1 serv	61	1	4	0	7	2	107

FOOD	PORTION	CALS	PROT	FAT	CHOL	CARB	FIBER	SOD
Cucumbers & Sour Cream	1 serv	90	2	7	22	6	1	122
Louisianne Bowl	1 serv	42	4	2	9	2	1	112
Mexican	1 serv	58	1	3	0	8	1	54
Piccadilly Bowl	1 serv	27	1	0	0	6	2	30
Piccadilly Fruit	1 serv	76	1	0	0	20	3	3
Shrimp Ramoulade	1 serv	521	31	29	410	33	5	871
Spring Bowl	1 reg serv	24	2	0	0	5	2	16
Tomato Cucumber & Onion	1 serv	44	1	0	0	10	1	106
Vegetable Combo w/ Cherry Tomatoes	1 serv	66	1	4	0	9	2	114
SOUPS								
Gumbo Chicken & Sausage No Rice	1 serv	224	12	15	39	10	1	649
Gumbo Chicken No Rice	1 serv	89	8	2	23	9	1	8463

PIZZA HUT
APPETIZERS

FOOD	PORTION	CALS	PROT	FAT	CHOL	CARB	FIBER	SOD
Breadstick	1	150	4	6	0	20	tr	220
Breadstick Cheese	1	200	7	10	15	21	tr	340
Breadstick Dipping Sauce	1 serv (3 oz)	50	1	0	0	11	2	270
Hot Wings	2 pieces	110	11	6	70	1	0	450
Mild Wings	2 pieces	110	11	7	70	tr	0	320
Wing Blue Cheese Dipping Sauce	1 serv (1.5 oz)	230	2	24	25	2	0	550
Wing Ranch Dipping Sauce	1 serv (1.5 oz)	210	tr	22	10	4	0	340
BEVERAGES								
Diet Pepsi	1 med (14 oz)	0	0	0	0	0	0	45
Mt. Dew	1 med (14 oz)	190	0	0	0	54	0	60
Pepsi	1 med (14 oz)	180	0	0	0	47	0	45
DESSERTS								
Apple Pizza	1 slice	260	4	4	0	53	1	250
Cherry Pizza	1 slice	240	4	4	0	47	1	250
Cinnamon Sticks	2	170	4	5	0	27	tr	170

FOOD	PORTION	CALS	PROT	FAT	CHOL	CARB	FIBER	SOD
White Icing Dipping Cup	1 serv (2 oz)	170	0	0	0	46	0	0
PIZZA								
Fit 'N Delicious Diced Chicken Mushroom Jalapeno	1 med slice	170	10	5	15	22	2	630
Fit 'N Delicious Diced Chicken Red Onion Green Pepper	1 med slice	170	10	5	15	23	2	460
Fit 'N Delicious Green Pepper Red Onion Diced Red Tomato	1 med slice	150	6	4	10	24	2	360
Fit 'N Delicious Ham Pineapple Diced Red Tomato	1 med slice	160	8	4	15	24	2	470
Fit 'N Delicious Ham Red Onion Mushroom	1 med slice	160	8	5	15	22	2	470
Fit 'N Delicious Tomato Mushroom Jalapeno	1 med slice	150	6	4	10	22	2	590
Hand Tossed Cheese	1 med slice	240	12	8	25	30	2	520
Hand Tossed Chicken Supreme	1 med slice	230	14	6	25	30	2	550
Hand Tossed Ham	1 med slice	220	12	6	20	29	2	550
Hand Tossed Meat Lover's	1 med slice	300	15	13	35	29	2	760
Hand Tossed Pepperoni	1 med slice	250	12	9	25	29	2	570
Hand Tossed Pepperoni Lover's	1 med slice	300	15	13	40	30	2	710
Hand Tossed Sausage Lover's	1 med slice	280	13	12	30	30	2	650
Hand Tossed Super Supreme	1 med slice	300	13	13	35	30	2	780

FOOD	PORTION	CALS	PROT	FAT	CHOL	CARB	FIBER	SOD
Hand Tossed Supreme	1 med slice	270	13	11	25	30	2	660
Hand Tossed Veggie Lover's	1 med slice	220	10	6	15	31	2	490
Marinara Dipping Sauce	1 serv (3 oz)	45	2	0	0	9	2	380
Pan Cheese	1 med slice	280	11	13	25	29	1	500
Pan Chicken Supreme	1 med slice	280	13	12	25	30	2	530
Pan Ham	1 med slice	260	11	11	20	29	1	540
Pan Meat Lover's	1 med slice	340	15	19	35	29	2	750
Pan Pepperoni	1 med slice	290	11	15	25	29	2	560
Pan Pepperoni Lover's	1 med slice	340	15	19	40	29	2	690
Pan Sausage Lover's	1 med slice	330	13	17	30	29	2	640
Pan Super Supreme	1 med slice	340	14	18	35	30	2	760
Pan Supreme	1 med slice	320	13	16	25	30	2	650
Pizone Classic	1	1220	66	42	100	142	6	2420
Pizone Pepperoni	1	1220	68	44	110	138	6	2560
Thin 'N Crispy Cheese	1 med slice	200	10	8	25	27	1	490
Thin 'N Crispy Chicken Supreme	1 med slice	200	13	7	25	23	2	520
Thin 'N Crispy Ham	1 med slice	180	9	6	20	21	1	530
Thin 'N Crispy Meat Lover's	1 med slice	270	13	14	35	21	2	740
Thin 'N Crispy Pepperoni	1 med slice	170	10	10	25	21	1	550
Thin 'N Crispy Pepperoni Lover's	1 med slice	260	13	14	40	21	2	690
Thin 'N Crispy Super Supreme	1 med slice	260	13	13	35	23	2	760
Thin 'N Crispy Supreme	1 med slice	240	11	11	25	22	2	640
Thin 'N Crispy Veggie Lover's	1 med slice	180	8	7	15	23	2	480

FOOD	PORTION	CALS	PROT	FAT	CHOL	CARB	FIBER	SOD
QUIZNO'S								
Cookie Oatmeal Chocolate Chip	1	360	5	17	25	48	1	120
Cookie w/ Reese's Pieces	1	360	6	17	20	48	1	130
Sub Honey Bourbon Chicken	1 sm	329	24	6	38	45	3	1494
Sub Sierra Turkey w/ Raspberry Chipotle Sauce	1 sm	350	23	6	25	53	3	1140
Sub Turkey Lite	1 sm	334	24	6	19	52	3	1909
Sub Tuscan Chicken Salad	1 sm	326	21	6	35	45	4	1271
RANCH 1								
MAIN MENU SELECTIONS								
Baked Potato w/ Broccoli	1 serv	510	12	1	0	117	12	50
Baked Potato w/ Cheese	1 serv	790	23	25	50	118	11	850
Baked Potato w/ Chicken	1 serv	610	30	4	55	114	11	135
Chicken Tenders	1 serv	370	52	15	140	7	0	620
Fajita Grilled Chicken	1	330	22	16	50	25	4	560
Fruit Cup	1 serv	90	3	1	0	21	2	20
Hot Pasta Grilled Chicken	1 serv	590	37	10	60	86	6	840
Platter Grilled Chicken & Vegetables	1 serv	790	54	7	105	129	16	270
Ranch Fries	1 reg	350	5	14	0	51	5	280
Ranch Fries	1 lg	420	6	17	0	62	7	340
Sandwich American Rancher	1	390	25	10	50	51	3	780
Sandwich Grilled Chicken Philly	1	450	28	14	50	53	3	500
Sandwich Ranch Classic	1	370	26	5	50	53	3	550

FOOD	PORTION	CALS	PROT	FAT	CHOL	CARB	FIBER	SOD
Sandwich Spicy Grilled Chicken	1	420	23	11	35	58	3	620
Sandwich Club	1	470	29	16	60	53	3	750
SALADS								
Gourmet Greens	1 serv	220	10	7	10	31	5	370
Gourmet Greens w/ Chicken	1 serv	350	32	11	70	31	5	470
Zesty Caesar	1 serv	180	8	3	5	31	4	350
Zesty Chicken Caesar	1 serv	290	26	6	50	31	4	440

RAX
MAIN MENU SELECTIONS

FOOD	PORTION	CALS	PROT	FAT	CHOL	CARB	FIBER	SOD
Baked Potato	1	207	–	0	0	60	–	9
Baked Potato w/ Butter	1	306	–	11	0	60	–	94
Baked Potato w/ Cheese	1 serv	270	–	tr	4	70	–	620
Baked Potato w/ Cheese Bacon	1 serv	336	–	19	82	70	–	876
Baked Potato w/ Cheese Broccoli	1 serv	281	–	tr	4	71	–	621
Baked Potato w/ Sour Topping	1 serv	257	–	4	0	62	–	29
BBQ Beef Sandwich	1	399	–	20	40	43	–	1030
Cheddar Melt	1	346	–	23	41	26	–	539
Deluxe Sandwich	1	521	–	34	68	34	–	785
Grilled Chicken Sandwich	1	526	–	33	69	32	–	994
Jr. Deluxe Sandwich	1	367	–	25	42	25	–	509
Mushroom Melt	1	599	–	37	104	35	–	1688
Philly Melt	1	537	–	32	79	35	–	1296
Regular Rax	1	388	–	22	54	31	–	708
Turkey Bacon Club	1	680	–	47	76	37	–	1898
Turkey Sandwich	1	484	–	32	50	32	–	1286
SALAD DRESSINGS								
1000 Island	1 serv	130	–	13	10	5	–	230
Blue Cheese	1 serv	145	–	16	25	1	–	300

FOOD	PORTION	CALS	PROT	FAT	CHOL	CARB	FIBER	SOD
Buttermilk Ranch	1 serv	175	—	20	0	1	—	240
Catalina Fat Free	1 serv	32	—	0	0	6	—	240
Creamy Caesar	1 serv	140	—	15	5	1	—	290
Honey French	1 serv	140	—	5	0	9	—	210
Italian Fat Free	1 serv	12	—	0	0	2	—	420
Ranch Fat Free	1 serv	30	—	0	0	6	—	300
Vinaigrette	1 serv	30	—	2	0	4	—	150
SALADS								
Garden	1 serv	220	—	9	5	12	—	840
Grilled Chicken	1 serv	160	—	5	50	6	—	1150
Side Salad	1 serv (19 oz)	40	—	4	0	2	—	90
SOUPS								
Chicken Noodle	1 serv	113	—	1	45	20	—	304
Chili	1 serv	158	—	9	31	11	—	421
Cream Of Broccoli	1 serv	95	—	4	1	14	—	512

RED LOBSTER

FOOD	PORTION	CALS	PROT	FAT	CHOL	CARB	FIBER	SOD
BEVERAGES								
Dannon Spring Water	1 glass	0	0	0	—	0	0	—
Diet Coke	1 serv	0	0	0	0	0	0	—
Hot Tea	1 cup	0	0	0	0	0	0	—
Iced Tea Unsweetened	1 glass	0	0	0	—	0	0	—
Michelob Ultra	1 glass	95	—	0	—	2	0	—
Perrier Water	1 glass	0	0	2	—	0	0	—
Sutter Home Cabernet Sauvignon	1 glass	138	—	0	—	5	0	—
Sutter Home Chardonnay	1 glass	147	—	0	—	5	0	—
MAIN MENU SELECTIONS								
Baked Potato Plain	1	170	—	2	—	36	4	—
Baked Potato w/ Pico De Gallo Topping	1 serv	185	—	2	—	37	5	—
Cheddar Bay Biscuit	1	160	—	9	—	17	0	—

FOOD	PORTION	CALS	PROT	FAT	CHOL	CARB	FIBER	SOD
Fresh Buttered Vegetables	1 serv	143	–	12	–	9	3	–
Garden Salad	1 serv	52	–	2	–	9	0	–
Light House Broiled Flounder	1 serv	240	–	5	–	0	0	–
Light House Grilled Chicken	1 serv	527	–	14	–	38	2	–
Light House Jumbo Shrimp Cocktail Dinner	1 serv	243	–	3	–	2	0	–
Light House King Crab Legs	1 serv	490	–	9	–	0	0	–
Light House Live Maine Lobster	1 serv	145	–	1	–	2	0	–
Light House Maine Lobster Tail	1 serv	104	–	5	–	2	0	–
Light House Rainbow Trout	1 lunch serv	273	–	14	–	2	0	–
Light House Rock Lobster Tail	1 serv	256	–	3	–	2	0	–
Light House Salmon	1 serv	578	–	31	–	0	0	–
Light House Salmon	1 lunch serv	258	–	12	–	0	0	–
Light House Snow Crab Legs	1 serv	262	–	5	–	0	0	–
Light House Tilapia	1 serv	346	–	10	–	0	0	–
Light House Tilapia	1 lunch serv	186	–	6	–	0	0	–
Seasoned Fresh Broccoli	1 serv	60	–	0	–	12	5	–
Shrimp Cocktail	1 jumbo	146	–	2	–	2	0	–
Wild Rice Pilaf	1 serv	2080	–	5	–	36	2	–
SALAD DRESSINGS AND TOPPINGS								
Large Cocktail Sauce	1 serv	68	–	0	–	17	0	–
Lemon Wedge	1 serv	8	–	0	–	2	0	–
Melted Butter	1 serv	183	–	21	–	0	0	–
Red Wine Vinaigrette	1 serv	49	–	3	–	5	0	–
Topping Petite Shrimp	1 serv	30	–	1	–	1	0	–

FOOD	PORTION	CALS	PROT	FAT	CHOL	CARB	FIBER	SOD

RUBIO'S
MAIN MENU SELECTIONS

FOOD	PORTION	CALS	PROT	FAT	CHOL	CARB	FIBER	SOD
Black Beans	1 serv	220	12	3	5	37	12	840
Burritos Baja Carne Asada	1	710	38	33	100	63	5	2270
Burritos Baja Carnitas	1	660	36	30	85	64	5	1950
Burritos Baja Chicken	1	640	42	28	85	61	5	1740
Burritos Carne Asada Especial w/ Black Beans	1	970	40	37	65	117	13	2740
Burritos Carne Asada Especial w/ Pinto	1	950	35	38	65	118	14	2530
Burritos Chicken Especial w/ Black Beans	1	920	42	32	50	116	13	2320
Burritos Chicken Especial w/ Pinto	1	900	37	32	50	116	14	2200
Burritos Fish	1	780	25	41	50	76	7	1220
Burritos HealthMax Chicken	1	520	33	11	40	75	9	1570
Burritos HealthMax Veggie	1	470	15	8	0	81	13	1100
Burritos Lobster	1	660	24	26	190	82	9	1630
Burritos Mahi	1	630	40	30	65	58	5	1070
Burritos Shrimp	1	650	26	25	170	77	6	1680
Carne Asada	1 serv	1430	54	87	170	114	19	2680
Chips	1 serv	430	5	22	0	56	7	480
Grilled Grande Bowl Asada Black Beans	1 serv	770	41	37	85	70	11	2350
Grilled Grande Bowl Asada Pinto	1 serv	760	38	37	85	70	12	2230
Grilled Grande Bowl Chicken Black Beans	1 serv	710	44	31	75	69	11	1930
Grilled Grande Bowl Chicken Pinto	1 serv	700	38	32	75	69	12	1810

FOOD	PORTION	CALS	PROT	FAT	CHOL	CARB	FIBER	SOD
Guacamole	1 sm	170	2	16	0	8	5	75
Nachos Grande	1 serv	1270	37	79	120	112	19	1790
Nachos Grande w/ Chicken	1 serv	1380	56	82	160	112	19	2280
Pinto Beans	1 serv	190	4	3	5	44	16	600
Quesadillas Carne Asada	1	1010	53	61	175	62	4	2340
Quesadillas Cheese	1	860	36	53	125	60	4	1450
Quesadillas Grilled Chicken	1	860	56	56	165	61	4	1820
Quesadillas Lobster	1	820	48	54	280	62	5	1820
Quesadillas Shrimp	1	810	48	54	285	61	4	1850
Salsa Picante	1 serv (1.5 oz)	30	1	2	0	3	2	290
Salsa Regular	1 serv (1.5 oz)	15	1	0	0	2	1	330
Salsa Verde	1 serv (1.5 oz)	5	0	0	0	1	1	230
Tacos Carne Asada	1	220	13	8	25	23	2	420
Tacos Fish	1	310	11	18	20	28	2	280
Tacos Fish Especial	1	370	14	21	35	38	3	360
Tacos Grilled Chicken	1	300	15	16	30	23	2	400
Tacos Grilled Fish	1	310	18	16	30	24	2	230
Tacos HealthMax w/ Chicken	1	170	12	3	15	23	2	270
Taquitos	3	310	16	11	45	37	5	310
SALADS AND SALAD DRESSINGS								
Grilled Chicken Chopped Salad	1 serv	540	33	33	75	33	5	1480
HealthMex Chicken	1 serv	220	22	4	40	27	2	890
Low Carb Chicken	1 serv	480	37	34	95	11	5	980
Serrano Grape Dressing	1 serv (1.3 oz)	10	0	0	0	2	0	160
RUBY TUESDAY'S								
Cajun Chicken Salad w/ Ranch Dressing	1 serv	636	—	46	—	16	—	—

FOOD	PORTION	CALS	PROT	FAT	CHOL	CARB	FIBER	SOD
Peppercorn Mushroom Sirloin	1 serv	947	–	57	–	19	–	–

SBARRO

FOOD	PORTION	CALS	PROT	FAT	CHOL	CARB	FIBER	SOD
Baked Ziti	1 serv (14 oz)	830	–	42	–	–	–	950
Meat Lasagna	1 serv (17 oz)	730	–	38	–	–	–	1660
Pizza Cheese	1 serv (6 oz)	450	–	14	–	–	–	990
Pizza Pepperoni	1 serv (6 oz)	510	–	21	–	–	–	1240
Pizza Sausage	1 serv (10 oz)	640	–	29	–	–	–	1560
Pizza Sausage & Pepperoni Stuffed	1 serv (11 oz)	880	–	44	–	–	–	2230
Pizza Spinach & Broccoli Stuffed	1 serv (11 oz)	710	–	26	–	–	–	1490
Pizza Supreme	1 serv (10 oz)	600	–	25	–	–	–	1580
Pizza Veggie Slice	1 serv (10 oz)	490	20	12	15	75	1	1350
Spaghetti w/ Sauce	1 serv (18 oz)	630	–	18	–	–	–	1260

SCHLOTZSKY'S DELI

SALADS AND SALAD BARS

FOOD	PORTION	CALS	PROT	FAT	CHOL	CARB	FIBER	SOD
Caesar	1 serv (7 oz)	150	–	8	–	–	–	510
Chicken Caesar	1 serv (9 oz)	250	–	10	–	–	–	940
Chinese Chicken	1 serv (9 oz)	150	–	3	–	–	–	450
Choice Potato Salad	1 serv (5 oz)	250	–	18	–	–	–	530
Country Style Cole Slaw	1 serv (4 oz)	230	–	16	–	–	–	290
Garden	1 serv (9 oz)	60	–	1	–	–	–	120
Greek	1 serv (12 oz)	220	–	12	–	–	–	560
Smoked Turkey Chef	1 serv (13 oz)	240	–	10	–	–	–	1280

FOOD	PORTION	CALS	PROT	FAT	CHOL	CARB	FIBER	SOD
SANDWICHES								
Light & Flavorful Albacore Tuna	1 (13 oz)	530	—	16	—	—	—	1660
Light & Flavorful Chicken Breast	1 (15 oz)	540	—	10	—	—	—	2370
Light & Flavorful Dijon Chicken	1 sm (10 oz)	330	—	4	—	—	—	1370
Light & Flavorful Dijon Chicken	1 (15 oz)	500	—	6	—	—	—	2090
Light & Flavorful Pesto Chicken	1 (14 oz)	510	—	9	—	—	—	1930
Light & Flavorful Santa Fe Chicken	1 (17 oz)	640	—	19	—	—	—	2300
Light & Flavorful Smoked Turkey Breast	1 (13 oz)	500	—	7	—	—	—	2120
Light & Flavorful The Vegetarian	1 (12 oz)	520	—	17	—	—	—	1330
Original Cheese	1 (14 oz)	850	—	44	—	—	—	2110
Original Ham & Cheese	1 (17 oz)	790	—	32	—	—	—	3430
Original Turkey	1 (17 oz)	1020	—	51	—	—	—	3740
Specialty Deli Albacore Tuna Melt	1 (16 oz)	820	—	40	—	—	—	2290
Specialty Deli BLT	1 (10 oz)	580	—	24	—	—	—	1550
Specialty Deli Chicken Club	1 (16 oz)	690	—	23	—	—	—	2400
Specialty Deli Corned Beef	1 (12 oz)	590	—	15	—	—	—	2490
Specialty Deli Corned Beef Reuben	1 (15 oz)	830	—	35	—	—	—	3510
Specialty Deli Pastrami & Swiss	1 (15 oz)	860	—	37	—	—	—	3720
Specialty Deli Pastrami Reuben	1 (16 oz)	920	—	43	—	—	—	3920
Specialty Deli Roast Beef	1 (14 oz)	620	—	17	—	—	—	1730

FOOD	PORTION	CALS	PROT	FAT	CHOL	CARB	FIBER	SOD
Specialty Deli Roast Beef & Cheese	1 (17 oz)	850	–	34	–	–	–	2450
Specialty Deli Texas Schlotzsky	1 (16 oz)	820	–	37	–	–	–	3360
Specialty Deli The Philly	1 (16 oz)	820	–	32	–	–	–	2190
Specialty Deli Turkey & Bacon Club	1 (17 oz)	870	–	40	–	–	–	3010
Specialty Deli Turkey Guacamole	1 (16 oz)	680	–	24	–	–	–	2680
Specialty Deli Turkey Reuben	1 (16 oz)	860	–	39	–	–	–	3890
Specialty Deli Vegetable Club	1 (13 oz)	580	–	24	–	–	–	1440
Specialty Deli Western Vegetarian	1 (12 oz)	650	–	33	–	–	–	1160
The Original	1 (14 oz)	940	–	50	–	–	–	3170

SEE'S CANDIES

FOOD	PORTION	CALS	PROT	FAT	CHOL	CARB	FIBER	SOD
Bridge Mix	14 pieces (1.4 oz)	200	2	12	10	24	1	45
Dark Chocolate Bordeaux	2 (1.4 oz)	170	tr	27	25	27	1	40
Dark Chocolates	2 (1.2 oz)	160	2	10	10	19	2	35
Marshmints	3 (1.4 oz)	140	tr	4	0	27	tr	10
Milk Chocolate Bordeaux	2 (1.4 oz)	170	1	8	15	27	tr	45
Milk Chocolate Butter	2 (1.4 oz)	190	1	9	15	27	tr	50
Milk Chocolate Buttercreams	2 (1.4 oz)	180	1	8	15	27	0	50
Milk Chocolate California Brittle	2 (1.3 oz)	220	3	16	25	19	0	115
Milk Chocolate Nuts & Chews	3 (1.7 oz)	250	4	16	15	26	2	60
Milk Chocolate Peanuts	3 (1.5 oz)	230	6	17	5	18	2	90

FOOD	PORTION	CALS	PROT	FAT	CHOL	CARB	FIBER	SOD
Milk Chocolate Soft Centers	2 (1.4 oz)	170	1	9	15	25	tr	40
Milk Chocolates	2 (1.2 oz)	160	2	9	10	20	tr	40
Nuts & Chews	3 (1.6 oz)	240	4	16	10	25	2	50
Peanut Brittle	1.5 oz	230	4	16	25	21	0	280
Pecan Buds	3 (1.7 oz)	270	3	21	10	22	tr	30
P-Nut Crunch	2 (1.4 oz)	220	4	15	10	21	1	80
Red Hot Swamp Goo	3 pieces (1.4 oz)	140	tr	4	0	27	tr	10
Soft Centers	2 (1.4 oz)	170	1	9	10	25	tr	40
Truffles Black or Gold	2 (1.4 oz)	180	2	11	10	22	1	25
Truffles Mint	3 (1.6 oz)	200	2	11	15	26	tr	30
Victoria Toffee	1.5 oz	250	4	19	20	19	1	115

SKIPPER'S

CHILDREN'S MENU SELECTIONS

FOOD	PORTION	CALS	PROT	FAT	CHOL	CARB	FIBER	SOD
Kids Catch Chicken Tenderloin + Chips & Kids Side	1 serv	560	20	11	30	79	1	1040
Kids Catch Fish Bites + Chips & Kids Side	1 serv	490	15	15	0	84	3	1270
Kids Catch Sandwich Grilled Cheese + Chips & Kids Side	1 serv	620	14	19	20	97	3	1150
Kids Catch Shrimp + Chips & Kids Side	1 serv	520	14	11	50	91	2	1150

MAIN MENU SELECTIONS

FOOD	PORTION	CALS	PROT	FAT	CHOL	CARB	FIBER	SOD
Baked Potato Plain	1	210	6	0	0	48	4	25
Basket Chicken & Fish + Chips & Slaw	1 serv	620	26	27	45	59	1	1650
Basket Chicken & Shrimp + Chips & Slaw	1 serv	760	33	25	120	84	1	2060
Basket Chicken + Chips & Slaw	1 pieces	730	33	25	70	60	0	1650

FOOD	PORTION	CALS	PROT	FAT	CHOL	CARB	FIBER	SOD
Basket Clam Strips + Chips & Slaw	1 serv	890	38	34	75	113	12	1670
Basket Clams & Fish + Chips & Slaw	1 serv	740	30	32	50	91	8	1720
Basket Original Recipe Shrimp + Chips & Slaw	1 serv	800	32	25	165	107	3	2470
Basket Popcorn Shrimp + Chips & Slaw	1 serv	750	33	25	180	96	2	2090
Basket Prawn & Fish + Chips & Slaw	1 serv	730	38	41	235	61	2	1600
Basket Prawn Seafood + Chips & Slaw	1 serv	720	36	40	280	52	tr	1200
Basket Shrimp & Fish + Chips & Slaw	1 serv	650	25	27	90	83	2	2060
Basket Shrimp Trio + Chips & Slaw	1 serv	1040	56	38	305	123	4	3020
Clam Chowder	1 cup	120	3	8	5	14	tr	600
Clam Strips	1 serv	270	17	6	30	39	6	490
Fish Bites + Chips & Slaw	6 pieces	490	7	17	0	94	7	1630
French Fries	1 reg	180	3	6	0	27	0	500
Grilled Veggies	1 serv	35	2	0	0	8	3	50
Halibut + Chips & Slaw	1 serv	580	23	30	45	51	0	1280
Homestyle Chicken Tenderloin	1 piece	190	15	2	30	13	0	480
Hush Puppies	3 pieces	240	3	9	0	47	3	820
Original Fish Fillet	1 piece	80	7	4	0	12	1	480
Original Fish + Chips & Slaw	2 pieces	510	18	29	15	59	2	1650
Original Shrimp	9 pieces	220	14	2	75	36	1	890
Sandwich Fish + Chips & Slaw	1 serv	800	22	34	20	105	4	1780

FOOD	PORTION	CALS	PROT	FAT	CHOL	CARB	FIBER	SOD
Sandwich Fried Chicken + Chips & Slaw	1	1260	52	49	105	117	3	2390
Sandwich Grilled Chicken + Chips & Slaw	1	1070	57	50	145	92	3	1510
Skipper's Platter + Chips & Slaw	1 serv	930	42	33	12	122	8	2550
SALADS								
Caesar	1 sm	150	2	13	5	8	2	300
Caesar w/ Chicken	1 sm	340	27	17	100	8	2	380
Caesar w/ Salmon	1 sm	350	35	19	80	8	2	380
Green Salad w/o Dressing	1 sm	25	1	0	0	5	2	20

SMOOTHIE KING

FOOD	PORTION	CALS	PROT	FAT	CHOL	CARB	FIBER	SOD
Activator Chocolate	1 (20 oz)	429	19	1	2	90	4	260
Activator Strawberry	1 (20 oz)	559	20	1	2	123	5	260
Activator Vanilla	1 (20 oz)	429	19	1	2	90	4	260
Banana Boat	1 (20 oz)	520	11	14	80	93	5	230
Coconut Surprise	1 (20 oz)	457	8	6	3	99	5	126
Coffee Smoothies Hazelnut	1 (20 oz)	118	6	tr	1	23	tr	124
Coffee Smoothies Amaretto	1 (20 oz)	118	6	tr	1	23	tr	124
Coffee Smoothies French Roast	1 (20 oz)	164	6	tr	1	35	tr	124
Coffee Smoothies French Vanilla	1 (20 oz)	118	6	tr	1	23	tr	124
Coffee Smoothies Irish Creme	1 (20 oz)	118	6	tr	1	23	tr	124
Coffee Smoothies Mocha	1 (20 oz)	206	8	1	1	42	1	215
HeaterZ Banana Nut	1	400	14	22	5	67	3	—
HeaterZ Blueberry Muffin	1	370	19	26	<5	15	9	—
HeaterZ Chocolate Peanut Butter Cup	1	380	23	13	5	48	6	—

FOOD	PORTION	CALS	PROT	FAT	CHOL	CARB	FIBER	SOD
HeaterZ Cinnamon Oatmeal Raisin	1	420	19	3	0	36	9	–
HeaterZ Coconut	1	440	17	13	5	3	3	–
HeaterZ Coffee Amaretto	1 (12 oz)	177	9	2	1	34	4	126
HeaterZ Coffee French Roast	1 (12 oz)	172	9	2	1	33	4	125
HeaterZ Coffee French Vanilla	1 (12 oz)	177	9	2	1	34	4	126
HeaterZ Coffee Hazelnut	1 (12 oz)	177	9	2	1	34	4	126
HeaterZ Coffee Irish Creme	1 (12 oz)	177	9	2	1	34	4	126
HeaterZ Coffee Mocha	1 (12 oz)	266	10	2	1	55	5	171
High Protein Almond Mocha	1 (20 oz)	402	31	13	17	45	4	245
High Protein Banana	1 (20 oz)	412	34	14	14	44	6	315
High Protein Chocolate	1 (20 oz)	401	31	13	17	45	4	244
High Protein Lemon	1 (20 oz)	390	29	13	12	41	3	177
High Protein Pineapple	1 (20 oz)	380	31	13	12	41	7	206
Hot Coffee Amaretto	1 (12 oz)	168	6	tr	1	35	tr	125
Hot Coffee French Roast	1 (12 oz)	164	6	tr	1	35	tr	124
Hot Coffee French Vanilla	1 (12 oz)	168	6	tr	1	35	tr	125
Hot Coffee Hazelnut	1 (12 oz)	168	6	tr	1	35	tr	125
Hot Coffee Irish Creme	1 (12 oz)	168	6	tr	1	35	tr	125
Hot Coffee Mocha	1 (12 oz)	209	7	1	1	44	1	169
Iced Coffee Amaretto	1 (20 oz)	168	6	tr	1	35	tr	125
Iced Coffee French Roast	1 (20 oz)	164	6	tr	1	35	tr	125
Iced Coffee French Vanilla	1 (20 oz)	168	6	tr	1	35	tr	125

FOOD	PORTION	CALS	PROT	FAT	CHOL	CARB	FIBER	SOD
Iced Coffee Hazelnut	1 (20 oz)	168	6	tr	1	35	tr	125
Iced Coffee Irish Creme	1 (20 oz)	168	6	tr	1	35	tr	125
Iced Coffee Mocha	1 (20 oz)	209	7	1	1	44	1	169
Kid Cup Berry Interesting	1	150	1	0	0	37	2	5
Kid Cup Choc-A-Laka	1	210	4	2	0	44	2	200
Kid Cup Gimmi-Grape	1	170	1	0	0	42	1	5
Kid Cup Smarti Tarti	1	150	1	0	0	36	0	5
Low Carb All Flavors	1 (20 oz)	225	35	6	6	4	2	207
Low Fat Angel Food	1 (20 oz)	330	6	1	2	79	4	71
Low Fat Blackberry Dream	1 (20 oz)	343	2	tr	0	86	3	39
Low Fat Carribean Way	1 (20 oz)	392	2	tr	0	96	5	18
Low Fat Celestial Cherry High	1 (20 oz)	285	1	tr	0	69	4	22
Low Fat Cherry Picker	1 (20 oz)	360	6	1	0	98	2	231
Low Fat Cranberry Supreme	1 (20 oz)	577	3	1	24	139	3	120
Low Fat Cranberry Cooler	1 (20 oz)	538	1	tr	0	132	3	95
Low Fat Grape Expectations	1 (20 oz)	399	3	tr	0	96	2	24
Low Fat Grape Expectations II	1 (20 oz)	529	4	tr	0	129	4	24
Low Fat Hearty Apple	1 (20 oz)	380	12	2	25	81	2	276
Low Fat Immune Builder	1 (20 oz)	333	5	1	24	80	4	47
Low Fat Instant Vigor	1 (20 oz)	359	2	1	0	87	2	38
Low Fat Island Treat	1 (20 oz)	334	2	1	0	81	5	29
Low Fat Lemon Twist Banana	1 (20 oz)	339	3	tr	0	82	2	24
Low Fat Lemon Twist Strawberry	1 (20 oz)	399	3	tr	0	97	2	23

FOOD	PORTION	CALS	PROT	FAT	CHOL	CARB	FIBER	SOD
Low Fat Light & Fluffy	1 (20 oz)	389	2	tr	0	98	4	12
Low Fat Mangofest	1 (20 oz)	320	1	0	0	78	2	50
Low Fat Muscle Punch	1 (20 oz)	339	6	1	2	80	4	75
Low Fat Muscle Punch Plus	1 (20 oz)	340	6	1	2	80	5	65
Low Fat Orange Ka-BAM	1 (20 oz)	320	2	0	0	104	3	200
Low Fat Peach Slice	1 (20 oz)	341	5	tr	2	80	3	93
Low Fat Pep Upper	1 (20 oz)	334	3	1	0	80	5	39
Low Fat Pineapple Pleasure	1 (20 oz)	331	2	tr	0	76	4	29
Low Fat Pineapple Surf	1 (20 oz)	440	8	1	3	104	4	190
Low Fat Raspberry Sunrise	1 (20 oz)	335	3	1	0	85	4	39
Low Fat Strawberry X-Treme	1 (20 oz)	370	3	0	0	91	4	40
Low Fat Strawberry Kiwi Breeze	1 (20 oz)	300	4	0	0	70	2	120
Low Fat Youth Fountain	1 (20 oz)	267	3	tr	0	65	5	40
Malts	1 (20 oz)	887	17	41	166	119	tr	370
Mo'cuccino	1 (20 oz)	420	9	12	75	71	1	190
Peanut Power	1 (20 oz)	502	15	21	2	72	4	88
Peanut Power Plus Grape	1 (20 oz)	703	16	21	2	119	4	87
Peanut Power Plus Strawberry	1 (20 oz)	632	15	21	2	104	5	87
Pina Colada Island	1 (20 oz)	550	16	11	5	102	6	300
Power Punch	1 (20 oz)	430	6	1	2	102	4	91
Power Punch Plus	1 (20 oz)	499	10	2	2	113	4	91
Shakes	1 (20 oz)	875	16	41	166	117	0	359
Slim-N-Trim Chocolate	1 (20 oz)	270	12	2	4	55	3	261
Slim-N-Trim Orange Vanilla	1 (20 oz)	199	5	1	0	43	1	150

FOOD	PORTION	CALS	PROT	FAT	CHOL	CARB	FIBER	SOD
Slim-N-Trim Strawberry	1 (20 oz)	357	7	1	2	79	3	149
Slim-N-Trim Vanilla	1 (20 oz)	227	6	1	2	51	2	150
Super Punch	1 (20 oz)	425	2	tr	0	95	6	179
Super Punch Plus	1 (20 oz)	516	2	tr	0	118	6	195
The Hulk Chocolate	1 (20 oz)	846	23	29	102	129	6	626
The Hulk Strawberry	1 (20 oz)	953	24	29	102	156	6	645
The Hulk Vanilla	1 (20 oz)	846	23	29	102	129	5	646
Yogurt D-Lite	1 (20 oz)	335	17	4	43	58	0	271

SONIC DRIVE-IN
ADD-ONS

FOOD	PORTION	CALS	PROT	FAT	CHOL	CARB	FIBER	SOD
Bacon	1 serv (0.5 oz)	80	5	7	15	0	0	330
Cheddar Cheese Shredded	1 serv (1 oz)	104	6	9	28	1	0	491
Cheese	1 serv (0.7 oz)	70	4	6	15	1	0	350
Chili	1 serv (1 oz)	52	2	4	8	1	0	59
Cone Coat Chocolate	1 serv (1 oz)	143	1	8	0	16	1	40
Green Chilies	1 serv (1 oz)	10	0	0	0	3	0	24
Hickory Barbecue Sauce	1 serv (1 oz)	41	–	0	–	10	–	429
Honey Mustard Dressing	1 serv (1.1 oz)	110	0	9	10	9	0	300
Jalapenos Nachos Sliced	1 serv (1 oz)	5	0	0	0	1	1	302
Malt	1 serv (1 oz)	104	4	1	0	22	–	23
Maraschino Cherry	1 serv (8 g)	10	0	0	0	3	0	0
Marinara Sauce	1 serv (1 oz)	15	0	0	0	3	1	260
Ranch Dressing	1 serv (1 oz)	147	0	16	5	2	0	215
Slaw	1 serv (0.9 oz)	45	0	3	0	4	1	45
Sweet Pickle Relish	1 serv (1.1 oz)	40	0	0	0	11	0	248
Syrup Blue Coconut	1 serv (1 oz)	65	0	0	0	16	0	23
Syrup Cherry	1 serv (1 oz)	64	0	0	0	16	0	0
Syrup Chocolate	1 serv (1 oz)	74	0	0	0	16	0	52

FOOD	PORTION	CALS	PROT	FAT	CHOL	CARB	FIBER	SOD
Syrup Grape	1 serv (1 oz)	63	0	0	0	16	0	19
Syrup Vanilla	1 serv (1 oz)	61	0	0	0	15	0	0
Syrup Watermelon	1 serv (1 oz)	71	0	0	0	18	0	28
Thousand Island Dressing	1 serv (1 oz)	150	0	15	10	3	0	170
Topping Pineapple	1 serv (1.5 oz)	108	0	0	0	28	0	27
Topping Strawberry	1 serv (1 oz)	101	1	4	0	16	0	39
Topping Strawberry	1 serv (1.2 oz)	38	0	0	0	10	1	0
BEVERAGES								
Barq's Root Beer	1 sm	160	0	0	0	43	0	35
Barq's Root Beer	1 lg	333	0	0	0	90	0	72
Coca-Cola	1 lg	291	0	0	0	81	0	27
Coca-Cola	1 sm	139	0	0	0	39	0	13
Diet Coca-Cola	1 lg	3	0	0	0	0	0	12
Diet Coca-Cola	1 sm	1	0	0	0	0	0	6
Diet Sprite	1 lg	8	0	0	0	0	0	0
Diet Sprite	1 sm	4	0	0	0	0	0	0
Dr Pepper	1 sm	144	0	0	0	39	0	50
Dr Pepper	1 lg	300	0	0	0	81	0	105
Float Or Flurry Blue Coconut Slush	1 reg	424	61	12	30	57	0	255
Limeade	1 lg	303	0	0	0	83	2	69
Limeade	1 sm	143	0	0	0	39	1	33
Limeade Cherry	1 lg	361	0	0	0	98	2	69
Limeade Cherry	1 sm	169	0	0	0	46	1	33
Limeade Strawberry	1 lg	341	0	0	0	93	2	69
Limeade Strawberry	1 sm	172	0	0	0	47	1	33
Slush Blue Coconut	1 lg	521	0	0	0	134	0	27
Slush Watermelon	1 lg	526	0	0	0	136	0	31
Sprite	1 sm	138	0	0	0	37	0	33
Sprite	1 lg	288	0	0	0	78	0	69
BREAKFAST SELECTIONS								
Breakfast Burrito	1	731	29	47	167	47	3	1535
Fruit Taquitos	1 serv	302	6	7	0	51	3	300
Sunrise	1 lg	368	0	0	0	100	2	72
Sunrise	1 reg	224	0	0	0	60	1	41

FOOD	PORTION	CALS	PROT	FAT	CHOL	CARB	FIBER	SOD
Toaster Bacon Egg & Cheese	1	500	28	20	156	40	2	1698
Toaster Ham Egg & Cheese	1	436	33	19	174	41	2	2079
Toaster Sausage Egg & Cheese	1	570	24	36	126	44	2	100
DESSERTS								
Banana Split	1 serv	467	6	11	23	75	3	224
Chocolate Covered Shake Banana	1 reg	625	10	25	46	66	2	383
Chocolate Covered Shake Cherry	1 reg	587	10	24	46	59	1	383
Chocolate Covered Shake Peanut Butter	1 reg	678	12	34	46	57	1	469
Chocolate Covered Shake Strawberry	1 reg	608	10	24	46	64	1	383
Cream Pie Shake Banana	1 reg	775	12	27	47	92	2	474
Cream Pie Shake Chocolate	1 reg	795	12	27	47	96	1	525
Cream Pie Shake Coconut	1 reg	721	11	26	47	79	1	474
Dish Of Vanilla	1 serv	265	5	11	26	24	0	212
Float Or Flurry Cherry Slush	1 reg	421	6	12	30	57	0	249
Float Or Flurry Coca-Cola	1 reg	379	6	12	30	47	0	246
Float Or Flurry Dr Pepper	1 reg	377	6	12	30	47	0	268
Float Or Flurry Grape Slush	1 reg	423	6	12	30	57	0	253
Float Or Flurry Orange Slush	1 reg	422	6	12	30	56	0	244
Float Or Flurry Rootbeer	1 reg	386	6	12	30	50	0	260
Float Or Flurry Watermelon Slush	1 reg	427	6	12	30	56	0	258
Ice Cream Cone	1	285	6	11	26	24	0	223

FOOD	PORTION	CALS	PROT	FAT	CHOL	CARB	FIBER	SOD
Shake Banana	1 reg	508	10	18	45	52	1	363
Shake Chocolate	1 reg	564	10	18	45	64	0	440
Shake Pineapple	1 reg	615	9	18	45	83	1	403
Shake Strawberry	1 reg	510	9	18	45	54	1	363
Shake Vanilla	1 reg	454	9	18	45	41	0	363
Sonic Blast Butterfinger	1 reg	636	13	26	46	59	1	436
Sonic Blast M&M	1 reg	641	11	27	50	64	1	387
Sonic Blast Oreo	1 reg	638	11	27	45	57	1	602
Sonic Blast Reese's	1 reg	658	13	30	47	56	1	478
Sundae Chocolate	1 serv	362	6	11	26	45	0	270
Sundae Hot Fudge	1 serv	392	6	15	27	44	0	255
Sundae Pineapple	1 serv	399	5	11	26	58	0	242
Sundae Strawberry	1 serv	322	6	11	26	37	1	213
MAIN MENU SELECTIONS								
Ched'R'Peppers	1 serv	256	8	12	28	29	4	1056
Cheese Fries	1 lg	322	7	19	15	31	5	1108
Cheese Fries	1 reg	265	6	17	15	23	4	998
Cheese Tater Tots	1 reg	329	4	22	15	28	3	1396
Cheese Tots	1 lg	435	4	27	15	41	4	1708
Chicken Strip Dinner	1 serv	749	32	32	47	86	5	1973
Chicken Strip Snack	1 serv	272	19	13	35	22	0	760
Chicken Strips	2	184	13	9	23	15	0	507
Chili Cheese Fries	1 lg	357	8	22	22	32	5	1062
Chili Cheese Fries	1 reg	299	8	19	22	24	4	952
Chili Cheese Tater Tots	1 reg	363	5	25	22	28	3	1350
Chili Cheese Tots	1 lg	547	9	36	37	43	5	1844
Corn Dog	1	262	6	17	15	23	1	480
Extra Long Coney Cheese	1	666	23	42	87	47	2	1648
Extra Long Coney Plain	1	483	14	27	50	44	1	1182
French Fries	1 lg	252	3	13	0	30	5	758
French Fries	1 reg	195	2	11	0	22	4	648
Fritos Chili Pie	1 serv	611	18	44	53	36	36	816
Hot Dog Plain	1	262	8	16	30	22	1	657
Jr. Burger	1	353	14	21	45	27	1	1294
Mozzarella Sticks	1 serv	382	20	19	50	35	0	1300

FOOD	PORTION	CALS	PROT	FAT	CHOL	CARB	FIBER	SOD
No.1 Hamburger	1	577	14	36	37	43	2	753
No.1 Sonic Cheeseburger	1	647	18	42	52	44	2	1103
No.2 Hamburger	1	481	14	25	29	43	2	761
No.2 Sonic Cheeseburger	1	551	18	31	44	44	2	1111
Onion Rings	1 reg	331	8	23	0	66	7	311
Onion Rings	1 lg	507	12	35	0	102	10	486
Regular Coney Cheese	1	366	13	24	52	24	1	962
Regular Coney Plain	1	262	8	16	30	22	1	657
Sandwich Breaded Chicken	1	582	28	23	53	66	2	427
Sandwich Country Fried Steak	1	748	24	47	60	56	2	804
Sandwich Grilled Chicken	1	343	27	13	70	31	2	829
Super Sonic No.1	1	929	28	66	964	45	2	1476
Super Sonic No.2	1	839	28	56	88	46	3	1571
SuperSonic Onion Rings	1 serv	706	16	10	1	141	11	788
SuperSonic Tots	1 serv	485	0	28	0	53	5	1570
SuperSonic Fries	1 serv	358	5	18	0	44	7	963
Tater Tots	1 reg	259	0	16	0	27	3	1046
Tater Tots	1 lg	365	0	21	0	40	4	1358
Toaster Sandwich Bacon Cheddar Burger	1	675	26	38	59	60	4	1786
Toaster Sandwich BLT	1	581	19	41	47	42	3	1307
Toaster Sandwich Chicken Club	1	675	39	29	85	75	3	1458
Toaster Sandwich Country Fried Steak	1	708	26	45	60	55	3	944
Toaster Sandwich Grilled Cheese	1	282	12	12	15	39	2	830
Wrap Chicken Strip	1	574	20	29	28	55	2	1071

FOOD	PORTION	CALS	PROT	FAT	CHOL	CARB	FIBER	SOD
Wrap Grilled Chicken	1	539	29	27	70	40	2	1035
Wrap w/o Ranch Chicken Strip	1	428	20	13	23	53	2	856
Wrap w/o Ranch Grilled Chicken	1	393	29	12	65	38	2	820

SOUPLANTATION
BREADS AND MUFFINS

FOOD	PORTION	CALS	PROT	FAT	CHOL	CARB	FIBER	SOD
Bread Low Fat Sourdough	1 slice	150	9	1	0	27	0	240
Breads Indian Grain Low Fat	1 slice	200	11	2	15	35	0	260
Cornbread Buttermilk Low Fat	1 piece	140	3	2	10	27	2	270
Focaccia Big Hearth Pizza	1	140	5	6	10	16	1	220
Focaccia Bruschetta	1 piece	130	4	6	5	15	1	260
Focaccia Pepperoni	1 piece	160	5	7	15	19	1	340
Focaccia Roasted Potato	1 piece	150	6	6	10	17	2	220
Focaccia Sauteed Vegetables	1 piece	150	3	7	10	18	1	230
Focaccia Tomatillo	1 piece	140	5	6	10	16	1	270
Focaccia Low Fat Garlic Parmesan	1 piece	100	2	3	0	15	1	170
Muffin Apple Cinnamon Bran 96% Fat Free	1	80	2	1	0	17	1	110
Muffin Apple Raisin	1	150	2	7	10	22	1	190
Muffin Banana Nut	1	150	2	7	10	22	1	190
Muffin Big Blue Blueberry	1	310	5	12	20	46	2	380
Muffin Black Forest	1	230	2	9	10	36	1	190
Muffin Cappuccino Chip	1	160	3	4	25	28	1	160
Muffin Caribbean Key Lime	1	170	2	6	10	28	1	210
Muffin Cherry Nut	1	150	2	7	10	22	1	190

FOOD	PORTION	CALS	PROT	FAT	CHOL	CARB	FIBER	SOD
Muffin Chocolate Brownie	1	170	3	8	10	22	1	190
Muffin Chocolate Chip	1	170	3	8	10	22	1	190
Muffin Country Blackberry	1	170	2	6	15	27	1	190
Muffin French Quarter Praline	1	290	4	15	20	38	2	100
Muffin Georgia Peach Poppyseed	1	150	2	6	10	20	1	210
Muffin Lemon	1	140	2	4	10	24	1	190
Muffin Macadamia Nut Spice	1	220	3	9	20	33	1	260
Muffin Maple Walnut	1	230	3	10	5	33	1	230
Muffin Nutty Peanut Butter	1	170	4	8	10	21	1	210
Muffin Pumpkin Raisin	1 piece	150	2	6	10	25	1	210
Muffin Strawberry Buttermilk	1	140	2	6	10	21	1	210
Muffin Sweet Orange & Cranberry	1	200	2	7	5	33	1	220
Muffin Taffy Apple	1	160	2	6	10	25	1	190
Muffin Tropical Papaya Coconut	1	180	2	7	10	28	1	210
Muffin Zucchini Nut	1	150	2	7	10	22	1	190
Muffin 96% Fat Free Cranberry Orange Bran	1	80	2	1	0	17	1	110
Muffin 96% Fat Free Fruit Medley Bran	1	80	2	1	0	17	1	110
Muffin Low Fat Chile Corn	1	140	3	3	10	27	2	320
DESSERTS								
Cobbler Apple	½ cup	350	2	10	0	64	1	160
Cobbler Blissful Blueberry	½ cup	380	3	10	0	70	3	230
Cobbler Cherry	½ cup	340	2	10	0	61	2	180

FOOD	PORTION	CALS	PROT	FAT	CHOL	CARB	FIBER	SOD
Cobbler Cranberry Apple	½ cup	370	3	10	0	58	3	210
Cobbler Peach	½ cup	360	2	10	0	65	2	220
Cookie Chocolate Chip	1 sm	70	1	3	5	10	0	90
Fat Free Apple Medley	½ cup	70	1	0	0	18	1	5
Fat Free Banana Royale	½ cup	80	1	0	0	20	1	5
Fat Free Frozen Yogurt Chocolate	½ cup	95	3	0	0	21	0	80
Jello Fat Free All Flavors	½ cup	80	1	0	0	20	0	40
Jello Fat Free Sugar Free All Flavors	½ cup	10	1	0	0	0	0	10
Pudding Banana	½ cup	160	4	4	10	27	1	220
Pudding Vanilla	½ cup	140	4	4	10	24	0	160
Pudding Low Fat Butterscotch	½ cup	140	4	3	10	24	0	160
Pudding Low Fat Chocolate	½ cup	140	4	3	10	23	0	220
Pudding Low Fat Rice	½ cup	110	3	2	10	20	1	50
Soft Serve Reduced Fat Vanilla	½ cup	140	3	4	20	22	0	70
Tapioca Low Fat	½ cup	140	4	3	10	24	0	160
MAIN MENU SELECTIONS								
Alfredo Broccoli w/ Basil	1 cup	380	12	17	40	45	1	790
Alfredo Fettuccine	1 cup	390	15	18	50	41	2	580
Alfredo Four Cheese	1 cup	390	19	13	30	50	3	690
Alfredo Roasted Garlic & Asiago	1 cup	330	13	11	25	45	2	650
Alfredo Roasted w/ Rosemary	1 cup	380	19	14	35	44	2	850
Alfredo Southwestern	1 cup	350	10	16	50	42	1	420
Beef Stroganoff	1 cup	340	9	21	75	28	2	590
Carbonara Pasta	1 cup	280	10	8	20	43	2	250

FOOD	PORTION	CALS	PROT	FAT	CHOL	CARB	FIBER	SOD
Chili Arizona	1 cup	220	14	8	20	25	7	690
Chili Longhorn Beef	1 cup	190	10	6	20	25	4	790
Chili Rock N' Mole	1 cup	240	7	13	25	22	5	690
Chili Santa Fe Black Bean Low Fat	1 cup	190	9	3	0	26	8	580
Chili Texas Red	1 cup	240	14	8	20	30	7	680
Chili Three Bean Turkey Low Fat	1 cup	140	9	3	20	19	5	560
Chili Vegetarian	1 cup	150	5	3	0	25	6	770
Chili Cheatin' Heart	1 cup	300	18	19	60	23	6	800
Chili Deep Kettle House Low Fat	1 cup	230	15	3	15	26	7	560
Creamy Herb Chicken	1 cup	310	8	17	80	32	2	360
Creamy Pepper Jack	1 cup	290	6	15	50	35	2	360
Garden Vegetable w/ Italian Sausage	1 cup	300	12	10	20	42	3	540
Garen Vegetable w/ Meatballs	1 cup	270	11	7	10	42	3	460
Greek Mediterranean	1 cup	290	10	8	15	45	2	520
Italian Vegetable Beef	1 cup	270	10	6	10	43	4	470
Italian Sausage w/ Red Pepper Puree	1 cup	250	6	10	45	35	2	380
Lemon Cream & Asparagus	1 cup	230	6	9	0	34	1	470
Linguini w/ Clam Sauce	1 cup	380	16	10	40	56	1	890
Low Fat Oriental Green Bean & Noodle	1 cup	240	7	3	0	45	2	780
Macaroni & Cheese	1 cup	260	10	6	15	40	2	480
Nutty Mushroom	1 cup	390	12	20	45	42	2	410
Pasta Florentine	1 cup	360	18	10	15	54	7	920
Penne Arrabbiatta	1 cup	340	18	10	20	43	3	710
Pesto Cilantro Lime	1 cup	370	9	21	20	36	2	760
Roasted Eggplant Marinara	1 cup	340	18	10	20	43	3	700

FOOD	PORTION	CALS	PROT	FAT	CHOL	CARB	FIBER	SOD
Smoked Salmon & Dill	1 cup	360	13	16	45	41	2	390
Tuscany Sausage w/ Capers & Olives	1 cup	240	10	10	15	29	2	920
Vegetable Ragu	1 cup	250	9	5	10	41	3	480
Vegetarian Marinara w/ Basil	1 cup	260	10	4	10	44	3	750
Walnut Pesto	1 cup	310	10	9	10	42	2	610
SALAD DRESSINGS								
Bacon	2 tbsp	120	1	11	0	5	0	320
Balsamic Vinaigrette	1 tbsp	180	0	19	0	1	0	190
Basil Vinaigrette	2 tbsp	160	0	17	0	1	0	160
Blue Cheese	1 tbsp	140	1	14	10	3	0	230
Creamy Italian	2 tbsp	120	0	13	10	1	0	300
Fat Free Honey Mustard	2 tbsp	45	0	0	10	10	0	160
Honey Mustard	2 tbsp	150	0	13	10	8	0	230
Italian Fat Free	2 tbsp	20	0	0	0	5	0	340
Kahlena French	2 tbsp	120	0	9	0	10	0	520
Parmesan Pepper Cream	2 tbsp	160	1	17	5	2	0	330
Ranch	2 tbsp	130	1	13	10	1	0	180
Ranch Fat Free	2 tbsp	50	1	0	0	2	0	180
Reduced Calorie Cucumber	2 tbsp	80	0	7	0	4	0	290
Roasted Garlic	2 tbsp	140	1	14	5	2	0	300
Thousand Island	2 tbsp	110	0	11	5	3	0	250
SALADS								
Ambrosia w/ Cocount	½ cup	170	1	6	5	30	2	80
Antipasto w/ Peppered Salami	1 cup	140	5	10	10	6	2	370
Artichoke Rice	¼ cup	160	3	8	3	21	2	780
Aunt Doris' Red Pepper Slaw Fat Free	½ cup	70	1	0	0	18	3	480
Baja Bean & Cilantro Low Fat	½ cup	180	9	3	0	29	5	190

FOOD	PORTION	CALS	PROT	FAT	CHOL	CARB	FIBER	SOD
Bartlett Pear & Walnut	1 cup	180	4	12	5	13	2	220
BBQ Julienne Chopped	1 cup	190	5	10	20	20	3	430
BBQ Smokehouse w/ Bacon & Peanuts	1 cup	190	6	10	10	19	3	530
Caesar Asiago	1 cup	190	5	14	10	10	1	280
California Cobb	1 cup	180	3	8	25	4	2	190
Carrot Ginger w/ Herb Vinaigrette	½ cup	150	1	12	0	9	3	40
Carrot Raisin Low Fat	½ cup	90	1	3	5	17	2	80
Chinese Krab	½ cup	160	5	8	3	19	3	260
Citrus Noodle w/ Snow Peas	½ cup	140	3	6	0	19	2	240
Country French w/ Bacon	1 cup	210	10	18	20	7	2	420
Ensalada Azteca	1 cup	130	6	9	15	7	4	230
Field Corn & Very Wild Rice	½ cup	170	4	9	0	19	3	420
Greek	1 cup	120	3	9	10	4	2	230
Greek Couscous w/ Feta	½ cup	170	6	9	4	19	3	480
Indian Summer Spinach	1 cup	200	6	15	15	11	6	220
Italian Garden Vegetable	½ cup	110	1	8	0	9	2	240
Italian Sub Salad w/ w/ Turkey & Salami	1 cup	260	9	17	20	18	2	470
Italian White Bean	½ cup	140	6	5	0	19	4	480
Joan's Blue BLT	1 cup	250	6	16	25	20	3	600
Joan's Broccoli Madness	½ cup	180	2	14	10	11	3	250
Lemon Rice w/ Cashews	½ cup	160	2	7	0	23	1	290
Mandarin Noodles w/ Broccoli Low Fat	½ cup	120	3	3	0	19	2	380

FOOD	PORTION	CALS	PROT	FAT	CHOL	CARB	FIBER	SOD
Mandarin Shells w/ Almonds	½ cup	120	3	3	0	19	2	360
Mandarin Spinach w/ Carmelized Walnuts	1 cup	170	3	11	0	14	3	150
Marinated Summer Vegetables Fat Free	½ cup	80	1	0	0	19	4	210
Mediterranean	1 cup	150	4	11	5	9	4	430
Monterey Blue w/ Peanuts	1 cup	200	3	12	5	20	2	330
Moroccan Marinated Vegetables Low Fat	½ cup	90	2	3	0	9	2	230
Old Fashioned Macaroni Salad w/ Ham	½ cup	180	4	11	10	15	3	360
Oriental Ginger Slaw w/ Krab Low Fat	½ cup	70	2	3	2	8	4	80
Penne w/ Chicken In Citrus Vinaigrette Low Fat	½ cup	130	5	3	5	20	2	380
Pesto Orzo w/ Pinenuts	1 cup	220	4	17	10	14	2	320
Pesto Pasta	½ cup	160	4	7	2	18	2	320
Pineapple Coconut Slaw	½ cup	150	1	10	15	14	2	190
Poppyseed Coleslaw	½ cup	120	1	9	10	9	3	130
Potato BBQ	½ cup	160	2	8	5	20	2	270
Potato Dijon w/ Garlic Dill Vinaigrette	½ cup	150	1	12	0	9	3	40
Potato German	½ cup	120	2	3	0	18	2	260
Potato Jalapeno	½ cup	140	2	5	0	20	2	490
Potato Picnic	½ cup	150	3	7	80	19	2	320
Potato Southern Dill Low Fat	½ cup	120	4	3	5	20	2	300
Ragin' Cajun	1 cup	200	7	14	15	12	2	450

FOOD	PORTION	CALS	PROT	FAT	CHOL	CARB	FIBER	SOD
Ranch House BLT Salad w/ Turkey	1 cup	180	6	11	15	10	6	390
Red Potato & Tomato	½ cup	120	2	10	5	8	3	540
Roasted Vegetables w/ Feta & Olives	1 cup	140	2	11	10	5	4	340
Roasted Potato Salad w/ Chipotle Chili Vinaigrette	½ cup	140	3	6	0	18	4	250
Roma Tomatoes Mozzarella & Basil	1 cup	120	4	9	10	7	1	180
San Francisco Herb Rice	½ cup	170	4	5	5	25	1	380
Shrimp & Seafood	½ cup	200	5	11	20	20	2	380
Smoked Turkey & Spinach w/ Almonds	1 cup	190	6	10	15	20	2	480
Sonoma Spinach w/ Honey Dijon Vinaigrette	1 cup	210	5	14	10	16	2	270
Southern Black Eyed Pea	½ cup	130	2	6	0	18	3	220
Southwestern Rice & Beans	½ cup	90	1	3	0	15	3	480
Spiced Pecans & Roasted Vegetables	1 cup	180	5	11	15	15	2	390
Spicy Southwestern Pasta Low Fat	½ cup	130	5	3	0	21	4	350
Spinach Gorgonzola w/ Spiced Pecans	1 cup	210	5	19	10	5	4	430
Strawberry Fields w/ Caramelized Walnuts	1 cup	130	3	8	0	15	3	75
Summer Barley w/ Black Beans Low Fat	½ cup	110	4	3	0	19	4	280
Summer Lemon w/ Spiced Pecans	1 cup	220	2	15	10	18	2	250

FOOD	PORTION	CALS	PROT	FAT	CHOL	CARB	FIBER	SOD
Thai Noodle w/ Peanut Sauce	½ cup	170	5	8	0	17	3	310
Three Bean Marinade	½ cup	170	4	6	0	27	3	320
Tomato Cucumber Marinade	½ cup	80	0	5	0	8	1	220
Traditional Spinach w/ Bacon	1 cup	160	5	11	40	7	3	310
Tuna Tarragon	½ cup	240	6	14	10	21	3	480
Turkey Chutney Pasta	½ cup	230	14	9	30	21	2	310
Watercress & Orange	1 cup	90	1	4	0	12	2	90
Wild Rice & Chicken	½ cup	300	5	22	20	20	1	490
Won Ton Chicken Happiness	1 cup	150	6	8	10	12	2	220
Zesty Tortellini	½ cup	190	4	15	10	18	2	460
SOUPS								
Albino Bean Chicken	1 cup	190	14	6	40	18	4	990
Albondigas Locas	1 cup	210	10	10	30	19	2	860
Autumn Root Vegetable w/ Wild Rice	1 cup	80	1	0	0	18	2	970
Baked Potato & Cheese w/ Bacon	1 cup	290	11	18	50	22	2	670
Be Wild With Mushroom	1 cup	220	4	16	50	14	2	830
Big Chunk Chicken Noodle Low Fat	1 cup	160	15	3	20	17	2	480
Black Bean Sausage Fling	1 cup	350	14	23	60	21	5	1900
Black Bean & Chorizo	1 cup	230	11	9	15	27	6	830
Bombay Lentil Low Fat	1 cup	160	8	3	0	25	9	880
Broc On	1 cup	220	3	18	60	13	2	930
Broccoli Cheese	1 cup	280	11	20	50	15	2	810
Butternut Squash	1 cup	140	3	6	17	15	4	670

FOOD	PORTION	CALS	PROT	FAT	CHOL	CARB	FIBER	SOD
Cheese Stuffed Cappelletti	1 cup	130	5	4	10	20	1	1580
Chesapeake Corn Chowder	1 cup	280	7	16	35	30	2	750
Chicken Got Smoked	1 cup	350	11	21	85	28	2	750
Chicken Tortilla w/ Jalapeno Chiles & Tomatoes Low Fat	1 cup	100	12	3	20	5	1	990
Chunky Potato Cheese w/ Thyme	1 cup	210	10	10	30	19	2	480
Classical French Onion	1 cup	130	2	5	5	16	2	1280
Classical Minestrone Low Fat	1 cup	120	4	2	0	20	3	510
Classical Shrimp Bisque	1 cup	240	9	16	70	15	1	230
Country Corn & Red Potato Chowder	1 cup	160	3	6	15	24	4	330
Cream Of Broccoli	1 cup	210	4	15	25	14	7	960
Cream of Mushroom	1 cup	290	10	21	30	15	2	820
Cream Of Rosemary Potato	1 cup	270	3	19	50	22	2	790
Cream Of Chicken	1 cup	260	8	18	55	17	1	770
Creamy Vegetable Chowder	1 cup	200	6	10	20	23	3	610
Devotion To The Ocean	1 cup	220	13	12	100	14	2	800
El Paso Lime & Chicken	1 cup	160	7	4	15	24	2	1250
Field Of Creams Cauliflower w/ Cheese	1 cup	260	5	20	40	15	1	990
Field Of Creams Celery	1 cup	210	2	15	30	15	2	800
Field Of Creams Spinach	1 cup	280	4	22	45	18	2	950
Field Of Creams Tomato Basil	1 cup	220	3	15	30	20	2	990

FOOD	PORTION	CALS	PROT	FAT	CHOL	CARB	FIBER	SOD
Fire Roasted Green Chili & Corn Chowder	1 cup	230	5	14	25	21	1	670
Garden Fresh Vegetable Low Fat	1 cup	110	4	1	0	22	4	890
Garlic Kickin Roasted Chicken	1 cup	140	10	6	30	10	3	310
Hungarian Vegetable Low Fat	1 cup	120	2	2	0	20	2	520
Irish Potato Leek	1 cup	250	5	15	35	23	1	940
Living On The Veg	1 cup	90	2	1	0	15	3	380
Manhattan Clam Chowder	1 cup	130	7	4	20	16	2	990
Mulligatawny	1 cup	210	8	12	40	18	2	690
Navy Bean w/ Ham	1 cup	340	35	10	40	30	6	980
Neighbor Joe's Gumbo	1 cup	280	14	8	50	36	3	850
Posole	1 cup	150	12	6	35	8	2	980
Ratatouille Provencale Fat Free	1 cup	110	2	0	0	25	2	600
Roasted Mushroom w/ Sage	1 cup	320	5	25	50	20	1	910
Spicy Sausage & Pasta	1 cup	310	15	12	30	36	5	1270
Split Pea w/ Ham	1 cup	350	36	10	40	32	6	980
Tomato Chipolte Bisque	1 cup	240	5	16	40	21	2	1140
Tomato Parmesan & Vegetables Low Fat	1 cup	120	4	3	5	18	3	460
Toot Your Horn For Crab & Corn	1 cup	290	10	20	90	18	2	750
Vegetarian Lentils & Brown Rice Low Fat	1 cup	130	6	1	0	25	6	740
Yankee Clipper Clam Chowder w/ Bacon	1 cup	330	18	20	80	21	2	630

FOOD	PORTION	CALS	PROT	FAT	CHOL	CARB	FIBER	SOD

STARBUCKS
BAKED SELECTIONS

FOOD	PORTION	CALS	PROT	FAT	CHOL	CARB	FIBER	SOD
Baby Bundt Cake Chocolate	1	330	5	15	25	45	4	380
Bagel	1	430	15	1	0	92	3	660
Bagel Cinnamon Raisin	1	440	13	1	0	96	3	570
Bagel Sesame	1	440	16	3	0	92	6	630
Bar Caramel Apple	1	310	3	16	40	38	2	150
Bar Carrot Cake	1	420	4	25	85	46	tr	440
Bar Lemon	1	310	4	14	140	44	0	130
Bar Oreo Dream	1	420	5	30	65	33	2	200
Bar Toffee Crunch	1	430	4	21	50	56	1	420
Biscotti Chocolate Hazelnut	1	110	2	5	25	15	1	80
Biscotti Vanilla Almond	1	110	2	5	25	15	1	75
Brownie Caramel	1	580	5	36	100	60	2	230
Brownie Enrobed Espresso	1	430	5	25	75	48	3	140
Brownie Espresso	1	370	4	21	85	43	2	115
Brownie Milk Chocolate Peanut Butter	1	460	6	29	50	45	2	170
Bundt Cake Lemon Yogurt	1 serv	350	4	13	55	56	tr	250
Caramel Pecan Sticky Roll	1	730	10	40	40	75	7	860
Cinnamon Roll	1	620	9	29	45	80	3	740
Cinnamon Twist	1	320	5	17	25	37	1	280
Coffee Cake	1 serv	570	7	28	75	75	2	310
Coffee Cake Apple Walnut	1 serv	320	4	17	55	41	1	330
Coffee Cake Blueberry Walnut	1 serv	340	4	18	60	43	1	360
Coffee Cake Cinnamon Walnut	1 serv	360	4	18	65	46	1	390
Coffee Cake Crumble Berry	1 serv	520	6	26	75	69	2	350

FOOD	PORTION	CALS	PROT	FAT	CHOL	CARB	FIBER	SOD
Coffee Cake Hazelnut	1 serv	630	9	35	125	74	2	460
Coffee Cake Sour Cream	1 serv	420	5	25	95	43	1	260
Cookie Black And White	1	430	4	17	50	68	2	210
Cookie Double Chocolate Chunk	1 serv	430	5	21	15	58	3	350
Cookie Oatmeal Raisin	1	390	6	15	15	65	3	340
Cookie White Chocolate Macadamia Nut	1	470	6	27	15	54	2	350
Crisp Cinnamon Twist	1	60	0	2	0	9	0	25
Croissant Almond	1	330	6	18	30	39	2	230
Croissant Butter w/ Apricot Glaze	1	320	5	17	25	37	1	280
Croissant Raspberry & Cream Cheese	1	260	4	12	30	34	1	270
Crumb Cake	1 serv	670	8	32	115	89	1	360
Crumb Cake Key Lime	1 serv	550	8	27	190	71	1	370
Danish Apple w/ Mocha Swirls	1	370	5	19	25	44	2	330
Danish Cheese w/ Mocha Swirls	1	460	7	28	50	44	1	400
Danish Raspberry w/ Mocha Swirls	1	370	5	19	25	45	1	380
Graham Dark Chocolate	1	140	2	8	<5	17	tr	60
Graham Milk Chocolate	1	140	2	8	<5	17	tr	60
Madeline	1	80	1	4	25	11	0	30
Muffin Blueberry	1	380	5	19	70	49	1	380
Muffin Chocolate Cream Cheese	1	450	5	24	80	53	1	420

FOOD	PORTION	CALS	PROT	FAT	CHOL	CARB	FIBER	SOD
Muffin Cranberry Orange	1	410	5	20	70	53	2	400
Muffin Morning Sunrise	1	330	5	12	35	54	2	550
Pound Cake Banana	1 serv	360	4	18	100	47	1	380
Pound Cake Cranberry Walnut	1 serv	390	6	21	110	45	1	310
Pound Cake Iced Carrot	1 serv	540	5	13	35	101	3	320
Pound Cake Iced Lemon	1 serv	500	6	23	145	69	tr	390
Pound Cake Marble	1 serv	400	6	21	130	49	tr	370
Pound Cake Orange Poppy	1 serv	490	8	27	140	55	2	380
Pound Cake Pumpkin	1 serv	310	5	12	65	47	2	360
Pound Cake Zucchini	1 serv	370	5	19	55	47	2	250
Pullman Banana	1 serv	400	5	17	65	57	2	320
Pullman Chocolate	1	380	5	17	55	54	2	270
Pullman Cranberry Walnut	1	360	5	15	25	53	2	240
Pullman Lemon Glazed	1	370	5	15	90	55	tr	180
Pullman Marble Chocolate Chip	1	440	6	20	95	61	1	250
Pullman Orange Poppy Cheese	1	450	7	22	110	55	1	290
Pullman Pumpkin	1	370	4	17	60	51	2	340
Scone Blueberry	1	460	5	18	50	68	3	400
Scone Butterscotch Pecan	1	520	7	27	50	64	2	390
Scone Cinnamon Chip w/ Icing	1	510	6	23	50	71	2	480
Scone Maple Oat w/ Icing	1	490	7	22	45	69	2	430
Scone Apricot Currant	1	450	7	17	60	67	3	360
Scone Raspberry	1	440	7	18	50	65	2	360

FOOD	PORTION	CALS	PROT	FAT	CHOL	CARB	FIBER	SOD
Shortbread	1	100	1	6	15	12	0	65
BEVERAGES								
Apple Juice	1 grande	230	0	0	0	57	0	20
Blended Coffee Of The Week	1 grande	10	0	0	0	2	0	0
Cafe Americano	1 grande	150	1	0	0	3	0	15
Cafe Au Lait Nonfat Milk	1 grande	90	9	0	<5	13	0	120
Cafe Au Lait Soy Milk	1 grande	110	6	3	0	15	tr	90
Cafe Latte Whole Milk	1 grande	260	14	14	55	21	0	200
Cafe Misto Cafe Au Lait Whole Milk	1 grande	140	8	8	30	11	0	115
Cafe Mocha Whip Whole Milk	1 grande	400	13	22	80	42	2	160
Caffe Latte Soy Milk	1 grande	210	11	6	0	28	2	160
Caffe Mocha No Whip Whole Milk	1 grande	300	13	12	40	41	2	150
Caffe Mocha No Whip Nonfat Milk	1 grande	230	14	2	5	43	2	160
Caffe Mocha No Whip Soy Milk	1 grande	260	10	6	0	46	3	120
Caffe Mocha Whip Nonfat Milk	1 grande	330	14	12	45	44	2	170
Caffe Mocha Whip Soy Milk	1 grande	360	10	16	40	48	3	125
Caffee Latte Nonfat Milk	1 grande	160	16	0	10	24	0	220
Cappuccino Nonfat Milk	1 grande	100	9	0	<5	14	0	125
Cappucino Soy Milk	1 grande	120	6	3	0	17	tr	90
Caramel Mocha No Whip Soy Milk	1 grande	340	10	6	0	66	3	120
Caramel Macchiato Nonfat Milk	1 grande	230	14	2	15	40	0	200
Caramel Macchiato Soy Milk	1 grande	300	9	8	5	49	1	160

FOOD	PORTION	CALS	PROT	FAT	CHOL	CARB	FIBER	SOD
Caramel Macchiato Whole Milk	1 grande	320	12	14	55	37	0	190
Caramel Mocha Whip Soy Milk	1 grande	440	10	16	40	68	3	125
Caramel Apple Cider No Whip	1 grande	300	0	0	0	72	0	15
Caramel Apple Cider Whip	1 grande	410	0	10	40	76	0	30
Caramel Mocha No Whip Whole Milk	1 grande	370	13	11	35	61	2	140
Caramel Mocha Whip Nonfat Milk	1 grande	410	14	12	45	65	2	160
Caramel Mocha Whip Whole Milk	1 grande	470	13	21	75	63	2	150
Caramel Mocha Whip Nonfat Milk	1 grande	300	14	3	5	63	2	150
Chocolate Nonfat Milk	1 grande	240	16	2	10	45	2	200
Chocolate Whole Milk	1 grande	340	15	15	50	42	2	—
Cinnamon Spice Mocha No Whip Nonfat Milk	1 grande	250	14	1	5	47	tr	180
Cinnamon Spice Mocha No Whip Whole Milk	1 grande	330	13	12	45	45	tr	170
Cinnamon Spice Mocha Whip Nonfat Milk	1 grande	350	14	11	45	49	tr	190
Cinnamon Spice Mocha Whip Milk	1 grande	430	13	22	85	47	tr	180
Cinnamon Spice No Whip Soy Milk	1 grande	290	10	6	0	51	2	130
Cinnamon Spice Whip Soy Milk	1 grande	390	10	15	40	53	2	140
Espresso Decaf Coffee Of The Week	1 grande	10	0	0	0	2	0	0

FOOD	PORTION	CALS	PROT	FAT	CHOL	CARB	FIBER	SOD
Frappuccino Blended Coffee	1 grande	230	5	3	10	46	0	220
Frappuccino Blended Coffee Mocha Coconut Whip Whole Milk	1 grande	400	7	10	15	75	2	310
Frappuccino Caramel Blended Coffee No Whip	1 grande	280	5	4	15	57	0	250
Frappuccino Caramel Blended Coffee Whip	1 grande	430	6	16	65	61	0	270
Frappuccino Chocolate Blended Creme Whip	1 grande	530	18	19	55	75	1	420
Frappuccino Chocolate Blended Creme No Whip	1 grande	400	18	7	<5	73	1	410
Frappuccino Chocolate Brownie Blended Coffee No Whip	1 grande	370	7	9	15	69	2	310
Frappuccino Chocolate Brownie Blended Coffee Whip	1 grande	510	7	22	65	72	2	320
Frappuccino Chocolate Malt Blended Creme No Whip	1 grande	470	15	10	15	87	2	420
Frappuccino Chocolate Malt Blended Creme Whip	1 grande	610	15	22	65	90	2	430
Frappuccino Mocha Blended Coffee No Whip	1 grande	290	6	4	15	58	0	250
Frappuccino Mocha Blended Coffee Whip	1 grande	420	6	16	65	61	0	260

FOOD	PORTION	CALS	PROT	FAT	CHOL	CARB	FIBER	SOD
Frappuccino Mocha Coconut Blended Coffee Whip	1 grande	550	7	22	65	80	2	320
Frappuccino Mocha Malt Blended Coffee No Whip	1 grande	430	14	7	20	91	1	390
Frappuccino Mocha Malt Blended Coffee Whip	1 grande	570	14	20	75	95	1	400
Frappuccino Tazo Chai Creme Blended Tea No Whip	1 grande	370	15	5	<5	69	0	370
Frappuccino Tazo Chai Creme Blended Tea Whip	1 grande	500	15	17	55	72	0	380
Frappuccino Tazoberry Blended Tea	1 grande	190	tr	0	0	49	tr	40
Frappuccino Tazoberry Creme Blended Tea No Whip	1 grande	330	6	2	0	74	tr	180
Frappuccino Tazoberry Creme Blended Tea Whip	1 grande	460	6	14	50	76	tr	190
Frappuccino Vanilla Blended Creme No Whip	1 grande	350	15	5	<5	64	0	370
Frappuccino Vanilla Blended Creme Whip	1 grande	480	15	17	55	66	0	380
Frappuccino White Chocolate Mocha Blended Coffee No Whip	1 grande	320	6	5	15	62	0	280

FOOD	PORTION	CALS	PROT	FAT	CHOL	CARB	FIBER	SOD
Frappuccino White Chocolate Mocha Blended Coffee Whip	1 grande	450	6	17	65	65	0	290
Hot Chocolate No Whip Whole Milk	1 grande	340	15	15	50	42	2	190
Hot Chocolate No Whip Nonfat Milk	1 grande	240	16	2	10	45	2	200
Hot Chocolate Whip Nonfat Milk	1 grande	340	16	12	45	47	2	210
Hot Chocolate Whip Whole Milk	1 grande	440	15	24	90	44	2	200
Ice Caffe Mocha Whip Milk	1 grande	350	9	20	75	37	2	105
Iced Cafe Latte Whole Milk	1 grande	160	8	8	30	13	0	120
Iced Cafe Mocha Whip Nonfat Milk	1 grande	310	9	14	55	38	2	110
Iced Cafe Mocha Whip Soy Milk	1 grande	330	7	17	50	40	3	85
Iced Caffe Americano	1 grande	20	1	0	0	3	0	15
Iced Caffe Mocha No Whip Whole Milk	1 grande	220	9	8	25	35	2	95
Iced Caffe Latte Nonfat Milk	1 grande	100	9	0	<5	14	0	130
Iced Caffe Latte Soy Milk	1 grande	120	6	5	0	17	tr	95
Iced Caffe Mocha No Whip Nonfat Milk	1 grande	180	9	2	<5	36	2	100
Iced Caffe Mocha No Whip Soy Milk	1 grande	200	7	5	0	38	3	75
Iced Caramel Macchiato Nonfat Milk	1 grande	100	11	1	10	36	0	160

FOOD	PORTION	CALS	PROT	FAT	CHOL	CARB	FIBER	SOD
Iced Caramel Macchiato Soy Milk	1 grande	230	7	5	<5	39	1	120
Iced Caramel Macchiato Whole Milk	1 grande	270	10	10	40	34	0	150
Iced Shaken Coffee	1 grande	80	0	0	0	20	0	5
Iced Tazo Chai Nonfat Milk	1 grande	230	8	0	0	50	0	120
Iced Tazo Chai Whole Milk	1 grande	270	7	7	25	48	0	110
Iced White Chocolate Mocha No Whip Soy Milk	1 grande	340	9	8	<5	59	tr	190
Iced White Chocolate Mocha No Whip Whole Milk	1 grande	360	11	11	25	56	0	210
Iced White Chocolate Mocha Whip Nonfat Milk	1 grande	450	11	18	55	59	0	220
Iced White Chocolate Mocha Whip Soy Milk	1 grande	470	9	20	55	61	tr	200
Iced White Chocolate Mocha Whip Whole Milk	1 grande	490	11	24	75	58	0	220
Iced White Chocolate No Whip Nonfat Milk	1 grande	320	11	6	5	57	0	210
Milk Nonfat	1 grande	160	16	0	10	23	0	230
Steamed Apple Cider	1 grande	230	0	0	0	57	0	20
Steamed Nonfat Milk	1 grande	160	16	0	0	23	0	230
Steamed Whole Milk	1 grande	270	15	15	60	21	0	220
Tazo Chai Whole Milk	1 grande	290	8	7	30	50	0	120
Tazo Chai Nonfat Milk	1 grande	230	8	0	5	51	0	125

FOOD	PORTION	CALS	PROT	FAT	CHOL	CARB	FIBER	SOD
Tazo Iced Tea	1 grande	80	0	0	0	20	0	0
Tazo Tea Lemonade	1 grande	120	0	0	0	31	0	15
Vanilla Creme Whip Nonfat Milk	1 grande	340	16	9	50	44	0	230
Vanilla Creme Whip Whole Milk	1 grande	440	14	24	95	42	0	220
Vanilla Creme No Whip Nonfat Milk	1 grande	240	16	0	10	43	0	230
Vanille Creme No Whip Whole Milk	1 grande	340	14	14	60	40	0	210
White Chocolate Mocha No Whip Nonfat Milk	1 grande	340	16	5	10	58	0	260
White Chocolate Mocha No Whip Whole Milk	1 grande	410	14	15	45	56	0	250
White Chocolate Mocha Whip Nonfat Milk	1 grande	440	16	14	45	60	0	270
White Chocolate Mocha Whip Milk	1 grande	510	14	24	80	58	0	260
White Chocolate No Whip Soy Milk	1 grande	370	12	14	0	62	1	220
White Chocolate Whip Soy Milk	1 grande	440	13	15	20	65	1	250
White Hot Chocolate No Whip Nonfat Milk	1 grande	390	18	6	10	66	0	320
White Hot Chocolate No Whip Whole Milk	1 grande	480	17	18	55	63	0	300
White Hot Chocolate Whip Nonfat Milk	1 grande	490	18	15	50	68	0	330
White Hot Chocolate Whip Whole Milk	1 grande	580	17	28	95	65	0	310
Whole Milk	1 grande	270	15	15	60	21	0	220

FOOD	PORTION	CALS	PROT	FAT	CHOL	CARB	FIBER	SOD
TOPPINGS								
Caramel	1 tbsp	15	0	1	0	2	0	5
Chocolate	1 tsp	5	0	0	0	1	0	0
Flavored Sugar Free Syrup	1 pump	0	0	0	0	0	0	0
Flavored Syrup	1 pump	20	0	0	0	5	0	0
Mocha Syrup	1 pump	25	1	1	0	6	0	0
Sprinkles	1 serv	0	0	0	0	tr	0	0
STEAK ESCAPE								
BEVERAGES								
Coca-Cola	12 oz	110	0	0	0	29	—	10
Coca-Cola	44 oz	430	0	0	0	118	—	40
Diet Coke	44 oz	0	0	0	0	0	0	75
Diet Coke	12 oz	0	0	0	0	0	0	20
Hi-C Fruit Punch	44 oz	452	0	0	0	123	—	60
Hi-C Fruit Punch	12 oz	116	0	0	0	30	—	15
Lemonade	44 oz	488	0	0	0	130	—	2
Lemonade	12 oz	126	0	0	0	34	—	0
Sprite	44 oz	430	0	0	0	114	—	157
Sprite	12 oz	110	0	0	0	28	—	40
CHILDREN'S MENU SELECTIONS								
Kids Fries	1 serv	249	4	13	0	34	—	205
Kids Tenders	2 pieces	240	15	11	35	21	—	1050
Sandwich Chicken	1	205	12	7	32	32	—	470
Sandwich Ham	1	183	6	1	13	32	—	765
Sandwich Steak	1	210	9	3	13	31	—	445
Sandwich Turkey	1	183	6	1	13	32	—	765
MAIN MENU SELECTIONS								
12 Inch Sandwich Grand Cobbler	1	680	49	4	60	116	—	3094
12 Inch Sandwich Grand Escape	1	776	55	12	100	108	—	1590
12 Inch Sandwich Grandest Chicken	1	770	61	10	110	110	—	1914
12 Inch Sandwich Great Escape	1	776	55	12	100	108	—	1590
12 Inch Sandwich Hambrosia	1	684	47	4	60	119	—	3090

FOOD	PORTION	CALS	PROT	FAT	CHOL	CARB	FIBER	SOD
12 Inch Sandwich Ragin' Cajun	1	756	59	10	110	108	—	1965
12 Inch Sandwich Turkey Club	1	675	52	4	70	111	—	3430
12 Inch Sandwich Vegetarian	1	524	18	2	0	109	—	1053
12 Inch Sandwich Wild West BBQ	1	841	55	12	100	126	—	2092
7 Inch Sandwich Grand Cobbler	1	380	26	2	30	67	—	1842
7 Inch Sandwich Grand Escape	1	435	30	6	50	64	—	892
7 Inch Sandwich Grandest Chicken	1	425	32	5	55	64	—	1052
7 Inch Sandwich Great Escape	1	428	29	6	50	63	—	890
7 Inch Sandwich Hambrosia	1	382	25	2	30	69	—	1640
7 Inch Sandwich Ragin' Cajun	1	418	31	5	55	63	—	1107
7 Inch Sandwich Turkey Club	1	390	30	2	40	65	—	1980
7 Inch Sandwich Vegetarian	1	302	10	1	0	64	—	622
7 Inch Sandwich Wild West BBQ	1	469	29	6	50	72	—	1141
Fries	1 serv (12 oz)	498	8	26	0	67	—	409
Fries	1 serv (32 oz)	996	16	52	0	134	—	818
Fries Loaded Bacon & Cheddar	1 serv	905	18	44	29	88	—	1587
Fries Loaded Ranch & Bacon	1 serv	1044	18	71	39	84	—	1398
Smashed Potatoes Loaded Bacon & Cheddar	1 serv	636	13	26	24	91	—	827

FOOD	PORTION	CALS	PROT	FAT	CHOL	CARB	FIBER	SOD
Smashed Potatoes Loaded Ranch & Bacon	1 serv	692	14	34	29	87	—	501
Smashed Potatoes Plain	1 serv	246	11	0	0	53	—	43
Smashed Potatoes w/ Chicken	1 serv	318	33	4	55	56	—	475
Smashed Potatoes w/ Ham	1 serv	336	27	2	30	59	—	1065
Smashed Potatoes w/ Steak	1 serv	391	31	5	50	56	—	313
Smashed Potatoes w/ Turkey	1 serv	336	27	2	30	59	—	1065
SALAD DRESSINGS AND TOPPINGS								
American Cheese	1 slice	101	6	9	26	3	—	437
Bacon	1 serv (1 oz)	80	5	7	10	0	0	374
BBQ Sauce	1 serv (1 oz)	40	0	0	0	9	—	252
Black Olives	1 serv (1 oz)	32	0	3	0	2	—	248
Brown Mustard	1 serv (1 oz)	0	0	0	0	0	0	340
Cheddar Cheese	1 slice	116	8	9	30	1	—	179
Dressing Italian	1 serv (0.5 oz)	51	0	5	0	1	—	248
Dressing Ranch	1 serv (0.5 oz)	83	0	9	5	0	0	137
Lettuce	1 serv (1 oz)	2	1	0	0	0	—	2
Margarine	1 serv (1 oz)	203	0	23	0	0	0	306
Mayonnaise	1 serv (1 oz)	101	0	11	5	0	—	76
Peppers Jalapeno	1 serv (1.5 oz)	11	0	0	0	2	—	415
Peppers Mild	1 serv (1.5 oz)	11	0	0	0	4	—	500
Provolone Cheese	1 slice	80	5	6	15	0	—	190
Sour Cream	1 serv (1 oz)	61	1	6	13	1	—	15
Swiss Cheese	1 slice	100	8	8	26	1	—	60
Tomatoes	1 serv (2 oz)	24	2	0	0	2	—	5
SALADS								
Grilled Salad w/ Chicken	1 serv	175	25	5	55	11	—	652
Grilled Salad w/ Ham	1 serv	130	19	2	30	8	—	1042
Grilled Salad w/ Steak	1 serv	185	23	6	50	11	—	292

FOOD	PORTION	CALS	PROT	FAT	CHOL	CARB	FIBER	SOD
Grilled Salad w/ Turkey	1 serv	130	19	2	30	8	–	1042
Side	1 serv	40	3	5	0	8	–	20

SUBWAY
BEVERAGES
FOOD	PORTION	CALS	PROT	FAT	CHOL	CARB	FIBER	SOD
Fruizle Smoothie Berry Lishus	1 sm (13 oz)	113	1	0	15	28	1	30
Fruizle Smoothie Berry Lishus w/ Banana	1 sm (17 oz)	221	1	1	15	56	4	30
Fruizle Smoothie Peach Pizazz	1 sm (12 oz)	103	1	0	0	26	0	25
Fruizle Smoothie Pineapple Delight w/ Banana	1 sm (17 oz)	241	1	1	0	61	4	25
Fruizle Smoothie Pineapple Delite	1 sm (13 oz)	133	1	0	0	33	1	25
Fruizle Smoothie Sunrise Refresher	1 sm (12 oz)	119	1	0	0	29	1	20

COOKIES
FOOD	PORTION	CALS	PROT	FAT	CHOL	CARB	FIBER	SOD
Chocolate Chip	1	215	2	10	13	30	1	160
Chocolate Chunk	1	217	2	10	12	30	1	105
Double Chocolate	1	209	2	10	15	30	1	170
M&M	1	215	2	10	13	30	1	105
Oatmeal Raisin	1	210	3	8	14	30	2	180
Peanut Butter	1	221	4	12	12	26	1	200
Sugar	1	227	2	12	17	28	0	135
White Macadamia Nut	1	221	2	11	15	28	1	160

SALAD DRESSINGS
FOOD	PORTION	CALS	PROT	FAT	CHOL	CARB	FIBER	SOD
Fat Free French	1 serv (2 oz)	70	0	0	0	17	0	390
Fat Free Italian	1 serv (2 oz)	20	0	0	0	4	0	610
Fat Free Ranch	1 serv (2 oz)	60	0	0	0	14	0	530

SALADS AND SALAD BARS
FOOD	PORTION	CALS	PROT	FAT	CHOL	CARB	FIBER	SOD
BMT	1 serv	275	16	19	55	11	3	1590
Cold Cut Trio	1 serv	234	14	15	57	11	3	1370
Ham	1 serv	112	11	3	25	11	3	1070
Meatball	1 serv	320	17	20	56	17	4	1050

FOOD	PORTION	CALS	PROT	FAT	CHOL	CARB	FIBER	SOD
Roast Beef	1 serv	117	12	3	25	10	3	720
Roasted Chicken Breast	1 serv	130	18	3	50	9	3	630
Seafood & Crab	1 serv	197	9	11	24	17	4	970
Steak & Cheese	1 serv	181	17	8	37	12	4	890
Subway Club	1 serv	146	17	4	33	12	3	1110
Subway Melt	1 serv	203	17	10	44	11	3	1410
Tuna	1 serv	238	13	16	42	10	3	880
Turkey Breast	1 serv	105	11	2	20	11	3	820
Turkey Breast & Ham	1 serv	117	13	3	26	11	3	1030
Veggie Delight	1 serv	50	2	1	0	9	3	310
SANDWICHES								
6 Inch Steak & Cheese	1	362	23	13	37	41	4	1200
6 Inch Subway Melt	1	384	23	15	44	40	3	1720
6 Inch Sub BMT	1	456	21	24	55	40	3	1890
6 Inch Sub Cold Cut Trio	1	415	19	20	57	40	3	1670
6 Inch Sub Ham	1	261	17	5	25	39	3	1260
6 Inch Sub Meatball	1	501	23	25	56	46	4	1350
6 Inch Sub Roast Beef	1	267	17	5	20	39	3	900
6 Inch Sub Roasted Chicken Breast	1	291	21	5	46	40	3	990
6 Inch Sub Seafood & Crab	1	378	14	16	24	46	3	1270
6 Inch Sub Subway Club	1	296	22	5	33	40	3	1290
6 Inch Sub Tuna	1	419	18	21	42	39	3	1180
6 Inch Sub Turkey Breast	1	254	17	4	20	39	3	1000
6 Inch Sub Turkey Breast & Ham	1	267	18	5	26	40	3	1210
6 Inch Sub Veggie Delight	1	200	7	3	0	37	3	500
American Cheese Triangles	2	41	2	4	10	0	0	200
Asiago Caesar Sauce	1.5 tbsp	110	1	11	10	2	0	230

FOOD	PORTION	CALS	PROT	FAT	CHOL	CARB	FIBER	SOD
Bacon Strips	2	45	3	4	8	0	0	180
Breakfast Bacon & Egg	1	321	14	16	184	34	3	520
Breakfast Cheese & Egg	1	317	14	15	187	34	3	550
Breakfast Ham & Egg	1	338	21	14	201	34	3	1100
Breakfast Western Egg	1	300	14	12	182	36	3	540
Cheddar Triangles	2	59	4	5	15	0	0	95
Cucumber Slices	3	2	0	0	0	0	0	0
Deli Ham	1	210	11	4	12	35	3	770
Deli Roast Beef	1	223	13	5	13	35	3	660
Deli Tuna	1	325	13	16	26	36	3	830
Deli Turkey Breast	1	215	13	4	13	36	3	730
Deli Style Roll	1	165	6	3	0	32	3	280
Dijon Horseradish	1.5 tbsp	91	0	10	8	1	0	160
Dijon Horseradish Melt	6 inch	465	25	22	52	47	4	1620
Fat Free Red Wine Vinaigrette	1.5 tbsp	29	0	0	1	6	0	340
Fat Free Sweet Onion	1.5 tbsp	38	0	0	0	9	0	85
Green Pepper Strips	3 (0.2 oz)	2	0	0	0	0	0	0
Hearty Italian Bread	6 inch	207	8	3	0	41	3	340
Honey Mustard	1.5 tbsp	28	0	0	0	7	0	140
Honey Mustard Ham	6 inch	311	18	5	25	52	4	1260
Honey Oat Bread	6 inch	249	10	4	0	48	4	380
Italian Bread	6 inch	178	7	2	0	33	2	350
Lettuce	1 serv (0.7 oz)	3	0	0	0	0	0	0
Mayonnaise	1 tbsp	111	0	12	9	0	0	80
Mayonnaise Light	1 tbsp	46	0	5	6	1	0	100
Moneterey Cheddar Bread	6 inch	235	10	6	10	39	3	400
Mustard	2 tsp	7	0	0	0	1	0	115
Olive Oil Blend	1 tsp	45	0	5	0	0	0	0
Olive Rings	3 (3 g)	3	0	tr	0	0	0	25
Onions	1 serv (0.5 oz)	5	0	0	0	1	0	0

FOOD	PORTION	CALS	PROT	FAT	CHOL	CARB	FIBER	SOD
Parmesan Oregano Bread	6 inch	211	8	4	0	40	3	530
Pepperjack Cheese Triangles	2	40	2	4	11	0	0	210
Pickle Chips	3 pieces (0.3 oz)	1	0	0	0	0	0	125
Provolone Circles	2 halves	51	4	4	11	0	0	125
Red Wine Vinaigrette Club	6 inch	350	24	6	33	53	4	1520
Roasted Garlic Bread	6 inch	225	8	3	0	45	4	1210
Sourdough Bread	6 inch	208	8	3	0	41	3	210
Southwest Sauce	1.5 tbsp	86	0	9	7	2	0	190
Southwest Turkey Bacon	6 inch	407	21	17	35	48	4	1230
Sweet Onion Chicken Teriyaki	6 inch	374	26	5	50	59	4	1090
Swiss Triangles	2	53	4	4	13	0	0	30
Tomato Slices	3 (1.2 oz)	7	0	0	0	2	0	0
Vinegar	1 tsp	1	0	0	0	0	0	0
Wheat Sub	6 inch	186	7	2	0	36	3	360
Wrap Chicken Bacon Ranch w/ Swiss	1	480	–	27	–	19	–	–
Wrap Turkey Bacon Melt	1	430	–	25	–	22	–	–
SOUPS								
Black Bean	1 cup	180	9	5	5	27	15	1160
Brown & Wild Rice w/ Chicken	1 cup	190	6	11	20	17	2	990
Cheese w/ Ham & Bacon	1 cup	230	8	16	20	13	2	1270
Chicken & Dumplings	1 cup	130	7	5	30	16	1	1030
Cream Of Broccoli	1 cup	130	4	7	15	12	1	890
Cream Of Potato w/ Bacon	1 cup	210	5	12	20	20	4	970
Golden Broccoli Cheese	1 cup	180	6	12	10	12	9	910

FOOD	PORTION	CALS	PROT	FAT	CHOL	CARB	FIBER	SOD
Hearty Chili Beef	1 cup	250	15	7	20	31	9	1450
Minestrone	1 cup	70	3	1	5	11	0	1030
New England Clam Chowder	1 cup	140	5	5	15	19	1	900
Potato Cheese Chowder	1 cup	210	7	10	25	22	2	1010
Roasted Chicken Noodle	1 cup	90	7	4	20	7	1	1180
Tomato Bisque	1 cup	90	1	3	0	15	3	750
Vegetable Beef	1 cup	90	5	2	5	14	2	1340

TACO CABANA

FOOD	PORTION	CALS	PROT	FAT	CHOL	CARB	FIBER	SOD
Black Beans	1 serv (4 oz)	111	6	tr	–	21	–	–
Borracho Beans	1 serv (4 oz)	108	4	3	–	17	–	–
Breakfast Taco Bacon & Egg	1	246	13	12	–	22	–	–
Breakfast Taco Barbacoa	1	307	22	15	–	2	–	–
Breakfast Taco Chorizo & Egg	1	248	12	12	–	22	–	–
Breakfast Taco Potato & Egg	1	234	10	10	–	27	–	–
Burrito Bean & Cheese	1	710	28	27	–	85	–	–
Burrito Beef	1	653	30	24	–	76	–	–
Burrito Black Bean	1	559	16	11	–	95	–	–
Burrito Chicken	1	665	31	26	–	74	–	–
Calabacita	1 serv (4 oz)	78	2	5	–	6	–	–
Chips	1 serv (2 oz)	285	5	14	–	36	–	–
Elotes	1	220	7	11	–	26	–	–
Fajitas Beef	1 serv (4 oz)	245	31	12	–	3	–	–
Fajitas Chicken Dark	1 serv (4 oz)	236	33	11	–	2	–	–
Fajitas Chicken White	1 serv (4 oz)	191	30	6	–	3	–	–
Grilled Chicken Dark	1 serv (4.5 oz)	298	33	18	–	1	–	–
Grilled Chicken Dark No Skin	1 serv (3.4 oz)	170	26	7	–	1	–	–

FOOD	PORTION	CALS	PROT	FAT	CHOL	CARB	FIBER	SOD
Grilled Chicken White	1 serv (5 oz)	295	42	14	–	1	–	–
Grilled Chicken White No Skin	1 serv (3.8 oz)	167	35	3	–	tr	–	–
Guacamole	1 serv (1 oz)	48	tr	4	–	2	–	–
Queso	1 serv (3 oz)	184	9	12	–	7	–	–
Refried Beans	1 serv (4 oz)	171	7	6	–	21	–	–
Sour Cream	1 serv (1 oz)	57	1	5	–	1	–	–
Spanish Rice	1 serv (4 oz)	181	3	5	–	30	–	–
Taco Bean & Cheese	1	292	12	12	–	35	–	–
Taco Black Bean	1	216	8	5	–	37	–	–
Taco Carne Guisada	1	202	14	8	–	20	–	–
Taco Crispy Beef	1	148	9	7	–	13	–	–
Taco Soft Chicken	1	217	13	9	–	21	–	–
Tortilla Corn	1 6-inch	70	2	1	–	11	–	–
Tortilla Flour	1 6-inch	129	3	3	–	22	–	–
Tortilla Soup	1 lg	371	33	13	–	32	–	–
Tortilla Soup	1 sm	249	18	8	–	26	–	–

TACO JOHN'S

DESSERTS

FOOD	PORTION	CALS	PROT	FAT	CHOL	CARB	FIBER	SOD
Apple Grande	1 serv	240	5	9	5	36	0	220
Choco Taco	1 serv	300	4	15	15	38	1	110
Churro	1 serv	230	2	11	10	31	1	120
Cinnamon Mini Swirl	1 piece	10	0	0	0	3	0	0

MAIN MENU SELECTIONS

FOOD	PORTION	CALS	PROT	FAT	CHOL	CARB	FIBER	SOD
Burrito Bean	1	380	15	12	15	53	10	830
Burrito Beefy	1	430	22	20	55	41	8	870
Burrito Chicken & Potato	1	460	18	19	35	54	8	1470
Burrito Combination	1	400	18	16	35	47	9	850
Burrito Meat & Potato	1	490	15	23	30	55	9	1190
Burrito Super	1	450	19	20	40	49	10	920
Crispy Taco	1 serv	180	9	10	25	13	3	270
Mexican Rice	1 serv	250	5	5	0	45	2	860
Nachos	1 serv	380	6	23	10	38	tr	970

FOOD	PORTION	CALS	PROT	FAT	CHOL	CARB	FIBER	SOD
Potato Oles	1 lg	790	7	47	0	86	8	2290
Potato Oles	1 sm	440	4	26	0	48	5	1270
Potato Oles Bravo	1 serv	580	9	36	20	55	6	1760
Potato Oles Super	1 serv	980	22	62	60	82	10	2950
Potato Oles w/ Nacho Cheese	1 serv	550	7	35	10	52	5	2000
Quesadilla Cheese	1	480	20	28	50	39	6	960
Quesadilla Chicken	1	540	29	29	75	41	7	1430
Refried Beans	1 serv	400	18	14	15	50	11	1110
Sierra Taco Beef	1	430	17	23	45	38	4	980
Sierra Taco Chicken	1	390	21	17	50	37	3	1350
Softshell Taco	1	220	11	10	25	21	4	470
Softshell Taco Chicken	1	190	14	6	30	19	4	760
Super Nachos	1 serv	830	22	51	60	73	5	1730
Super Nachos Chicken	1 serv	780	31	45	90	62	3	2250
Taco Bravo	1 serv	340	15	14	25	30	8	650
Taco Burger	1	280	14	12	35	28	3	600
Texas Chili	1 serv	270	15	12	35	26	4	1400
SALAD DRESSINGS AND TOPPINGS								
Bacon Ranch Dressing	1 serv (3 oz)	250	2	19	20	21	0	740
Barbecue Sauce	1 serv (2 oz)	70	0	0	0	15	0	490
Chipotle Cream Sauce	1 serv (3 oz)	450	—	45	30	6	0	1020
Creamy Italian Dressing	1 serv (3 oz)	260	0	29	0	6	0	600
Guacamole	1 serv (2 oz)	90	0	9	0	6	—	360
Hot Sauce	1 serv (1 oz)	5	0	0	0	1	0	135
House Dressing	1 serv (3 oz)	140	0	15	0	5	tr	540
Jalapenos	1 serv (2 oz)	15	1	1	0	3	1	950
Mild Sauce	1 serv (1 oz)	5	0	0	0	1	0	140
Nacho Cheese	1 serv (3 oz)	120	4	9	10	5	0	740
Pico De Gallo	1 serv (2 oz)	15	1	0	0	4	tr	160
Ranch Dressing	1 serv (3 oz)	280	3	31	45	6	0	710
Salsa	1 serv (2 oz)	20	0	0	0	5	0	390
Sour Cream	1 serv (2 oz)	120	2	12	25	2	0	30
Super Hot Sauce	1 serv (1 oz)	10	1	0	0	2	tr	25

FOOD	PORTION	CALS	PROT	FAT	CHOL	CARB	FIBER	SOD
SALADS								
Chicken Festiva w/o Dressing	1 serv	400	24	23	70	24	4	830
Chicken Taco w/o Dressing	'	530	27	27	70	45	3	1330
Side w/o Dressing	1 serv	80	3	5	5	6	1	50
Taco w/o Dressing	1 serv	580	23	32	60	46	4	960
TACOTIME								
DESSERTS								
Cinnamon Crustos	1 serv	373	9	15	0	47	–	86
Fruit Filled Empanada	1 serv	250	5	9	0	37	–	46
MAIN MENU SELECTIONS								
Burrito Beef Bean & Cheese	1 serv	617	39	23	63	66	18	1343
Burrito Casita	1 serv	647	40	31	89	54	16	1233
Burrito Chicken & Black Bean	1 serv	400	19	18	36	45	5	580
Burrito Chicken BLT	1 serv	580	23	39	50	36	5	1020
Burrito Crisp Bean	1 serv	427	15	18	12	53	9	453
Burrito Crisp Chicken	1	422	17	25	54	32	2	795
Burrito Crisp Meat	1 serv	552	34	30	58	39	7	1000
Burrito Soft Bean	1	380	16	10	15	58	13	715
Burrito Soft Meat	1 serv	491	31	21	56	48	12	1197
Burrito Veggie	1 serv	491	21	16	24	70	10	643
Burrito Big Juan Beef	1 serv	640	34	25	60	71	15	1120
Burrito Big Juan Chicken	1 serv	620	34	24	65	69	12	1230
Cheddar Fries	1 lg	704	16	48	–	54	–	1862
Cheddar Fries	1 sm	352	6	24	–	27	–	931
Cheddar Melt	1 serv	205	11	11	30	17	1	255
Mexi-Fries	1 sm	266	3	17	–	27	–	799
Mexi-Fries	1 lg	532	6	34	–	54	–	1598
Mexi-Rice	1 serv	159	3	2	0	30	1	530
Nachos	1 serv	680	26	38	78	61	11	1250
Nachos Deluxe	1 serv	1048	46	57	109	91	17	2252

FOOD	PORTION	CALS	PROT	FAT	CHOL	CARB	FIBER	SOD
Refritos Cheese Sauce Chips	1 serv	326	18	10	22	44	13	525
Stuffed Fries	1 sm	490	6	37	20	34	3	1400
Stuffed Fries	1 lg	990	16	73	35	88	6	2580
Taco Cheeseburger	1	633	31	36	66	48	7	1291
Taco Crisp	1	295	22	17	48	16	5	609
Taco Soft	1 serv	316	24	15	48	23	5	599
Taco Soft ½ lb	1 serv	512	33	23	63	46	12	1111
Taco Soft ½ lb Chicken	1 serv	387	21	16	48	41	7	933
Taco Super Soft	1 serv	510	29	23	60	50	11	590
SALAD DRESSINGS AND TOPPINGS								
1000 Island Dressing	1 serv (1 oz)	120	0	12	5	3	0	120
Green Sauce	1 serv (1 oz)	5	0	0	0	2	tr	115
Original Hot Sauce	1 serv (1 oz)	10	0	0	0	2	0	120
Salsa Fresca	1 serv (1 oz)	65	0	0	0	16	0	3508
SALADS								
Chicken Fiesta	1 serv	390	20	19	45	35	4	840
Taco	1 reg	479	30	28	63	30	7	895
Taco Salad Chicken	1 serv	370	19	21	48	27	3	861
Tostada	1 serv	628	36	33	82	48	13	1004

TGI FRIDAY'S

FOOD	PORTION	CALS	PROT	FAT	CHOL	CARB	FIBER	SOD
Sizzling Chicken & Broccoli	1 serv	700	–	40	–	15	–	–
Sizzling NY Strip Steak w/ Blue Cheese & Broccoli	1 serv	684	–	36	–	15	–	–

TIM HORTONS
BAGELS AND CREAM CHEESE

FOOD	PORTION	CALS	PROT	FAT	CHOL	CARB	FIBER	SOD
Blueberry	1	200	11	2	0	59	3	520
Cinnamon Raisin	1	300	11	2	0	58	4	390
Cream Cheese	1.5 oz	150	3	12	40	3	0	230
Cream Cheese Light	1.5 oz	90	4	7	20	5	0	200
Cream Cheese Plain	1.5 oz	140	3	14	45	1	0	140
Everything	1	300	12	2	0	57	3	560
Multigrain	1	300	12	3	0	58	6	655
Onion	1	295	11	2	0	58	3	530
Plain	1	290	11	2	0	57	3	800

FOOD	PORTION	CALS	PROT	FAT	CHOL	CARB	FIBER	SOD
Poppy Seed	1	300	11	3	0	58	4	500
Sesame Seed	1	300	11	3	0	57	4	570
Whole Wheat & Honey	1	300	11	2	0	59	6	590
BAKED SELECTIONS								
Biscuit Southern Country Cranberry	1	470	7	19	0	68	2	1050
Biscuit Southern Country Raspberry	1	470	7	19	0	68	2	1050
Cake Black Forest	1 serv	500	4	21	0	75	3	790
Cake Celebration	1 serv	500	4	16	5	85	1	530
Cake Chocolot Fantasy	1 serv	420	5	15	35	72	3	630
Cake Shadow	1 serv	430	4	19	35	63	2	470
Cookie Chocolate Chip	1	150	2	7	20	21	1	140
Cookie Macaroon	1	140	1	8	0	14	3	60
Cookie Oatcakes	1	190	2	10	0	22	1	150
Cookie Oatmeal Raisin	1	150	2	6	15	22	1	140
Cookie Peanut Butter	1	170	3	10	20	17	1	190
Cookie Peanut Butter Chocolate Chunk	1	170	3	10	15	18	1	190
Croissant Butter	1	210	5	11	30	25	1	370
Croissant Cheese	1	240	6	12	20	27	1	370
Danish Cherry Cheese	1	380	7	23	45	33	1	410
Donut Apple Fritter	1	300	5	14	0	40	2	280
Donut Chocolate Dip	1	230	4	10	0	33	0	270
Donut Chocolate Glazed	1	360	3	22	10	36	1	340
Donut Dutchie	1	280	4	13	0	39	1	240
Donut Honey Dip	1	230	4	10	0	32	0	250
Donut Maple Dip	1	250	4	10	0	36	0	280
Donut Old Fashion Glazed	1	270	3	12	15	39	0	280

FOOD	PORTION	CALS	PROT	FAT	CHOL	CARB	FIBER	SOD
Donut Old Fashion Plain	1	220	3	12	15	24	0	260
Donut Sour Cream Plain	1	280	3	18	20	25	0	230
Donut Sugar Twist	1	230	5	10	0	32	0	280
Donut Walnut Crunch	1	320	5	18	10	36	2	410
Donut Filled Angel Cream	1	280	4	13	0	36	0	280
Donut Filled Blueberry	1	220	4	8	0	33	0	280
Donut Filled Boston Cream	1	230	4	8	0	36	0	320
Donut Filled Canadian Maple	1	230	4	8	0	36	0	320
Donut Filled Strawberry	1	220	4	8	0	33	0	310
Donuts Honey Stick	1	280	4	15	30	34	0	350
Muffin Blueberry Bran	1	300	5	9	10	51	5	690
Muffin Carrot Whole Wheat	1	410	5	22	10	52	4	580
Muffin Chocolate Chip	1	390	5	15	20	62	2	580
Muffin Oatbran Carrot 'n Raisin	1	340	5	11	0	57	4	390
Muffin Oatbran 'n Apple	1	350	5	12	0	58	4	430
Muffin Oatmeal Raisin	1	430	6	11	20	80	3	520
Muffin Raisin Bran	1	380	6	10	10	66	6	750
Muffin Wild Blueberry	1	330	4	11	15	54	2	520
Muffin Low Fat Carrot	1	260	5	2	0	60	6	620
Muffin Low Fat Cranberry	1	260	5	2	0	60	6	610
Muffin Low Fat Honey	1	290	6	2	0	66	6	700

FOOD	PORTION	CALS	PROT	FAT	CHOL	CARB	FIBER	SOD
Pie Apple	1 serv	540	4	31	0	62	3	230
Pie Banana Cream	1 serv	440	2	26	0	50	1	135
Pie Cherry	1 serv	570	4	31	0	70	2	320
Pie Chocolate Cream	1 serv	490	2	31	10	52	1	170
Tart Fresh Strawberry	1 serv	220	1	9	0	36	2	140
Tart Raisin Butter	1 serv	330	3	11	15	54	1	200
Tea Biscuit Plain	1	220	5	6	0	36	1	590
Tea Biscuit Raisin	1	250	5	6	0	47	2	570
Timbits Chocolate Glazed	1	70	1	3	5	9	0	95
Timbits Dutchie	1	60	1	2	0	10	0	90
Timbits Honey Dip	1	50	1	1	0	10	0	70
Timbits Old Fashion Plain	1	45	1	2	5	7	0	70
Timbits Filled Banana Cream	1	45	1	1	0	8	0	70
Timbits Filled Lemon	1	50	1	2	0	9	0	75
Timbits Filled Spiced Apple	1	80	1	1	0	9	0	75
Timbits Filled Strawberry	1	50	1	1	0	9	0	80
BEVERAGES								
Apple Juice	1 (9 oz)	140	0	0	0	36	0	16
Cafe Mocha	1 (10 oz)	250	3	10	0	34	0	330
Cappuccino English Toffee	1 (10 oz)	130	3	5	0	20	0	120
Cappuccino French Vanilla	1 (10 oz)	130	3	5	0	20	0	120
Cappuccino Iced	1 (16 oz)	430	3	23	80	54	0	50
Chocolate Milk	1 (14 oz)	280	15	5	15	46	0	270
Coffee Decaffeinated + Sugar & Cream	1 (10 oz)	80	1	4	12	10	0	20
Coffee + Sugar & Cream	1 (10 oz)	80	1	4	12	10	0	20
Coke	1 (14 oz)	170	0	0	0	44	0	12
Diet Coke	1 (14 oz)	1	0	0	0	0	0	20
Fruit Punch	1 (10 oz)	150	0	0	0	38	0	10

FOOD	PORTION	CALS	PROT	FAT	CHOL	CARB	FIBER	SOD
Hot Chocolate	1 (10 oz)	200	2	6	0	44	0	370
Iced Tea	1 (14 oz)	130	0	0	0	34	0	0
Milk 2%	1 (14 oz)	210	14	6	30	20	0	210
Orange Juice	1 (10 oz)	140	2	0	0	36	0	14
Sprite	1 (14 oz)	160	0	0	0	41	0	40
Tea + Sugar & Milk	1 (10 oz)	45	1	0	0	9	0	20
SANDWICHES								
Albacore Tuna Salad	1 serv	350	21	8	15	49	3	1100
Black Forest Ham & Swiss	1 serv	640	33	27	75	53	2	1540
Chunky Chicken Salad	1 serv	380	23	10	45	50	3	770
Fireside Roast Beef	1 serv	470	22	19	36	48	2	1470
Garden Vegetable	1 serv	460	12	24	45	50	3	730
Harvest Turkey Breast	1 serv	470	22	18	30	53	2	1460
SOUPS								
Barley & Wild Rice	1 serv	120	22	2	6	22	1	330
Chicken Noodle	1 serv	100	8	3	14	15	1	710
Chili	1 serv	320	29	9	65	32	8	960
Cream Of Broccoli	1 serv	190	7	7	6	27	1	1120
Cream of Mushroom	1 serv	195	4	10	8	21	1	900
Hearty Vegetable	1 serv	130	3	2	0	27	2	830
Minestrone	1 serv	125	4	2	1	25	2	910
Potato Bacon	1 serv	195	4	7	5	29	1	1100
Vegetable Beef Barley	1 serv	110	5	2	9	14	2	840
T.J. CINNAMONS								
Cinnachips	1 bag (10 oz)	1130	–	50	42	157	3	700
Cinnamon Twist	1	260	–	13	5	33	10	190
Coffee Black	1 (12 oz)	0	0	0	0	0	0	0
Mocha Chill w/ Whipped Cream	1 (12.5 oz)	310	–	6	25	49	10	190
Mocha Chill w/o Whipped Cream	1 (12.5 oz)	260	–	4	15	48	10	190
Original Roll w/o Icing	1	500	–	17	30	81	0	370

FOOD	PORTION	CALS	PROT	FAT	CHOL	CARB	FIBER	SOD
Original Roll w/ Cream Cheese Icing	1	651	—	37	40	103	0	420
Pecan Sticky Roll	1	690	—	28	32	97	0	400

TOGO'S
SALAD DRESSINGS

FOOD	PORTION	CALS	PROT	FAT	CHOL	CARB	FIBER	SOD
1000 Island	1 serv (2.3 oz)	231	1	22	30	9	0	532
Caesar	1 serv (2.3 oz)	241	2	23	20	8	0	633
Oriental	1 serv (2.3 oz)	221	0	14	5	24	0	512
Ranch	1 serv (2.3 oz)	321	2	33	15	5	0	643
Reduced Calorie Italian	1 serv (2.3 oz)	60	0	5	0	4	0	693
Reduced Calorie Ranch	1 serv (2.3 oz)	191	1	16	25	10	0	603

SALADS AND SALAD BARS

FOOD	PORTION	CALS	PROT	FAT	CHOL	CARB	FIBER	SOD
Caesar Salad	1 serv	471	30	31	72	23	2	1189
Garden Salad	1 serv	256	12	10	214	31	2	579
Oriental Salad	1 serv	499	25	21	41	49	3	1062
Taco Salad	1 serv	943	29	59	71	76	11	1623

SANDWICHES

FOOD	PORTION	CALS	PROT	FAT	CHOL	CARB	FIBER	SOD
Albacore Tuna	1 sm	701	32	30	67	78	3	1653
Avocado & Turkey	1 sm	675	27	28	80	80	6	1606
Avocado Cucumber & Alfalfa Sprouts	1 sm	637	16	28	85	85	7	1150
Bar-B-Q Beef	1 sm	724	39	22	88	94	3	2120
California Roasted Chicken	1 sm	510	36	15	65	73	3	1768
Cheese Swiss American Provolone	1 sm	859	42	46	107	77	3	2196
Chunky Chicken Salad	1 sm	636	40	26	42	72	3	1562
Egg Salad w/ Cheese	1 sm	728	29	35	456	76	3	1765
Ham & Cheese	1 sm	661	33	26	68	76	3	2900

FOOD	PORTION	CALS	PROT	FAT	CHOL	CARB	FIBER	SOD
Hot Pastrami	1 sm	705	34	26	72	85	3	2260
Hummus	1 sm	668	20	21	9	102	4	1510
Italian Salami & Cheese	1 sm	770	42	33	118	78	3	3288
Italian Salami Capicolla Mortadella Cotto & Provolone	1 sm	736	31	32	85	74	3	2191
Meatballs w/ Pizza Sauce & Parmesan	1 sm	707	36	28	97	78	4	1602
Pastrami Reuben	1 sm	875	44	45	111	85	2	2460
Roast Beef Hot & Cold	1 sm	552	42	11	84	73	3	1537
Turkey & Cranberry	1 sm	623	30	13	49	96	4	1904
Turkey & Bacon Club	1 sm	667	37	26	81	73	3	2108
Turkey & Cheese	1 sm	638	34	23	71	75	3	2277
Turkey & Ham w/ Cheese	1 sm	670	37	25	76	76	3	2772

WENDY'S
BEVERAGES

FOOD	PORTION	CALS	PROT	FAT	CHOL	CARB	FIBER	SOD
Cola	11 oz	130	0	0	0	36	0	10
Diet Cola	11 oz	0	0	0	0	0	0	15
Frosty Junior	6 oz	170	4	4	20	26	0	100
Frosty Medium	16 oz	440	11	11	50	73	0	260
Frosty Small	12 oz	330	8	8	35	56	0	200
Lemon-Lime Soda	11 oz	130	0	0	0	34	0	30

CHILDREN'S MENU SELECTIONS

FOOD	PORTION	CALS	PROT	FAT	CHOL	CARB	FIBER	SOD
French Fries Kid's Meal	1 serv (3.2 oz)	270	4	13	0	35	3	85
Kid's Meal Cheeseburger	1 (4.2 oz)	310	17	12	45	33	2	800
Kid's Meal Hamburger	1 (3.9 oz)	270	14	9	30	33	1	620
Kid's Meal Chicken Nuggets	4 pieces (2.1 oz)	190	9	13	25	9	0	380

MAIN MENU SELECTIONS

FOOD	PORTION	CALS	PROT	FAT	CHOL	CARB	FIBER	SOD
¼ lb Hamburger Patty	1 (2.6 oz)	200	19	14	65	0	0	290

FOOD	PORTION	CALS	PROT	FAT	CHOL	CARB	FIBER	SOD
2 oz Hamburger Patty	1 (1.3 oz)	100	9	7	30	0	0	150
American Cheese	1 slice (0.6 oz)	70	4	6	15	0	0	260
American Cheese Jr.	1 slice (0.4 oz)	45	3	4	10	0	0	170
Bacon	1 strip (4 g)	20	1	2	5	0	0	90
Big Bacon Classic	1 (9.9 oz)	580	34	30	100	46	3	1460
Breaded Chicken Fillet	1 (3.5 oz)	230	22	11	50	13	0	390
Cheddar Shredded	2 tbsp (0.6 oz)	70	4	6	15	1	0	110
Chicken Breast Filet Sandwich	1 (7.3 oz)	430	27	16	56	46	2	750
Chicken Club Sandwich	1 (7.6 oz)	470	30	20	65	47	2	940
Chicken Nuggets	5 pieces (2.6 oz)	230	11	16	30	11	0	470
Chili	1 lg (12 oz)	310	23	10	45	32	7	1190
Chili	1 sm (8 oz)	210	15	7	30	21	5	800
Classic Single w/ Everything	1 (7.6 oz)	410	25	19	70	37	2	920
French Fries	1 Biggie (5.6 oz)	470	7	23	0	61	6	150
French Fries	1 med (5 oz)	420	6	20	0	50	5	130
French Fries	1 Great Biggie (6.7 oz)	570	8	27	0	73	7	180
Grilled Chicken Fillet	1 (2.9 oz)	110	19	3	55	1	0	400
Grilled Chicken Sandwich	1 (6.6 oz)	300	24	7	56	36	2	740
Honey Mustard Reduced Calorie	1 tsp (7 g)	25	0	2	0	2	0	40
Hot Stuffed Bake Potato Plain	1 (10 oz)	310	7	0	0	72	6	25

FOOD	PORTION	CALS	PROT	FAT	CHOL	CARB	FIBER	SOD
Hot Stuffed Baked Potato Bacon & Cheese	1 (12.6 oz)	530	16	18	25	78	7	820
Hot Stuffed Baked Potato Broccoli & Cheese	1 (14.4 oz)	470	9	14	5	80	9	470
Jr. Bacon Cheeseburger	1 (5.8 oz)	380	20	19	55	34	2	870
Jr. Cheeseburger	1 (4.5 oz)	310	17	12	45	34	2	800
Jr. Cheeseburger Deluxe	1 (6.3 oz)	360	18	16	50	36	2	860
Kaiser Bun	1 (2.5 oz)	200	6	3	0	38	2	340
Ketchup	1 tsp (7 g)	10	0	0	0	2	0	80
Lettuce	1 leaf (0.5 oz)	0	0	0	0	0	0	0
Mayonnaise	1½ tsp (9 g)	30	0	3	5	1	0	60
Mustard	½ tsp (5 g)	5	0	0	0	0	0	50
Nuggets Sauce Barbeque	1 pkg (1 oz)	45	1	0	0	10	0	160
Nuggets Sauce Honey Mustard	1 pkg (1 oz)	130	0	12	10	6	0	220
Nuggets Sauce Sweet & Sour	1 pkg (1 oz)	50	0	0	0	12	0	120
Onion	4 rings (0.5 oz)	5	0	0	0	1	0	0
Pickles	4 slices (0.4 oz)	0	0	0	0	0	0	140
Saltines	2 (0.2 oz)	25	1	1	0	4	0	80
Sandwich Bun	1 (2 oz)	160	5	2	0	31	1	300
Spicy Chicken Fillet	1 (3.6 oz)	210	22	9	60	10	0	920
Spicy Chicken Sandwich	1 (7.5 oz)	410	28	14	65	43	2	1280
Tomatoes	1 slice (0.9 oz)	5	0	0	0	1	1	0
Whipped Margarine	1 pkg (0.5 oz)	70	0	7	0	0	0	115
SALAD DRESSINGS								
Blue Cheese	1 pkg (2 oz)	360	2	36	30	1	0	350
French	1 pkg (2 oz)	250	0	21	0	13	0	670

FOOD	PORTION	CALS	PROT	FAT	CHOL	CARB	FIBER	SOD
Hidden Valley Ranch	1 pkg (2 oz)	200	1	20	25	3	0	410
Hidden Valley Ranch Reduced Fat Reduced Calorie	1 pkg (2 oz)	120	1	11	20	4	0	470
Italian Reduced Fat Reduced Calorie	1 pkg (2 oz)	80	0	7	0	6	0	690
Italian Caesar	1 pkg (1.5 oz)	230	1	24	25	1	0	350
Thousand Island	1 pkg (2 oz)	260	1	25	20	7	0	380
SALADS AND SALAD BARS								
Ceasar Side Salad w/o Dressing	1 (3.2 oz)	110	9	5	15	6	1	360
Deluxe Garden Salad w/o Dressing	1 (9.5 oz)	110	7	6	0	10	4	320
Grilled Chicken Salad w/o Dressing	1 (11.9 oz)	200	27	7	55	10	4	780
Side Salad w/o Dressing	1 (5.4 oz)	60	4	3	0	5	2	160
Soft Breadstick	1 (1.5 oz)	130	4	3	5	23	1	250
Taco Chips	15 (1.5 oz)	210	3	9	0	28	2	160
Taco Salad w/o Dressing	1 (16.4 oz)	380	26	19	65	28	8	1040

WHATABURGER
BAKED SELECTIONS

FOOD	PORTION	CALS	PROT	FAT	CHOL	CARB	FIBER	SOD
Cinnamon Roll	1	860	12	34	50	126	4	320
BEVERAGES								
Cherry Coke	1 sm (20 oz)	169	0	0	0	46	0	7
Cherry Coke	1 lg (44 oz)	343	0	0	0	92	0	13
Coca-Cola Classic	1 sm (20 oz)	161	0	0	0	44	0	10
Coca-Cola Classic	1 lg (44 oz)	327	0	0	0	89	0	20
Coffee	1 sm (8 oz)	30	0	1	0	4	0	5
Creamer Nondairy	1 pkg	15	0	1	0	1	0	0
Diet Coke	1 sm (20 oz)	0	0	0	0	0	0	16
Diet Coke	1 lg (44 oz)	0	0	0	0	0	0	34
Diet Dr Pepper	1 sm (20 oz)	0	0	0	0	0	0	73
Dr Pepper	1 sm (20 oz)	147	0	0	0	42	0	49

FOOD	PORTION	CALS	PROT	FAT	CHOL	CARB	FIBER	SOD
Fanta Strawberry	1 sm (20 oz)	177	0	0	0	47	0	13
Fanta Strawberry	1 lg (44 oz)	360	0	0	0	96	0	26
Fruit Drink	1 lg (44 oz)	244	0	0	0	63	0	92
Fruit Drink	1 sm (20 oz)	121	0	0	0	31	0	46
Lemonade	1 sm (20 oz)	158	0	0	0	42	0	67
Lemonade	1 lg (44 oz)	320	0	0	0	86	0	135
Lipton Iced Tea	1 med	0	0	0	0	0	0	0
Milk 2%	8 oz	120	8	5	20	11	0	115
Orange Juice	1 serv	140	2	0	0	33	0	0
Orange Soda	1 lg (44 oz)	350	0	0	0	96	0	0
Orange Soda	1 sm (20 oz)	173	0	0	0	47	0	0
Shake Chocolate	1 sm (20 oz)	616	13	17	61	100	0	325
Shake Strawberry	1 sm (20 oz)	620	12	16	61	101	0	296
Shake Vanilla	1 sm (20 oz)	559	13	17	65	82	0	301
Sprite	1 sm	158	0	0	0	42	0	36
Sprite	1 lg (44 oz)	320	0	0	0	86	0	73
CHILDREN'S MENU SELECTIONS								
Kid's Justaburger	1	306	16	15	40	27	1	682
Kid's Chicken Strips	1 serv	382	19	24	33	22	4	705
MAIN MENU SELECTIONS								
Biscuit Buttermilk	1	300	5	16	0	34	0	470
Biscuit w/ Bacon	1	375	10	22	12	34	0	788
Biscuit w/ Bacon Egg & Cheese	1	476	17	29	252	35	0	875
Biscuit w/ Egg & Cheese	1	446	15	27	250	35	0	777
Biscuit w/ Sausage	1	517	16	35	35	34	1	947
Biscuit w/ Sausage Egg & Cheese	1	663	26	46	285	35	1	1254
Biscuit w/ Sausage Gravy	1	491	8	33	19	47	tr	1249
Breakfast Platter w/ Bacon	1 serv	698	23	43	466	52	3	1362
Breakfast Platter w/ Sausage	1 serv	840	29	56	489	52	4	1521
Breakfast On A Bun Ranchero w/ Bacon	1	404	20	23	262	29	3	1183

FOOD	PORTION	CALS	PROT	FAT	CHOL	CARB	FIBER	SOD
Breakfast On A Bun Ranchero w/ Sausage	1	546	27	36	285	29	3	1342
Breakfast On A Bun w/ Bacon	1	398	20	23	262	28	2	965
Breakfast On A Bun w/ Sausage	1	540	27	36	285	28	2	1124
Chicken Strips	2	382	19	24	33	22	4	705
Croutons Njoy Seasoned	1 pkg	35	0	2	0	4	0	90
French Fries	1 lg	514	9	26	0	66	5	413
French Fries	1 sm	257	4	13	0	33	3	207
Grape Jelly	1 pkg	35	0	0	0	9	0	5
Gravy White Peppered	1 serv	53	0	5	0	8	0	345
Hashbrown Sticks	1 serv	140	0	8	0	16	3	440
Honey	1 pkg	25	0	0	0	7	0	0
Hot Apple Pie	1	240	2	12	5	31	1	290
Justaburger	1	309	17	15	40	28	1	682
Ketchup	1 pkg	40	1	0	0	8	0	350
Margarine	1 pkg	23	0	3	0	0	0	39
Onion Rings	1 med	201	3	11	0	23	1	477
Pancake Syrup	1 pkg	120	0	0	0	31	0	25
Pancakes	1 serv	614	19	8	0	118	3	2250
Pancakes w/ Bacon	1 serv	689	24	13	12	118	3	2568
Pancakes w/ Sausage	1 serv	831	30	27	35	118	5	2727
Picante Sauce	1 serv	5	0	0	0	1	0	110
Sandwich Egg	1	323	16	17	250	28	1	647
Sandwich Grilled Chicken	1	473	30	20	82	49	4	1167
Sandwich Grilled Chicken Not Bun	1	190	22	7	73	10	1	609
Sandwich Whatacatch	1	473	20	26	59	45	2	936
Sandwich Whatachick'n	1	523	28	21	49	63	5	1524
Strawberry Jam	1 pkg	40	0	0	0	10	0	5
Taquito Bacon & Egg	1	387	19	22	352	25	1	839

FOOD	PORTION	CALS	PROT	FAT	CHOL	CARB	FIBER	SOD
Taquito Potato & Egg	1	382	14	20	340	33	4	741
Taquito Sausage & Egg	1	389	17	26	354	26	1	675
Taquito w/ Bacon Egg & Cheese	1	432	21	25	362	25	1	1059
Taquito w/ Potato Egg & Cheese	1	427	17	24	350	33	4	961
Taquito w/ Sausage Egg & Cheese	1	434	19	27	364	26	1	895
Texas Toast	1 serv	328	8	15	0	42	2	540
Whataburger	1	607	31	30	75	53	3	1158
Whataburger Double Meat	1	857	51	48	150	53	3	1297
Whataburger Double Meat No Bun	1	520	41	36	150	4	1	487
Whataburger Jr.	1	315	16	16	40	29	2	685
Whataburger No Bun	1	270	21	18	75	4	1	348
Whataburger Triple Meat	1	1107	71	66	225	53	4	1435
Whataburger w/ Bacon & Cheese	1	810	42	45	113	54	3	2065
Whatacatch	2 pieces	814	28	65	147	38	2	1360
SALAD DRESSINGS								
Low Fat Ranch	1 pkg	66	2	4	19	9	2	605
Low Fat Vinaigrette	1 pkg	35	0	2	0	6	0	890
Ranch	1 pkg	310	1	33	20	3	0	470
Thousand Island	1 pkg	150	0	13	20	11	0	490
SALADS								
Chicken Strips	1 serv	419	21	25	33	29	7	744
Chicken Strips w/ Cheddar Cheese	1 serv	600	31	39	76	32	8	957
Chicken Strips w/ Cheddar Cheese & Bacon	1 serv	675	36	45	88	33	8	1275
Garden Salad	1	49	3	1	0	10	4	49
Garden w/ Cheddar Cheese	1 serv	218	13	15	43	10	4	252

FOOD	PORTION	CALS	PROT	FAT	CHOL	CARB	FIBER	SOD
Garden w/ Cheddar Cheese & Bacon	1 serv	293	18	20	55	11	4	570
Grilled Chicken	1 serv	229	25	7	73	19	5	653
Grilled Chicken w/ Cheddar Cheese	1 serv	398	34	21	115	19	4	855
Grilled Chicken w/ Cheddar Cheese & Bacon	1 serv	473	39	27	127	19	5	1173

WHITE CASTLE
BEVERAGES

FOOD	PORTION	CALS	PROT	FAT	CHOL	CARB	FIBER	SOD
Coca-Cola	16 oz	200	0	0	0	54	–	15
Coffee Black	1 sm	6	0	0	0	1	–	5
Diet Coke	16 oz	0	0	0	0	0	0	20
Iced Tea	16 oz	90	0	0	0	24	–	35
Shake Chocolate	16 oz	250	9	15	30	37	–	160
Shake Vanilla	16 oz	260	9	15	30	40	–	170

MAIN MENU SELECTIONS

FOOD	PORTION	CALS	PROT	FAT	CHOL	CARB	FIBER	SOD
Bacon Cheeseburger	1	200	10	13	25	12	3	430
Cheese Sticks	3	250	10	14	25	22	2	750
Cheeseburger	1	160	7	9	15	11	2	250
Chicken Rings	6	210	11	14	50	10	0	420
Double Cheeseburger	1	290	14	18	30	16	5	430
Double Hamburger	1	240	11	14	20	16	4	200
French Fries	1 sm	115	–	6	–	15	2	15
Hamburger	1	140	6	7	10	11	2	135
Onion Rings	6	260	4	13	0	31	3	520
Sandwich Breakfast	1	340	14	25	130	17	0	900
Sandwich Chicken	1	190	6	8	20	21	–	360
Sandwich Chicken Ring	1	180	8	8	25	20	0	370
Sandwich Fish	1	180	7	7	10	27	1	390

WINCHELL'S DONUTS

FOOD	PORTION	CALS	PROT	FAT	CHOL	CARB	FIBER	SOD
Chocolate Bar	1	240	4	16	–	29	–	125
Chocolate Round	1	240	4	16	–	29	–	125
Chocolate Twist	1	240	4	16	–	29	–	125

FOOD	PORTION	CALS	PROT	FAT	CHOL	CARB	FIBER	SOD
Croissant	1	260	5	17	–	28	–	280
Glazed Round	1	230	2	15	–	27	–	120
Glazed Twist	1	230	2	15	–	27	–	120
Iced Chocolate	1	230	2	15	–	28	–	220
Traditional	1	215	2	14	–	26	–	215

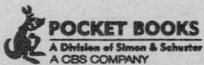
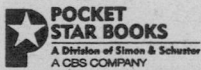